Editors

Erin A. McGill, MA, NASM-CPT, CES, PES, FNS
Ian N. Montel, NASM-CPT, CES, PES

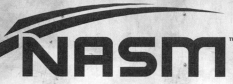

NATIONAL ACADEMY OF SPORTS MEDICINE

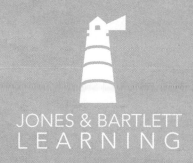

NASM ESSENTIALS OF
PERSONAL FITNESS TRAINING

FIFTH EDITION

JONES & BARTLETT
LEARNING

World Headquarters
Jones & Bartlett Learning
5 Wall Street
Burlington, MA 01803
978-443-5000
info@jblearning.com
www.jblearning.com

National Academy of Sports Medicine
1750 East Northrop Boulevard
Suite 200
Chandler, AZ 85286
800-460-6276
www.nasm.org

Jones & Bartlett Learning books and products are available through most bookstores and online booksellers. To contact Jones & Bartlett Learning directly, call 800-832-0034, fax 978-443-8000, or visit our website, www.jblearning.com.

Substantial discounts on bulk quantities of Jones & Bartlett Learning publications are available to corporations, professional associations, and other qualified organizations. For details and specific discount information, contact the special sales department at Jones & Bartlett Learning via the above contact information or send an email to specialsales@jblearning.com.

Production Credits

Sr. Director of Product Development, NASM: Erin A. McGill
Director of Vendor Management: Amy Rose
Director of Marketing: Andrea DeFronzo
VP, Manufacturing and Inventory Control: Therese Connell
Project Management and Composition: S4Carlisle Publishing Services
Production Editor: Kristen Rogers
Text Design: Jacqueline Werner

Cover Design: Nick Bradshaw
Associate Director of Rights & Media: Joanna Lundeen
Rights & Media Specialist: Merideth Tumasz
Media Development Editor: Shannon Sheehan
Cover Image: © Blair Bunting
Printing and Binding: RR Donnelley
Cover Printing: RR Donnelley

Library of Congress Cataloging-in-Publication Data

Library of Congress Cataloging-in-Publication Data unavailable at time of printing.

6048

Printed in the United States of America
20 19 18 17 16   10 9 8 7 6 5 4 3 2

Table of Contents

Foreword   iv
Contributors   v
Acknowledgments   vi
New Content   vii

1	Introduction to the Fitness Profession	1
2	Career Directions in Sport, Health, and Fitness	17
3	Disciplines of Functional Biomechanics	39
4	The Human Movement System in Fitness	85
5	Client-Based Nutrition Sciences	141
6	Concepts of Integrated Training	177
7	Navigating the Professional Fitness Environment	215
8	Client Acquisition and Consultations	237
9	Executing Formal Fitness Assessments	281
10	Initializing Program Design	325
11	The Optimum Performance Training™ (OPT™) Model: Applying Stabilization	373
12	The Optimum Performance Training™ (OPT™) Model: Applying Strength	405
13	The Optimum Performance Training™ (OPT™) Model: Applying Power	441
14	The Optimum Performance Training™ (OPT™) Model: Every Day	473
15	Exercise Technique	529
16	Behavior Change Strategies for Client Results	651

Appendix A   Exercise Library   689
Appendix B   Nutritional Concepts   729
Appendix C   Additional Objective Assessment Information   737
Appendix D   The Kinetic Chain   749
Glossary   779
Index   799

Foreword

Congratulations on making the decision to begin a career devoted to improving the quality of life for others, and thank you for choosing the National Academy of Sports Medicine (NASM) to be your education provider. Fitness professionals are in demand now more than ever before, and your future clients will trust you to help them achieve their health and fitness goals both safely and effectively.

For nearly 30 years, NASM has been the authority in certification, continuing education, and career development for health and fitness professionals. As the world's foremost resource for fitness and sports medicine information, NASM continues to elevate industry standards by providing outstanding educational programs and quality certification courses for our members.

Scientific research and techniques also continue to evolve, and, as a result, you must stay on the cutting edge to remain competitive. Designed exclusively by NASM, the Optimum Performance Training (OPT) model is the industry's first scientific, evidence-based training system. Along with our OPT model, NASM seeks to provide the most up-to-date science, research, and proven practices to best prepare you to work with people of all ages, disciplines, and requirements. Designed to fit the needs and learning styles of the adult learner, this textbook will help you evolve from student to fitness professional.

Leading experts across the country collaborated to author this text with the primary goal of elevating the standards of entry-level education for professional fitness trainers. The authors carefully examined occupational outcomes in the fitness industry to provide an authentic learning experience that will allow you to more easily transition to your position as a fitness professional.

As an educator, practitioner, and advocate of the sound and progressive methodologies of NASM's OPT model, I am thrilled to introduce you to all that the fifth edition of NASM's *Essentials of Personal Fitness Training* has to offer. You are about to embark on an extraordinary journey in a rewarding career, where you will be highly regarded for the credentials you receive. I look forward to watching you shape the future of fitness with NASM. Welcome to the NASM family!

Sincerely,
Dr. Mike Clark, DPT, MS, CES, PES
Founder & CEO, Fusionetics

Contributors

Managing Editors

Erin A. McGill, MA, NASM CPT, CES, PES, BCS
Scottsdale, Arizona

Ian Montel, MS, NASM CPT, CES, PES, CSCS
Gilbert, Arizona

Instructional Designers

Casey DeJong, MEd, MBA
Mesa, Arizona

Jeri Dow, MS
Gilbert, Arizona

Editors

Andrew Payne, MS, NASM CPT, CES
Phoenix, Arizona

Kristen Radaich, NASM CPT
Mesa, Arizona

Contributing Authors

Susan J. Hewlings, PhD, RD
Cudjoe Key, Florida

Adam Horak, MBA, BS, NASM CPT, PES, CES
Houston, Texas

Douglas S. Kalman, PhD, RD, FISSN, FACN
Miami, Florida

Brett Klika, BS, CSCS
San Diego, California

Scott Lucett, MS, NASM CPT, PES, CES
Oxnard, California

Pete McCall, MS, NASM CPT, PES
San Diego, California

Marty Miller, DHSc, ATC, NASM CPT, CES, PES, MMACS
Palm Beach Gardens, Florida

Matthew Rhea, PhD, CES, PES, CSCS*D
St. George, Utah

Richard Richey, MS, LMT, NASM CPT, CES, PES
New York, New York

Mabel J. Robles, MS, PES, CES, FNS, WFS, WLS, NASM CPT
Gilbert, Arizona

Kyle Stull, DHSc, MS, LMT, NASM CPT, CES, PES
Austin, Texas

Craig Valency, MA, CSCS
San Diego, California

Robert Weinberg, PhD, CC-AASP
Cincinnati, Ohio

Acknowledgments

Dr. Mike Clark, DPT, MS, CES, PES
Atlanta, Georgia

Aaron Drogoszewski LMT, NASM- CPT, CES, PES, MMACS
Brooklyn, New York

Joshua Gonzalez, BS, CPT, CES, PES, TPI-L1, PCS-Master Coach
Gladewater, Texas

Natalie McCoy, MS, ATC, LAT, PES, CMES, USAF PTL
Colorado Springs, Colorado

Crystal Reeves, BA, NASM Master Trainer, CPT, CES, PES, FNS,
    BCS, WLS, WFS, YFS, GPTS
Scottsdale, Arizona

Prentiss Rhodes, DC, BS, NASM Master Instructor, CPT, CES,
    PES, CSCS, FMS, SFG, Level 1 & 2 Kettlebell Instructor
Scottsdale, Arizona

Alan Russell, MS, ATC, PES, CES
Frisco, Texas

Karl Sterling, NASM MT, EBFA MI, CPT, CES, PES, FNS, GFS
New York, New York

Joshua J. Stone, MA, ATC, CSCS, PES, CES
Champaign, Illinois

Russell Wynter, NASM Master Trainer, CPT, CES, PES, GFS, FNS,
    GPTS, BCS, MMACS, WLS
Scottsdale, Arizona

Additional contributions by: Christopher R. Mohr, C. Alan Titchenal, Cherilyn McLester, Christian Thompson, Fabio Comana, Geoff Lecovin, Jenna A. Bell, Jill E. Gaukstern, Jim Thornton, Jordan R. Moon, Joseph Marsit, Karen G. Roos, Kenneth Miller, Kyle Stull, Lisa Borho, Mark Spreizer, Melanie L. McGrath, Mike Fantigrassi, Ronald Merryman, Scott Roberts, Steve Myers, Theresa Miyashita, Tony Ambler-Wright, Wendy Batts, Yusuf Boyd

New Content

The new edition of *Essentials of Personal Fitness Training* has been revised to meet the needs of the fitness industry by producing a more highly qualified and employable personal trainer, based on market feedback from NASM personal trainers in addition to other industry professionals and employers. The text is sequenced to create a learning experience that exposes students to concepts as they would be relevant in the natural education and development process seen in the industry, thus creating a logical progression from student to professional.

NASM recognizes the need for fitness professionals to feel confident in taking and passing their exam, as well as ensuring that they have an application-based foundation of knowledge to transform science to real-world scenarios. Common industry challenges related to the onboarding of new professional trainers are addressed in detail within this new edition. Some of these challenges include client soft skills, business development and sales exposure, accurate assessment/ corresponding program design, and performing technically sound exercises. Each chapter has an increased focus on the career relevance of the material presented, providing a link between the required science and its application to succeed as a professional within the fitness industry.

In the new edition of this text, students will have exposure to over two full chapters dedicated to business development, as well as four full chapters focused specifically on the rationale, implementation, and appropriate execution of program design. A chapter has also been devoted solely to exercise execution. This addresses the industry need of viewing each exercise as having a distinct purpose and opportunity for movement assessment, thereby increasing the rate of results while aiming to reduce movement dysfunction. This chapter includes a multitude of modalities, robust technique descriptions, explanations of muscle action surrounding the joints, and best practices for modifications. Finally, an updated chapter on behavior change highlights not only the way in which an individual moves through making lifestyle modifications, but also provides an in-depth look at the influences on human behavior and specific tactics that can be applied throughout the training and coaching process. Additionally, the chapter on behavior change provides a more detailed approach to goal setting that has been proven through research.

New Pedagogical Features

This edition of *Essentials of Personal Fitness Training* employs strategic learning features that not only make the content more digestible, but also turn theory into practice. Chapter progression threads science throughout the entire text, rather than all at once, in order to enhance learning and contextual understanding. The new features are as follows:

◆ **Memory Tips**: Tips and trick for trainers to easily remember complex terms without the extended effort of rote memorization.
◆ **Trainer Tips**: Inside-the-industry application tips from experts with years of experience.
◆ **Check It Out**: Quick tips and facts that have an apparent application and real-world usability. This feature enables the reader a quick insight and application to the concepts read.
◆ **Caution**: Distinct things trainers should be aware of as they relate to scope of practice and potential pitfalls.
◆ **Case Scenarios**: Chapter openings and closings that present a relevant situation a personal trainer might come across, along with recommendations for how a fitness professional should address the situation. In addition, the case scenarios help explain real-life situations relevant to the concepts read and help facilitate critical thinking and deeper levels of understanding.

CHAPTER 1

INTRODUCTION TO THE FITNESS PROFESSION

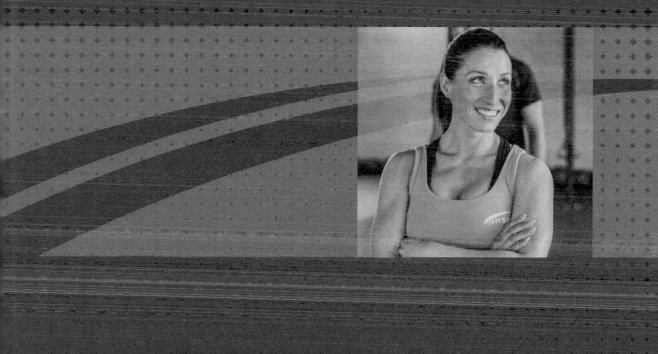

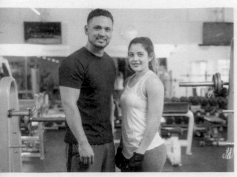
© antoniodiaz/Shutterstock

Case Scenario

You've been thinking about it for some time and have finally taken the steps to begin the journey to becoming a fitness professional. Because of your love for exercise, you feel that making it your profession is a logical decision. However, you have paid little attention to the fitness professionals in the gym you regularly attend, and you feel that it's important to understand what a personal trainer actually does. You want to find out what their duties are and the role they play within the fitness industry.

While in the gym the following week, you make a point to watch a few of the fitness professionals to gain insight into what they do. As you complete your workout, you have listed three concepts that you feel define a fitness professional: science, customer service, and sales. Based on your observations, you feel that further exploration of these three characteristics is needed to fully understand what fitness professionals are and how they fit within the fitness industry.

How do fitness professionals secure a path for success using the concepts of science, customer service, and sales with their clientele?

Welcome to the Fitness Industry

With numerous career pathways and a wide variety of training settings available, the National Academy of Sports Medicine (NASM) Certified Personal Trainer (CPT) has the opportunity to achieve high job satisfaction and career longevity. Personal training provides clients with a valuable service, and health improvement is only one of the many benefits. Additionally, personal training is projected to be a career with a high level of growth potential. Government agencies, businesses, and insurance organizations are continuing to recognize the benefits that health and fitness programs can provide employees. Thus, they are providing their employees with incentives to get fit, and stay fit. Some organizations even provide exercise facilities onsite in an effort to promote the wellness of their employees and to increase productivity. This is expected to help increase the demand for personal trainers and group fitness instructors, leading to a bright career path for the aspiring fitness professional!

The fitness industry plays an important role in the health of the country. Physical activity can promote weight loss and improve body fat composition, which, in turn, can help minimize risk factors for some major chronic diseases. Physical activity can help elevate mood, concentration, and cognitive function. However, many individuals do not know where to start or what to do when it comes to becoming more physically active. Fortunately, fitness facilities provide individuals with solutions they may not be able to find at home. From motivation and assistance to equipment and innovative programs, the fitness industry has made joining a health club or fitness center more appealing than ever. The International Health, Racquet and Sports Club Association (IHRSA) reported that 54.1 million Americans belonged to at least one health club

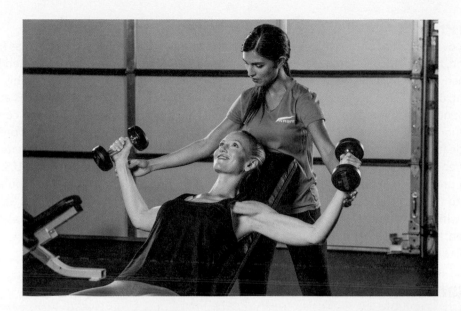

nationwide through 2014. And in that same year there were 144.7 million members utilizing more than 180,000 health clubs; generating $84 billion in revenue worldwide (IHSRA, n.d.).

The Modern State of Health and Fitness

The Industrial Revolution of the early 1900s resulted in the advancement of new technologies that replaced many jobs which previously required physical activity. This major change resulted in a decrease in physical activity in the population as many people adopted a more sedentary urban lifestyle. By the 1950s and 1960s conditions linked to sedentary lifestyles, such as cardiovascular disease, type 2 diabetes, and cancer, were identified as leading causes of death. Since then, efforts have been made to encourage individuals to be more physically active, with national initiatives set in motion to promote healthy lifestyles. Regular exercise has been shown to significantly reduce the risk of heart disease, type 2 diabetes, high blood pressure, some cancers, fractures caused by osteoporosis, and age-related dementia and Alzheimer's disease (Hoeger & Hoeger, 2016). In 2008, the U.S. Department of Health and Human Services issued the Physical Activity Guidelines for Americans, which complement recommendations provided by organizations such as the World Health Organization (WHO) and the American Heart Association (AHA).

Obesity

The condition of being considerably overweight; a person who has a BMI of at least 30 or is at least 30 pounds over the recommended weight for his or her height.

The Prevalence of Obesity

Being overweight or obese creates a predisposition to major health risk factors such as hypertension, hyperlipidemia, and type 2 diabetes, and is a leading determinant for increased levels of inactivity for an affected individual. **Obesity** is the condition of being considerably overweight, and refers to a person with a body mass index (BMI) of 30 or higher or who is at least 30 pounds over the recommended weight for their height (Must et al., 1999). It is a complex condition that increases the risk of death from chronic diseases and is a major cause of preventable death (Centers for Disease Control and Prevention [CDC], 2016). In the United States, the occurrence of obesity in the population varies by state and territory. As of 2014, no U.S. state had a prevalence of obesity below 20%, and in three states 35% or more of the populations fell into this high-risk category (CDC, 2014). Overall, the rate of obesity in the United States is high, with approximately one-third of adults and one-fifth of children being classified as obese (Ogden, Kit, & Flegal, 2014).

History of the Fitness Industry

In the 1950s, health clubs consisted of bodybuilders, power lifters, Olympic lifters, and athletes. It was a male-dominated environment in which men trained with free weights to increase muscle size and strength. Then, in 1951 Jack LaLanne began hosting America's first televised fitness show, *The Jack LaLanne Show*, which aired until 1984. Jack's workouts consisted mainly of calisthenics intermixed with tips on counting calories, weight training, and nutrition. Yet before pioneering a TV show, at the age of 21 Jack LaLanne opened his first health club in Oakland, California, in 1936 where he invented the cable pulley weight training system and the Smith weightlifting machine. Today, both of these implements are still actively used in most fitness centers around the world.

In the 1960s, women's fitness centers, or "figure salons," became a popular trend. Unlike male-oriented gyms, where the focus was on developing muscle size and strength, women's fitness centers typically focused on weight loss and physique improvement. Instead of barbells and dumbbells, most exercise machines in women's fitness centers were passive and focused on "spot reduction." For example, a rolling machine was used to "roll away fat" or a mechanical

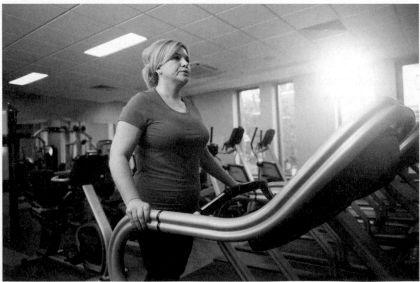

© gpointstudio/Shutterstock

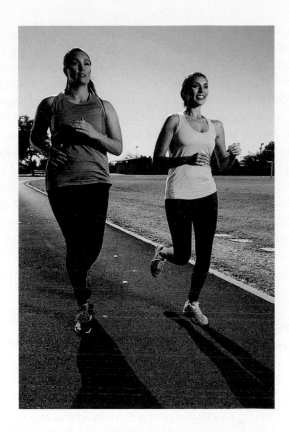

oscillating belt supposedly helped vibrate fat from the thighs and midsection. These techniques have since been proven wholly ineffective.

In the early 1960s, President John F. Kennedy changed the name of the President's Council on Youth Fitness to the President's Council on Physical Fitness in order to address not only children but adults as well. President Kennedy's public support of fitness and exercise had a significant impact on generating greater awareness of health, and spawned tremendous interest in jogging and running. In 1966, Bill Bowerman, the head track coach for the University of Oregon, published a book titled *Jogging*, which helped launch the jogging/running boom in the United States.

By the 1970s, joining a health club or exercising outdoors was becoming more socially acceptable, and soon men and women of all ages were exercising side by side. Joining a health club provided a way of achieving social interaction and health simultaneously. Health clubs began offering an alternative to participating in team sports, which often involve high levels of skill and endurance before the activity can be enjoyed, and also require a more competitive nature. Health clubs became an outlet for anyone to enjoy, regardless of physical ability, which could be used year-round, day or night. The growth in popularity of health clubs was a sign that the general population was becoming more conscious of their health and appearance, and that both could, in turn, be improved through exercise.

The Role of the Fitness Professional

As interest in personal fitness continued to flourish throughout the 1970s, fitness facilities became the desired location for people looking for ways to begin exercising for the first time. Due to the lack of qualified staff during the early days of the health club industry, the majority of new members would often seek out advice from a perceived expert. By default, these "fitness gurus" were the individuals who had been training the longest, appeared to be the most fit, or were the strongest. Oftentimes, novice members would offer money in exchange for training knowledge and guidance, and thus the personal training profession was born.

The 1980s and 1990s saw the formation of various organizations that were solely dedicated to fitness education, as well as the evolution of more formalized education for personal and group fitness trainers. The understanding and application of human movement science began to take precedence, and nutrition content was incorporated more frequently into formal educational programs. As the role of the personal trainer became more prominent within the health club setting, more was required of the individuals filling these positions. More education was required; more job training was required; and, ultimately, more responsibility was required. In today's fitness industry, trainers are becoming highly educated fitness professionals, providing a valuable service to millions of people in need of individualized guidance. Studies show that exercising under the direction of a qualified fitness professional results in greater benefits compared to working out alone (Gentil & Bottaro, 2010; Loughead, Patterson, & Carron, 2008).

Evolution of the Fitness Professional

As fitness professionals become more prominent within the industry, they are being asked to take on more job responsibilities, including sales and ultimately great customer service. Today, the role of a fitness professional includes numerous tasks – on top of simply rendering personal training services – such as providing group instruction, searching for new clients and selling various services sustaining client relationships, maintaining and cleaning equipment, and sometimes even managing other employees. It is important for the new fitness professional to understand that as the fitness industry continues to evolve, so must the traditional job role of the personal trainer.

The role of the fitness professional has also begun to encompass coaching and counseling. It is now extremely important to understand the role that behavior change plays within a successful exercise program. Correctly employing behavior change strategies for clients may be vital to the success or failure of their fitness programs. A great program can be developed with solid scientific backing, but if the client's behaviors are not addressed, and solutions are

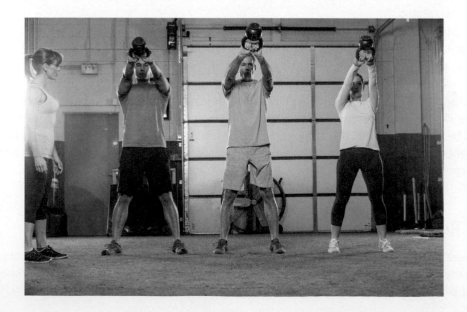

not enacted, then the goals will never be achieved. Not only do fitness professionals serve the fitness needs of their clients, they are also the driving force motivating their clients to succeed.

In recent years, a hybrid role combining personal training and group fitness instruction has become common: group personal training. Fitness professionals looking to serve more clients, and clients looking to reduce the per-session costs of training, have prompted the evolution of the group personal training service. As the trend of participation in group personal training has continued to grow, new challenges have emerged for the fitness professional. Fitness professionals must develop the unique skills needed to meet these challenges and develop the coaching skills necessary to provide individual direction in a group setting.

Welcome to NASM

For more than 20 years, NASM has provided certification, continuing education, solutions, and tools for health, fitness, sports performance, and sports medicine professionals. NASM provides evidence-based health and fitness solutions that optimize physical performance and allow individuals to achieve a variety of fitness-related goals. In addition to the many training and certification programs for experts, NASM empowers individuals to live healthy lives through the use of systematic evidence-based fitness programs. Though NASM may be thought of as an educational provider for the fitness industry, the organization has also been on the forefront of the application of science for the fitness professional. Through the instruction of scientific fitness principles in an easily applicable way, NASM has made it easier for fitness professionals to apply their understanding of the human body in a safe and effective manner. Additionally, NASM is an advocate for the fitness profession, actively participating in events around the world, and forming strategic partnerships with select organizations that also promote health and fitness.

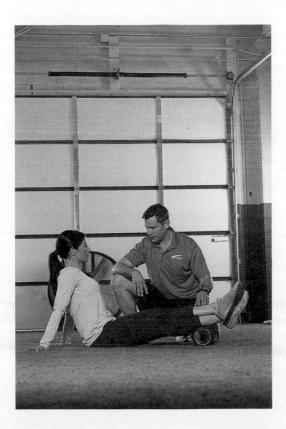

The NASM Certified Personal Trainer Certification

The focus on scientific principles makes NASM's systems and methodologies safe and effective for implementation into a program for any client. Understanding the implementation of these methodologies requires a comprehensive knowledge of human movement science, functional anatomy, physiology, and kinesiology, as well as functional assessments and program design. The NASM CPT certification will provide the basic understanding of scientific principles individuals will need in order to begin a career as a fitness professional. It should be understood that gaining this credential is only the beginning of a path that will require continued growth and education in order to remain successful. Fitness professionals need to enter this career knowing that their professional practice will have to continue to develop, as the science will continually evolve. Changing with the science will also help ensure that the fitness professional is always in a position to safely and effectively change the lives of clients for the better.

Evidence-Based Practice

Science is a fundamental component of the fitness industry. By definition, *science* is the systematic study of something through observation and experimentation. In order for a result to be scientifically sound it must be valid, reliable, and repeatable. A new form of exercise may allegedly produce significant results, but if it is not supported by scientific research it becomes a questionable trend. It is important that fitness professionals have a strong foundation in scientific areas in order to provide solid education to clients, to develop safe and effective training programs, and to help clients reach their goals.

Through a deep understanding of integrated training principles, NASM has made it easier for fitness professionals to apply evidence-based practices to their own careers. It is important for professionals to maintain their current and scientifically based knowledge. It is also important to implement that knowledge in order to provide safe and effective programs for clients. The professional must be able to translate what is learned from the scientific research presented in education programs into actions that will acutely affect the fitness and health of clients. This evidence-based practice is what will ultimately make a program successful.

Musculoskeletal system

The combined, interworking system of all muscles and bones in the body.

Deconditioned

A state of lost physical fitness, which may include muscle imbalances, decreased flexibility, and a lack of core and joint stability.

Muscle imbalance

Alteration of muscle length surrounding a joint.

Integrated Training and the OPT Model

Exercise training programs need to address all components of health-related physical fitness using scientifically recognized training principles. Unfortunately, many training programs and fitness modalities are based on unsound principles and guidelines. It is vital to train essential areas of the body for a safe and effective exercise training program, such as the stabilizing muscles of the hips and the upper and lower back. The strength and stability of a person's **musculoskeletal system** is directly related to the potential risk of injury; that is to say, the more **deconditioned** a person is, the greater the risk of injury becomes (Barr, Griggs, & Cadby, 2005). It is important to note that *deconditioned* does not simply mean that a person is out of breath when climbing a flight of stairs, or that he or she is simply overweight. It is a state in which a person may have **muscle imbalances**, decreased flexibility, or a lack of core and joint stability. All of these conditions can greatly inhibit the ability of the human body to produce proper movement, and can eventually lead to injury.

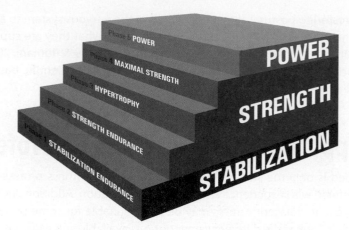

FIGURE 1.1 The OPT Model.

The personal training industry is growing dramatically, especially in regards to the ability of fitness professionals to work with individuals with chronic health conditions or musculoskeletal impairments. Many clients who seek out personal training services are physically inactive and have poor overall functional capacities. However, most training programs do not emphasize movements in all planes of motion or in an environment that challenges an individual's stability and balance, both of which are essential aspects of fitness that cannot be overlooked. The new mindset in fitness should be to create programs that address overall functional capacity as part of a program designed specifically for each individual. In other words, training programs must consider a client's goals, needs, and abilities in a dynamic and systematic fashion. This is best achieved by introducing an approach that integrates multiple components of fitness to not only design a program that is safe and effective, but one that is both challenging and enjoyable.

NASM addressed the need for this integrated approach to training by developing the Optimum Performance Training (OPT) model (**Figure 1.1**). The OPT model was conceptualized as a training program for a society that has more structural imbalances and susceptibility to injury than ever before. It is a process of programming that systematically progresses any client to any fitness goal. The OPT model is built on a foundation of principles that progressively allows any client to achieve optimal levels of physiological, physical, and performance adaptations. The luxury of the OPT model is that it is flexible, so it can be applied to any client, with any fitness need, in virtually any environment. It is comprised of three levels: stabilization, strength, and power; with the strength level broken down into three unique phases. These five phases of training build upon one another culminating in the eventual development of functional power.

Postural Assessments

By observing an individual's posture, both with and without movement, the fitness professional can identify areas of a client's body that need to be focused on in order to produce more efficient movement patterns. Optimal posture allows for correct joint motion, as well as effective absorption and distribution of forces throughout the body. If the body is better able to move and absorb forces, the potential for injury is reduced. Because of the importance of correct posture, the starting point for the development of any program within the OPT model is postural assessment. Posture can either be static (no movement) or dynamic (with movement). Both static and dynamic assessments provide information about how a client's body may function and set a baseline to provide guidance for the direction of a program. Dynamic assessments are vital for identifying areas of movement dysfunction that may affect a client. The goal of these movement assessments is to provide a guide for the fitness professional to assist a client in restoring postural alignment, allowing the nervous system to accurately communicate with the muscular system so that the muscles do what they are supposed to do at the right time (Janda, 1993; Kendall, McCreary, Provance, Rodgers, & Romani, 2005; Sahrmann, 2002). It is important for fitness professionals to understand the scientific basis for these assessments so they can provide the best service for their clients.

Career Opportunities for the Fitness Professional

Becoming certified is only the starting point for a career as a fitness professional. Skills will continue to be refined with experience and continued education. Additionally, multiple career paths are possible, and adjacent careers may be more suitable for some people. New fitness professionals should look at the different career options available and evaluate which one they would like to pursue. From there, they can then put an educational and career development plan into place to achieve their individual professional goals.

Fitness Careers

Many career opportunities exist within the fitness industry, and the newly certified fitness professional is ready to embark on a rewarding career. Employment as a personal trainer in a fitness center is typically where most individuals start their journey as a fitness professional. Other times, they may begin as group exercise instructors, membership representatives, sales associates, or front desk attendants already working in and around the health club setting, and who are looking to branch out to working directly with clients. Regardless of where someone decides to start, the foundation for embarking on a career in the fitness industry is a passion for helping others. Ultimately, the fitness professional may have a desire to grow into a department manager, general manager, or even run his or her own business. These goals will require added dedication and professional development, as these positions have increased responsibilities. It is important that fitness professionals who are looking to advance their careers in this way develop strong managerial, leadership, and business skills.

Adjacent Fitness Careers

Some fitness professionals may decide they want to continue growing their career into a licensed profession, such as a physical therapist or athletic trainer. These licensed professions require education and specialized training that may take several years to obtain. These professions work with and alongside clinical staff and serve the medical community with the ability to diagnose and treat ailments and injuries. As the industry continues to evolve, personal trainers are becoming more prevalent working alongside these licensed professions. Although a career in a licensed occupation may not be the fitness professional's end goal, there may still be opportunities to work with and alongside these clinicians if the necessary knowledge, skills, and abilities are demonstrated.

Places of Employment

Personal training can occur in several different settings. Each venue is unique and requires special skills to be successful. The most accessible health club market is with large-scale national chain fitness centers, where fitness professionals may work exclusively for one corporate employer.

Medium-sized fitness centers, small group training facilities, and high-end boutique health clubs are also on the rise, and all present their own unique challenges and requirements. Furthermore, many fitness professionals will go into business for themselves, offering the flexibility of working from their own homes or homes of clients, in public open spaces, or out of multiple fitness centers as independent contractors. To ensure success in a personal training career, fitness professionals should develop the skills necessary to function effectively in a variety of employment settings.

Succeeding in the Fitness Industry

Knowledge of the science, the ability to apply that knowledge, and being certified are only some key aspects of being a fitness professional. In order to secure the path for a successful career in personal training, the social and business aspects of working in the fitness industry must be addressed. It is imperative to learn about marketing; building relationships; sales; and providing quality, professional customer service. Building a long-lasting career will take time, determination, and preparation, and true success as a fitness professional will be realized from the fusion of three simple things: science, service, and sales.

Incorporating Science

Earning a certification from a recognized and accredited organization is highly important, and should be one of the first goals of an aspiring fitness professional. Having a foundational understanding of the scientific principles of health and wellness will allow the professional to properly assess and instruct clients through safe and effective workouts. No matter what new exercise is utilized with a client, it is important to always question the efficacy of the exercise. The fitness professional must be sure that an exercise can be rationalized based on scientific principles. The exercises chosen for a client should be applied for a specific purpose, in a way that complements that client's individual abilities and goals. Exercises should not be chosen simply because others are performing them or because they look challenging. If the question "What is the purpose of the exercise for the client?" cannot be answered and explained, the fitness professional should consider removing the exercise from the workout.

It is also important to note that the way a professional learns exercise science will not be the way it should be explained to clients, as most clients will not understand complicated scientific terms. As the science behind exercise is learned, it is important to think of creative ways in which the concepts could be explained to a client. The application of the science should also be considered. Scientific concepts are not just facts to be learned, but techniques that must be understood and applied.

Quality Service

Ultimately, the fitness industry is highly dependent on relationships. Fitness professionals will need to develop their social skills in order to effectively connect with clients. Sometimes having a genuine conversation about how an individual's day is going can add tremendous value to the professional–client relationship. This will allow the fitness professional to find out what the client wants and needs, as well as why it is important to the client. These goals can then be incorporated into the planning process, helping the client to move toward achievements in health and fitness while providing the highest levels of service possible.

Quality customer service is driven by maintaining a professional attitude and appearance. It is not only important for the fitness professional to think of how a client's goals can be met,

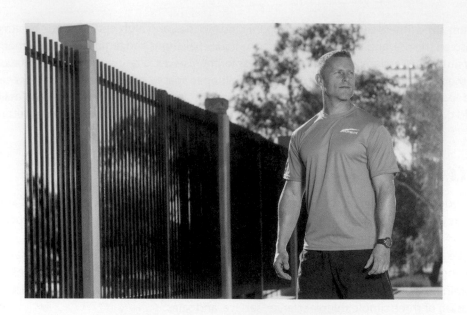

but to do so in a manner that makes the client comfortable and builds trust and credibility. Fitness professionals should actively listen to their clients, find ways to relate to them, and build a rapport that enables the clients to rely on the advice and guidance that is being provided. Similarly, the fitness professional should never project negative feelings onto the client or reveal too much personal information. Although everyone has bad days, fitness professionals' clientele are the core of their business and livelihood, and should always be treated with the utmost professional courtesy. The fitness professional should convey a positive, welcoming, professional attitude that will be apparent to everyone around. This will enhance the fitness professional's reputation, as well as that of the brand or facility represented.

An additional aspect of providing high-quality professional service is record keeping. Assessments should be performed in an ongoing manner throughout the client's fitness program, and the results of the different assessments should be well documented. This process should also be used for tracking the progression of acute variables of each exercise in a client's program. This allows fitness professionals to establish and record a baseline for clients, enabling them to track client progress and provide accurate feedback along the way. Each place of employment will have its own internal system for client management, so it is imperative that new fitness professionals familiarize themselves with the facility's record keeping process right away to provide the best professional service to clients.

Introduction to Sales

Earning an accredited certification provides the scientific knowledge, and an individual's professional attitude, combined with a passion for fitness and helping others, will always lead to excellent service for clients. However, a thorough understanding of the sales process and applicable selling techniques is what will get clients in the door, earn their business, and retain them as clients for the long term. Sales acumen is a must in the fitness industry, because it will ultimately determine how many clients a fitness professional works with and directly drive earning potential. Clients will not often readily commit financially in the name of fitness alone. Many potential clients will need some extra convincing to overcome objections and fully buy in to a personal training regimen. Furthermore, fitness facilities consider the sales process an

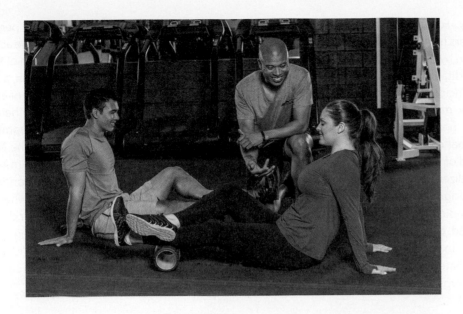

integral part of the personal training workday, often formally evaluating employees on their sales performance. One of the major difficulties facing fitness industry managers today is finding and retaining top-quality fitness professionals who not only know the science and service, but can also master the sales process and drive revenue.

The sales process is not just about asking a potential customer for business and presenting a sales pitch. It is about fully demonstrating the value of personal training services. The potential outcomes for the client should be the focus point, because one cannot put a price on enhanced quality of life. One common technique is to use the science and service to make the sale. This will often be accomplished through a complimentary training session, with the professional taking the potential client through a series of lifestyle evaluations and assessments. These sessions will serve to show the interested individual just how valuable working with a fitness professional can be and allow the fitness professional to demonstrate high levels of credibility to assist in building trust and rapport, strengthening the potential for buy-in to a personal training regimen.

Scope of Practice for the Fitness Professional

Much debate has taken place within the fitness industry with regard to a distinct **scope of practice** for all fitness professionals. Scope of practice serves to define how services should be delivered, the minimum responsibilities of those providing the services, who can receive such services, and, in some instances, the setting in which the services are delivered. In general, the scope of practice for a professional describes the actions, procedures, and processes that he or she is permitted to undertake in meeting the set terms of the professional's license or credential. If a procedure is out of the professional's scope of practice, then taking action should be avoided, and the client should be referred out to another professional.

The concept of scope of practice has traditionally been used within the medical professions, almost all of which require a license in order to practice in individual states. Personal trainers do not currently occupy a role that requires registry of state licensure. However, because fitness professionals interact with apparently healthy individuals and also offer a pay-for-service relationship, it became essential to create a set level of standards to help ensure the safety of the

Scope of practice

The actions, procedures, and processes that a professional is allowed to undertake in keeping with the terms of the professional's license or credential.

public. For this reason, in 2003 the IHRSA recommended that certifying agencies of personal trainers have their exam validated by an independent third party and voluntarily pursue accreditation by the National Commission for Certifying Agencies (NCCA). Thus, as a condition of NCCA accreditation, each organization is required to document a definition of the profession, as well as principles of professionalism, such as standards of professional conduct and a code of ethics.

The modern fitness professional serves to provide guidance to help clients achieve their personal, health, fitness, and performance goals via the implementation of exercise programs, nutritional recommendations, and suggestions in lifestyle modification. According to the NASM Board of Certification, a CPT is defined as a health and fitness professional who performs individualized assessments and designs safe, effective, and individualized exercise and conditioning programs that are scientifically valid and based on clinical evidence for clients who have no medical or special needs. It is not appropriate to diagnose or treat areas of pain or disease. Instead, clients should be referred to other health professionals or practitioners when appropriate. In addition, CPTs are required to hold a current cardiopulmonary resuscitation (CPR) and automated external defibrillator (AED) certification in order to be able to respond appropriately in emergency situations.

Conclusion

Starting this course is the first step toward building a career as a fitness professional. The journey through the fitness industry is both rewarding and life changing. Joining a passionate group of professionals looking to change the lives of those around them is a responsibility that should be taken with great respect. It is important that the new fitness professional be open to learning and gaining as much knowledge as possible in order to guide clients to success. Welcome to the fitness industry!

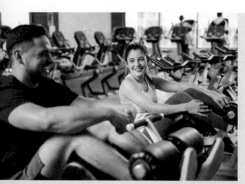
© antoniodiaz/Shutterstock

Case in Review

As you look further into what makes a successful fitness professional, you learn that there is so much more than what you originally thought. From your observations, you have determined the following:

In order for personal trainers to be successful they must be able to provide great service to potential clients and existing clients. This will require focus and personalized attention in all aspects of the job, as well as follow-up. I may even have to do things that I would normally consider someone else's job, such as cleaning equipment, getting a towel for someone, or helping them to get their TV on the right channel. Providing this level of service will make the sales part of the career easier, but I cannot overlook it. In order to build a base of clients and keep clients I have to develop my skillset in order to effectively sell my services. I know that I will have to present packages for people to purchase and try to get them to look past obstacles that may prevent them from purchasing services. Finally, I will have to use a high level of knowledge in order to get the client to meet their goals safely and effectively. If I can do this with great service in mind, the sales will be easier as the clients will fully understand the importance of what they are purchasing from me!

References

American Heart Association. (2015). Heart disease and stroke statistics: 2015 Update. Accessed March 15, 2016. Available at: circ.ahajournals.org/content/131/4/e29.full

Barr, K., Griggs, M., & Cadby, T. (2005). Lumbar stabilization: Core concepts and current literature, Part 1. *American Journal of Physical Medicine and Rehabilitation, 84*(6), 473–480.

Centers for Disease Control and Prevention. (2014). Data, trends, and maps. Accessed March 15, 2016. Available at: www.cdc.gov/obesity/data/prevalence-maps.html

Centers for Disease Control and Prevention. (2016). Characteristics of physician office visits for obesity by adults aged 20 and over: United States, 2012. Accessed March 15, 2016. Available at: www.cdc.gov/nchs/products/databriefs/db237.htm#ref1

Gentil, P., & Bottaro, M. (2010). Influence of supervision ratio on muscle adaptations to resistance training in nontrained subjects. *Journal of Strength and Conditioning Research, 24*(3), 639–643.

Hoeger, W., & Hoeger, S. (2016). *Principles and labs for fitness and wellness.* Boston, MA: Wadsworth, Cengage Learning.

International Health, Racquet and Sportsclub Association. (n.d.). About the industry: Health club industry overview. Accessed March 15, 2016. Available at: www.ihrsa.org/about-the-industry

Janda, V. (1993). Muscle strength in relation to muscle length, pain and muscle imbalance. In: H. Ringdahl (Ed.), *Muscle strength* (pp. 83–91). New York, NY: Churchill-Livingstone.

Kendall, F., McCreary, E., Provance, P., Rodgers, M., & Romani, W. (2005). *Muscles: Testing and function with posture and pain.* Baltimore, MD: Lippincott Williams & Wilkins.

Loughead, T. M., Patterson, M. M., & Carron, A. V. (2008). The impact of fitness leader behavior and cohesion on an exerciser's affective state. *International Journal of Sport and Exercise Psychology, 6*(1), 53–68.

Must, A., Spadano, J., Coakley, E. H., Field, A. E., Colditz, G., & Dietz, W. H. (1999). The disease burden associated with overweight and obesity. *Journal of the American Medical Association, 282*(16), 1523–1529.

Ogden, C. L., Kit, B. K., & Flegal, K. M. (2014). Prevalence of childhood and adult obesity in the United States, 2011–2012. *Journal of the American Medical Association, 311*(8), 806.

Robert Wood Johnson Foundation. (2007). *Recess rules: Why the undervalued playtime may be America's best investment for healthy kids and healthy schools.* Princeton, NJ: Author. Available at: www.rwjf.org/content/dam/web-assets/2007/09/recess-rules.

Sahrmann, S. (2002). *Diagnosis and treatment of movement impairment syndromes.* St. Louis, MO: Mosby.

CHAPTER 2

CAREER DIRECTIONS IN SPORT, HEALTH, AND FITNESS

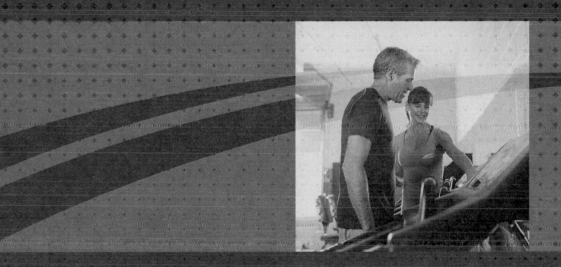

OBJECTIVES

After studying this chapter, you will be able to:

1. **Describe** careers adjacent to the traditional personal trainer.

2. **Detail** the profiles of adjacent careers.

3. **Compare** the scope of practice for various health and fitness careers.

4. **Identify** the educational and experiential requirements associated with adjacent health and fitness careers.

5. **Create** and implement a personal career path that requires personal trainer credentialing.

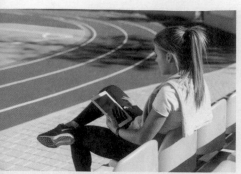

© Dean Drobot/Shutterstock

Case Scenario

You have made the commitment to become a fitness professional due to your love of fitness and healthy living, and feel it is a career choice that provides many great opportunities and avenues to grow as a professional. Without wasting any time, you make it a priority to map out and truly understand how you want to grow professionally within the fitness industry. However, before you begin this process, you realize that there are a few key acknowledgments to be made before you can begin executing your career plan. You have listed the following questions to help you further explore how you plan to grow your career as a fitness professional:

- What are the adjacent careers that can help my career growth within the fitness industry? How do I plan to leverage scope of practice among the various careers adjacent to personal training to build and retain clientele?

- What are some of the educational opportunities that I can take advantage of to develop my career as a fitness professional? How and when will I use these opportunities to become a more successful and specialized personal trainer?

- How will I align networking strategies to my career plan? What steps will I take in order to begin the networking process?

Introduction

Throughout a fitness professional's career, numerous avenues of professional development and advancement will be presented. Oftentimes, these may be in the form of industry requirements that all like-certified professionals are held to. The National Academy of Sports Medicine (NASM) requires Certified Personal Trainers (CPTs) to adhere to a 2-year cycle of continuing education in order to ensure that NASM fitness professionals stay at the cutting-edge of industry advancements and research. With that educational responsibility also comes other requirements that the CPT must adhere to, such as the NASM Professional Code of Conduct and the necessary certifications to respond in an emergency with a client. Continuing education allows fitness professionals to not only stay current within the industry, but to expand their practice in numerous exciting directions. Through the utilization of networking and professional mentors, combined with an understanding of the characteristics of each available career path, fitness professionals will be able to successfully identify the career direction that best suits their individual needs.

Employment Opportunities and Educational Requirements

NASM's CPT certification is an entry-level credential, providing high-quality entry-level skills for the aspiring fitness professional. This certification should be viewed as the launching point for the development of a profession, not the culmination of the necessary education to sustain a long-term career. If fitness professionals stop learning, they will stop progressing, so education is an important part of the fitness career lifecycle. Continued learning is not only a requirement for the maintenance of a certification, but it is also a vital component to career growth and advancement. According to the U.S. Department of Labor, Bureau of Labor Statistics (BLS), fitness trainers and instructors are projected to have a job growth outlook that is on par with the national average, with a current median income of $34,980 per year (BLS, 2015). Numerous avenues of employment are available within the fitness industry, as well as options for fitness professionals to take their careers in adjacent directions.

Fitness Employment Opportunities

As a fitness professional, an individual will have the opportunity to work in a variety of health and wellness settings. These can range from personal training at a large-scale fitness club to assisting licensed medical professionals in a clinical setting. Regardless of their desired career path, new fitness professionals should be familiar with the various options that are available in order to determine which one will be the best fit for them.

Large-Scale Clubs

Many fitness professionals will find themselves working in a large-scale club at some point in their career. These facilities offer numerous amenities to their clientele that are not commonly found in traditional gym environments. These may include spas, restaurants and juice bars, recreational programming, climbing walls, tennis courts, swimming pools, and other offerings in order to provide an all-inclusive family experience for members.

In a large-scale facility, the fitness professional will be able to find work in several different capacities. These positions can include personal trainers, group trainers, group fitness instructors, managers, and membership advisors. Some may also provide space for licensed professionals such as athletic trainers, physical therapists, and registered dieticians in a partnership capacity. These professionals may provide services to members at discounted rates while expanding their practice to individuals who they would not normally reach.

Medium-Sized Fitness Centers

Similar career opportunities for fitness professionals exist in medium-sized fitness centers. These types of facilities are smaller than their large-scale counterparts, focusing more on the fitness portion of a club and less on the all-inclusive family experience. Similar to the fitness opportunities of a large-scale club, a smaller gym may provide personal trainers, group trainers, group fitness instructors, managers, and membership advisors, depending on the size of the facility. These facilities may also partner with licensed professionals for services but on a smaller scale.

Clinical Settings

A clinical setting is generally reserved for those professionals who are licensed. Physicians, athletic trainers, and physical therapists will all work within a clinical practice. Fitness professionals can work alongside many of these licensed professionals in a complementary role. Oftentimes, these individuals may not have time to monitor the prescribed exercise programs given to their patients. Qualified fitness professionals are sometimes utilized to assist the licensed professional in applying the prescribed workouts for patients, as well as helping with the patient's postclinical workouts. The licensed professional does not always have the expertise or time to assist with the design of a postrehabilitation exercise program. A well-trained and well-educated fitness professional can therefore assist by developing and applying effective integrated programming.

Sports Performance

Sports performance centers are focused on the development of the athlete. Although the focus is on developing speed, agility, quickness (SAQ), power, and athletic movement, these facilities may also offer physical therapy and licensed athletic training services as well. A fitness professional with knowledge and experience in the niche areas of high-performance sports can develop a career at a sports performance center. Advanced levels of education and knowledge will be needed to meet the needs of the athletes. In this setting, the fitness professional may assist in the development and/or delivery of a workout regimen. In some cases, the fitness professional may be able to develop into a sports performance coach and train athletes of their own or lead their own group training sessions.

Profiles of Adjacent Careers

Fitness professionals are traditionally understood to work within a gym or club setting by the general public. They are also traditionally looked at as professionals who will help someone develop desired improvements in physique and achieve weight loss goals. As the fitness industry grows and the level of education demanded for these positions increases, a broader understanding of what these professionals can do is beginning to be realized.

Fitness professionals now have the opportunity to grow into or work alongside professionals in adjacent careers. These are careers that may require advanced levels of education and training. However, fitness professionals may be able to either assist with one of these professions, or may even have a desire to grow into one of the occupations themselves. Demand for fitness professionals to not only understand but to also actively develop relationships with these professionals is growing due to the needs of patients and clients. Fitness professionals need to understand the differences between these careers and how they can develop working relationships that are mutually beneficial.

Athletic Trainer

Athletic trainers work directly with sports teams. Some may work out of a standalone facility and contract with local schools and sports teams while still providing athletic training services to individual athletes out of their own private practice. Athletic trainers may serve as emergency responders at sporting events, including games, tournaments, and practices. They will also work closely with injured athletes for rehabilitation purposes and return-to-play protocols. Athletic trainers will also serve as a point of evaluation, providing details on the physical condition of the athlete.

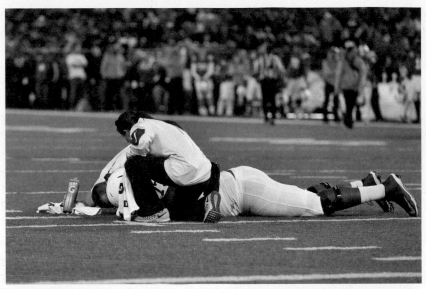

© Aspen Photo/Shutterstock

Traditionally, the athletic training career has required a bachelor's degree. However, the field is now beginning to move towards a master's degree point of entry. This is a licensed profession; by law, candidates are required to sit for and pass a licensure exam in order to practice. The education of an athletic trainer will include the core sciences, along with more advanced athletic training courses. Courses in diagnostic imaging and pharmacology are also included in the overall education of the athletic trainer. According to the BLS, the median income for athletic trainers is $43,370 per year, with a faster than average projected job growth through 2024 (BLS, 2016).

A certified fitness professional can find a very rewarding niche in assisting athletic trainers. Athletic trainers may have several teams and/or athletes they are providing care for. This may not allow them the time needed to oversee every program being carried out at one time. Fitness professionals can assist by overseeing the protocols and ensuring the athlete is performing the prescribed exercises correctly.

Good networking with an athletic trainer can also provide a great benefit to the fitness professional as athletes prepare to return to normal workouts and the field of play. Fitness professionals' knowledge will enable them to provide proper periodization and programming protocols for the further development of the athlete. This is especially important at the high school level, as these athletic trainers do not always have the availability to provide continued guidance once the athlete is cleared to return to normal activity and participation levels.

The scope of practice of the athletic trainer is important for the fitness professional to understand for two reasons. The first is to ensure that the fitness professional is not performing the work of an athletic trainer without the advanced level of knowledge and licensing required by the profession. The second is so that the fitness professional knows what licensed professional to refer a client to when issues emerge outside of the fitness professional's own scope of practice. One of the most common misunderstandings of the general population is the difference between an athletic trainer and personal trainer. It needs to be understood that an athletic trainer is responsible for the following (National Athletic Trainers' Association, 2010):

- Providing emergency services at sports practices and sporting events.
- Providing preventive care, diagnosis, treatment, and rehabilitation of injuries in an athletic setting.
- Coordinating care with physicians and other healthcare professionals.

Fitness professionals should not serve as first responders for athletic events or diagnose and treat athletic injuries unless they have been trained and licensed to do so.

Physical Therapist

Physical therapy is similar to athletic training in that it is a licensed profession; however, it requires doctoral-level education for entry. This career path will require several years of specialized schooling in order to enter the profession. Physical therapists may choose to specialize in a specific area, such as geriatrics, neurology, or pediatrics. In order to specialize, an advanced certification must be sought and acquired by the physical therapist.

The main focus of the physical therapist is to continually assess and reassess in order to ensure the full rehabilitation of each patient. Physical therapists focus on the development of correct movement patterns to ensure proper functioning of the interrelated movement systems of the body. These licensed professionals will utilize hands-on manipulation of the limbs in order to achieve optimal results for the patient as well. Physical therapists will generally work out of a clinic and may partner with other professionals, organizations, or facilities to provide an extended variety of services. Over the next 10 years, occupations in physical therapy are projected to see a much faster than average job growth, with a current median salary of $82,390 (BLS, 2016).

Similar to athletic trainers, fitness professionals may be able to provide assistance to physical therapists by carrying out exercise protocols that are part of a patient's prescribed rehabilitation program. The fitness professional can also provide extended services by providing fitness programming and continued support in postrehabilitation efforts for patients. This will include programing that further assists clients in returning to their preinjury functional capacity, as well as preventing future injury.

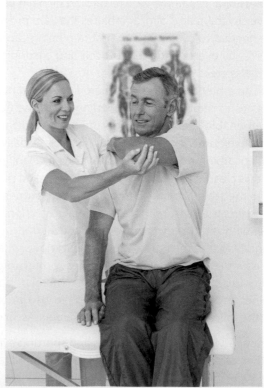

© wavebreakmedia/Shutterstock

It is important for the fitness professional to understand the scope of practice of physical therapists in the same way they understand the scope of practice of athletic trainers. Although athletic trainers and physical therapists often have similar functions, they are distinct professions governed by different scopes of practice and licensure. The fitness professional should understand this differentiation so it is known who to refer to, or from whom a referral is coming. The scope of practice of a physical therapist covers the following (American Physical Therapy Association, 2014):

- Examining of individuals in order to determine a diagnosis, prognosis, and intervention.
- Alleviating impairment and functional limitation through therapeutic interventions.
- Preventing injury and limitation while promoting the maintenance of health, wellness, and fitness.
- Determining return-to-play for athletes.
- Engaging in consultation, education, and research.

These individuals work in clinical settings and, along with consultation and diagnosis, also provide prognoses for patients. They are an integral part of the allied health team for the rehabilitation and prevention of all injuries, surgeries, and diseases that affect patients' ability to function in daily life.

Registered Dietician

Fitness professionals who wish to specialize in the nutritional and dietary considerations of clients may want to consider becoming a registered dietician. A thorough understanding of nutrition science will allow fitness professionals to better market themselves as health and wellness experts. However, if fitness professionals want to provide detailed meal planning, as well as nutritional guidance for those who have special dietary needs, they will need to seek the educational pathway that leads to registered dietician licensure.

As with other licensed professions, a registered dietician will need to meet the educational requirements in order to sit for and pass the professional licensing exam. This career field requires a master's degree for entry. The education will cover advanced concepts in chemistry and biochemistry to develop a complete understanding of the interactions of nutrients within the

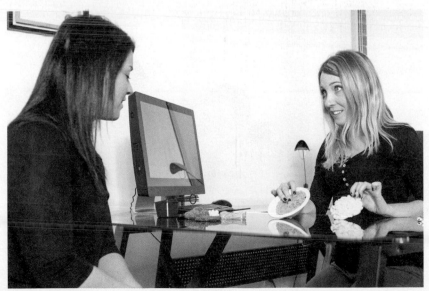

© Lopolo/Shutterstock

body as well as to describe the many clinical concerns that affect the body's ability to maintain a healthy nutritional balance. Registered dieticians currently earn a median salary of $56,950 and have a much faster than average job growth outlook (BLS, 2016).

Fitness professionals can benefit from networking with registered dieticians by providing fitness training services to the dieticians' clients. The fitness professional will also have a resource to refer clients to who may want more specific nutritional guidance or who have special dietary considerations. Dieticians are a valuable resource that fitness professionals should include in their network.

A registered dietician must also follow a strict scope of practice. It is especially important for fitness professionals to understand this scope of practice so they can ensure that they are not crossing over into the realm of a licensed professional. It is very easy to end up providing nutritional guidance that would otherwise fall under the scope of practice of a registered dietician, leading to legal and ethical issues for the fitness professional. The scope of practice for a registered dietitian includes the following (Academy of Nutrition and Dietetics, 2013):

◆ Performing comprehensive nutrition assessments.
◆ Determining nutritional diagnoses.
◆ Designing and implementing nutritional intervention plans.

The fitness professional can evaluate a client's eating habits and provide general advice that is available to the public, such as government-approved guidelines on how to improve nutritional intake. However, utilizing his or her expertise in order to provide extensive nutritional plans, without understanding potential clinical risks, will put the fitness professional outside of his or her scope of practice.

Facility Owner

Some fitness professionals may want to own their own business at some point in their career. Owning a club or gym requires a high level of entrepreneurial acumen. Fitness professionals pursuing this route will not only need to continue to grow their understanding of the fitness industry as a whole, but they will need to obtain advanced education on business and business law. Depending on the size of the facility the fitness professional wishes to own, the fitness

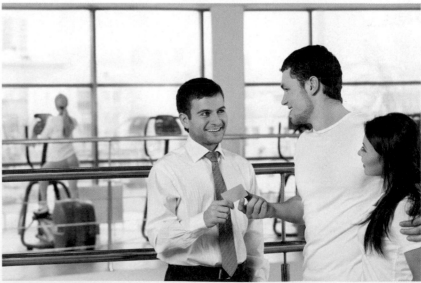

© LuckyImages/Shutterstock

professional may also need to work on developing a partnership with investors in order to start the business. Once a business is up and running, however, the earning potential for the fitness entrepreneur is limited only by his or her dedication and drive to succeed.

As a club owner, the fitness professional will need to understand industry trends and what clients are looking for from a fitness facility. Just as the fitness professional may want to develop his or her knowledge, skills, and abilities to address a niche market, gyms and clubs do the same. The owner will need to decide what the niche market of the facility is in order to provide services and equipment to meet the needs of that clientele.

The club owner will also have to gain a deeper understanding of available equipment and equipment maintenance practices. A fitness professional can obtain this understanding by working in gyms and clubs and observing what the owner is responsible for. The owner will be responsible for ensuring that the right equipment is purchased from reputable manufacturers and that it is properly maintained over time. This will require the development of relationships with equipment sales and service representatives and an understanding of the differences between manufacturers.

Group Fitness

A group fitness instructor has historically been referred to as an *aerobics instructor*. With the growth of the group fitness instructor industry, and expansion into areas such as cycling, suspension training, and fight sports–type classes, the term *group fitness instructor* has replaced the traditional "aerobics" moniker. The group fitness instructor has a unique role in the fitness industry and can be a very valuable resource. Many group fitness instructors have a large following, and therefore a platform to develop relationships with several clients at one time. This gives group fitness instructor an excellent starting point for a client base if they are looking to move into the personal training space. Group fitness instructors can expect a similar median income and job outlook as other fitness professionals.

The fitness professional should make a point of developing relationships with group fitness instructors. Not only will this provide an opportunity to help personal training clients discover beneficial classes they may not have explored on their own, but a good symbiotic relationship

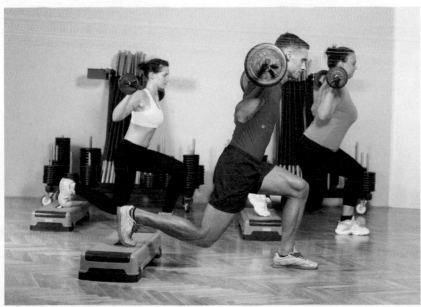

with a group fitness instructor may be reciprocated. For example, if a trainer has a client who needs to increase her level of activity but lacks a high level of motivation, the trainer may suggest she attend a class with high-intensity interval training (HIIT) based in sports performance exercises. If the fitness professional has a good relationship with the group fitness instructor of the class, the fitness professional may receive a referral back the next time the group fitness instructor has a participant who is looking for more one-on-one training. Developing an understanding of different classes and instructors is vital for the fitness professional to provide better service for clients, and to build a larger client base.

Management

The manager of a club or gym serves as the day-to-day leader of the team. Managers may be in charge of a specific team (personal trainers, group fitness instructors, sales, etc.), several teams, or the entire facility. The educational pathway for managers is not clearly defined, although some facilities have minimum educational and experience requirements. Managers will need to have a solid understanding of the fitness industry and of the club's target clientele, as well as a good understanding of customer service and business practices. Managers should also develop strong leadership skills.

Managers will be in charge of pushing their assigned area of the club to success. They will need to develop client-focused processes, programs, and services and mentor and train their employees. Managers are in charge of all staffing issues, including hiring, firing, training, and disciplining employees. Some managers may also be required to provide some of the same services as their staff members. Managers may work more defined hours than their staff, though they may also be the last resort to fill in if an assigned staff member is unavailable. Although salaries vary greatly across different industries, as well as by facility size and type within the fitness industry, general and operations managers can expect annual salaries ranging from $40,000 to over $100,000 (BLS, 2016).

A fitness professional with career aspirations to become a manager needs to understand the added responsibility that comes with the position. The fitness professional should also work closely with the current manager and administration to gain an understanding of club operations and what the job requirements and expectations are for the facility.

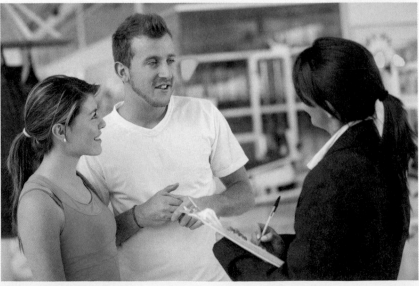

© Andresr/Shutterstock

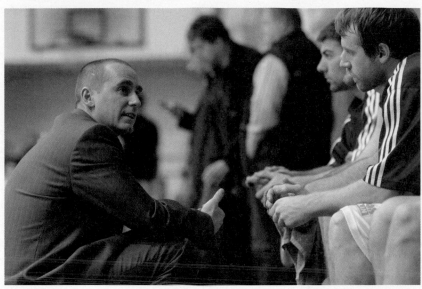

© muzsy/Shutterstock

Sports Coach

Sports coaches are those who are involved in the instruction and training of an individual or team of athletes. Sports coaches have generally participated in, or are passionate about, the sport they coach. The pathway to becoming a sports coach does not always require a formalized path of education, rather it requires experience. Many sports coaches will have spent time taking courses in sports management programs. Similar to fitness professionals, sports coaches have a job growth outlook that is on par with the national average, and currently see a median annual salary of $30,640 across all levels of athletics (BLS, 2016).

Sports coaches can work with athletes of all ages, from youth programs through the professional levels of sports. Coaches at the high school level will often provide services as both a sports coach and as a trainer in developing workout programs for athletes. If sports coaches do not feel confident in their abilities to provide a safe and effective training program for athletes, they may employ the services and expertise of a fitness professional who understands the needs and demands of student athletes in a specific sport.

Strength and Conditioning Coach

Strength and conditioning coaches are certified professionals who have gone through educational pathways that provide the background necessary to work with high-performance athletes. This career requires credentials specifically in the niche of sports performance. Some positions will demand higher levels of education, including formal degrees. Other positions may require certain credentials and experience.

Strength and conditioning coaches may work with a single team, single athlete, or several teams. They will be required to evaluate the success of athletes, develop and oversee athlete-specific programs, and work with the coaching staff and sports medicine faculty to ensure that the athletes are receiving the needed care and developing in a way that is conducive to their success. These athlete-specific coaches will see a job growth and earning potential similar to other fitness professionals.

The fitness professional looking to work in this capacity needs to seek out the advanced certifications and educational opportunities specifically for sports performance. They will also need to become a student of the specific game of the athletes they are looking to work with. Without a deep understanding of the demands, movements, and requirements of the sport,

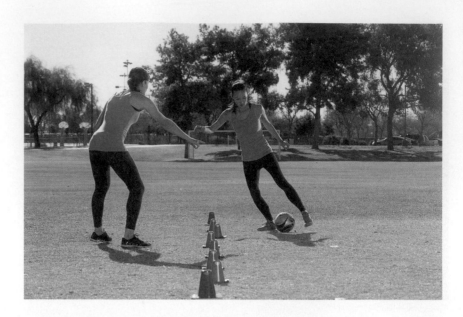

the professional will be unable to provide a clear and effective training program. Although not a requirement, a deep passion for the development of the athlete will help the success of the fitness professional who chooses this career pathway.

Licensed Massage Therapist

Licensed massage therapists are individuals who have completed a formal education program from an accredited massage school. Most U.S. states require specific licensing that can be obtained once the educational program has been completed. Programs for certifying as a licensed massage therapist are usually 500–1,000 hours in length and cover a wide range of topics, such as anatomy and physiology, kinesiology, massage techniques, and legal and ethical issues surrounding the practice. Numerous massage types and methods are available to massage therapists, with many focusing specifically on sports and fitness applications.

Individuals interested in massage therapy must not only be passionate about helping others, but highly comfortable with the human body and direct interaction with clients. Furthermore, as fitness professionals expand their education and practice into advanced areas such as corrective exercise, they will recognize the benefits of obtaining licensing as a massage therapist so that they can manipulate their clients' bodies directly. Dedicated licensed massage therapists are projected to see a much faster than average job growth over the next decade, and currently have a median salary of $37,180 across the profession (BLS, 2016).

Fitness professionals will benefit from developing a professional relationship with a licensed massage therapist. Many areas covered in a fitness professional's scope of practice, such as flexibility, posture, and muscle imbalances, are areas a massage therapist will also directly assist clients with. Furthermore, massage therapy can offer excellent relief from the soreness associated with intense training.

Continuing education

Any of a variety of course offerings that serve the purpose to keeping professionals up-to-date with their knowledge and skills.

Educational Responsibilities

Fitness professionals should spend a substantial part of their practicing career in **continuing education**. With the rise of the internet and the accompanying information age, today people are able to access more industry content than ever before. In the fitness world, there is a great deal of

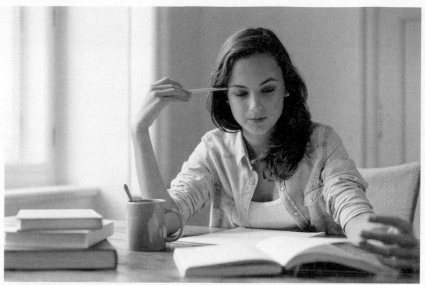

© CandyBox Images/Shutterstock

good information, just as there is a great deal of bad information. As people attempt to decipher what is right and wrong in the conflicting reports, they will look to fitness professionals as the experts, helping them to determine what information is most accurate. Fitness professionals should use continuing education to arm themselves with knowledge in order to address common misconceptions and remain at the forefront of industry changes in order to better meet their clients' needs.

Evolving research also continues to show new best practices. **Best practices** are the techniques and processes that have been shown to be the safest and most effective for a given situation. New research may show that some training techniques are no longer relevant, or that they are now shown to be contraindicated. The fitness professional has an obligation to ensure that the most up-to-date practices and knowledge are identified and employed with clients. Fitness professionals need to align their personal techniques and styles with the available evidence. Research should not just be read, but rather be actively implemented into the fitness professional's daily practice. This will ensure that safe and effective training practices are in place at all times. Fitness professionals should also seek out the best practices that will most benefit the specific client they are currently working with. If a client falls under the classification of a **special population** or requires the accomplishment of a unique goal, the fitness professional should look for continuing education opportunities that will provide the knowledge, skills, and abilities to successfully work with that particular client.

The fitness professional should take the time to evaluate the different learning and **continuing education unit (CEU)** options available. Beginning this search process is as simple as looking at the preapproved CEU providers that align with NASM. In order to maintain the NASM CPT certification, the fitness professional will need to obtain 2.0 CEUs every 2 years. The CEUs are counted by contact hour of training, with each contact hour equaling 0.1 CEUs. This means that a NASM-certified professional needs 20 contact hours of continuing education every 2 years to maintain the certification.

CEUs should not be viewed as a last-minute requirement for the fitness professional to obtain in order to remain certified. Instead, they should be viewed as an opportunity for fitness professionals to grow, learn, and add value to their services on a consistent basis. The fitness industry is large, with several options a fitness professional can specialize in. Continuing education supplies the necessary knowledge to provide services to a more diverse group of clients, and allows fitness professionals to further define their career path.

Best practices
Professional procedures that are considered to be correct, safe, or most effective.

Special population
Individuals who will require modifications or specialized training.

Continuing education unit (CEU)
A measure used in continuing education courses that is designed for professionals to maintain a certification or licensure.

TRAINER TIPS

Make sure to frequently visit the NASM.org website for the most up-to-date recertification requirements and continuing education options.

CHECK IT OUT

The following are a few questions a fitness professional can use to evaluate CEU courses:

- *How do I learn best?* CEUs are offered in a variety of ways. Fitness professionals should evaluate their own learning style and find the CEU offerings that best match their learning style.
- *What area do I need to grow in/review?* It is important that a fitness professional become well-rounded in many different areas to address the needs of several different clients. Fitness professionals should be willing to look at their own level of knowledge and address any knowledge gaps through continuing education opportunities. Many fitness professionals feel that they have an inadequate amount of knowledge in the area of nutrition to fully address the questions their clients have. A course in nutrition may be able to help address these particular knowledge gaps.
- *What needs do my clients have?* Clients are going to have different needs and/or requirements. A good fitness professional will look at ways in which these needs can be addressed. Oftentimes, it may be through CEU courses. For example, a course devoted to women's fitness will be important for a fitness professional who has a growing clientele of prenatal clients.
- *What niche do I want to have?* As fitness professionals become more established in their careers and develop a solid client base, they may want to focus on a specific niche. Some fitness professionals enjoy working with older adults. They may work in an area that has a growing senior population that needs fitness opportunities. A course that addresses the needs of the senior population would be a good fit for these professionals.
- *What are my interests?* Fitness professionals should also look at courses that are interesting to them. If a fitness professional is interested in sports and athletes, a CEU course in sports performance may be the perfect fit.

CEU Courses

CEU courses are delivered through a variety of different means. Many are delivered through an online format that offers the fitness professional access to videos, activities, and downloadable reading materials. These courses will generally have a capstone quiz or test to evaluate the professional's level of understanding of the content. Upon completion of the course with a passing score, the professional is awarded the CEUs from the course. Some courses may also be offered with a video or book that is mailed to the professional. If the course is not offered online, the organization may require a mail-in or fax-in answer sheet to obtain the CEUs. Further, if the CEU provider is not NASM preapproved, the professional will be required to submit the course information to NASM for approval in order to receive CEUs toward their recertification.

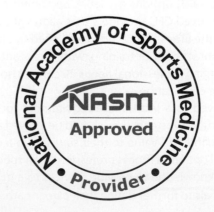

Traditional Advanced Education

Traditional educational pathways are an excellent way to grow and gain CEUs. Collegiate degrees will increase the marketability of the fitness professional, similar to earning an advanced credential, which may lead to career advancement within the industry. And continuing a formal education is now more convenient than ever, with options delivered completely online, hybrid programs that are both online and in classrooms, and traditional programs delivered in person on a campus. They range from 6-month associate degrees to doctoral programs (e.g., PhD), and any credit hours earned in collegiate courses that relate directly to health, wellness, and fitness can be applied as CEUs.

As with any major decision, the choice to continue one's education through traditional means should be made with care. Formal school will require time, dedication, and resources that many other CEU opportunities will not require. Further, to complete an educational program, fitness professionals may also need to take time off from the direct development of their career to focus on higher learning. It should also be noted that the career path of a fitness professional may define whether advanced education is necessary. For example, some positions and careers will directly require an undergraduate degree in order to gain the necessary skills for entry, whereas others may simply prefer that certain certifications are obtained to ensure greater levels of marketability for the facility. Although traditional schooling is not a requirement to become a successful fitness professional, it should not be ruled out as a viable or necessary option for continuing education.

Live Events

Live events can encompass several different types of CEU opportunities and are offered at various locations. They range from single-day intensive seminars to week-long conferences that offer multiple educational opportunities. Oftentimes, these events will require travel and overnight lodging. CEUs are awarded to the fitness professional based on his or her attendance at the event. Some may offer onsite testing for specializations or certifications during the event. Not only are live events an excellent opportunity to obtain hands-on learning and direct contact with teaching professionals, but they offer an excellent opportunity for networking with other fitness professionals from around the globe.

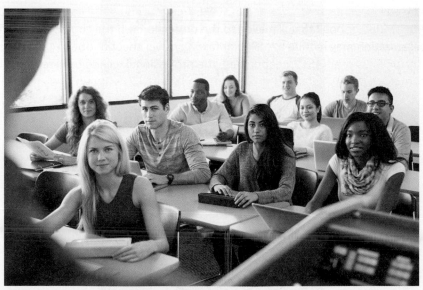

© Monkey Business Images/Shutterstock

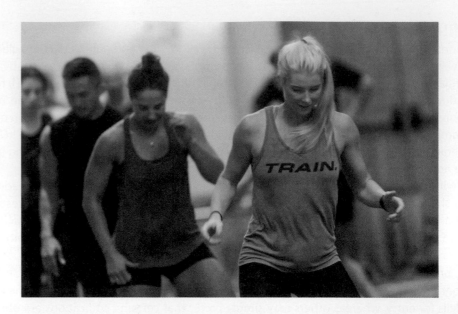

Publications

One of the best ways for a fitness professional to gain quick access to the most up-to-date research is through publications. The fitness industry is served by several types of publications, ranging from digital magazines to peer-reviewed research journals. Some will offer quizzes based on one of the articles in the publication, which the fitness professional can then mail/fax in for CEUs upon successful completion.

When selecting publications, fitness professionals must be vigilant in selecting only those that are based on valid research. Some publications may provide statements based on opinion or industry myth rather than scientific research. Having an understanding of who the authors are, as well as who the publisher is, will define the credibility of the article and help the professional determine which publications to choose.

In the same respect, fitness professionals must be able to read, understand, and apply scientific research when selecting publications. Peer-reviewed journals provide scientific

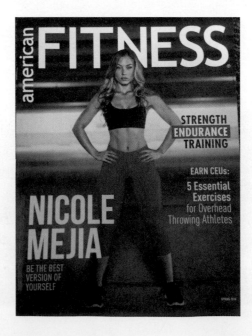

research studies that require an understanding of research and statistical practices. Without this prerequisite understanding, the fitness professional may not understand the applicability of the research to fitness practice. Other publications provide not only the research, but also the practical application of the research. These types of publications will be better options for those fitness professionals who do not have a formal background in statistics or research studies.

Growing Professionally

The fitness industry has several different career pathways that the fitness professional can embark upon. Each of these pathways will force the fitness professional to continue to grow and learn in order to maintain professional licensure or certification. Education is a vital component in career growth. However, working with experienced fitness professionals can provide valuable experience and insight that educational pathways cannot. Finding mentors and networking are two ways this can be accomplished.

Mentors

Mentors are an invaluable resource for the new fitness professional. These are experienced individuals who will provide advice and guidance to less experienced individuals. Good mentors will provide life and career experience not always found within the structure of educational courses. They will also give the mentored individual continual feedback on different situations as they are encountered.

The fitness professional who is seeking a mentor should look to those who have successfully achieved similar career aspirations. Mentors should be those who are delivering messages in line with the same philosophies carried by the fitness professional. This may require fitness professionals to look beyond their own community. Some mentors are willing to provide guidance through phone calls, email, and video chats. A single fitness professional may seek the advice of several different mentors from different backgrounds. Some of these mentors may even be outside of the fitness industry.

Mentor
A trusted advisor in a specific area.

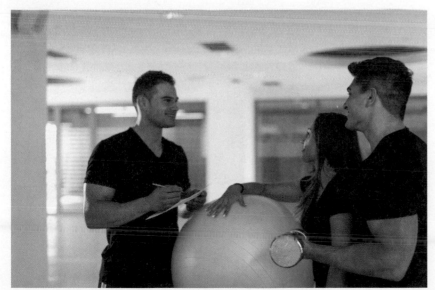

© Jasminko Ibrakovic/Shutterstock

When working with a mentor, the fitness professional should understand that he or she is building a relationship with the mentor. It may take some time to get comfortable with communication and asking the right questions. Mentored individuals need to approach the relationship from a mindset of listening and learning. Being open minded and willing to hear hard advice will help the fitness professional grow. In the same way, fitness professionals should seek out mentors who challenge them in a professional manner.

Note that some mentors may charge money for their mentoring services. In these instances, fitness professionals should evaluate the opportunity in a similar way they would the educational opportunities in the industry. Having a mentor is an investment of time, and potentially money, to the future success of their career.

Networking

An important part of advancement in any career is networking. Networking is the active development of professional relationships that will result in the exchange of information or services to advance one's career. In any profession, the development of relationships with those who are both in and out of the industry is a vital component in continued business opportunities and growth.

Fitness professionals need to be willing to extend themselves to engage with other professionals in order to develop trust in the relationship. One of the quickest ways to begin developing a network and building these relationships is to discuss the industry with other professionals. Sharing industry information, including discussions on the latest trends, research, and methodologies, will show a willingness to grow professionally as well as reflect the fitness professional's strong background in, and understanding of, science-based training. The conversation should approach a level of discussion similar to speaking with a colleague or friend. People will hold those in their professional network as relevant and equal peers. These discussions should be held in person, if possible, and not via email or cold calls.

Professionals should also be selective about who they allow into their professional network. These individuals should be made up of professionals who can serve as referral resources. Developing a strong network of trusted massage therapists, chiropractors, physical therapists, athletic trainers, dieticians, personal trainers, group fitness instructors, and others will provide a trusted pool of individuals that the fitness professional can not only learn from, but also

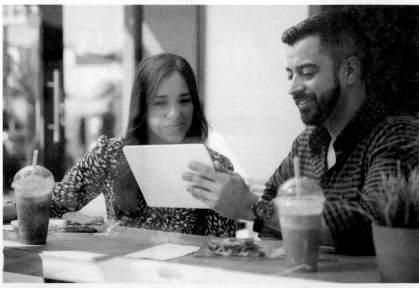

© antoniodiaz/Shutterstock

send clients to as needed. Referrals are a reciprocal relationship from which new clients can be gained.

Building a strong network can also provide support and insight into the industry that may not otherwise be available. Networks provide a group of professionals who can be turned to for job recommendations, inside information on industry or community trends, and guidance for certain client conditions. The fitness professional should work diligently to build a trusted network of professionals that can be relied upon for professional support and camaraderie.

Scope of Practice and Professional Limitations

Scope of practice refers to the knowledge, skills, abilities, processes, and limitations that a practitioner in a specific industry should be held accountable for. It sets the guidelines as to what certain professionals can legally do in their professional practice. The scope of practice for a fitness professional lies within the knowledge gained from the combined educational advancements an individual has made, including professional certifications and credentials. Fitness professionals should not recommend anything to clients that they have not been properly trained in. This defines the limitations that the fitness professional will be held to. Some individuals will have advanced levels of education that allow them to perform procedures that fall outside the traditional scope of practice for a fitness professional. The NASM scope of practice is as follows:

◆ CPTs are health and fitness professionals who perform individualized assessments and design safe, effective, and individualized exercise and conditioning programs that are scientifically valid and based on clinical evidence to clients with no medical or special needs.
◆ CPTs provide guidance to help clients achieve their personal health, fitness, and performance goals via the implementation of exercise programs, nutritional recommendations, and suggestions in lifestyle modification
◆ CPTs hold a current emergency cardiopulmonary resuscitation (CPR) and automated external defibrillator (AED) certification and respond appropriately in emergency situations.
◆ CPTs do not diagnose and/or treat areas of pain or disease and will refer clients to other healthcare professionals/practitioners, when appropriate.
◆ CPTs abide by NASM's code of professional conduct at all times.

Referring Clients

"Certified Personal Trainers . . . will refer clients to other healthcare professionals/ practitioners when appropriate."

The fitness professional should remain within the scope of practice at all times. If a situation occurs where the fitness professional is unsure about whether a situation falls within his or her scope of practice, the best thing to do is to refer the client to a more qualified professional This may happen with certain nutritional discussions. It is good for fitness professionals to have nutritional resources that they can guide the client to if the discussion reaches a point outside of the fitness professional's knowledge.

Referrals may also occur if a physical limitation or impairment is exposed or becomes a problem for a client. Referring a client to a licensed medical professional should become common practice in incidences where further medical evaluation is necessary. If a client is experiencing joint pain after rehab, a referral to a physical therapist will be needed. If a client has difficulty when breathing after running, a referral to a physician may be warranted.

The fitness professional should also be willing to refer a client to a colleague of the same profession if the situation or needs of the client makes the fitness professional feel uncomfortable. Some clients may have conditions the fitness professional has not heard of or worked with previously. Referring the client to someone who has experience working with the condition will ensure the safety and effectiveness of a program for that individual. It is important for the fitness professional to continue learning; however, the fitness professional should remain aware of his or her limitations and be willing to get clients in touch with those who can best help them.

Diagnosing

"Certified Personal Trainers do not diagnose and/or treat areas of pain or disease."

Diagnosing occurs when there is an identification of a medical condition (pain or disease) based on the examination of symptoms. The only professionals who should be making diagnoses are those who are licensed clinical professionals. These professions are those that require the individual to take a state or federally mandated examination in order to provide professional services (e.g., physicians, chiropractors, athletic trainers, physical therapists, etc.).

Fitness professionals who are not licensed (e.g., personal trainers, group fitness instructors, etc.) should not diagnose any condition based on symptoms a client or participant is showing. The fitness professional should refer the client/participant to speak with a professional who can better address his or her needs. The fitness professional should avoid any language that may lead the individual to believe that he or she has a medical condition, such as "it sounds similar to a torn ACL" or "you may have diabetes." Instead the fitness professional should guide the participant to speak to a licensed professional about the symptoms in order to receive a proper diagnosis.

Prescribing

"They provide the guidance to help clients achieve their personal health, fitness, and performance goals via the implementation of exercise programs, nutritional recommendations, and suggestions in lifestyle modification."

Similar to diagnosing, prescribing treatments or protocols for disease or injury is something that only a licensed professional should be performing. Prescribing is authorizing the use of medicine or a treatment for someone to overcome a specific ailment. Generally, fitness professionals are not put into situations in which they will be prescribing treatments for clients or participants. The fitness professional should be providing workout programs for clients, rather than "prescribing" workouts.

Many fitness professionals will find themselves in a gray area of prescription when it comes to nutrition. Registered dieticians are licensed professionals who are legally allowed to prescribe specific meal plans and dietary programs for individuals who have special dietary needs. Fitness professionals can speak to scientifically valid nutritional information, but should not provide specific meal plans that direct individuals to eat set amounts of food at specific times. These types of discussions and materials should be left to the registered dietician to handle.

Conclusion

With a solid understanding of the requirements needed to maintain the NASM CPT certification, fitness professionals now have the roadmap to continue their education and further steer their desired career paths to meet their individual desires. Understanding the scope of practice for fitness professionals, as well as those of adjacent health and wellness professions, will enable the fitness professional to practice safely with their clients, as well as avoid any unwanted legal liability. Note that any job functions that lie outside the scope of practice of a fitness professional should be referred to the correct licensed practitioner. So long as the overarching requirements and guidelines are met, fitness professionals will be ready to certify, and then begin to network and work with mentors to take their careers as far as their ambition will allow.

Case in Review

After taking the time to research the fitness industry further, you have made some notable findings that will be used to help define your career path as a fitness professional. Having an understanding of the professional direction you need to take will help you to grow your career and ensure you stay competitive in the industry. From the questions you had asked yourself initially, you have compiled some answers to help better define the direction you plan to grow as a fitness professional.

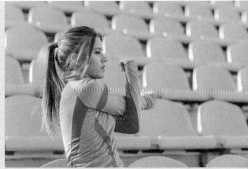

© Dean Drobot/Shutterstock

Educational opportunities that will help me grow as a professional	**CEU courses**: After I become certified, I will research areas and potential CEU opportunities that interest me. This will begin with talking to NASM and some of my professional mentors.
	Live events: I am going to look into industry events and live events offered by NASM. I will choose ones that seem interesting and are nearby to save on travel. I will begin attending these events before I complete my certification because I want to understand what I am learning more.
	Mentors: I will talk to my professional mentors to get their recommendations for how to succeed professionally. I will do this immediately to supplement what I am learning in my course.

Adjacent careers that can help reach potential clientele	**Physical therapist:** I can work with a physical therapist to recommend clients to and get referrals from. I can also seek mentoring on tasks that are within my scope from the physical therapist.
	Athletic trainer: I can work with an athletic trainer and learn from them. I can also seeking referrals from them as their athletes work in the off-season or outside of rehab.
	Registered dietician: I can work with the registered dietician for referrals. I could even partner with the registered dietician to provide comprehensive packages that would include both nutrition and training.
Adjacent careers that I can build a network with to help provide an inclusive service experience	**Physical therapist:** I will locate a physical therapist close to my gym and walk in to introduce myself, drop off a card, and see if I can set up some time with them to discuss the development of a referral network. I will set them up with a free training session so they can see my expertise.
	Athletic trainer: I will locate a local high school with an athletic trainer and ask if I can shadow a practice or game they are working. I will discuss the knowledge that each of us has and provide an overview of what I can offer athletes. I will ask if I can run their athletes through a free training session so they can see my expertise.
	Registered dietician: I will locate a registered dietician close to my gym and ask to meet with them to get an idea of what services they offer. I would discuss my service offerings, scope of practice, and why I think a partnership would be valuable.

References

Academy of Nutrition and Dietetics. (2013). Academy of Nutrition and Dietetics: Scope of practice for the registered dietitian. *Journal of the Academy of Nutrition and Dietetics*, *113*(6, Suppl 2), S17–S28.

American Physical Therapy Association. (2014). Guidelines: Physical therapist scope of practice. Accessed March 15, 2016. Available at: www.apta.org/uploadedFiles/APTAorg/About_Us/Policies/Practice/ScopePractice.pdf

Bureau of Labor Statistics, U.S. Department of Labor. (2015). *Occupational Outlook Handbook, 2014–2024*. Accessed March 15, 2016. Available at: www.bls.gov./ooh/personal-care-and-service/fitness-trainers-and-instructors.htm

National Athletic Trainers' Association. (2010). An overview of skills and services performed by certified athletic trainers. Accessed March 15, 2016. Available at: www.nata.org/sites/default/files/guide_to_athletic_training_services.pdf

CHAPTER 3

DISCIPLINES OF FUNCTIONAL BIOMECHANICS

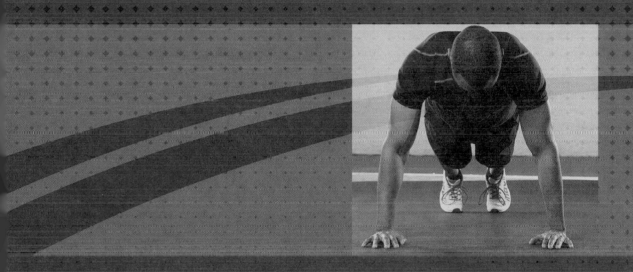

OBJECTIVES

After studying this chapter, you will be able to:

1. **Explain** biomechanics and the role it plays in the development of a personal training program.

2. **Apply** basic biomechanics principles.

3. **Explain** the function of the muscle action spectrum.

4. **Use** biomechanics terminology to explain functional muscle anatomy.

5. **Explain** the influence of dysfunctional muscles on the function of the kinetic chain.

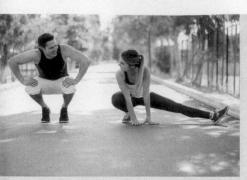

© antoniodiaz/Shutterstock

Case Scenario

After making the decision to begin a career in fitness, you have researched professions that align with your goal of becoming a fitness professional. By now you have a strong grasp on how becoming a certified personal trainer aligns with your personal and professional goals.

Before you begin a daily run with a friend, you begin to express your excitement for this new career path you have chosen by explaining the importance and benefits of understanding human motion. Your friend, a fitness enthusiast as well, is finding what you have begun to say interesting, and wants to know more about the functions of the Human Movement System and how they can be explained in everyday movements.

Identify three common movements done on a daily basis and explain to your friend the biomechanics involved in a manner that he or she will be able to understand, while also discussing:

- Planes of motion

- Joint actions

- Muscle movements

Role of Biomechanics

It is important for the fitness professional to fully analyze and discuss the functions of the body, or Human Movement System (kinetic chain), including the role of biomechanics. This chapter explains biomechanics and basic principles that relate to the function of the muscle action spectrum. Knowledge of biomechanics principles allows for a common understanding and language in the fitness profession. This information will serve as the foundation for more complex concepts involved in fitness assessments, program design, and exercise implementation.

Kinesiology
The study of human movement.

Basics of Biomechanics

Biomechanics
The study of how forces affect a living body.

Kinesiology and **biomechanics** are two subdisciplines under the umbrella of human movement analysis. In Greek, *kenesis* means "to move" and the term *logy* means "to study" (Neumann, 2010). Similarly, *bio* means "life" and *mechanics* is a physics term involving the study of how forces affect a living body (Hall, 2014). For example, muscles have to exert an internal force in order to lift a heavy object off the ground. An external force is the resistance of the body's weight as gravity pulls it toward the earth's center (Watkins, 2014). The ground also produces an external force called a **ground reaction force**, and it is felt at the feet when walking. In a ground reaction force, an equal and opposite force is exerted back onto the body with each step. Whether muscular or gravitational, forces affect the body depending on their magnitude, direction, and duration (Hall, 2014; Levangie & Norkin, 2001).

When analyzing human motion, biomechanical analysis can be both quantitative and qualitative (Hall, 2014; Hamil, Knutzen, & Derrick, 2015). **Qualitative analysis** involves applying principles of proper technique and combining them with observations in order to make an educated evaluation. Qualitative analysis is the primary focus for the fitness professional, because observations are integral to working with clients effectively. **Quantitative analysis**, in contrast, involves taking physical measurements and making mathematical computations to reach a conclusion. This can be seen in certain assessments, such as body composition testing.

Anatomic Locations

To ensure universal communication, human movement terminology requires the use of a standardized posture as a frame of reference. This standard posture is called the **anatomic position**. In the anatomic position, the body stands upright with the arms beside the trunk, the palms face forward, and the head faces forward. This position will be used as the frame of reference when discussing anatomic locations, planes of motion, and naming conventions for joint actions.

When describing the position or the spatial orientation of a feature on a body part, the following directional terms are commonly used to identify anatomic locations in relation to posture **Figure 3.1**.

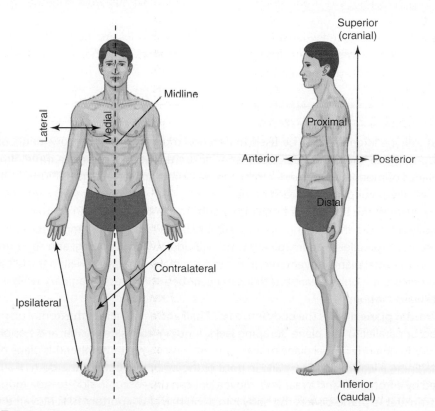

FIGURE 3.1 Anatomic locations.

Ground reaction force

An equal and opposite external force that is exerted back onto the body by the ground.

Qualitative analysis

Applying principles of proper technique and combining them with observations in order to make an educated evaluation.

Quantitative analysis

Taking physical measurements and making mathematical computations to reach a conclusion.

Anatomic position

Standard posture wherein the body stands upright with the arms beside the trunk, the palms face forward, and the head faces forward.

TRAINER TIPS

Keep in mind that this terminology will often be unfamiliar to clients. Try to use digestible language such as, "tuck your hips under to reduce the arch in your back," versus "posteriorly rotate your pelvis so we can fix your anterior tilt."

Anterior is the word used when a body part is either toward or on the front side of the body.
- In an anterior pelvic tilt, the iliac crest (upper part of the pelvis) tilts toward the front of the body.

Posterior is the word used when a body part is either toward or on the back side of the body.
- The gluteus maximus and latissimus dorsi are located on the body's posterior.

Superior is the word used when a body part is located above a landmark or closest to the head.
- The knee is superior to the ankle.

Inferior is the word used when a body part is located toward or closest to the bottom part of the body.
- The hip joint is inferior to the shoulder joint.

Proximal is the word used when a body part is located closest to the center of the body or a landmark.
- The fracture is proximal to the head of the humerus.

Distal is the word used when a body part is located farthest from the center of the body or a landmark.
- Some populations are more susceptible to distal femur (thigh bone) fractures.

Medial is the word used when a body part is located toward or closest to the **midline** of the body. The midline of the body is considered to be that which is contained within an imaginary line that splits the body into equal halves.
- The nose is medial to the ear.

Lateral is the word used when a body part is located away or farthest from the midline of the body.
- The ear is lateral to the nose.

Contralateral is the word used when a body part is located on the opposite side of the body.
- The latissimus dorsi and contralateral gluteus maximus work together to stabilize the hip.

Ipsilateral is the word used when a body part is located on the same side of the body.
- The gluteus medius and ipsilateral adductors work together to stabilize the body during side-to-side movements.

Planes and Axes of Motion

The anatomic position can also be used to describe multidimensional movements produced by the body. Three imaginary reference planes divide the body to produce three dimensions. These planes of motion are termed frontal, sagittal, and transverse planes (**Figure 3.2**). Movements typically occur parallel to each of the planes.

The **sagittal plane** bisects the body into a right half and a left half. Predominantly, sagittal plane movements are those that move forward and backward. Because movements in the sagittal plane occur parallel to an imaginary window pane, walking, cycling, and squatting are all examples of sagittal plane movements. In the sagittal plane, imagine a wall to the left and right side of a person; the only movement that can occur between these imaginary walls is forward and backward motion.

The **frontal plane** divides the body into a front half and a rear half. In the frontal plane, movements occur parallel to this plane. Jumping jacks, lunging from side to side, and hopping laterally are predominantly frontal plane movements. An easy way to remember this plane of motion is by imagining a wall or window pane in front of the body and behind the body. If a person is restricted by a front wall and a rear wall, movement can only occur in side-to-side motions.

The **transverse plane** bisects the body into a top half and a bottom half. Movements in the transverse plan occur parallel to this plane, and also include rotational motions. Examples of

Midline

That which is contained within an imaginary line that splits the body into equal halves.

Sagittal plane

An imaginary plane that bisects the body into equal halves, producing a left half and a right half.

Frontal plane

An imaginary plane that bisects the body into equal halves, producing a front half and a back half.

Transverse plane

An imaginary plane that bisects the body into equal halves, producing a top half and a bottom half.

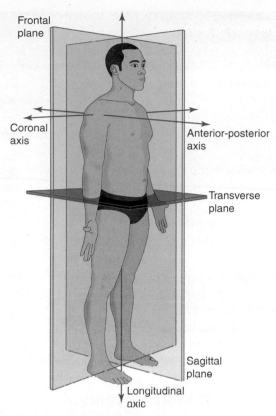

FIGURE 3.2 Planes and axes of motion.

movements in the transverse plane include a dancer's pirouette or a cable rotation. When an individual reaches for a laptop on the back seat of a car, he or she must rotate and extend at least one of the arms backward. These also are transverse plane movements.

In addition to the three planes of reference, there also are three axes of reference used to describe human movement. These axes are called medial-lateral, anterior-posterior, and longitudinal. Each of these axes represents an imaginary line that passes through the body and is perpendicular to each associated plane. Specific movements rotate around each of the three axes similar to the way a wheel on a bicycle rotates around its axle.

In the sagittal plane, rotation happens around a medial-lateral axis. The medial-lateral axis consists of an imaginary straight line that cuts through the body laterally from side to side. Think of a long pin that crosses the neck from one side of the shoulder to the other. Nodding the head forward and backward is a movement that occurs around a medial-lateral axis and in the sagittal plane.

The **anterior-posterior axis** consists of a straight line that cuts through the body from front to back. Think of a long pin that that is crossing the shoulder joint from front to back (anterior-posterior). Rotation of the shoulder joint will occur around that axis. For example, raising the arm laterally is a frontal plane movement that happens around an anterior-posterior axis.

The **longitudinal axis** is where an imaginary long straight line cuts through the body from the top to bottom. This imaginary plumb line that hangs from the head and runs downward to where the feet are can also be thought of when referring to the longitudinal axis. Rotation around a longitudinal axis takes place in the transverse plane. Spinal rotation with twisting of the trunk is an example of rotation around a longitudinal axis. See **Table 3.1** for more information.

Anterior-posterior axis
A straight line that cuts through the body from front to back.

Longitudinal axis
An imaginary long, straight line that cuts through the body from top to bottom.

TABLE 3.1 Planes and Axes of Reference			
Plane	**Axis**	**Examples of Joint Movements**	**Examples of Exercises**
Sagittal	Medial-lateral (coronal)	Flexion Extension	Biceps curl Squat Calf raise Running
Frontal	Anterior-posterior	Abduction Adduction Lateral flexion Eversion Inversion	Lateral arm raise Side step Side lunge Side shuffle
Transverse	Longitudinal	Pronation Supination Internal rotation External rotation Horizontal adduction Horizontal abduction	Turning a doorknob Trunk rotation Throwing a baseball Swinging a bat

Naming Conventions for Joint Movements

Naming conventions for joint movements are best learned in terms of the planes of motion. A joint action occurs when the surface of one joint moves in relation to another (Hall, 2014). All body segments begin their range of motion at zero degrees when in the anatomic position, except for movements in the transverse plane (Hall, 2014). **Range of motion** (ROM) is the term used to define the amount of motion produced by one or multiple joints (Hall, 2014). ROM can be quantitatively measured in a 0 to 180 degree system with a tool called a goniometer, which measures the angle created at a joint. ROM can also be analyzed qualitatively. How high the arms are raised to catch a fly ball at a baseball game demonstrates the range of motion at each joint of the arm. The inability to perform a yoga pose may be a limitation in range of motion. The names of joint actions are largely dependent on the plane in which they occur and the direction in which the movement occurs.

Sagittal Plane Motions

Joint actions in the sagittal plane include flexion, extension, hyperextension, dorsiflexion, and plantar flexion. **Flexion** is the bending at a joint where the relative angle between two adjoining segments decreases (Hall, 2014). Flexion also occurs when a body segment is moving away from zero degrees (starting position) into a positive direction. This is seen when raising the arm from the side to up over the head in shoulder flexion. Flexion occurs in an anterior direction for the following body segments (**Figures 3.3–3.7**):

- ◆ Ankle
- ◆ Hip
- ◆ Trunk
- ◆ Upper extremity
- ◆ Neck

Range of motion

The amount of movement produced by one or multiple joints.

Flexion

A bending at a joint where the relative angle between two adjoining segments decreases.

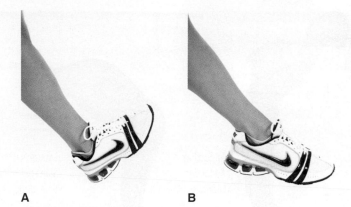

A   **B**

FIGURE 3.3 A. Dorsiflexion. B. Plantar flexion.

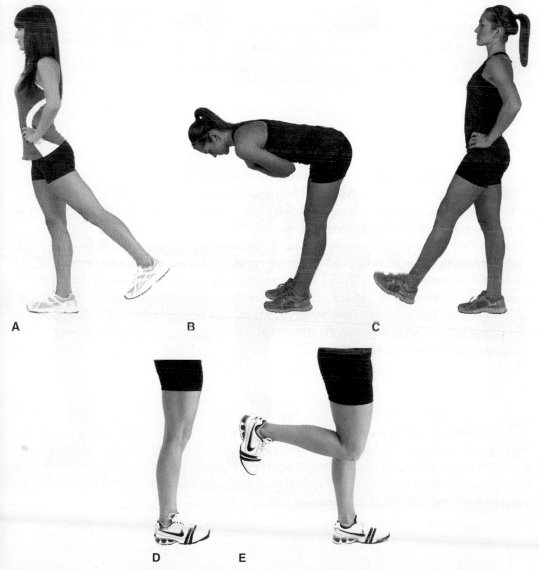

A   B   C

D   E

FIGURE 3.4 A. Hip extension. B. Hip flexion: pelvic-on-femoral rotation. C. Hip flexion: femoral-on-pelvic rotation. D. Knee extension. E. Knee flexion.

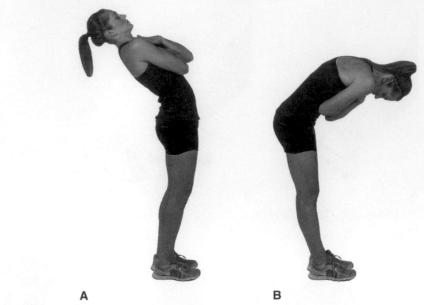

FIGURE 3.5 A. Trunk: spinal extension. B. Trunk: spinal flexion.

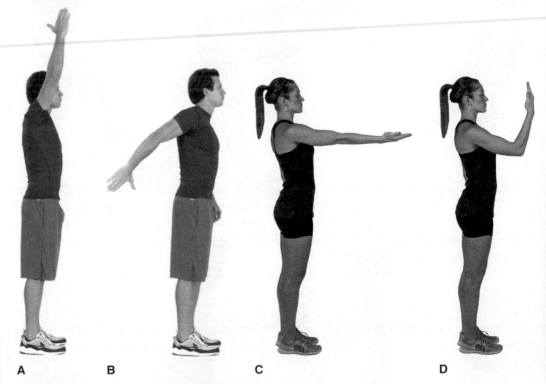

FIGURE 3.6 Upper extremity. A. Shoulder flexion. B. Shoulder extension. C. Elbow extension. D. Elbow flexion.

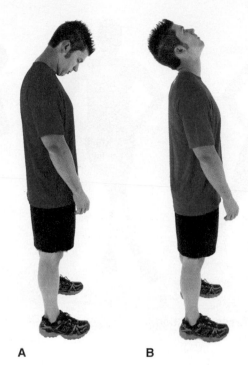

A   B

FIGURE 3.7 A. Cervical flexion. B. Cervical extension.

Flexion occurs in a posterior direction for the following body segments:

◆ Knee
◆ Ankle
◆ Toes

The easiest example is elbow flexion, such as when placing a fork in the mouth to eat. The angle formed between the upper arm and forearm decreases as the hand gets closer to the mouth. Another example of flexion occurring in the anterior direction is when raising the arm. Flexion at the shoulder begins at zero degrees in the anatomic position and increases in a positive direction as the arm is raised anteriorly.

Conversely, **extension** is the movement in the opposite direction. It is more of a straightening motion where the relative angle between two adjoining segments increases. For example, when standing up from a chair, the hip joint goes into extension as the angle formed by the torso and the upper leg bone increases. Extension also occurs when a body segment is returning to zero degrees from a flexed position, as occurs during shoulder extension.

Extension

A bending at a joint where the relative angle between two adjoining segments increases.

Frontal Plane Motions

Joint actions in the frontal plane include abduction and adduction, lateral flexion at the spine, and eversion and inversion of the foot. Shoulder elevation and depression as well as upward and downward rotation of the shoulder blade are also frontal plane movements

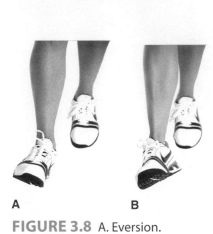

A   **B**

FIGURE 3.8 A. Eversion.
B. Inversion.

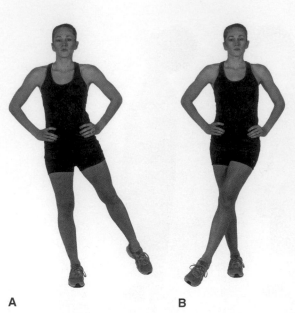

A   **B**

FIGURE 3.9 A. Hip abduction.
B. Hip adduction.

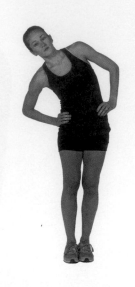

FIGURE 3.10 Lateral flexion.

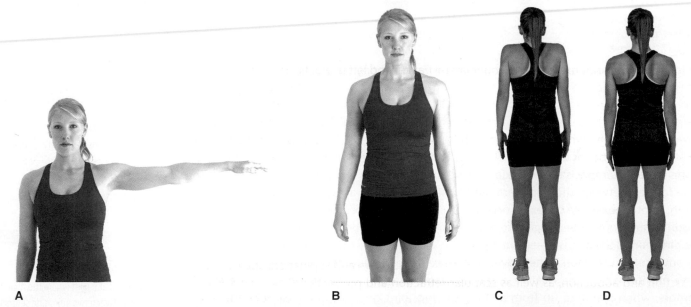

A   **B**   **C**   **D**

FIGURE 3.11 Upper extremity. A. Shoulder abduction. B. Shoulder adduction. C. Shoulder elevation. D. Depression.

Abduction

A body segment is moving away from the midline of the body.

(Figures 3.8–3.12). Remember, movements in the frontal plane are not front to back but rather side to side. **Abduction** means a body segment is moving away from the midline of the body. For example, laterally raising an arm or a leg is abduction of that body part. Conversely, **adduction** means a body segment is moving toward the midline of the body. An example is the lowering of a laterally raised arm back to resting position. The terms abduction and

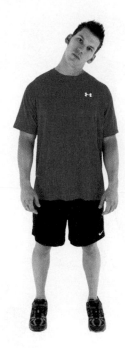

FIGURE 3.12 Neck. Lateral flexion.

Adduction

A body segment is moving toward the midline of the body.

Internal rotation

Rotation of a limb or body segment toward the midline of the body.

External rotation

Rotation of a limb or body segment away from the midline of the body.

Pronation

A triplanar movement that is associated with force reduction.

Supination

A triplanar motion that is associated with force production.

adduction can be confusing because they sound similar. Movements in the frontal plane that involve abduction or adduction include side lunges and side stepping, as well as raising the leg laterally.

Another set of joint movements is right lateral flexion and left lateral flexion of the spine. As the names suggest, the spine can bend sideways toward either the right or the left. Eversion and inversion are related to movements of the foot. With eversion, the bottom of the foot rotates outward, such as seen when feet flatten. With inversion, the bottom of the foot rotates inward, such as seen when creating an arch in the foot (Hall, 2014). Elevation of the shoulder girdle refers to superior movement of the shoulder blades. Depression of the shoulder girdle means inferior movement of the scapulae (shoulder blades).

Transverse Plane Motions

Movements in the transverse plane either occur parallel to the plane or rotate around a longitudinal axis and include internal and external rotation, pronation and supination, and horizontal abduction and adduction, as well as scapular retraction and protraction (Levangie & Norkin, 2001; Neumann, 2010). **Internal rotation**, also known as medial rotation, refers to the inward rotation of a limb or body segment. **External rotation**, also known as lateral rotation, refers to the outward rotation of a limb or body segment. When referring to the forearm, it is appropriate to use the terms pronation and supination. **Pronation** means the forearm is rotated inward, and **supination** means the forearm is rotated outward.

Horizontal abduction is a lateral movement away from the midline of the body with the movement beginning with flexion at either the shoulder or hip joint to an anterior position. Horizontal adduction is the movement from a lateral to an anterior position with the shoulder or hip joint in an anteriorly flexed position. Rotational movements are shown below (**Figure 3.13**).

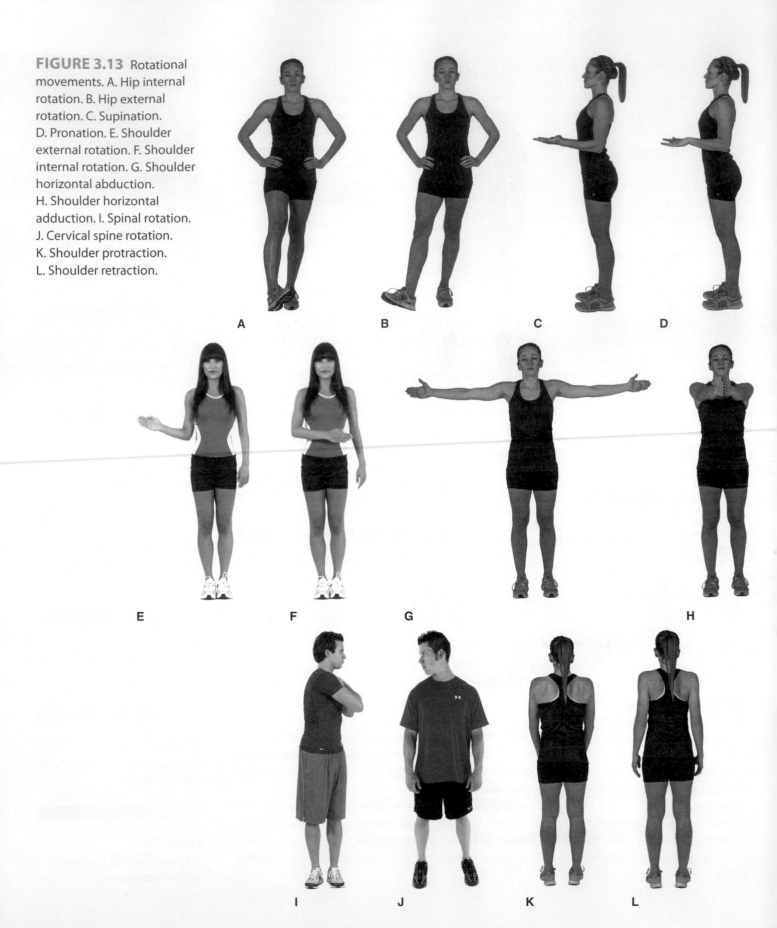

FIGURE 3.13 Rotational movements. A. Hip internal rotation. B. Hip external rotation. C. Supination. D. Pronation. E. Shoulder external rotation. F. Shoulder internal rotation. G. Shoulder horizontal abduction. H. Shoulder horizontal adduction. I. Spinal rotation. J. Cervical spine rotation. K. Shoulder protraction. L. Shoulder retraction.

Application of Biomechanics

Knowledge of anatomic locations and joint actions in relation to spatial orientation is fundamental to the application of biomechanics. There are times when basic biomechanics terms facilitate the naming of muscles, exercises, and training programs. An introduction to the naming conventions of muscles, exercises, and programs can help students better remember terminology.

Through the qualitative analysis of anatomy, muscles have been classified into functional groups (Knudson, 2007). These functional groups are based on the actions that occur at various joints. Examples of functional muscle groups include:

- **Flexors** and **extensors**
- **Abductors** and **adductors**
- **Pronators** and **supinators**

Muscles are called flexors when they produce flexion of a limb at a joint, whereas extensors are muscles that produce extension of a limb at a joint. Similar naming conventions apply for the rest of the groups.

A system of functional grouping can serve to judge the relevance of exercises (Knudson, 2007; Neumann, 2010). An exercise such as a *back extension* is exactly as its name suggests—extension of the spine. This sagittal plane exercise serves to activate spinal extensors such as the erector spinae and can be performed on a specialized bench or **prone** (Figure 3.14) on the floor. An exercise such as a *triceps extension* involves extension at the elbow joint and is also a sagittal plane movement that can be performed in a variety of positions such as while lying with the face upward or **supine** (Figure 3.15) on a bench. Some exercises involve movements where more than one joint is involved. A simple *sagittal plane lunge* is a multijoint exercise that requires flexion at the hip, knee, and ankle, also known as **triple flexion** (Figure 3.16), during the first phase of the movement. The second phase requires extension at the hip, knee, and ankle, or **triple extension** (Figure 3.17).

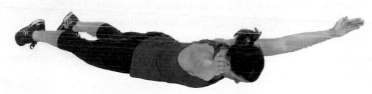

FIGURE 3.14 Prone.

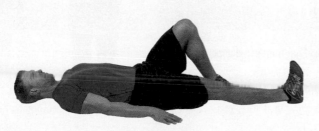

FIGURE 3.15 Supine.

Flexors
A muscle that produces flexion of a limb or joint.

Extensors
A muscle that produces extension of a limb or joint.

Abductors
A muscle that produces abduction of a limb or joint.

Adductors
A muscle that produces adduction of a limb or joint.

Pronators
A muscle that produces pronation of a limb or body segment.

Supinators
A muscle that produces supination of a limb or body segment.

Prone
Body position where one is lying with the face downward.

Supine
Body position where one is lying on the back and face is upward.

Triple flexion
A multijoint exercise that involves flexion at the hip, knee, and ankle.

Triple extension
A multijoint exercise that involves extension at the hip, knee, and ankle.

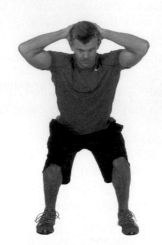

FIGURE 3.16 Triple flexion.

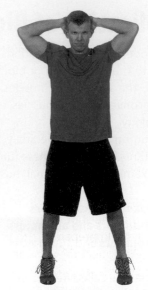

FIGURE 3.17 Triple extension.

Static posture

The starting point from which an individual moves.

Multiplanar

Occuring in more than one plane of motion.

Studying the structure and function of the human body in a **static posture** is the basis for studying dynamic postures (Hall, 2014). Think about dynamic movement that occurs in everyday life and how that might affect the kinetic chain. Functional biomechanics can be described in terms of everyday activities such as walking or getting out of a car. An activity as simple as walking can be quite complex when broken down into its biomechanical components.

In another example, getting out of a car involves stepping onto a potentially unstable and unpredictable environment. It requires joint actions such as external hip rotation and rotation of the spine. Additionally, lifting groceries out of a shopping cart and placing them into the trunk of a car requires joint actions such as the ability to flex and extend the spine, as well as being able to move in multiple planes. Exercises that prepare individuals for movements such as the ones described here can all be considered functional. The commonality of all these movements is they involve multiple joints, they are **multiplanar** (i.e., occurring in more than one plane of motion), and they may be performed on unstable as well as unpredictable environments. As fitness professionals, clients are best served if training is more specific so that it carries over from exercise into everyday life.

CHECK IT OUT

When first learning about human movement, joints are described as occurring in one plane of motion. Common gym movements such as biceps curls, triceps extensions, knee extensions, and calf raises isolate one joint and predominantly occur in one plane of motion. However, outside of the gym, this is not how people move. Joints move in all three planes of motion, so exercises should incorporate multiple joints and be multiplanar.

Common Gym Movements

Common gym exercises can translate into functional activities of daily living. The more a fitness professional can learn about how the Human Movement System functions, the more capable he or she is in creating variations of common gym movements. This empowers the professional to be creative in ways that are more functional for the client.

The first common exercise to discuss is an overhead shoulder press, predominantly a frontal plane movement. This exercise includes shoulder abduction/adduction and elbow extension/flexion. A functional movement that mimics the biomechanics of an overhead shoulder press would be lifting a heavy box above the shoulders.

Another common gym movement is the chest press and its variations. This movement predominantly occurs in the sagittal plane of motion. This exercise involves horizontal adduction/abduction at the shoulder and elbow extension/flexion. Consider a chest pass during a basketball game. In preparation to pass the ball to another basketball player, the individual must horizontally abduct the arms and activate the biceps brachii to produce flexion at the elbows. As the ball is released, the arms horizontally adduct and the elbows extend.

Some pulling movements, such as a seated cable row, bench row, and even supine pull-up, are predominantly sagittal plane exercises. To perform the exercise, the shoulders extend, the elbows flex, the shoulder blades retract, and the shoulder joint medially rotates as the upper arms are pulled backward. This is functionally seen when opening a heavy door and when bending over to pick up a heavy object.

Other pulling movements, such as a seated cable pulldown or a pull-up, are predominantly frontal plane exercises. In a traditional seated cable pulldown, an individual begins the exercise from a seated position. The shoulders are both flexed and abducted, the elbows are extended, and the wrists are pronated in order to achieve an overhand grip on the pulldown bar. The exercise is performed as the bar is pulled down toward the chest. To perform this movement, the shoulders are adducted, the elbows are flexed, and some degree of retraction occurs at the shoulder blades.

Common gym exercises for the lower body include various forms of squats and lunges. Both of these movements occur predominantly in the sagittal plane. The squat is an example of triple flexion because the hip, knee, and ankle joints flex in a controlled manner until the upper leg is parallel to the floor (Gullett, Tillman, Gutierrez, & Chow, 2009). The hip, knee, and ankle joints then extend until reaching the starting position, which is also an example of triple extension. Similarly, lunging also involves triple flexion as an individual lunges forward. Pushing off the front foot and back onto the back leg to the starting position involves triple extension. This is common in everyday living such as getting out of a car, kneeling down to pick something up, and any form of jumping in a sport.

Although many common gym movements incorporate multiplanar joint actions, they tend to occur predominantly in one plane of motion. The beginning professional should ask how functional an exercise is and how it translates into the activities of daily living for a client to set them up for long-term success. Furthermore, when creating exercise programs, the professional should focus on incorporating exercises that challenge the body through multijoint and multiplanar training (**Table 3.2**). Specific exercise mechanics, applications, and techniques will be discussed in greater detail later in the text.

Exercise Naming Conventions

Exercise names should closely represent what the movement does. There are no standardized conventions for naming exercises used within the industry. Some exercises have commonly used names, and others have more than one name. For this reason, it is a best practice to name

TRAINER TIPS

Rather than training specific body parts that only focus on one plane at a time, consider exercises that mimic total body movements which are functional in nature.

TABLE 3.2 Multijoint vs. Multiplanar	
Multijoint Exercises (Predominantly Single Plane)	**Multijoint and Multiplanar Exercises**
Lunge	Lunge with rotation
Squat	Squat to rotational lift
Push-up	Push-up with rotation
Chest press	Rotational chest pass

TABLE 3.3 Planes of Motion	
Plane of Motion	**Example**
Frontal plane	Lateral lunge
Sagittal plane	Reverse lunge
Transverse plane	Transverse plane lunge
Multiplanar	Multiplanar lunge

exercises based on a set of criteria. This allows a greater number of individuals to know what an exercise is, based on its name. In general, the following are some of the criteria used when an exercise is named:

- ◆ Plane of motion
- ◆ Body position
- ◆ Type of resistance training modality used
- ◆ Joint action
- ◆ Primary muscle targeted

When learning the names of exercises, it is helpful to break down a name into its separate elements. This can help with determining what is involved in the movement. The following are examples of stems used to name an exercise and how they are used.

Planes of Motion

When an exercise can be performed in multiple planes, it is helpful to indicate the plane. For example, a *lunge to balance* exercise can be performed in the sagittal, frontal, or transverse plane. Thus, it is best to specify the plane in which an exercise should be performed. If all the planes of motion will be used, then it is best to use the word *multiplanar*. See **Table 3.3** for more information.

Body Position

Some exercises can be performed in different body positions such as supine, prone, kneeling, standing, two leg, single leg, two arm, or single arm. For example, an exercise popularly known as the *plank* is also called *prone iso-abs*. As *prone iso-abs*, the exercise name indicates the exercise is to be performed in a prone position and that it is an exercise to isolate the abdominals. See **Table 3.4** for more information.

TABLE 3.4 Body Positions

Position	Example
Supine	Supine marching
Prone	Prone iso-abs
Quadruped	Quadruped leg raise
Kneeling	Kneeling hip flexor stretch
Standing	Standing cable row
Single leg	Single-leg squat touchdown
Staggered stance	Staggered-stance cable chest press
Two arm	Two-arm overhead press
Alternating arms	Alternating-arm biceps curl
Single arm	Single-arm triceps extension

TABLE 3.5 Resistance Modality Exercises

Modality	Example
Stability ball	Ball wall squat
Machine	Leg press machine
Machine pad	Single-leg balance on balance pad
Balance Disc	Single-leg balance disc lift and chop
Suspension	Suspension trainer push-up
Cable	Standing cable row
Tubing or band	Tube walking
Barbell	Barbell squat
Dumbbell	Two-arm dumbbell overhead press
Medicine ball	Front medicine ball oblique throw
Kettlebell	Two-arm kettlebell swing
Whole body vibration	WBV step-up to balance

Resistance Modality Used

Additionally, the type of resistance training modality or piece of equipment used may also be included in the name of an exercise. Modalities may include a barbell, cable apparatus, tubing, band, medicine ball, or kettlebell. For example, a *ball crunch* indicates the exercise is to be performed on a stability ball. **Table 3.5** provides examples of how exercises may be named based on the modality used to perform the exercise.

TABLE 3.6 Joint Action Exercises

Joint Action	Example
Flexion	Medicine ball squat with arm flexion and extension
Extension	Back extension; Triceps extension
Abduction	Prone iso-abs with hip abduction
Adduction	Standing adductor stretch
Rotation	Single-leg hip rotation; Walking lunge with rotation

TABLE 3.7 Primary Muscle Targeted

Muscle Group	Example
Chest	Bench chest press
Shoulder	Overhead shoulder press
Biceps	Biceps curl
Triceps	Triceps extension
Abdominals	Prone iso-abs
Back	Back extension
Legs	Leg press
Hamstring	Hamstring curl
Quadriceps	Quadriceps extension
Calf	Calf raise

Joint Action

Sometimes a joint action is indicated in the name of an exercise. For example, a *single-leg hip rotation* incorporates both internal and external rotation at the hip joint. **Table 3.6** shows examples of how exercises may be named based on joint action.

Primary Muscle Targeted

Exercises can also be named based on the primary muscle that is targeted. In a *barbell triceps extension*, the triceps are the primary muscles targeted when performing the exercise. Similarly, in a *bench chest press*, the exercise primarily targets the chest muscles. See **Table 3.7** for more examples.

Putting It All Together

After identifying some of the elements used in naming an exercise, it is possible to see how stems are used and combined. Some exercise names may seem long and cumbersome to use on

TABLE 3.8 Simplifying Modality Names

Modality	Example
Stability ball	Ball
Balance pad	BP
Balance disc	BD
Tubing	TB
Barbell	BB
Dumbbell	DB
Kettlebell	KB
Whole body vibration	WBV
Single-leg	SL
Medicine ball	MB
Extension	EXT

programming sheets or with clients. However, fitness professionals must keep in mind that these naming conventions are useful during the beginning stages of learning human movement and that they provide universal understanding. Nevertheless, exercise names should not confuse colleagues or clients. Once professionals become familiar with commonly used naming conventions, they can shorten the names of some stems to help facilitate the development of programming templates. One way to do this is through the use of acronyms. **Table 3.8** provides examples of ways to shorten stem names in order to simplify the names of exercises.

Muscular Function and Application

Knowing the various functions of muscles allows the fitness professional to implement specific training strategies to prevent injury and increase endurance, strength, and power. This information and eventual application is founded in the muscle action spectrum, functions of muscles, and kinetics.

Muscle Action Spectrum

Muscle action is a product of communication and coordination from the nervous system to the muscular system. This leads to movement or stabilization of the musculoskeletal system (Knudson, 2007). Just as the gears and breaks on a bicycle aid movement during cycling on varying terrains, the muscle action spectrum facilitates joint actions via the different types of muscle activation. The muscle action spectrum includes three major types of activation:

- Concentric
- Isometric
- Eccentric

Concentric activation

The production of an active force when a muscle develops tension while shortening in length.

Active force

Muscle tension that is generated by its contractile elements.

Isometric activation

The production of an active force when a muscle develops tension while maintaining a constant length.

Eccentric activation

The production of an active force when a muscle develops tension while lengthening.

Isolated function

(1) A muscle's primary function.
(2) A muscle action produced at a joint when a muscle is being concentrically activated to produce acceleration of a body segment.

Eccentric function

Action of a muscle when it is generating an eccentric contraction.

Concentric activation means that a muscle is producing an **active force** as it shortens. An active force refers to tension generated by contractile elements in the muscle. During this type of activation the force generated is sufficient to overcome a load, and two bones are pulled toward each other. One way to remember concentric activation is by learning the meaning of its root words. The word *concentric* can be broken into two root words, the prefix *con* and the suffix *centric*. In Latin, the term *con* means "together," and the term *centric* means "toward the center." Concentric activation can be used to accelerate or increase the rate of speed for a movement. This can be thought of in how a car works when the gas pedal is pressed. By pressing on the gas pedal, one accelerates the movement of the car. This is how concentric activation works.

Isometric activation means that a muscle is producing an active force while it maintains the same length; no visible movement occurs during this time. The tension produced by a muscle is equal to the force of an external load that is being applied. Additionally, this type of muscle action does not produce joint movement. Static exercises do not involve mechanical work and typically require isometric activation of one or more muscles to stabilize the body.

Eccentric activation means a muscle is producing an active force while lengthening in order to resist an external force. For example, when lowering the arm after a biceps curl, the biceps eccentrically decelerate elbow extension. The biceps become activated in order to resist the force of gravity and the force of any weight being held by the hand, otherwise the arm would just fall straight without control. Examples of eccentric muscle activation include jogging or walking downhill and the lowering portion of a squat because an individual has to resist the force of gravity. Additionally, muscles can produce more force eccentrically than they can concentrically or isometrically (Brooks, Fahey, & Baldwin, 2005). It is helpful to think of eccentric muscle actions as a braking mechanism, much like the brakes on a bicycle. Applying the brakes by pressing them serves to slow down or decelerate the bicycle's movement. Eccentric training can produce more soreness because there is more tension-induced damage with these types of contractions. It is important to understand that eccentric activation is common to all muscles and almost all human movement (Knudson, 2007).

Muscle Function

Each muscle has a role or function within the body. **Isolated function** refers to a muscle's primary function. Although there are eccentric and integrated functions, learning and memorizing the isolated function of each muscle is helpful when first learning functional anatomy. The isolated function is a muscle action produced at a joint when a muscle is being concentrically activated to produce acceleration of a body segment. A muscle's isolated function produces an intended movement. For example, if the intended movement is to flex the elbow, the body recruits the biceps muscles to perform that muscle action. Concentrically accelerating elbow flexion is the isolated function of the biceps muscle.

Eccentric function refers to the action of a muscle when it is generating an eccentric contraction. A muscle that eccentrically decelerates the action of a primary mover is reducing the speed of the movement in order to maintain control and avoid injury.

As previously mentioned, eccentric function is important when going down a flight of stairs, walking or running downhill, and lowering a weight such as a heavy box. Hamstring strains frequently occur in activities that involve sprinting during eccentric activation of the hamstrings (Brooks et al., 2005; Kisner & Colby, 2007). Knowing this is important because it can be useful in training and preventive strengthening. Recall that eccentric activation has the potential to produce more force than isometric or concentric activation. Thus, a muscle strain can happen if an eccentrically active muscle is suddenly overcome by an unexpected force in a client who is fatigued or not conditioned to experience repetitive eccentric actions. It is for these reasons that clients should be conditioned to experience both concentric and eccentric activation during exercise. Incorporating exercises that challenge a muscle's eccentric function in a variety of parameters may help prevent injury during many functional movements.

Integrated function refers to the muscle actions produced at various joints. Muscles rarely act alone, even though they have an isolated function. Over time, it will become easier to define the integrated function of muscles, after knowledge of isolated function is automatic. During functional movements, all three muscle actions play a role in coordinating movement and protecting the body from injury. Integrated function includes isometric and eccentric functions when a muscle is concentrically activating. A muscle's integrated function refers to its function when it works together with other muscles to produce a movement. Think of integrated function as an orchestra that is directed by a conductor. The conductor is the nervous system, and the orchestra is the musculoskeletal system. The nervous system conducts or controls muscle actions to ensure they work harmoniously and in synchrony. An easy way to remember integrated function is to think of integrated function as being inclusive of all muscle functions (concentric, isometric, eccentric).

Force, Torque, and Levers

Kinetics is a biomechanics term that involves the study of forces. This is important to fitness professionals because forces play a role in the movement of the body, and it is how resistance training works. **Force** can be thought of as a push or a pull that can create, stop, or change movement (Neumann, 2010). The amount of force produced is dependent on an object's mass multiplied by how fast it is moving. The following equation can assist in the visualization of this concept:

$$\text{Force} = \text{Mass} \times \text{Acceleration}$$

Mass is the amount of **matter** in an object, and **acceleration** is the rate at which an object is increasing in speed. When a substance takes up space, it can be regarded as matter. This information is applicable to the human body. When a muscle with a relatively large amount of mass moves quickly, it will most likely apply a larger amount of force. It is important to note that mass is different from weight. **Weight** is a force; it is the amount of force that gravity has on the body and is measured in pounds (lbs). **Gravity** is another force; it accelerates downward, toward the earth's center. Forces can be internal, such as those produced by muscles to move limbs, or they can be external, such as those of mass, weight, and gravity. It is possible to manipulate these external forces to challenge clients during exercise programming. For example, mass can be added in the form of a barbell, dumbbell, or kettlebell during an exercise. Some exercises can simply be bodyweight exercises. These challenge a client through the pull of gravity. Suspension training is another alternative that manipulates bodyweight and gravity to challenge the client during exercise.

Levers are another important biomechanical concept as shown in **Figure 3.18**. Bones and muscles act as levers. A **lever** is a relatively rigid rod or bar that rotates around a fulcrum, or pivot point. Think of a fulcrum much like an axis around which a joint rotates. There are three different types or classes of levers where an effort or force and a resistance are applied.

With a first-class lever, a force is applied on one side and a resistance is applied on the other side. A frequently used example is that of a playground seesaw with an individual sitting on each end. As one side falls toward the ground, the other is raised yet still applies a resistive force because of the person sitting on that side of the seesaw. In the human body, think of agonist and antagonist muscles on opposite sides of a joint. The agonist provides the effort force, and

Integrated function

The coordination of muscles to produce, reduce, and stabilize forces in multiple planes for efficient and safe movement.

Kinetics

Biomechanics term that involves the study of forces.

Force

(1) A push or a pull that can create, stop, or change movement. (2) Force = Mass × Acceleration.

Mass

The amount of matter in an object or physical body.

Matter

A substance that has mass and takes up space.

Acceleration

The rate at which an object is increasing in speed.

Weight

The amount of force that gravity has on the body.

Gravity

A force that accelerates an object or mass downward toward the earth's center.

Lever

A relatively rigid rod or bar that rotates around a fulcrum.

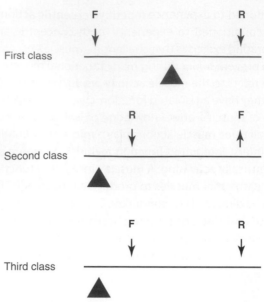

FIGURE 3.18 The three types of levers.

the antagonist provides the resistive force as it decelerates the movement of the agonist. This movement occurs around a joint as the axis or fulcrum.

With a second-class lever, the fulcrum is toward the end of one side. The fulcrum can be located on either side of the lever. Both the applied force and the resistance are on the same side. With this type of lever, the resistance is applied closer to the fulcrum. Moving a loaded wheelbarrow is a classic example. There are limited examples of second-class levers within the musculoskeletal system. A calf raise is one example of a second-class lever where the ball of the foot acts as the fulcrum, the weight of the body is the resistance, and the calf muscle applies the force.

With third-class levers, the fulcrum is toward the end of one side (either side). Both the applied force and the resistance are on the same side. However, with this type of lever the applied force is closer to the fulcrum. Using a shovel to scoop up gravel is an example of a third-class lever when the top hand does not apply force. The top hand is the fulcrum as the other hand applies a force to pick up the gravel. The gravel provides the resistance. Most body segments act as third-class levers when concentric actions are involved (Hall, 2014; Neumann, 2010). An example is a dumbbell biceps curl where the elbow joint acts as the fulcrum, the biceps brachii concentrically activates to apply the force, and the resistance is the load provided by the dumbbell. In this scenario, it is important to note that the applied force is on the same side as the resistance because the distal attachment of the biceps brachii muscle is actually on the radius.

CHECK IT OUT

Functional training that includes components of stabilization and flexibility are just as important as those that assist with building muscle and getting stronger. A system of levers demonstrates that the body is also designed for speed and range of motion. Second-class levers provide the capacity to produce more force at the expense of speed and range of motion. Third-class levers allow for greater speed and range of motion at the expense of force.

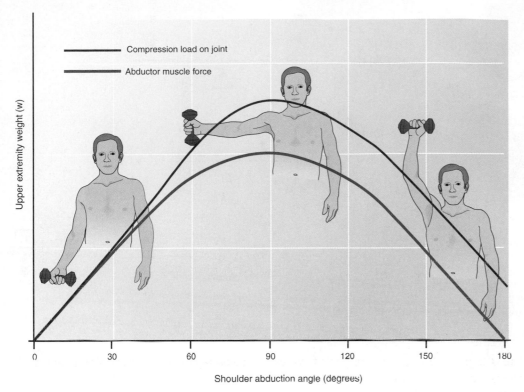

FIGURE 3.19 Torque.

Levers use torque to assist in the moving of objects. A force that acts on a lever arm such as a limb to create rotation at a joint is known as torque in biomechanics terminology. **Torque** is the rotary or rotational effect that a force has around an axis (**Figure 3.19**).

A joint action occurs around an axis of rotation, or rather the point where two bones connect. When the amount of torque increases at a joint, the more likely that joint is to rotate. In the body, muscles of the shoulder girdle produce the internal force that is needed to create torque at the shoulder joint in order to move a limb such as the arm. When thinking of torque, think of the effect a wrench has on a bolt. The amount of torque can be increased by either having a longer lever arm or by applying more force. Additionally, force is most effective in producing torque when it is applied perpendicular to the wrench. Similarly, during a biceps curl, it is easier to move a dumbbell when the elbow is flexed at a 90-degree angle as opposed to when the elbow is fully extended. Also, bending the wrist shortens the lever, decreasing the amount of torque a client can produce at the elbow joint by the biceps. This is one more reason as to why proper form is important when a client performs an exercise. If the goal is to increase

Torque
The rotary or rotational effect that a force has around an axis.

CHECK IT OUT

Manipulate the principles of torque to help muscles be more efficient at moving. Strengthening a muscle will help it to increase its ability to produce force, and in turn produce a joint action. Force is also most effective when it is applied perpendicular to the lever. This is why the hamstrings can produce the most force when the knee is flexed at a 90-degree angle, such as when performing a hamstring curl.

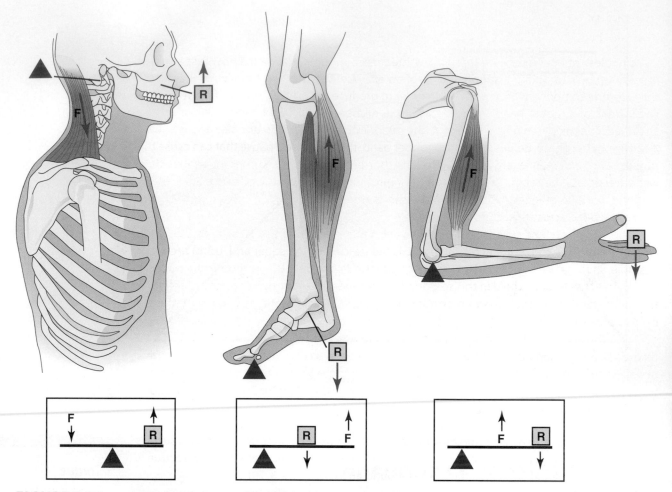

FIGURE 3.20 First class, second class, and third class levers.

movement, then the principles of torque can be manipulated to help a muscle be more efficient at moving a body part. Maximizing the amount of torque that a muscle can generate optimizes that muscle's ability to be strengthened. The stronger a muscle is, the greater the amount of force a muscle can create, and the greater the amount of torque that can be produced to move a lever on the body such as an arm or leg during strength-training exercises (**Figure 3.20**).

Application of Tempo

During exercise, the tempo used for each repetition affects the amount and type of demand placed on the body. **Tempo** controls the amount of time that muscle is actively producing tension during exercise movements. **Repetition tempo** refers to the speed with which each repetition is performed. When creating an exercise program, it is important to consider and include repetition tempo, as will be discussed later. A three-digit notation is used to indicate the tempo a repetition should be performed. Here are some of the ways that tempo can be written:

- 4/2/1
- 4-2-1
- 4:2:1

Tempo
The amount of time that muscle is actively producing tension during exercise movements.

Repetition tempo
The speed at which each repetition is performed.

- (4-2-1)
- [421]

Regardless of how repetition tempo is written, each number represents how fast a movement is performed during a specific phase of an exercise. The first number always represents the eccentric component of an exercise. In order to produce force, muscles must first be lengthened. Think of a rubber band. In order to shoot a rubber band across a room, it must first be stretched. The middle number represents the midpoint, or pause, of an exercise and is known as the isometric phase. Before shooting a rubber band, there may be a pause that can cause the rubber band's potential energy to dissipate. The shorter the pause, the farther the rubber band will travel across the room. The third number represents the concentric phase of an exercise. Letting go of a lengthened rubber band releases its stored energy, producing enough force to propel the band across the room.

To better understand how tempo works, it helps to see how it is used. For example, when a client performs a squat, the eccentric phase is the descent of the squat and, using the 4/2/1 example, should take 4 seconds. Pausing in the squatted position is the isometric phase where stabilizers activate, and is held in this scenario for 2 seconds. The concentric phase occurs when the client stands from the squatting position in 1 second. Not all exercises begin with the eccentric phase, but tempo will always be written in the same sequence. In a dumbbell biceps curl, for example, it begins with the concentric phase as the biceps concentrically accelerates elbow flexion and supination of the radioulnar joint in order to curl the weight. A pause in the middle of the exercise is the isometric phase, and bringing the weight back down is the eccentric phase as the triceps brachii eccentrically decelerates elbow flexion. Different applications of tempos to achieve desired results will be discussed in later chapters

Biomechanics as a Language

A common challenge when studying human movement analysis is the vocabulary. It can feel like learning a new language because most anatomic structures are not in common English terminology. However, many medical terms come from Latin and Greek root words, so it should be no surprise that anatomic terminology also comes from foreign words (Saladin, 2007). Fortunately, having knowledge of fundamental biomechanics can assist in the comprehension of how muscle anatomy works. This section will focus on the English equivalents and is meant to provide students with insights and learning tips for understanding the structure and function of muscles.

Location of Muscles: Origin and Insertion

Which motion a muscle performs is highly dependent on its location relative to the joint it is attached to (Levangie & Norkin, 2001). Additionally, the direction in which a muscle is pulled is known as the **line of pull** (Figure 3.21) and is dependent on its attachments, as well as the arrangement of its muscle fibers. Essentially, muscle fibers are arranged in straight lines and pull on the bones during contraction. The direction in which a bone is pulled can help determine which way a limb will move, the movement that will occur, as well as muscle action. Both attachment sites and the line of pull affect the way a muscle will function. Muscles are attached to body segments in at least two places, and a muscle must cross at least one joint in order to create a joint action. In general, muscles crossing the anterior aspect of a joint on areas of the body such as the upper extremity, the trunk, and the hip are flexors. In contrast, the muscles

Line of pull
The direction in which a muscle is pulled.

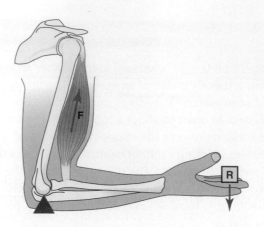

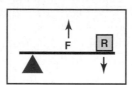

FIGURE 3.21 Line of pull.

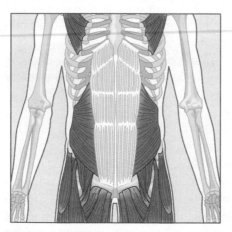

FIGURE 3.22 Parallel muscle.

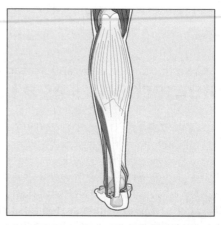

FIGURE 3.23 Pennate muscle.

Parallel muscle

Muscle with fibers that are oriented parallel to that muscle's longitudinal axis.

Pennate muscle

Muscle with fibers that are oriented at an angle to the muscle's longitudinal axis.

crossing the posterior aspect of these same joints are typically extensors. Knowing where a muscle's attachments are located can usually provide information as to what it does.

Muscle fiber arrangement influences muscle function because the fibers of a muscle tend to pull in the direction that those fibers are arranged. So, if a muscle's fibers run vertically like a plumb line does, then the muscle will pull either up or down, depending on its attachment sites. In general, muscles will pull toward their center. The two general types of muscle fiber arrangements are **parallel** (**Figure 3.22**) and **pennate** (**Figure 3.23**) (Hall, 2014). Most muscle fibers in parallel arrangement are oriented parallel to that muscle's longitudinal axis. Muscles such as the biceps brachii and the rectus abdominis are considered to have a parallel muscle fiber arrangement (**Table 3.9**). The arrangement of pennate muscle fibers is at an angle to the muscle's longitudinal axis. Each of the fibers of a muscle with a pennate arrangement is attached to one or multiple tendons that can span the length of the muscle. Think of the orientation of these fibers much like those of a feather, angled on two different ends.

TABLE 3.9 Muscle Fiber Arrangement	
Muscle Fiber Arrangement	**Examples**
Parallel	Sternocleidomastoid, biceps brachii, rectus abdominis
Pennate	Deltoid, rectus femoris, gastrocnemius

Location of muscle attachments also affects the function of a muscle. Typically, a muscle attaches to a relatively stationary attachment on one end of a body segment such as a bone. This is called the **origin**. On the other end, the muscle attaches to a relatively mobile attachment called the **insertion** (Hamil et al., 2015; Saladin, 2007). Also a muscle's origin is proximal to the midline and the insertion tends to be distal from it.

A muscle will pull on all the segments to which it is attached when it produces force. A muscle can shift between creating movement at one end of an attachment to its other end, based on the activity being performed. For example, many muscles cross multiple joints and have the ability to produce more than one movement at multiple body segments. The psoas is one of those muscles. It originates at part of the thoracic spine and crosses the hip joint by inserting into the anterior aspect of the femur. The psoas concentrically flexes the hip during a single-leg raise or it can concentrically extend the lumbar spine (raise the trunk) during back extension.

Muscles can also be attached to a **tendon** or an **aponeurosis**. For example, an aponeurosis is considered as the origin and a tendon is the point of insertion when a muscle is extended between the aponeurosis and the tendon. Note that there are exceptions to the definition of origin and insertion. It is for this reason that some anatomists prefer to avoid the use of origin and insertion terminology and instead refer to attachments as being proximal and distal or superior and inferior.

Isolated Function

Knowing a muscle's isolated function is important because this helps a fitness professional determine which muscle is doing what during different movements. Consider what must happen when standing up from a seated position. The hips must extend in order to be able to stand, and this happens because of muscles that concentrically produce hip extension. The gluteus maximus is a powerful hip extensor. It is the primary mover for movements requiring hip extension for several reasons, one of those being its location. It originates on the pelvis and inserts onto the femur. When it concentrically develops tension, the gluteus maximus shortens and brings the femur closer to the pelvis, thus accelerating hip extension. One way of remembering a muscle's isolated function is by learning its concentric muscle action.

Analyzing the Names of Muscles

Anatomic terminology has become standardized internationally with the help of the Federative Committee on Anatomical Terminology, an international group of anatomists. Their work is published in a book called the *Terminologia Anatomica* and provides Latin names as well as their English equivalents (Saladin, 2007). Its intention was to resolve the confusion created by having different names for the same structures. Terms are typically composed of various word

Origin
The relatively stationary attachment site where skeletal muscle attaches begins.

Insertion
The relatively mobile attachment site.

Tendons
Connective tissues that attach muscle to bone and provide an anchor for muscles to produce force.

Aponeurosis
A white tendinous sheet that attaches muscle to bone.

MEMORY TIPS

When thinking about the movement of a muscle, think about what happens when a muscle concentrically develops tension: it shortens when contraction occurs. By shortening, the insertion moves toward the origin. As the insertion moves toward the origin, it produces a muscle action. This determines a muscle's function.

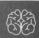

MEMORY TIPS

One way of remembering a muscle's isolated function is by learning its concentric muscle action.

elements. Learning the meanings of at least some of these word elements provides the tools to partially understand the structure and function of many muscles. In addition, learning to "dissect" a word by breaking it down into its elements helps with pronunciation, spelling, and memorization. In general, scientific terminology is made up of one or more of the following elements:

- A root word
- Combining vowels
- A prefix
- A suffix

As an example, consider the word *sternocleidomastoid*, a muscle of the neck. This term breaks down into *sterno/cleido/mast/oid*:

- *sterno*—meaning "sternum"
- *cleido*—meaning "clavicle"
- *mast*—meaning "chest"
- *oid*—a suffix meaning "resembling"

The understanding of human movement can be facilitated by knowing the names of muscles, their location, as well as their functions. Rote memorization is unnecessary when the name of a muscle itself can provide information about its location or movement. Knowing how muscles are typically named can assist with this endeavor.

Skeletal muscles are typically named based on the following criteria (Behnke, 2012):

- Action
- Attachment
- Direction
- Location
- Structure
- Size
- Shape

Action

Some muscles are named based on their action or function (**Table 3.10**). These are the easiest muscles to remember because the name of the muscle tells you what it does. As previously discussed, for example, an extensor is a muscle that extends. The term *levator* refers to a muscle that elevates or pulls up. One of the functions of the *levator scapulae* is elevation of the scapulae. Exercises that are named based on the action being performed include back extension and triceps extension.

Attachment

Where a muscle is attached with respect to the bone of its origin is another way some muscles are named. Muscles with long names tend to reside in this category. As discussed earlier, the name *sternocleidomastoid* can be broken down into various parts, with each part having a meaning that provides information about the nature of the muscle. For this muscle, the first two parts represent the bones of its origin sites and the last part represents its insertion site. The sternocleidomastoid has two heads, with one originating at the sternum and the other at the clavicle, hence the *sterno* and *cleido* elements. Finally, the muscle inserts into the mastoid process, which is an area located at the base of the skill; thus, the term *mastoid* is the last element in the name:

- *sterno*—originates at the sternum
- *cleido*—originates at the clavicle
- *mastoid*—inserts into the mastoid process

TABLE 3.10 Example Root Words: Action

Term	Meaning	Example
Extensor	Muscle that extends	Extensor digiti minimi
Flexor	Muscle that flexes	Flexor carpi ulnaris
Levator	Muscle that elevates	Levator scapulae
Depressor	Muscle that lowers or depresses	Depressor anguli oris
Abductor	Muscle that pulls bone away from midline	Abductor magnus
Adductor	Muscle that pulls bone toward midline	Adductor brevis
Pronator	Muscle that pronates; downward rotation of the palm	Pronator teres
Supinator	Muscle that supinates; upward rotation of the palm	Supinator brevis

TABLE 3.11 Example Root Words: Direction

Term	Meaning	Example
Oblique	Diagonal	Internal oblique
Rect-	Straight; parallel	Rectus abdominis
Transverse	Perpendicular; across	Transverse abdominis

Direction

Muscles are also named based on the direction of their muscle fibers or fascicles relative to the body's midline (**Table 3.11**). The term *trans* is the Latin root word for "across," so the *transverse abdominis* is so named because its fibers run perpendicular to the midline. Another example includes both the internal and external oblique muscles, which receive their name after the term *oblique*, which means "slanted" or "diagonal." The muscle fibers for both of these muscles run diagonally, each in a different direction.

Location

A muscle can be named based on its location relative to a body part or bone (**Table 3.12**). A muscle may be located on top of a bone or in between bones, as indicated by their root words. Muscles with the root *brachi* refer to muscles of the upper arm, such as in the biceps brachii. Similarly, the rectus femoris lies over the femur. A root word can provide the exact location of a muscle; some of them highly resemble their English equivalents. For example, the root word *abdominis* in the muscle name *rectus abdominis* sounds very similar to the English word *abdomen*, which is exactly where the rectus abdominis is located.

Structure

Muscles can be named based on their number of origins (**Table 3.13**). The mid-region in between the origin and insertion is called the **muscle belly**. Some muscles have more than one

Muscle belly
The mid-region in between the origin and insertion.

TABLE 3.12 Examples of Root Words: Location

Term	Meaning	Example
Abdominis	Abdomen	Rectus abdominis
Brachi-	Upper arm	Biceps brachii; brachialis
Digiti	Finger or toe (singular)	Extensor digiti minimi
Femoris	Over the femur; thigh region	Biceps femoris
Gluteus	Buttock	Gluteus maximus
Intercostal	In between the ribs	External intercostal
Lumborum	Lower back	Quadratus lumborum
Pectoralis	Chest	Pectoralis major
Peroneus	Fibula	Peroneus longus
Scapulae	On top of scapula or shoulder	Levator scapulae
Superficialis	Superficial	Flexor digitorum superficialis
Supra-	Above	Supraspinatus
Infra-	Inferior	Infraspinatus

TABLE 3.13 Example Root Words: Structure

Term	Meaning	Example
Bicep	Two origins	Biceps brachii
Tricep	Three origins	Triceps brachii
Quadricep	Four origins	Quadriceps

belly, which is also called a *head*. *Bi* means "two," and *cep* is from the Latin root word *caput*, which means "head." The term *ceps* is plural. Thus, *bi-ceps* means "two heads." For example, the biceps brachii has two bellies or heads, a long head and a short head. Each head originates from a different location, one being the scapula and the other on the humerus. Similarly, the quadriceps is a group of muscles made up of four heads. Although all four have the same insertion site, each has a different origin.

Size
Muscles can also be named according to their size relative to other muscles in the same group (**Table 3.14**). For example, there are three gluteus muscles, yet each one is named based on its size. The gluteus maximus is the largest in size, followed by the gluteus medius, and finally the gluteus minimus, which is the smallest of the three. The pectoralis muscles are named in a similar way.

TABLE 3.14 Example Root Words: Size

Term	Meaning	Example
Maximus	Large	Gluteus maximus
Medius	Medium; intermediate	Gluteus medius
Minimus	Small	Gluteus minimus
Brevis	Short	Fibularis brevis
Longus	Long	Fibularis longus
Vastus	Huge	Vastus lateralis
Latissimus	Widest; very broad	Latissimus dorsi
Major	Large	Pectoralis major
Minor	Small	Pectoralis minor
Magnus	Large	Adductor magnus
Gastrocnemius	Large belly of the leg	Gastrocnemius

Shape

Finally, some muscles are named according to the shape they resemble (**Table 3.15**). If the deltoid muscle were laid out flat on a table, it would resemble a triangle. Similarly, the trapezius muscle was named as such because it resembles the shape of a trapezoid. A muscle such as the gracilis received its name because it is a very slender muscle. The gracilis is a hip adductor that is located on the inner thigh. A muscle such as the serratus anterior received the first part of its name because the word *serratus* refers to a serrated or jagged edge, describing the appearance the muscle's origin.

TABLE 3.15 Example Root Words: Shape

Term	Meaning	Example
Deltiod	Triangular	Posterior deltoid
Gracilis	Slender	Gracilis
Orbicularis	Circular	Orbicularis oculi
Rhomboid	Diamond shaped	Rhomboid major
Serratus	Serrated; jagged edge	Serratus anterior
Teres	Cylindrical	Teres major
Trapezius	Trapezoidal	Middle trapezius

Common Muscles that Become Dysfunctional

Certain muscles, as will be addressed multiple times in subsequent chapters, are prone to becoming dysfunctional. Muscles become dysfunctional either because they are overactive or underactive, which can place undue stress on the body during movement. While learning all the muscles is beneficial in the role of a fitness professional, knowing the problematic muscles is imperative for continued learning in assessments, program design, and implementation.

Common Muscle Imbalances

Muscle imbalances can result from changes in muscle length, strength, and neuromuscular activity, creating static and dynamic **malalignment** (Kisner & Colby, 2007; Sahrmann, 2002; Kendall, McCreary, Provance, Rodgers, & Romani, 2005). Muscles tend to have an effect on the joints they cross. Faulty alignment of the joints while standing or moving can have an effect throughout the kinetic chain. Factors such as poor posture, repetitive movement, immobilization, and even aging can affect the muscles surrounding a joint and lead to dysfunctional neuromuscular control and create malalignment, or incorrect alignment of the joints. Consequently, this can lead to altered joint actions, and eventually injury.

When referring to muscle imbalances, it is important to distinguish between the terms *overactive* and *underactive*. The term **overactive** refers to the state of having disrupted neuromuscular recruitment patterns that lead a muscle to be more active during a joint action. Conversely, the term **underactive** refers to the state of having disrupted neuromuscular recruitment patterns that lead a muscle to be less active during a joint action. In general, an overactive muscle is considered as being shortened, tight, and strong. A muscle is generally considered underactive when it is lengthened and weak. However, there may also be circumstances where these terms may not seem to apply.

Common Overactive and Underactive Muscles of the Foot and Ankle

A number of specific muscles tend to be implicated as problematic in the foot and ankle complex. **Extrinsic** muscles of the foot and ankle have proximal attachments on the leg (femur, fibula, and smaller tibia), whereas the **intrinsic** muscles of the foot and ankle have proximal and distal attachments within the foot itself (**Figure 3.24**) (Miller, Whitcome, Lieberman, Norton, & Dyer, 2014). Both groups of muscles provide control, create movement, and absorb shock. By learning the muscle actions of the intrinsic and extrinsic muscles of the foot and ankle, the fitness professional can learn how to help his or her clients strengthen these muscles. Extrinsic muscles of the foot and ankle that may become either overactive or underactive include those

CHECK IT OUT

It is important to understand that inhibition is not a complete shutdown but rather a decrease in activity, much like the way a light dimmer can decrease the amount of light being produced.

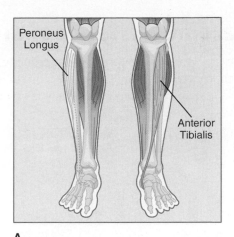
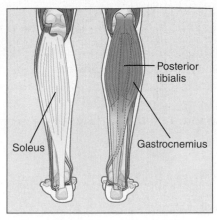

FIGURE 3.24 Muscles of the foot and ankle. A. Intrinsic muscles. B. Extrinsic muscles.

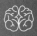
of the posterior leg, such as the soleus and lateral and medial gastrocnemius, as well as the posterior tibialis. On the anterior side of the leg is the anterior tibialis and on the lateral side are the peroneal muscles. The following are common overactive and underactive muscles of the foot and ankle.

Common overactive muscles:

◆ Soleus
◆ Lateral gastrocnemius
◆ Peroneus longus and brevis (peroneals)

Common underactive muscles:

◆ Medial gastrocnemius
◆ Anterior tibialis
◆ Posterior tibialis

Common Overactive and Underactive Muscles of the Knee

Several muscles cross the knee, meaning that they have attachments at both the thigh and lower leg bones. The primary function of these muscles is to flex, extend, adduct, or abduct the knee. These muscles include the adductors, abductors, quadriceps, and hamstring complex (**Figure 3.25**). There are also two-joint muscles that have attachments at the hip and the thigh bone that can have an effect on the actions of the knee. The following are common overactive and underactive muscles of the knee.

CHECK IT OUT

An interest in strengthening the intrinsic muscles of the foot has led to a rise in the popularity of minimalist shoes and even barefoot training. Although some studies suggest that these can strengthen the muscles of the foot, there is not enough evidence to support that they improve performance and reduce injuries (Jenkins & Cauthon, 2011; Miller et al., 2014).

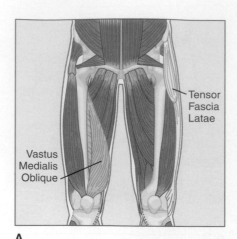 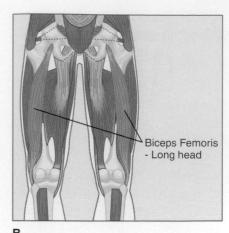

FIGURE 3.25 Muscles of the knee. A. Anterior. B. Posterior.

Common overactive muscles:

◆ Biceps femoris (short head)
◆ Tensor fascia latae (TFL)

Common underactive muscles:

◆ Vastus medialis oblique (VMO)

Common Overactive and Underactive Muscles of the LPHC

The lumbo-pelvic-hip complex, or LPHC, can be highly susceptible to muscle imbalances due to the number of muscles that cross the hip (**Figure 3.26**). The following are common overactive and underactive muscles of the LPHC.

Common overactive muscles:

◆ Hip flexors (TFL, rectus femoris, psoas)
◆ Adductors
◆ Abdominals (rectus abdominis, external obliques)
◆ Erector spinae

Common underactive muscles:

◆ Gluteus maximus
◆ Gluteus medius
◆ Hamstrings
◆ Intrinsic core stabilizers
◆ Erector spinae

Intrinsic core stabilizers

Deep inner muscles behind the superficial abdominals that have a direct effect on stabilizing the lumbo-pelvic-hip complex.

Intrinsic core stabilizers include the transverse abdominis and the internal obliques. These are deep inner muscles behind the superficial abdominals that have a direct effect on stabilizing the LPHC. The transverse abdominis lies beneath the rectus abdominis and the internal obliques are underneath the external obliques. By itself, the transverse abdominis supports the internal organs or viscera behind the abdomen via compression. When working together with the internal obliques, the transverse abdominis isometrically stabilizes the LPHC. Think of these muscles much like a supportive elastic brace that covers the internal organs. As the brace

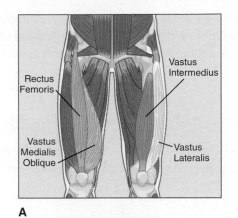

A

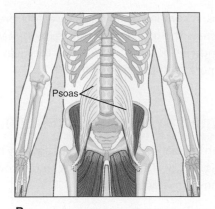

B

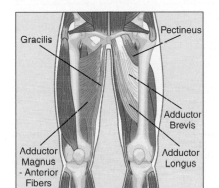

C

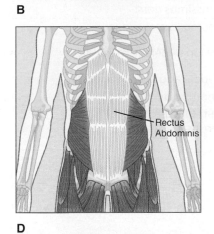

D

E

F

G

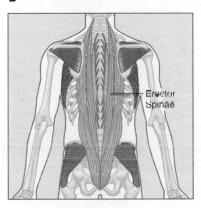

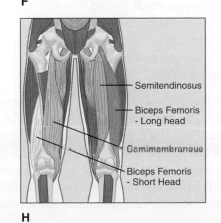

H

FIGURE 3.26 Common overactive and underactive muscles of the LPHC. A. Quadriceps. B. Psoas. C. Adductors. D. Rectus Abdominis. E. External Oblique. F. Erector Spinae. G. Gluteus Medius and Gluteus Maximus. H. Hamstring complex.

tightens, it compresses and increases the pressure on the contents inside. This compression also stiffens the back to a certain extent, making it more rigid and not as easily bent. When these muscles become underactive, they leave the abdomen, internal organs, and lower back much more susceptible to injury.

Common Overactive and Underactive Muscles of the Shoulder

When an imbalance exists, some muscles may have a negative effect on the stability of the shoulder (**Figure 3.27**). The following are common overactive and underactive muscles of the shoulder.

Common overactive muscles:

- Latissimus dorsi
- Pectoralis major/minor

Common underactive muscles:

- Middle and lower trapezius
- Rhomboids
- Rotator cuff

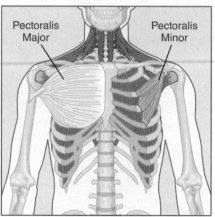

A

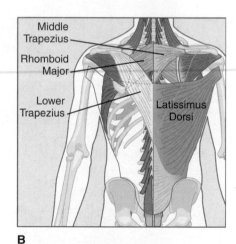

B

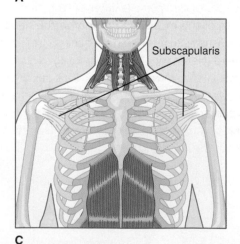

C

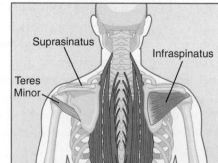

D

FIGURE 3.27 Common overactive and underactive muscles of the shoulder. A. Anterior. B. Posterior; Rotator cuff. C. Anterior. D. Posterior.

Common overactive muscles of the shoulder include the latissimus dorsi as well as the pectoralis major and minor. The latissimus dorsi is a broad and powerful muscle of the back that extends, adducts, and can internally rotate the shoulder when concentrically activated.

Common underactive muscles of the shoulder include the middle and lower trapezius, rhomboids, and the rotator cuff. The middle trapezius is the primary producer of retraction due to its ideal location right over the shoulder blades (Neumann, 2010). **Retraction** refers to the adduction of the shoulder blades where the shoulder blades move toward the spine.

The rotator cuff consists of four different muscles. All four muscles share attachments on the scapula and on the humerus, forming a cuff. To better understand what a cuff is, think of the thicker material at the end of a sleeve on a shirt. The cuff on a sleeve can add a protective layer that prevents the ends from fraying. The muscles of the rotator cuff stabilize the scapulae by helping compress the humeral head into the glenoid fossa. The rotator cuff includes the following four muscles:

- Supraspinatus
- Infraspinatus
- Teres minor
- Subscapularis

Retraction
Adduction of the shoulder blades where the shoulder blades move toward the spine.

MEMORY TIPS

You can easily remember these muscles by the acronym SITS: Supraspinatus, Infraspinatus, Teres minor, and Subscapularis.

CHECK IT OUT

To better understand what a cuff is, think of the thicker material at the end of a sleeve on a shirt. The cuff on a sleeve can add a protective layer that prevents the ends from fraying. The muscles of the rotator cuff stabilize the scapulae by helping compress the humeral head into the glenoid fossa.

Common Overactive and Underactive Muscles of the Head and Neck

Postures where the shoulders remain elevated for prolonged periods or where the head excessively protracted forward can produce imbalances of the muscles surrounding the head and neck (**Figure 3.28**). Engaging in slouched sitting postures to view a computer can create adaptive shortening of the muscles supporting the head (Neumann, 2010). If prolonged, over time such postures may cause lengthening of such muscles and weaken them. This can place an individual at risk of damage to the cervical spine. Note that some lordosis of the cervical spine is normal, meaning that there is a natural inward curvature of the cervical spine. Faulty postures in addition to other factors may disrupt the normal structure of the cervical spine. The following are common overactive and underactive muscles of the head and neck.

Common overactive muscles:

- Upper trapezius
- Sternocleidomastoid
- Levator scapulae

Common underactive muscles:

- Deep cervical flexors

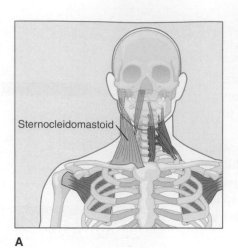
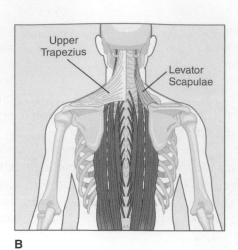
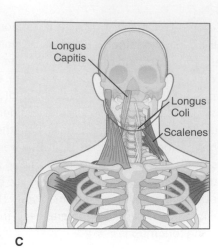

A   B   C

FIGURE 3.28 Muscles of the Cervical Spine. A. Anterior. B. Posterior; C. Deep Cervical Flexors.

The extensors of the neck hold the head upright or bring it back from a protruding position. The upper trapezius muscle is a superficial extensor of the neck, and it has the ability to extend the head back past the shoulders and toward the back (Saladin, 2007). The upper trapezius may become adaptively shortened or mechanically lengthened, depending on the posture of the individual.

Excessive neck extension may shorten the sternocleidomastoid muscle on the anterior side of the neck and make it overactive when combined with overactivity of the upper trapezius. As the prime mover for neck flexion, the sternocleidomastoid also concentrically rotates and laterally flexes the head and neck.

The levator scapulae is a posterior muscle that originates on the first few vertebrae of the cervical spine and inserts into the top border of the scapula. When concentrically activated, this muscle extends, adducts, and produces ipsilateral rotation of the neck when the shoulder blades are stationary.

With regards to underactivity, the deep cervical flexors are commonly involved. The deep cervical flexors are small intrinsic muscles that are located on the anterior and lateral side of the neck. Located underneath the sternocleidomastoid muscle, they include the longus capitus and longus coli.

Biomechanics and Kinetic Chain Disruption

Dysfunctional muscles play a significant role in the functioning of the kinetic chain. They can disrupt the communication between the nervous system and the muscles. This changes the length and tension of muscles, placing articular structures out of alignment and creating patterns of dysfunction throughout the body. Kinetic chain disruption is not just an isolated event in most cases, but rather one part of a chain reaction involving a number of dysfunctional muscles, leading to compensations and adaptations that may lead to pain and injury (Clark, 2001).

Take a simple yet functional dynamic movement such as a squat as an example. During the descent portion of a squat, a lack of dorsiflexion (sagittal plane movement) at the ankle due to overactivity or tightness of the gastrocnemius and soleus can force the LPHC into a forward flexed position in order to alter the body's center of gravity to maintain balance. This can place too much stress on the lower back as it acts as the effort force in an attempt to resist the force

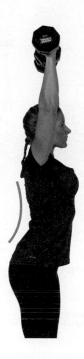

FIGURE 3.29 LPHC dysfunction.

of gravity. If the erector spinae and gluteus maximus are underactive, they may be unable to overcome the resistive force of gravity as they attempt to keep the trunk in an upright position, ultimately producing a compensation in the form of an excessive forward lean. Such compensation may also result in low back pain (Cholewicki et al., 2005; Cholewicki & Van Vliet, 2002; Radebold, Cholewicki, Polzhofer, & Greene, 2001). In addition, underactivity of the gluteus maximus may cause synergistic dominance of the latissimus dorsi muscle, making it overactive or tight as it attempts to extend the spine and stabilize the LPHC. Overactivity or tightness of the latissimus dorsi may also anteriorly rotate the pelvis (anterior pelvic tilt), creating excessive extension of the lumbar spine (**Figure 3.29**). This, in turn, can lead to synergistic dominance of the hamstrings or adductors and may lead to hamstring or groin strains (Sahrmann, 2002). The latissimus dorsi can also alter the rotation of the shoulder blade (scapula) or of the shoulder joint (humeral head), thus leading to compensations at the shoulder complex in the form of limited range of motion in any of the three planes. This may lead to injuries of the upper extremity such as impingement, tendonitis, and strain.

Muscle tightness or overactivity of muscles such as the pectoralis major and minor can decrease stabilization of the shoulder blades as well as the shoulder joint, leading to **shoulder impingement** (**Figure 3.30**) (Clark, 2001). This may lead to a loss of control of the shoulder blades, encouraging them to protract and elevate. Changes to the normal movement of the shoulder blades can increase neuromuscular activity of the upper trapezius (Ludewig & Cook, 2000). This creates an imbalance the production of force between the upper and lower portions of the trapezius muscles. Excessive extension from a protruding of the neck further encourages excessive protraction of the shoulder blades if the head protrudes forward to obtain a better view of the computer screen. Furthermore, prolonged extension of the neck places excess stress on the muscles of the neck (cervical spine), such as the upper trapezius and levator scapulae, making them overactive. This can contribute to shoulder instability, create neck strain, or even cause headaches (Sahrmann, 2002).

Shoulder impingement

When the space between the bone on top of the shoulder (acromion) and the tendons of the rotator cuff rub against each other during arm elevation.

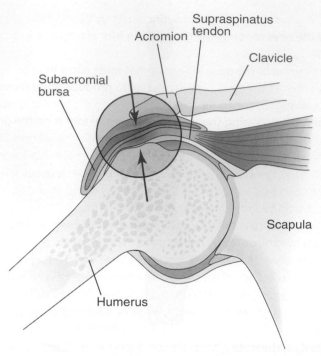

FIGURE 3.30 Shoulder impingement.

CHECK IT OUT

Shoulder impingement occurs when the space between the bone on top of the shoulder (acromion) and the tendons of the rotator cuff rub against each other during arm elevation. A lubricating sac (bursa) exists to help the tendons glide freely during movement. However, in the event of shoulder impingement, the acromion rubs or pinches against both the tendon and the bursa, causing irritation, inflammation, and even pain. With enough pinching, the tendons may fray, causing inflammation, or they may tear, resulting in a rotator cuff tear. People who do a lot of repetitive overhead lifting or tasks such as assembly-line, construction, and welding, paint, and steel work are especially susceptible to shoulder injuries such as impingement. Incorporate exercises that strengthen the muscles of the rotator cuff when creating a shoulder routine as a preventive measure. This is especially important if a client is known to engage in repetitive overhead work or has experienced shoulder injuries in the past.

Biomechanics to Explain the Observance of Kinetic Chain Disruption

The kinetic chain adapts during functional movements so the body can maintain its center of gravity, even over a changing base of support. This is why a change in alignment of one joint can cause other joints to change their alignment. For example, turning the kneecap (patella) inward (internal or medial rotation) then outward (external or lateral rotation) causes an obligatory effect from the heel (subtalar joint) to the hips (pelvis). Similarly, externally rotating the feet will cause an obligatory effect from the heel, knee, and hip joints. To better understand this concept, consider what happens during a functional, dynamic, and multiplanar movement such as walking. As the heel contacts the ground, the foot pronates, causing internal rotation of the tibia, femur, and pelvis. **Pronation of the foot** is a combination of dorsiflexion, eversion, and abduction. Recall some of the muscle actions that must occur in order to eccentrically decelerate to control as well as concentrically accelerate to produce these movements.

Acting as a shock absorber, the foot pronates in order to reduce the ground reaction force that the body sustains by increasing the amount of time the foot is on the ground. During the midstance phase of walking, the forefoot makes contact with the ground as the body briefly balances on one leg. Normally, the foot supinates, causing external rotation of the tibia, femur, and pelvis. **Supination of the foot** is a combination of plantar flexion, inversion, and adduction. This is when the body bears all of its weight and the demand for a stable surface is high, so weight distribution should be spread over the ball of the foot.

The foot then transitions from being a shock absorber to being an effective lever in order to propel the body forward. Propulsion occurs once the heel leaves the ground. The transition from pronation to supination at midstance is also the time when injury is most likely to occur. Poor neuromuscular control of any of these muscle actions places the kinetic chain in a position where it cannot function properly. Muscles of the foot and ankle must be able to eccentrically decelerate pronation in an efficient manner. A weak or inhibited anterior tibialis may not be strong enough to dorsiflex the foot during pronation after heel strike and may not be strong enough to eccentrically decelerate plantar flexion during propulsion. Likewise, muscles of the foot and ankle (**Table 3.16**) must be capable of concentrically accelerating supination so that propulsion can happen. A disruption in the kinetic chain can lead to compensations that can contribute to injuries that occur at the foot all the way up the kinetic chain. The ability to properly stabilize isometrically is just as important. All of the muscles of the foot and ankle described here play some role in stabilizing the foot during movements where the foot is planted on a surface. The ability to stabilize is needed so that an individual does not sprain their ankle during the transition from pronation to supination.

The example of what happens during walking is significant to the fitness professional because it illustrates what can happen during dynamic movement when there is a disruption in the kinetic chain. Recall that a disruption at one part of the kinetic chain can create disruptions at other kinetic chain checkpoints. It is important for the fitness professional to provide the best service, which means including an injury prevention component in client programs. Understanding functional anatomy and multiplanar biomechanics can assist with the identification of compensations that may lead to injury. This information can be used both during the assessment process and when selecting exercises for clients. Once compensations have been

Pronation of the foot
A combination of dorsiflexion, eversion, and abduction.

Supination of the foot
A combination of plantar flexion, inversion, and adduction.

TABLE 3.16 Foot and Ankle: Muscles and Functions

Muscle	Concentrically Accelerates	Eccentrically Decelerates
Anterior tibialis	Dorsiflexion; inversion	Plantar flexion; eversion
Posterior tibialis	Plantar flexion; inversion	Dorsiflexion; eversion
Soleus	Plantar flexion	Dorsiflexion
Gastrocnemius	Plantar flexion	Dorsiflexion
Peroneus longus	Plantar flexion; eversion	Dorsiflexion; inversion

identified in a client, the fitness professional can select the most appropriate exercises to safely assist the client in reaching his or her goals. It is imperative to set up a program where clients are graduated into new levels of training to prepare them to move efficiently, with the right force, and at the right time. This will help them prevent injury, progress them towards their goals, and help them break plateaus, as needed.

Biomechanics to Reverse Kinetic Chain Dysfunction

Becoming familiar with how muscle is structured and how it functions allows for troubleshooting when there is a disruption in the kinetic chain. Fortunately, fitness professionals can use functional anatomy and biomechanics to reverse kinetic chain dysfunction. The first step is to identify compensations the client has at each of the kinetic chain checkpoints. Observing posture as the client stands still (static posture) is one way to achieve this. All kinetic checkpoints must be adequately aligned in order for the body to produce the greatest amount of force during exercise.

Muscles that cross the joints at each of these kinetic chain checkpoints have the potential of becoming overactive or tight. Muscles that are tight from adaptive shortening can be lengthened in order to help them achieve an optimal length–tension relationship. One way to create length is by using a muscle's eccentric function to create a lengthening exercise. Recall that during eccentric activation a muscle actively lengthens while creating tension. Knowing a muscle's concentric function and its eccentric function is imperative to reversing kinetic chain dysfunction. For example, a client with a tight gastrocnemius (ankle extensor) may inhibit the anterior tibialis (ankle flexor) from concentrically producing dorsiflexion. Using the eccentric function of the gastrocnemius, which is dorsiflexion, can help to lengthen the muscle. Another example is straightening the knee when trying to stretch the hamstrings. Knee flexion is the primary concentric function of the hamstrings, and knee extension is the muscle's eccentric function. When extending then knee, the hamstring muscles elongate yet still create some tension as they attempt to slow down that movement. This is eccentric deceleration at work.

Introduction to Flexibility and Activation

In order for the body to move efficiently, the joints require optimum neuromuscular control as they move through their full range of motion. They also need to have a certain level of flexibility. **Flexibility** can be defined as the normal extensibility of soft tissue, which allows a joint to be moved through its full range of motion.

Flexibility
The normal extensibility of soft tissue, which allows a joint to be moved through its full range of motion.

CHECK IT OUT

Elongating a muscle, or rather stretching it, begins with the contractile components of muscle. When sarcomeres shorten, the thick and thin filaments slide closer together to create overlap. When stretching occurs, this overlap decreases and allows muscle fibers to elongate. If and when these sarcomeres become fully stretched, the body can receive additional elongation from the surrounding connective tissue such as fascia and tendons to which the muscle is connected.

Flexibility training affects the neuromuscular system by improving the communication between the nervous system and the muscular system. The nervous system is sensitive to the intensity of a stretch and will respond accordingly based on how much a muscle is stretched, as well as for how long.

A comprehensive strategy to reverse kinetic chain dysfunction should also addresses underactive muscles via the implementation of corrective exercise. **Corrective exercise** is a programming process that identifies neuromuscular dysfunction, develops a plan of action, and implements a corrective strategy as a part of an exercise training program. Clients who demonstrate patterns of dysfunction through poor static or dynamic posture should be evaluated so imbalances can be identified. Once identified, overactive muscles should be lengthened and underactive muscles strengthened.

Neuromuscular Efficiency

In order for the body to work in the most efficient way, the neuromuscular system must allow all muscles surrounding a joint to concentrically produce force, eccentrically reduce force, and dynamically stabilize the kinetic chain in all three planes of motion. When this occurs, there is said to be **neuromuscular efficiency**. For example, when standing up from a seated position, the gluteus maximus (agonist) must be able to concentrically accelerate hip extension while the psoas (antagonist) eccentrically decelerates hip flexion. At the same time, muscles such as the transverse abdominus and deep erector spinae must dynamically stabilize the LPHC.

Thanks to neuromuscular efficiency, the body is also designed to take the path of least resistance. This means that while a client may have movement dysfunctions, his or her body is still going to move as efficiently as possible, even if it means doing so through altered movement patterns. This is called **relative flexibility**. For example, a client with poor flexibility at the ankle due to tight calf muscles may have limited dorsiflexion during the lowering phase of a squat. Consequently, the client may widen his or her stance and will externally rotate the feet in order to squat. This altered movement pattern demonstrates a lack of dorsiflexion and indicates probable weakness of the anterior tibialis, as well as probable overactivity or tightness of the calves. Altered movement patterns are indicative of neuromuscular efficiency that is not optimal.

Conclusion

A solid understanding of biomechanics and the Human Movement System will provide the fitness professional with the requisite skills and information to support client progress. In this chapter, the role of biomechanics and its basic application was discussed and important terms were defined. Using this information, fitness professionals can better speak to common issues such as muscular dysfunction and kinetic chain disruption.

Corrective exercise

The programming process that identifies neuromuscular dysfunction, develops a plan of action, and implements a corrective strategy as a part of an exercise training program.

Neuromuscular efficiency

When the neuromuscular system allows agonists, antagonists, and stabilizers to synergistically produce muscle actions in all three planes of motion.

Relative flexibility

The human movement system's way of finding the path of least resistance during movement.

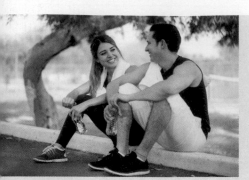
© antoniodiaz/Shutterstock

Case in Review

After you and your friend complete your run, you continue the conversation on the kinetic chain as it applies to everyday movements. In order to discuss the biomechanics behind common movements you must first understand the planes of motion, joint actions, and muscles associated with the movements. One common movement that we often overlook is standing up from sitting in a chair. Because your friend may not know the scientific terminology used to describe the biomechanics behind standing up from sitting on a chair, you use hand gestures to animate and support how you explain this movement to your friend.

In order to describe the movement of standing up from sitting in a chair, you explain that the sagittal plane that passes through the body, dividing the right and left sides. When discussing planes of motion, you use hand motions to show how this vertical plane passes through your body. While going through the movement, you show your friend the breakdown as you stand up from the chair, identifying the joint actions and muscle movements while explaining them in a way that minimizes the chance of confusing your friend.

The joint actions involved in this common movement include knee extension, hip extension, and ankle plantar flexion. Simply explaining this without showing where these joint actions occur will confuse your friend. Similar to the muscles associated with the movement, you can still use the scientific name but accompany the terminology with a description or name that is easily identified or understood. For example, one muscle associated with the movement of standing up from sitting on a chair is the gluteus maximus. Using gestures to show where this muscle is and how it is involved in the movement as well as using the general names it is called will aid in your friend's understanding.

As certified personal trainers, it is not the amount of scientific rationales we can inundate our clients with to build credibility, but our ability to explain the importance of these concepts in a manner that is relevant and usable by the client.

References

Behnke, R. (2012). *Kinetic anatomy* (3rd ed.). Champaign, IL: Human Kinetics.

Brooks, G., Fahey, T., & Baldwin, K. (2005). *Exercise physiology: Human bioenergetics and its applications* (4th ed.). New York, NY: McGraw-Hill.

Cholewicki, J., Silfies, S. P., Shah, R. A., Greene, H. S., Reeves, N. P., Alvi, K., & Goldberg, B. (2005). Delayed trunk muscle reflex responses increase the risk of low back injuries. *Spine, 30*, 2614–2620.

Cholewicki, J., & Van Vliet, J. J. (2002). Relative contribution of trunk muscles to the stability of the lumbar spine during isometric exertions. *Clinical Biomechanics, 17*, 99–105.

Clark, M. (2001). *A scientific approach to understanding kinetic chain dysfunction*. Thousand Oaks, CA: National Academy of Sports Medicine.

Gullett, J., Tillman, M., Gutierrez, G., & Chow, J. (2009). A biomechanical comparison of back and front squats in healthy trained individuals. *Journal of Strength and Conditioning Research, 23*, 284–292.

Hall, S. (2014). *Basic biomechanics* (7th ed.). New York, NY: McGraw-Hill Education.

Hamil, J., Knutzen, K., & Derrick, T. (2015). *Biomechanical basis of human movement* (4th ed.). Philadelphia, PA: Lippincott Williams & Wilkins.

Jenkins, D., & Cauthon, D. (2011). Barefoot running claims and controversies. *Journal of the American Podiatric Medical Association, 101*(3), 231–246.

Kendall, F., McCreary, E., Provance, P., Rodgers, M., & Romani, W. (2005). *Muscles: Testing and function with posture and pain* (5th ed.). Baltimore, MD: Lippincott Williams & Wilkins.

Kisner, C., & Colby, L. (2007). *Therapeutic exercise: Foundations and techniques* (5th ed.). Philadelphia, PA: F.A. Davis.

Knudson, D. (2007). *Fundamentals of biomechanics* (2nd ed.). New York, NY: Springer.

Levangie, P., & Norkin, C. (2001). *Joint structure and function: A comprehensive analysis* (3rd ed.). Philadelphia, PA: F.A. Davis.

Ludewig, P., & Cook, T. (2000). Alterations in shoulder kinematics and associated muscle activity in people with symptoms of shoulder impingement. *Physical Therapy, 80*(3), 276–291.

Miller, E., Whitcome, K., Lieberman, D., Norton, H., & Dyer, R. (2014). The effect of minimal shoes on arch structure and intrinsic foot muscle strength. *Journal of Sport and Health Science, 3*(2), 74–85.

Neumann, D. (2010). *Kinesiology of the musculoskeletal system: Foundations for rehabilitation* (2nd ed.). St. Louis, MO: Mosby/Elsevier.

Radebold, A., Cholewicki, J., Polzhofer, G. K., & Greene, H. S. (2001). Impaired postural control of the lumbar spine is associated with delayed muscle response times in patients with chronic idiopathic low back pain. *Spine, 26*, 724–730.

Sahrmann, S. (2002). *Diagnosis and treatment of movement impairment syndromes*. St. Louis, MO: Mosby.

Saladin, K. (2007). *Anatomy and physiology: The unity of form and function* (4th ed.). New York, NY: McGraw-Hill.

Watkins, J. (2014) *Fundamental biomechanics of sport and exercise*. New York, NY: Routledge.

CHAPTER 4

THE HUMAN MOVEMENT SYSTEM IN FITNESS

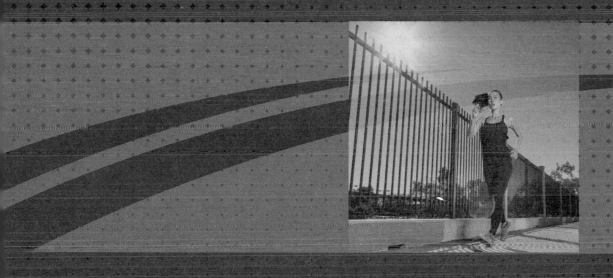

OBJECTIVES

After studying this chapter, you will be able to:

1. **Identify** the three systems of the kinetic chain.

2. **Explain** the roles and interactions of the systems of the kinetic chain.

3. **Apply** basic human movement concepts to determine the development of kinetic chain dysfunction.

4. **Identify** major areas of kinetic chain dysfunction common among clients.

5. **Analyze** influencers to movement dysfunction.

6. **Discuss** other systems related to human movement.

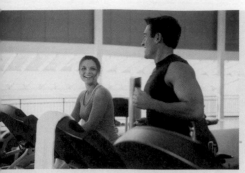

© Sean Locke Photography/Shutterstock

Case Scenario

You have been a fitness enthusiast for 5 years now, but you have never really taken the time to understand the fundamentals behind how and why you move the way you do. In the past, your personal trainer discussed the Human Movement System, its interrelationships with other systems, and the role it plays in the movements we take every day, but he never connected the dots to show how the Human Movement System was directly related to your fitness goals. He would refer to the five kinetic chain checkpoints, but he never explained them in a way that made sense to what you were doing at the moment. Now that you have become aware of the kinetic chain and how it works, you have begun to look further into the notion of dysfunction and optimizing movement as it relates to fitness. Looking back at your past experiences with your personal trainer, you feel that an understanding of the Human Movement System would have helped you to better define your fitness goals as a client.

Without conducting a formal fitness assessment, how would you educate a friend about the following in a way that is relevant to fitness and can be easily understood?

- What is the Human Movement System?

- What are the kinetic chain checkpoints?

- How do you identify kinetic chain dysfunction, examples of influencers, and its importance in optimal movement?

TRAINER TIPS ⟨⬡⟩

It is important to explain to clients the role the nervous system plays in human movement. Oftentimes, clients think that training only involves working with the muscular system.

Introduction to the Human Movement System

The Human Movement System, also known as the kinetic chain, comprises three different, intimately interwoven systems that allow our bodies to move. These three systems are the nervous, muscular, and skeletal systems.

To produce movement in the body, all of the components of the Human Movement System must work together. This chapter discusses the three major components of the Human Movement System and the importance of understanding how each system operates alone as well as part of an integrated system. In addition, kinetic chain dysfunction and its effect on client performance are explained. By understanding the systems involved in human movement and how they work together to form the kinetic chain, fitness professionals are better able to support their clients.

Nervous System

The **nervous system** is a key topic of study for fitness professionals; knowledge about the nervous system and its governing functions in human movement science is empowering as a professional. The nervous system functions as the software of the Human Movement System. It tells the hardware of the body when to move, in which direction, and at what speed. The nervous system activates and recruits muscles to create movement and stabilization forces within the skeletal framework. It collects all the sensory information, both internal and external, about the environment. After it integrates that information, it sends what it perceives as the appropriate movement responses for a specific outcome. When outcomes do not turn out favorably, like missing a shot from the free throw line in basketball, the nervous system can influence future outcomes through repetition. The nervous system, through practice, solidifies the ability to achieve a specified outcome. It is like the physical application of the adage "practice makes perfect."

The nervous system is divided into two distinctly different, yet interdependent, parts. The **central nervous system (CNS)** includes the brain and spinal cord, and its primary function is to coordinate activity of all parts of the body. The CNS is where interneurons are located. Interneurons receive impulses from afferent neurons and then conduct back out to provide the efferent response. The brain is where **motor control**, **motor learning**, and **motor development** are honed in order to produce skilled movement over time. The spinal cord is the connection between the peripheral nervous system and the brain. It is also controls the body's reflexes.

The nervous system can adapt to provide **structural efficiency** by coordinating proprioceptive movement for stability and balance. For example, it can adapt to enable a person to remain balanced on one foot, even with closed eyes. The nervous system also can adapt to inactivity. Sedentary habits, such as being in seated positions at work and home for multiple hours a day, can have negative effects on the nervous system.

Fitness professionals must start with a quality assessment that allows them to know where their clients' starting points are, and then follow with appropriate progressions in the development of personalized programs (this topic will be discussed in later chapters). Fitness professionals need to recognize that training the body includes training the nervous system, and motor patterns, to support their clients' functional demands.

Afferent and Efferent Neurons and Interneurons

The nervous system is made up of approximately 100 billion specialized nerve cells called **neurons**. Neurons are the functional unit of the nervous system. A neuron has three main parts: the cell body, an axon, and dendrites. The word **dendrite** comes from a Greek word meaning "tree." Dendrites act as branches reaching out from the cell body, feeling for impulses from other neurons or sensory receptors. The **cell body**, or *soma*, processes the information from the dendrite and sends it along to the axon. The **axon** conducts impulses away from the cell body.

The consecutive linking of neurons conducts electrochemical signals called **nerve impulses** that travel throughout the nerve fiber. Nerve impulses that move *toward* the spinal cord and brain from the periphery of the body are sensory in nature. These sensory neurons are known as **afferent neurons**. Afferent (sensory) neurons rely on sensory receptors to recognize environmental stimuli. Sensory receptors include:

- Mechanoreceptors (touch and position)
- Thermoreceptors (temperature)

Nervous system

A conglomeration of billions of cells specifically designed to provide a communication network within the human body.

Central nervous system (CNS)

The division of the nervous system comprising the brain and the spinal cord. Its primary function is to coordinate activity of all parts of the body.

Motor control

How the central nervous system integrates internal and external sensory information with pervious experiences to produce a motor response.

Motor learning

The integration of motor control processes with practice and experience that leads to relatively permanent changes in the body's capacity to produce skilled movements.

Motor development

The change in motor skill behavior over time throughout the lifespan.

Structural efficiency

The structural alignment of the muscular and skeletal systems that allows the body to maintain balance in relation to its center of gravity.

Neuron

The functional unit of the nervous system.

Dendrite

The portion of a neuron that is responsible for gathering information from other structures.

 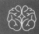
Cell body

The portion of the neuron that contains the nucleus, lysosomes, mitochondria, and Golgi complex.

Axon

A cylindrical projection from the cell body that transmits nerve impulses to other neurons or effector sites.

Nerve impulses

The consecutive linking of neurons by electrochemical signals that travel throughout the nerve fiber.

- ◆ Nociceptors (pain)
- ◆ Chemoreceptors (taste, smell)
- ◆ Photoreceptors (light)

Nerve impulses that move *away* from the brain and spinal cord are called **efferent neurons**. Efferent neurons stimulate muscle contraction, which is why they are also referred to as motor neurons—they create movement. **Interneurons** are only located within the spinal cord and brain and receive impulses from afferent (sensory) neurons and conduct back out to provide a motor (efferent) response.

Mechanoreceptors

Mechanoreceptors are specialized sensory receptors that respond to deformation of body tissues. *Deformation* simply refers to a change in position of the receptor, which generates a nerve impulse. Mechanoreceptors can be stimulated in response to touch, pressure, stretch, and motion. They also allow the brain to gauge body position. For instance, if a person closes her eyes, can she still touch the tip of her index finger to her nose? If so, the joint and body positioning mechanoreceptors allow her to know where her nose is, and her finger position in relation to it. It seems a nominal task, until one considers all of the body positions an individual goes into and out of that are not consciously thought about, yet done effortlessly. Proprioceptors (body positioning receptors) work consistently throughout the day, and even more so during athletic performance. **Proprioception** refers to the cumulative sensory input to the CNS from all the mechanoreceptors that sense body position and limb movement. This is an important component to consider when developing programs that aim to impact and improve the performance of the nervous system in human movement.

Muscle spindles are small mechanoreceptors found in the belly of skeletal muscles that measure the amount and rate of stretch. When the muscle is lengthened too much or too quickly the muscle spindle sends afferent impulses to the CNS, resulting in muscular contraction as a protective response. This happens when practicing static stretching in flexibility routines. When the muscle is stretched to a point the muscle spindles deem potentially dangerous, the muscle is triggered to contract, disallowing any movement that goes further into the stretch.

Golgi tendon organs (GTOs), or tendon organs, are located at the musculotendinous junction, which is where the muscle and tendon converge. The GTO measures the amount and rate of tension that develops within the muscle. If the tension developed is too much, or the onset of tension is too rapid, the GTO will cause the muscle to relax as a safety response. During flexibility training this happens after the muscle spindle causes the protective muscular contraction. This contraction creates the *tension* that the GTO measures in this circumstance. As the GTO monitors the muscular contraction, it will signal the muscle to relax after approximately 30 seconds of applied tension to the muscle. At that point the joint can be taken farther into its range of motion. This is the rationale behind why a static stretch is held for at least 30 seconds—to allow the GTO time to inhibit the muscle.

A common example of the GTO phenomenon is when weightlifters have completed an intense leg workout and the legs become sore. As they walk, one of their legs simply gives out for a fraction of a second. This is a reflex response of the GTO measuring the amount and rate of tension in the muscle and sending a protective inhibitory response.

Joint receptors are located within the joint capsule and respond to the amount and rate of joint movement, as well as pressure. They signal an inhibitory response during extreme joint positions or if too much pressure is placed on the joint, in order to prevent injury.

All of these mechanoreceptors are also called *proprioceptors*. Proprioceptors are classified by location. They are located in skeletal muscle, joint capsules, and tendons and provide information about body positioning. Mechanoreceptors are also classified by the stimulus detected, which in this case is the deformation of position. These are just two different ways of classifying the same thing.

Muscular System

The muscular system is part of the kinetic chain and is composed of three different types of muscles: smooth, cardiac, and skeletal. Smooth muscles are involuntary muscles, meaning that they are not consciously controlled. They are found in the walls of blood vessels and hollow organs. Cardiac muscles are the involuntary muscles that make up the heart. The fitness professional will certainly address physiological outcomes like heart rate, but there is little actual focus on the cardiac muscle beyond this. Skeletal muscles are voluntary, or consciously controlled, muscles that provide both locomotion and stability to the skeletal system. These are the muscles that fitness professionals focus on by helping clients achieve increased skeletal muscle activation, coordination, strength, size (or hypertrophy), and form during movement patterns.

Muscle Fiber Types

The two major categories of muscle fibers are type I and type II. These different muscle fiber types have specific purposes with regards to human movement. An understanding of the two types of muscle fibers is needed so that programs can be developed to achieve specific adaptations in the body.

Type I Fibers

Type I fibers are also known as *slow-twitch fibers* or *red fibers*. These fibers contain large numbers of capillaries, mitochondria, and myoglobin. Capillaries are small blood vessels where the exchange of oxygen and carbon dioxide takes place. Mitochondria are where food energy is converted into energy the cells can use. Myoglobin is a red-colored protein in the fluid of muscle cells that pulls in oxygen and temporarily holds it. Myoglobin contains a red pigment, which is why type I muscle fibers are often referred to as red fibers. These muscle fibers are considered highly aerobic for three reasons: (1) the excellent oxygen delivery system via capillaries, (2) myoglobin's ability to hold on to oxygen, and (3) the mitochondria's ability to metabolize in the presence of oxygen.

Type I fibers are considered slow twitch. A *twitch* is a single contraction of facilitated muscle. Type I fibers are slower to reach maximal contraction. Because of their slow twitch speed and high aerobic capacity, type I fibers are more resistant to fatigue. They are also smaller in size, produce less force, and do not respond as well to hypertrophy as type II fibers. These are excellent characteristics for stabilization muscles that help support posture against the continual gravitational stresses as well as provide the dynamic stabilization needed during functional movement patterns and activities of daily living.

Type II Fibers

Type II muscle fibers are also known as *fast-twitch fibers* or *white fibers*. They contain fewer capillaries, mitochondria, and myoglobin than type I fibers. Because there is little myoglobin, the fibers do not have a red pigment, causing the muscle to appear white—hence why they are called white fibers. Fewer capillaries means less oxygen delivery. Fewer mitochondria decreases

Afferent neurons

Nerve impulses that move toward the spinal cord and brain from the periphery of the body and are sensory in nature.

Efferent neurons

Efferent neurons are motor neurons that send a message for muscles to contract.

Interneurons

Only located within the spinal cord and brain; receive impulses from afferent (sensory) neurons and conduct back out to provide a motor (efferent) response.

Mechanoreceptors

Sensory receptors responsible for sensing distortion in body tissues.

Proprioception

The cumulative sensory input to the central nervous system from all mechanoreceptors that sense body position and limb movements.

Muscle spindles

Receptors sensitive to change in length of the muscle, and the rate of that change.

MEMORY TIPS

Mitochondria are nicknamed the "powerhouse of the cell."

TABLE 4.1 Muscle Fiber Types

Type	Characteristic
Type I (slow-twitch)	More capillaries, mitochondria, and myoglobin
	Increased oxygen delivery
	Smaller in size
	Less force produced
	Slow to fatigue
	Long-term contractions (stabilization)
	Slow twitch
Type II (fast-twitch)	Fewer capillaries, mitochondria, and myoglobin
	Decreased oxygen delivery
	Larger in size
	More force produced
	Quick to fatigue
	Short-term contractions (force and power)
	Fast twitch

Golgi tendon organs (GTOs)

Receptors sensitive to the change in tension of the muscle, and the rate of that change.

Joint receptors

Receptors in and around a joint that respond to pressure, acceleration, and deceleration of the joint.

the amount of oxygen uptake. Therefore, type II muscle fibers are considered to be more anaerobic with regard to their metabolic abilities. Because of this they can produce more speed and strength than type I fibers, but the burst of intensity will be short-lived.

Type II muscle fibers are subdivided into type IIa and type IIx based on their chemical and mechanical properties. Type IIx muscle fibers embody the type II characteristics listed above.

Type IIa muscle fibers are type II fibers, but they are considered to be intermediate fast-twitch fibers. They can use both aerobic and anaerobic metabolism almost equally to create energy. In this way, they are a combination of the type I and type IIx muscle fibers. See **Table 4.1** for a summary of the characteristics of type I and type II muscle fibers.

Behavioral Properties of Muscle

Muscle develops tension to allow movement at a joint and to exert a force on the bone it is trying to move. Muscle is the only tissue in the human body that can do this (Hall, 2014; Hamill, Knutzen, & Derrick, 2015; Knudson, 2007; Levangie & Norkin, 2001). Skeletal muscle allows the body to remain upright, to move its limbs, and to absorb shock from external forces. The nervous system controls the timing and rate of a muscle action. The nervous system must work together with the muscular system in order for these movements to occur efficiently. Having a general understanding of how muscle behaves can help fitness professionals better conceptualize how muscles will act when they develop tension during movement.

CHECK IT OUT

Can Chickens Fly?

Unexpectedly, the answer is yes; they just can't fly far! Chickens' bodies are not aerodynamic, so flying requires significant amounts of explosive work that can only be maintained for short bursts before fatigue sets in. The largest part of the chicken is the breast—the muscle responsible for flying. This muscle is prone to hypertrophy because of the type of muscle required for these explosive movements. An informed individual will also know that the chicken breast is considered to be white meat. All of these descriptions show a clear similarity to type IIx muscle fibers in humans.

Do Chickens Walk?

When chickens are allowed to roam freely, they do so by regularly walking about, looking for food and pecking at the ground. They have much more endurance in their legs, although they are not incredibly fast. The legs produce less force and are smaller in size. They have a high aerobic capacity with increased numbers of capillaries, mitochondria, and the red pigment protein myoglobin. This is the dark meat of the chicken. All of these similarities show a clear similarity to type I muscle fibers in humans.

It is important to note that human muscles and chicken muscles are not the same, and that the red and white muscle fibers in humans are distributed differently than in chickens.

Muscle has four behavioral properties:

- Extensibility
- Elasticity
- Irritability
- Ability to develop tension

The first behavioral property is extensibility. This is an important concept to understand because it relates to flexibility. Extensibility refers to the ability to be stretched or lengthened. A client lacking extensibility of a muscle will be limited in his or her ability to lengthen that muscle.

Elasticity refers to a muscle's ability to return to normal or resting length after it has been stretched. Muscle is elastic, much like a rubber band that can be elongated with stretching and can resume its original position after being released.

In addition, skeletal muscle has a **viscoelastic** property that allows it to extend and recoil with time. To better understand viscosity, think of the consistency of honey. Filling up a cup with honey takes longer than filling it up with a liquid such as water. This happens because honey is much more viscous than water.

Another behavioral property is irritability. Irritability means that a muscle is able to respond to a stimulus. In the case of muscle, a stimulus can be in the form of an action potential coming from an attached nerve or from the impact of an external force on the muscle.

Finally, a muscle has the ability to develop tension. Traditionally, a muscle's ability to develop tension has been known as *contraction*; however, this term must be understood and used with caution to avoid confusion. Although the term *contractility* implies the ability to shorten or draw together, in reality a muscle can remain the same length, as well as either increase or decrease in length, when it develops tension. Thus, the term *contraction* should be understood as the activation of a force within a muscle to produce an action at a joint (Brooks, Fahey, & Baldwin, 2005; Knudson, 2007; Neumann, 2010).

Viscoelastic
Ability to stretch linearly.

Because of these behavioral properties, individuals can improve their mobility and have the potential to improve their performance of activities of daily living. Extensibility and elasticity allow muscles to take joints through their full range of motion so that people can walk with fluidity as opposed to walking like stiff robots. Irritability of a muscle means that it is sensitive to neural stimulation so that an individual can move a limb at any time. Muscle is also sensitive to outside stimulation, such as stepping on a sharp object. The pain felt creates a reflex that causes one to quickly move one's foot in order to avoid injury. Lastly, the ability to develop tension in a muscle is what allows it to produce the force that moves a joint, which in turn moves a limb. An individual is able to grab a glass of water and take a drink thanks to the ability of muscles to develop tension.

Muscles as Movers

As discussed, muscles provide the human body with the ability to produce and reduce movement, as well as to stabilize forces. A muscle's particular function further categorizes it as an agonist, antagonist, synergist, or stabilizer.

Agonists are the prime movers. These muscles are the major force producer for a particular joint action. For some basic exercises it is very easy to figure out what the agonist is because of the exercise's name. For example, the biceps brachii is the agonist in a biceps curl; the latissimus dorsi is the agonist in a lat pulldown. The posterior deltoid is the agonist in a rear delt fly. The pectoralis major is the agonist in the chest fly.

Synergists are muscles that assist the prime mover in a given joint action. For example, a biceps curl uses the biceps brachii as the prime mover with the brachialis and brachioradialis working as synergists to assist in elbow flexion. The latissimus dorsi has a synergist at the shoulder joint called the teres major that works as a synergist in almost all the joint's actions. Because it is such a significant synergist of the latissimus dorsi, it is often referred to as the "lat's little brother."

Stabilizers are muscles that minimize unwanted ancillary movements. These are the muscles that keep the shoulder blades from shrugging while doing a biceps curl, or the muscles that keep the back from arching during a lat pulldown. The muscles of the core are also stabilizers in all movements, which is why it may be said that "every exercise is a core exercise." This is because the core stabilizers are required during functional movement patterns.

The **antagonist** opposes the prime mover. In a biceps curl the triceps brachii is the antagonist because it opposes elbow flexion. The deltoid muscle is the antagonist in a lat pulldown. The rear deltoid fly and the chest fly are done in the same horizontal/transverse plane of motion, but have opposing forces. The rear deltoids and the pectoralis major have an agonist/antagonist relationship in these exercises.

In a squat several joint actions are taking place. Pay attention to the lifting phase of the hip extension in the squat. The gluteus maximus is considered the agonist, or primary mover, in a hip extension. The hamstrings and posterior fibers of the adductor magnus are synergists in a hip extension, meaning that they assist the primary mover as the hips extend in the squat. As these muscles move the hips into extension other muscles stabilize the lumbar spine, pelvis, and hips (lumbo-pelvic-hip complex, or LPHC). The primary antagonist, or opposing muscle, of the hip extension is the iliopsoas muscle, which must minimize how much it contracts so that the hips can extend and the person can stand up from the squatted position.

The squat also includes knee extension. The primary mover in knee extension is the quadriceps group. There is no true synergist to the quadriceps in knee extension. The rotator cuff

Agonists

Muscles that works as the prime mover of a joint exercise.

Synergists

Muscles that assist the prime mover in a joint action.

Stabilizers

Muscles that minimize unwanted movement while the agonist and synergists work to provide movement at the joint.

Antagonists

Muscles that oppose the prime mover.

TABLE 4.2 Muscles as Movers

Muscle Type	Muscle Function	Exercise	Muscle(s) Used
Agonist	Prime mover	Chest press	Pectoralis major
		Overhead press	Deltoid
		Row	Latissimus dorsi
		Squat	Gluteus maximus, quadriceps
Synergist	Assist prime mover	Chest press	Anterior deltoid, triceps
		Overhead press	Triceps
		Row	Posterior deltoid, biceps
		Squat	Hamstring complex
Stabilizer	Stabilize while prime mover and synergist work	Chest press	Rotator cuff
		Overhead press	Rotator cuff
		Row	Rotator cuff
		Squat	Transversus abdominis
Antagonist	Oppose prime mover	Chest press	Posterior deltoid
		Overhead press	Latissimus dorsi
		Row	Pectoralis major
		Squat	Psoas

of the hip, transverse abdominus, internal obliques, and multifidi muscles are LPHC stabilizers during the squat. Finally, the hamstrings are the functional antagonists in knee extension because their primary joint action is knee flexion.

Table 4.2 provides a summary of the types of muscles based on their role in different types of movement.

Skeletal System

The skeletal system is composed primarily of bones and joints. Bones are rigid structures that muscles connect to via tendons. The junction where two or more bones join is called a *joint*, and it is the place where skeletal movement occurs. **Ligaments** are the strong connective tissues that connect bone to bone. **Tendons** are the connective tissues that attach muscle to bone.

The skeletal system serves five major roles in the body:

1. **Movement**. The skeletal system consists of the levers and pivot points the muscular system acts upon to create movement. Bones are the levers, and joints are the pivot points. The

TRAINER TIPS ⬛

The skeletal system provides more than just the framework for the client's body during exercise. Show your clients how their bones act as levers to help support proper movement.

Ligament
Strong connective tissue that connects bone to bone.

Tendon
Connective tissue that attaches muscle to bone.

fitness professional will work with joint actions as well as changes in lever length during fitness programs in order to modify exercises.

2. **Support**. Bones provide the framework for a body. Bones are the scaffolding that everything else in a body is built on top of or held within. They give shape. Posture has an effect on a skeletal system's functionality, so the fitness professional should take steps to reinforce the skeletal support system.

3. **Protection**. Bones encase vital organs and protect them from trauma. The brain is protected by the skull. The heart and lungs are protected by the rib cage. Athletes may use their skeletal system for protection in their sports; for example, a straight-arm block in football or covering up the face in boxing.

4. **Blood production**. Blood cells are formed in the bone marrow. Bone marrow is housed in the cavity of certain bones in the body.

5. **Mineral storage**. Minerals such as calcium and phosphorus are stored in bones.

Axial and Appendicular Skeletons

The skeletal system comprises 206 bones. The two main divisions of the human skeletal system are the axial skeleton and the appendicular skeleton.

The **axial skeleton** has 80 bones, including the skull, rib cage, and spinal column:

- ◆ Skull: 28 bones
- ◆ Hyoid bone: 1 bone
- ◆ Sternum and ribs: 25 bones
- ◆ Spinal column: 26 bones (including sacrum and coccyx)

Knowledge of the spinal column (aka the vertebral column) is important because fitness professionals will deal with spinal alignment/posture, stability, and movement. Although fitness professionals do not deal with pain management, they often field questions about back issues, so it is important to be informed on the subject.

The bones of the spinal column are divided into five major categories (**Figure 4.1**). From the top down they are as follows:

- ◆ Cervical vertebrae (C1–C7)
- ◆ Thoracic vertebrae (T1–T12)
- ◆ Lumbar vertebrae (L1–L5)
- ◆ Sacrum
- ◆ Coccyx

The first seven vertebrae, starting from the top of the column, are known as the *cervical vertebrae* or the *cervical spine*. Vertebrae are named based on their region ("C" for *cervical*) and are numbered from the top down, so they are named C1–C7. The top two vertebrae have special names. C1 is known as the *atlas* because it supports the whole weight of the head, just as the Greek mythological character Atlas supported the weight of the world. C2 is known as the *axis* because the atlas (C1) rotates around it. Another notable cervical vertebra is C7 because its large spinous process protrudes posteriorly prominently. C7 can be easily seen and felt at the base of the cervical region, particularly when the head drops down toward the chest. Overall, the cervical vertebrae are small, mobile spinal bones that form a flexible framework and provide support and motion for the head.

The next 12 vertebrae are known as the *thoracic spine* (T1–T12), *T-spine*, or *thoracic vertebrae*. They are larger than the cervical vertebrae and increase in size from the top down. Each

Axial skeleton

Portion of the skeletal system that consists of the bones of the skull, rib cage, and vertebral column.

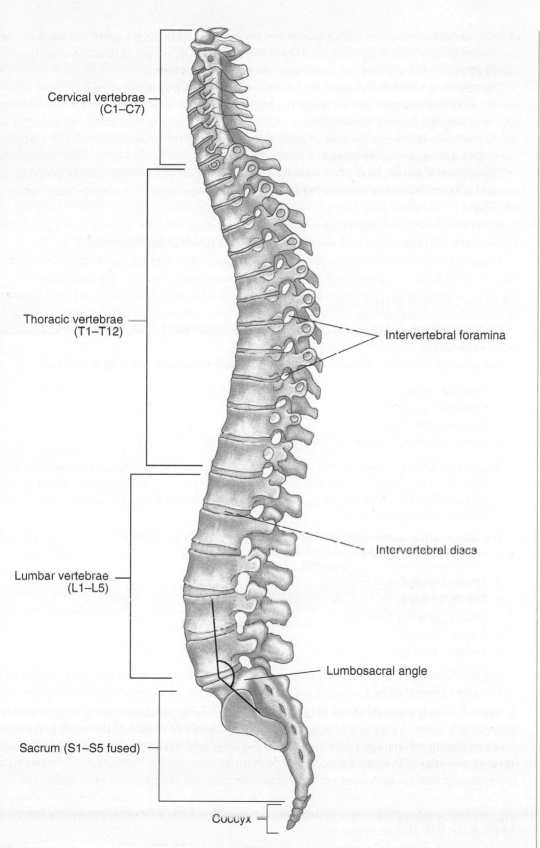

Cervical vertebrae
(C1–C7)

Thoracic vertebrae
(T1–T12)

Intervertebral foramina

Intervertebral discs

Lumbar vertebrae
(L1–L5)

Lumbosacral angle

Sacrum (S1–S5 fused)

Coccyx

FIGURE 4.1 Bones of the spinal column.

thoracic vertebra articulates with a pair of ribs on each side. Clients are generally weak in the surrounding musculature and lack mobility in this area. This is, in part, due to the chair-bound nature of today's society and the subsequent postural implications.

The adjoining series of five large vertebrae are known as the *lumbar spine* or *lumbar vertebrae* (L1–L5). They support the weight of the body and are the attachment site for many of the back muscles. The lumbar spine is often a location of pain for many individuals because this is where they carry the most amount of body weight, making the region subject to the largest forces and stresses along the spine.

The sacrum is a triangular bone located just inferior (below) the fifth lumbar vertebra. It consists of four to five sacral bones until about 25 years of age, when these bones fuse together into one.

At the bottom of the spinal column is the coccyx, often referred to as the tailbone. It is composed of three to five bones and, like the sacrum, fuses together in adulthood.

Between the bodies of each vertebra are intervertebral discs that are made up of fibrous cartilage and are designed to absorb shock and help increase spinal mobility. The specialized vertebral column allows humans to stand upright and maintain balance. It also supports the head and arms; provides attachment sites for muscles, ribs, and some organs; and protects the spinal cord.

The **appendicular skeleton** is composed of 126 bones and is divided into the upper and lower extremities.

The upper extremity is made up of 64 bones, including the shoulder girdle:

- Clavicle: 2 bones
- Scapula: 2 bones
- Humerus: 2 bones
- Radius: 2 bones
- Ulna: 2 bones
- Carpals: 16 bones
- Metacarpals: 10 bones
- Phalanges: 28 bones

The lower extremity is made up of 62 bones, including the pelvic girdle:

- Innominate (os coxa, hemi-pelvis): 2 bones
- Femur: 2 bones
- Patella: 2 bones
- Tibia: 2 bones
- Fibula: 2 bones
- Tarsals: 14 bones
- Metatarsals: 10 bones
- Phalanges: 28 bones

Without strong support from a stable axial skeleton, the appendages cannot produce force well. Or, as it is often said in the rehabilitative world, "one can't have distal mobility without proximal stability." The body relies on a well-supported axial skeleton as the base from which distal movements can occur.

Types of Bones

The bones of the skeletal system are categorized into five major categories based primarily on their shape.

Appendicular skeleton

Portion of the skeleton that includes the bones that connect to the spinal column including the upper extremities and lower extremities.

Long Bones

Long bones have a cylindrical body called a shaft, are longer than they are wide, and enlarge and widen at each end. Long bones can vary in size. In fact some long bones can be quite short. The distal phalanges (fingertip) is only about 21 mm (0.8 inches) in the average adult (Alexander & Viktor, 2010), yet it is categorized as a long bone, as is the femur bone of the thigh.

Long bones are made up of compact bone tissue and spongy bone tissue. This enables them to tolerate considerable leverage forces, support a large amount of weight, and absorb shock. Long bones oftentimes have a slight curve, both for efficiency and for better force distribution.

The following are the long bones of the upper body (**Figure 4.2**):

◆ Clavicle
◆ Humerus
◆ Radius
◆ Ulna
◆ Metacarpals
◆ Phalanges

The following are the long bones of the lower body (**Figure 4.3**):

◆ Femur
◆ Tibia
◆ Fibula
◆ Metatarsals
◆ Phalanges

Short Bones

Short bones are cube- or box-shaped bones that are nearly as wide as they are long (**Figure 4.4**). They are made up of mostly spongy bone tissue to maximize shock absorption.

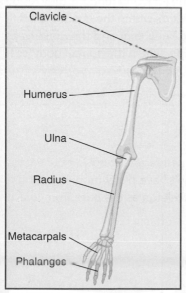

FIGURE 4.2 Long bones of the upper body.

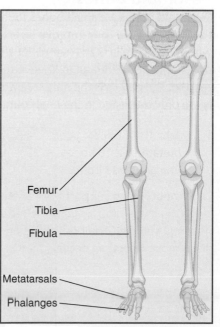

FIGURE 4.3 Long bones of the lower body.

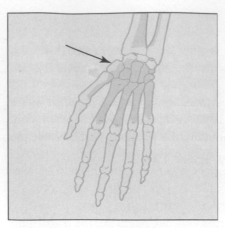

FIGURE 4.4   Short bones.

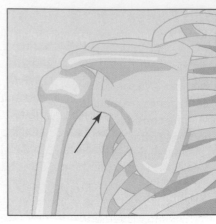

FIGURE 4.5   Flat bones.

Flat Bones

Flat bones are thin bones made up of two layers of compact bone tissue surrounding a layer of spongy bone tissue (**Figure 4.5**; Hamill & Knutzen, 2003; Tortora, 2001). These bones are involved in protection of internal structures and also provide broad attachment sites for muscles (Hamill & Knutzen, 2003). The flat bones include the sternum, scapulae, ribs, ilium, and cranial bones (Hamill & Knutzen, 2003; Luttgens & Hamilton, 2007; Tortora, 2001).

Irregular Bones

Irregular bones are bones of unique shape and function that do not fit the characteristics of the other categories (**Figure 4.6**). These include the vertebrae, pelvic bones, and certain facial bones (Hamill & Knutzen, 2003; Luttgens & Hamilton, 2007; Tortora, 2001).

Sesamoid Bones

Sesamoid bones are small bones found or developed within tendons close to the joint and in the joint capsule. They improve leverage and help to protect the joint and tendons they reside within. The patella is an example of a sesamoid bone that develops within the quadriceps tendon to provide leverage in knee extension and to protect the knee joint and the quadriceps tendon. The patella is the only sesamoid bone that is regularly present in the human body, so it is the only one listed in the final count of the skeletal system's 206 bones.

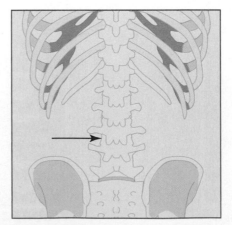

FIGURE 4.6   Irregular bones.

MEMORY TIPS

The sesamoid bones are named as such because they resemble sesame seeds in shape.

Joints

Joints are formed where one bone articulates with another bone (Tortora, 2001). They can be categorized by both their structure and their function (i.e. the way they move) (Norkin & Levangie, 2000; Tortora, 2001; Watkins, 1999).

Joint motion is referred to as **arthrokinematics**. The three major motions are roll, slide, and spin (Clark, 2001; Norkin & Levangie, 2000; Watkins, 1999). Note that motion rarely occurs, if ever, as an isolated, true motion. Variations and combinations of these joint motions take place during functional movement (Watkins, 1999).

In a rolling movement, one joint rolls across the surface of another, much like the tire of a bicycle rolls on the street (**Figure 4.7**). An example of a rolling movement in the body is the femoral condyles moving (rolling) over the tibial condyles during a squat.

In a sliding movement, one joint's surface slides across another, much like the tire of a bicycle skidding across the street (**Figure 4.8**). An example of slide in the human body is the tibial condyles moving (sliding) across the femoral condyles during a knee extension.

In a spinning movement, one joint surface rotates on another much like twisting the lid off of a jar (**Figure 4.9**). An example of a spin movement in the human body is the head of the radius (a bone of the forearm) rotating on the end of the humerus during pronation and supination of the forearm.

Classification of Joints

Synovial joints are the most common joints associated with human movement. They comprise approximately 80% of all the joints in the body and have the greatest capacity for motion (Hamill & Knutzen, 2003; Norkin & Levangie, 2000; Tortora, 2001; Watkins, 1999). Synovial joints have a synovial capsule (collagenous structure) of hyaline cartilage that pads the ends of the articulating bones. This design gives synovial joints their increased mobility (Norkin & Levangie, 2000). Synovial joints also have another unique quality in that they produce synovial fluid. Synovial fluid resembles egg whites and works much like engine oil. It is secreted within the joint capsule from the synovial membrane and is essential for lubricating the joint surfaces to reduce excessive wear and to nourish the cartilage cells that line the joint (Hammill & Knutzen, 2003; Norkin & Levangie, 2000; Tortora, 2001; Watkins, 1999).

Arthrokinematics
The motions of the joints in the body.

Synovial joints
Joints that are held together by a joint capsule and ligaments; type of joint most associated with movement in the body.

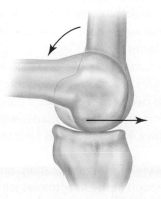

FIGURE 4.7 Rolling joint.

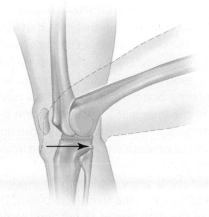

FIGURE 4.8 Sliding joint.

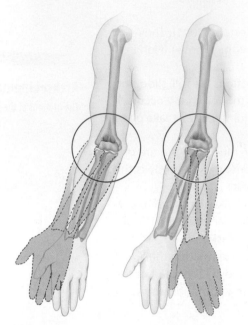

FIGURE 4.9 Spinning joint.

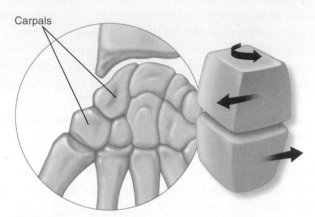

FIGURE 4.10 Gliding joint.

The body has several types of synovial joints. They include gliding (plane), condyloid (condylar or ellipsoidal), hinge, saddle, pivot, and ball-and-socket joints (Hammill & Knutzen, 2003; Tortora, 2001; Watkins, 1999). A gliding (plane) joint is a nonaxial joint that has the simplest movement of all joints (Hammill & Knutzen, 2003; Tortora, 2001). It moves either back and forth or side to side. Examples include the joint between the navicular bone and the second and third cuneiform bones in the foot or the carpals of the hand and in the facet (spine) joints (Figure 4.10; Hammill & Knutzen, 2003; Tortora, 2001; Watkins, 1999).

Condyloid (condylar or ellipsoidal) joints are termed so because the condyle of one bone fits into the elliptical cavity of another bone to form the joint (Tortora, 2001). Movement predominantly occurs in one plane (flexion and extension in the sagittal plane), with minimal movement in the others (rotation in the transverse plane; adduction and abduction in the frontal plane). Examples of condyloid joints are seen in the wrist between the radius and carpals and in the joints of the fingers (metacarpophalangeal) (Figure 4.11; Hammill & Knutzen, 2003).

A hinge joint is a uniaxial joint that allows movement predominantly in only one plane of motion, the sagittal plane. Joints such as the elbow, interphalangeal (toe), and ankle are considered hinge joints (Figure 4.12; Hammill & Knutzen, 2003; Tortora, 2001).

The saddle joint is named after its appearance. One bone looks like a saddle with the articulating bone straddling it like a rider. This joint is only found in the carpometacarpal joint in the thumb. It allows movement predominantly in two planes of motion (flexion and extension in the sagittal plane; adduction and abduction in the frontal plane) with some rotation to produce circumduction (circular motion) (Figure 4.13; Hammill & Knutzen, 2003; Tortora, 2001).

Pivot joints allow movement in predominantly one plane of motion (rotation, pronation, and supination in the transverse plane). These joints are found in the atlantoaxial joint at the base of the skull (top of spine) and the proximal radioulnar joint at the elbow (Figure 4.14; Hammill & Knutzen, 2003; Tortora, 2001).

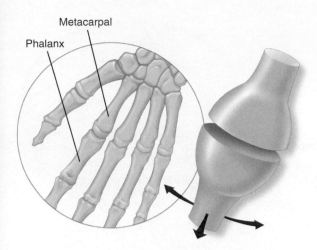

FIGURE 4.11 Condyloid joint.

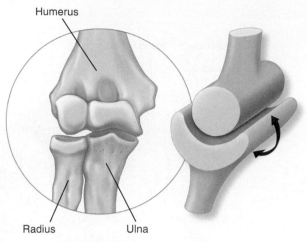

FIGURE 4.12 Hinge joint.

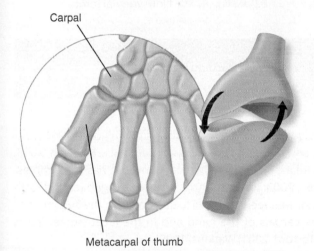

FIGURE 4.13 Saddle joint.

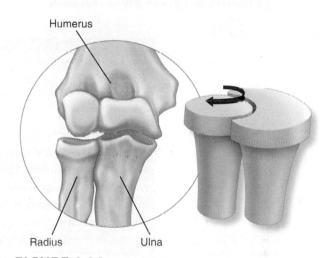

FIGURE 4.14 Pivot joint.

Ball-and-socket joints are the most mobile of the joints. They allow movement in all three planes. Examples of these joints are the shoulder and hip (**Figure 4.15**; Hammill & Knutzen, 2003; Tortora, 2001).

Nonsynovial joints are named as such because they have no joint cavity, fibrous connective tissue, or cartilage in the uniting structure. These joints exhibit little to no movement. Examples of this joint type are seen in the sutures of the skull, the distal joint of the tibia and fibula, and the symphysis pubis (pubic bones) (**Figure 4.16**; Norkin & Levangie, 2000; Tortora, 2001).

See **Table 4.3** for a full description of the characteristics of these types of joints and examples of each.

Nonsynovial joints
Joints that do not have a joint cavity, connective tissue, or cartilage.

Function of Joints

Joints serve numerous functional requirements of the musculoskeletal system; most importantly, joints allow for motion, and thus movement (Luttgens & Hamilton, 2007; Norkin & Levangie, 2000). Joints also provide stability, allowing for a desired movement to take place without unwanted movement.

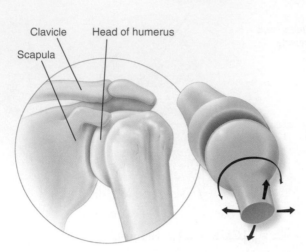

Clavicle   Head of humerus

Scapula

FIGURE 4.15 Ball-and-socket joint.

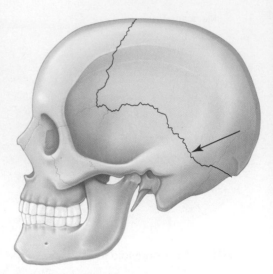

FIGURE 4.16 Nonsynovial joint.

TABLE 4.3	Types of Joints	
Joint	**Characteristic**	**Example**
Nonsynovial	No joint cavity and fibrous connective tissue; little or no movement	Sutures of the skull
Synovial	Produces synovial fluid, has a joint cavity and fibrous connective tissue	Knee
Gliding	No axis of rotation; moves by sliding side-to-side or back and forth	Carpals of the hand
Condyloid	Formed by the fitting of condyles of one bone into elliptical cavities of another; moves predominantly in one plane	Knee
Hinge	Uniaxial; moves predominantly in one plane of motion (sagittal)	Elbow
Saddle	One bone fits like a saddle on another bone; moves predominantly in two planes (sagittal, joint of thumb frontal)	Only: carpometacarpal
Pivot	Only one axis; moves predominantly in one plane of motion (transverse)	Radioulnar
Ball-and-socket	Most mobile of joints; moves in all three planes of motion	Shoulder

Types of Synovial

All joints in the human body are linked together, which implies that movement of one joint directly affects the motion of others (Clark, 2001; Norkin & Levangie, 2000). This is an essential concept for fitness professionals to understand because it creates an awareness of how the body functionally operates and is the premise behind kinetic chain movement (Clark, 2001; Norkin & Levangie, 2000).

The concept of kinetic chain movement is easy to demonstrate. First, start by standing with both feet firmly on the ground and then roll your feet inward and outward. Notice what your knees and hips are doing. Next, keep your feet stationary and rotate your hips, notice what your knees and feet are doing. Moving one of these joints will inevitably move the others. If you understand this concept, then you understand what kinetic chain movement is. It should also be easy to see that if one joint is not working properly it will affect other joints (Clark, 2001).

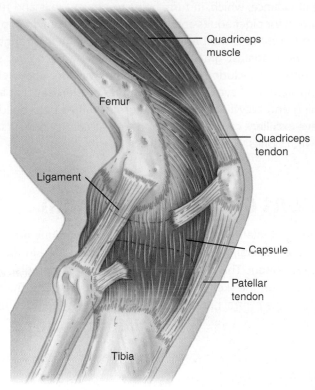

Quadriceps muscle

Femur

Quadriceps tendon

Ligament

Capsule

Patellar tendon

Tibia

FIGURE 4.17 Ligament.

Joint Connective Tissue

Ligaments are fibrous connective tissues that connect bone to bone and provide static and dynamic stability as well as input to the nervous system (proprioception) (**Figure 4.17**); (Alter, 1996; Gross, Fetto, & Rosen, 1996). Ligaments are primarily made up of a protein called collagen and varying amounts of a second protein called elastin. Collagen fibers are situated in a more parallel fashion to the forces that are typically placed on the ligament. Thus, they provide the ligament with the ability to withstand tension (tensile strength).

Elastin gives a ligament some flexibility or elastic recoil to withstand the bending and twisting it may have to endure. Not all ligaments will have the same amount of elastin; for example, the anterior cruciate ligament of the knee contains very little elastin and is predominantly composed of collagen. Because of this, it is much better suited for resisting strong forces and makes a good stabilizing structure of the knee (Alter, 1996; Gross et al., 1996). Finally, it is important to note that ligaments are characterized by having poor vascularity (or blood supply), meaning that ligaments do not heal or repair very well and may be slower to adapt to stresses placed on the body, such as stress caused by exercise (Alter, 1996; Gross et al., 1996; Nordin, Lorenz, & Campello, 2001; Solomonow et al., 1987).

Exercise and Its Effect on Bone Mass

Like muscle, bone is living tissue that responds to exercise by becoming stronger. Individuals who exercise regularly generally achieve greater peak bone mass (maximal bone density and strength) than those who do not. Exercise is crucial in maintaining muscle strength,

TRAINER TIPS -◻—◻-

Ligaments and tendons have a low blood supply; this is one reason why it can take up to 6 weeks for recovery from an injury.

coordination, and balance, which, in turn, helps to prevent falls and related fractures. This is especially important for older adults and people who have been diagnosed with osteoporosis.

Weight-bearing exercise is the best kind of exercise to help strengthen bones because it forces bones to work against gravity, and thus react by becoming stronger. Examples of weight-bearing exercises include resistance training, walking, bodyweight squats, push-ups, jogging, climbing stairs, and even dancing. Examples of exercises that are not weight-bearing include swimming and bicycling. Although these activities help build and maintain strong muscles and have excellent cardiovascular and weight-control benefits, they are not the best way to exercise your bones (National Institutes of Health, 2015).

Interactions of the Kinetic Chain

The kinetic chain, or Human Movement System, uses the unique attributes of three very different systems—the skeletal, muscular, and nervous systems—in an intricately interwoven way to produce movement. The nervous system acts on the muscular system to contract. The muscular system acts on the skeletal system to create movement. The skeletal system acts as a protective case for the central nervous system. The three systems complement, support, and protect each other.

Integrated Muscular Systems

As previously discussed, functional movements do not happen in isolation. A leg extension machine exercise is used for isolated resistance for the quadriceps. A movement in daily living that requires this isolated movement is rare, if it even exists. This indicates the need for multiple muscles to work in tandem to allow multiple joints to move together to function. The complexities of these movements require stabilization of some parts of the Human Movement System and synchronized activation from the nervous system to create and refine global movement patterns.

This section focuses on the interactions of the body's stabilization and movement systems. The movement system will be broken down into subsystems to further show how muscles work in groups, pairs, and force-couples to create patterns of movement in the human body. The origin, insertion, isolated function, isometric function, and integrated function of each muscle can found in the appendix.

Local Muscular (Stabilization) System

The local muscular system is also called the **stabilization system** (**Figure 4.18**). It is composed of muscles whose primary function is to provide joint support and stabilization (Bergmark, 1989; Crisco & Panjabi, 1991; Mooney, 1997; Panjabi, 1992; Richardson, Jull, Hodges, & Hides, 1999). These muscles are present throughout the spine to provide support for the vertebrae during functional movement. They stabilize the spine to allow peripheral movement so that there is a place to produce force from. In other words, there cannot be distal mobility without proximal stability. An individual cannot move one's arms or legs well unless supported by a stable core. The following are the principle core stabilization muscles (Bergmark, 1989; Crisco & Panjabi, 1991; Richardson et al., 1999; Schmidt & Lee, 1999):

- ◆ Transverse abdominus
- ◆ Multifidus

Stabilization system

The muscles whose primary function is to provide joint support and stabilization; also known as the *local muscular system*.

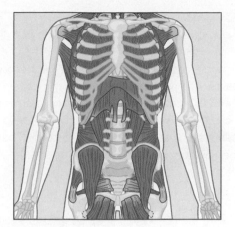

FIGURE 4.18 Local muscular system.

- Internal oblique
- Diaphragm
- Pelvic floor muscles

Local muscles are not limited to the spine. A number of muscles in the appendicular skeleton bear the primary responsibility of joint stability rather than movement.

In some cases particular fibers of a large movement system muscle are positioned in a way to produce stabilization forces. An example is the vastus medialis muscle of the quadriceps group that has a unique section of oblique fibers that are key stabilizers of the kneecap. This section of muscle is often called the vastus medialis oblique (VMO).

Global Muscular (Movement) System

The **global muscular system** is designed for larger muscles to work synergistically in larger movement patterns, such as a combination squat to row exercise. These movements involve a combination of axial and appendicular skeletal coordination that equalizes external loads and transfers and absorbs forces from the upper and lower extremities to the LPHC. The global muscular system has four subsystems: deep longitudinal, lateral, anterior oblique, and posterior oblique. Once the fitness professional knows these subsystems and how they work together synergistically to produce, reduce, and stabilize forces within the Human Movement System, exercise programming and movement-based training can be designed with emphasis on subsystems rather than just body parts.

A loss in function in one of the subsystems can affect the other subsystems. For instance, if the right gluteus medius, a segment of the lateral subsystem, experiences a loss of strength, there will likely be adduction and internal rotation of the hips, resulting in a knock-kneed position. This will shorten the adductors. These muscles are not only part of the lateral subsystem, but are also part of the anterior oblique subsystem. The knock-kneed position will lengthen the gluteus maximus, which will directly affect the posterior oblique subsystem. A common muscle that will become overactive when the gluteus maximus is not functioning correctly is the biceps femoris, which is a member of the deep longitudinal subsystem. One muscle can cause a domino effect in the Human Movement System, impacting all of the subsystems.

Deep Longitudinal Subsystem

The **deep longitudinal subsystem (DLS)** includes the peroneus longus, anterior tibialis, long head of the biceps femoris, sacrotuberous ligament, thoracolumbar fascia, and erector spinae

Global muscular system

System composed of four subsystems that are designed for larger muscles to work synergistically in larger movement patterns, such as a combination squat to row exercise.

Deep longitudinal subsystem (DLS)

Subsystem of the global movement system that includes the peroneus longus, anterior tibialis, long head of the biceps femoris, sacrotuberous ligament, thoracolumbar fascia, and erector spinae. These muscles work together to create a contracting tension to absorb and control ground reaction forces during gait.

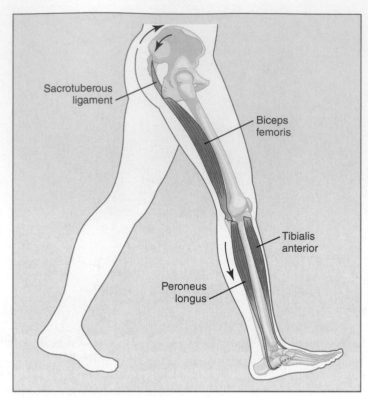

FIGURE 4.19 Deep longitudinal subsystem.

(**Figure 4.19**). Working together synergistically these muscles create a contracting tension to absorb and control ground reaction forces during gait.

Posterior Oblique Subsystem

The **posterior oblique subsystem (POS)** is made up of the latissimus dorsi and the contralateral gluteus maximus, with the thoracolumbar fascia creating a fascial bridge for the cross-body connection. **Figure 4.20** shows how these two muscles create a nearly straight line with each other across the sacroiliac joint. When they both contract they produce a pulling force across the thoracolumbar fascia and stabilization force at the sacroiliac joint (force closure). This system works concurrently with the DLS during gait.

Anterior Oblique Subsystem

The **anterior oblique subsystem (AOS)** is similar to the POS in that it also functions in the transverse plane, but it is on the anterior side of the body. The muscles include the internal and external obliques, the adductor complex, and the hip external rotators (**Figure 4.21**). The external obliques and contralateral adductors are the most common visualization of this subsystem because of the "X" pattern made across the front of the body, similar to the cross-body pattern the POS makes on the posterior. The synergistic coupling of the AOS creates stability from the trunk, through the pelvic floor, and to the hips. It contributes to rotational movements, leg swing, and stabilization (Basmajian, 1985; Inman, Ralston, & Todd, 1981; Innes, 1999). The AOS and POS work together in enabling rotational force production in the transverse plane.

Posterior oblique subsystem (POS)

Subsystem of the global movement system composed of the latissimus dorsi and the contralateral gluteus maximus, with the thoracolumbar fascia creating a fascial bridge for the cross body connection. These muscles create a nearly straight line with each other across the sacroiliac joint, and when they both contract they produce a pulling force across the thoracolumbar fascia and stabilization force at the sacroiliac joint (force closure). This system works concurrently with the DLS during gait.

Anterior oblique subsystem (AOS)

Subsystem of the global movement system composed of the internal and external obliques, the adductor complex, and the hip external rotators. The synergistic coupling of the AOS creates stability from the trunk, through the pelvic floor, and to the hips. It contributes to rotational movements, leg swing, and stabilization. The AOS and POS work together in enabling rotational force production in the transverse plane.

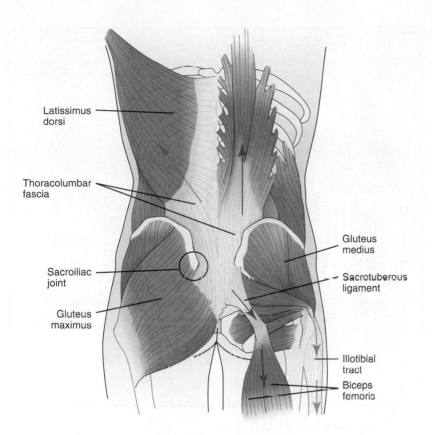

Latissimus dorsi

Thoracolumbar fascia

Sacroiliac joint

Gluteus maximus

Gluteus medius

Sacrotuberous ligament

Iliotibial tract

Biceps femoris

FIGURE 4.20 Posterior oblique subsystem.

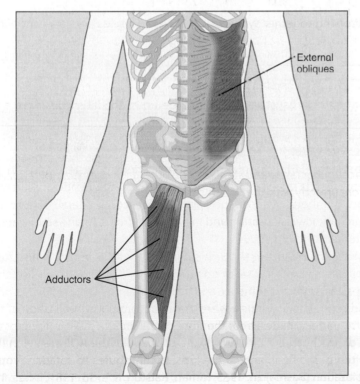

External obliques

Adductors

FIGURE 4.21 Anterior oblique subsystem.

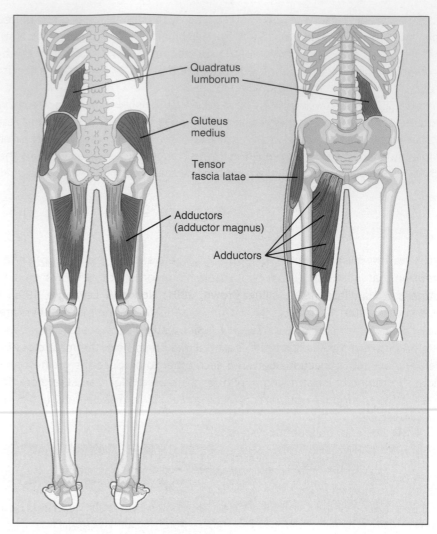

FIGURE 4.22 Lateral subsystem.

Lateral Subsystem

Lateral subsystem (LS)

Composed of the gluteus medius, tensor fascia, latae, adductor complex, and quadratus lumborum, all of which participate in frontal plane and pelvofemoral stability.

The **lateral subsystem (LS)**, or frontal plane stabilization subsystem, is made up of the gluteus medius, tensor fascia latae (TFL), the adductors on the same side (ipsilateral) of the body, and the quadratus lumborum (QL) on the opposite side (contralateral) (**Figure 4.22**). Together these muscles are tasked with creating and maintaining frontal plane stabilization of the LPHC movement patterns.

Reciprocal Inhibition

Reciprocal inhibition

The simultaneous contraction of one muscle and the relaxation of its antagonist to allow movement to take place.

The word *reciprocal* means "inverse" or "opposite." *Inhibition* means "inhibiting" or "restricting." Recall from the discussion of biomechanics that **reciprocal inhibition** is when the muscles on one side of a joint relax to allow the muscle on the other side to contract appropriately. Sometimes a muscle can become overactive, stealing neural drive, strength, and range of motion from the working muscle.

Consider how overactive hip flexors could reciprocally inhibit the ability of the gluteus maximus to produce hip extension. When a tight muscle, the hip flexor in this scenario, is stretched too far, or too quickly, a neural activation of the stretched muscle is facilitated. If this happens to the hip flexors while a person is running, jumping, or even squatting, the hyperfacilitation of the hip flexors impacts their ability to do their job.

Another example where this can easily be seen is with an active hamstring stretch. With the isolated knee-extension machine, the terminal range of motion is completed against resistance. However, many people when placed into an active 90/90 hamstring stretch cannot extend their knee completely. There is no weight providing the resistance to knee extension, only the neural drive of the stretching hamstring reciprocally inhibiting the opposing muscle—the quadriceps.

Length–Tension Relationship

The **length–tension relationship (LTR)** (**Figure 4.23**) refers to the resting length of a muscle and the tension that muscle can produce at that resting length (Fox, 1996; Hamill & Knutzen, 1995; Luttgens & Hamilton, 1997; Milner-Brown, 2001; Norkin & Levangie, 1992; Vander, Sherman, & Luciano, 2001; Watkins, 1999). The sarcomeres within the muscle fibers are where the actin and myosin filaments slide across each other, leading to muscular contraction. When these actin and myosin myofilaments are ideally aligned they have the most cross-bridging, and therefore the most connections between each other to produce the greatest amount of contraction. Shortening or lengthening minimizes the cross-bridges, and therefore decreases the muscle's ability to produce optimal contractile forces. Sarcomeres are discussed in greater detail in the appendix.

Length–tension relationship (LTR)

The resting length of a muscle and the tension the muscle can produce at that resting length.

CHECK IT OUT

Imagine a boxer trying to throw a powerful punch into a heavy bag, but he is standing too close or too far away to land it with optimal force. Visualize a baseball player who is "choking" up too far on the bat, which slows down his ability to swing optimally. Think about a basketball player jumping up to get a rebound by going into a deep squat prior to the jump, or a shallow bend of the knees and hips, barely allowing the player to leave the floor in either scenario. For each of these examples there is an optimal position from which the athlete can produce the greatest amount of force.

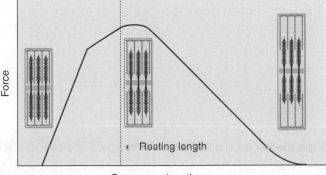

FIGURE 4.23 Length–tension relationship.

CHECK IT OUT

1. Make a fist as hard and tight as possible. Hold for 5 seconds. Then relax.
2. Flex your wrist, and maintain wrist flexion while trying to make a fist as tight as possible for 5 seconds. Is your fist as strong?
3. Extend your wrist, and try making a strong/tight fist while maintaining wrist extension. Is your fist as strong as it was in neutral position?
4. Try the same thing with radial and ulnar deviation. Is your fist weak?
5. If strength is affected that much with smaller muscles at the most distal portion of the upper extremity, consider the possible effects on strength more proximal joint musculature may experience with altered reciprocal inhibition.

There is a relationship between the length of a muscle and the tension that muscle can produce:

♦ If a muscle is too short, it is weakened.
♦ If a muscle is too long, it is weakened.
♦ A muscle at optimal length can produce optimal strength.

Fitness professionals should assess each client's static, transitional, and dynamic posture and positioning. Deviation from ideal alignment can indicate altered length–tension relationships.

Force-Couple Relationships

Force-couple relationship
Muscle groups moving together to produce movement around a joint.

Muscles often work together in synergist pairings. One type of synergistic pairing is a force couple. A **force-couple relationship** is when synergists work together to create a joint action by pulling from different vectors, thus creating divergent tension. Simply put, force couples are muscles moving together to produce movement around a joint.

An example of a force-couple relationship is the gluteus maximus and hamstrings muscle goups pulling down on the posterior of the pelvis, and the rectus abdominus pulling up on the anterior pelvis, thus developing forces from different angles to create a posterior pelvic tilt. This is divergent tension because it pulls from different directions to create the same joint action. An anterior pelvic tilt is the force-coupling of the iliopsoas as it pulls down on the anterior portion of the pelvis while the erectors pull up on the posterior portion of the pelvis.

Upward rotation of the scapula is a force-coupling of the upper traps pulling up (superior) on the lateral border of the spine of the scapula, the lower traps pulling down (inferior) on the medial border of the spine of the scapula, and the serratus anterior pulling the medial border toward the chest (**Figure 4.24**). These three angles of pull create upward rotation of the scapula.

Creation of Efficient Movement (Motor Behavior)

Motor output
Response to stimuli that activates movement in organs or muscles.

The creation of efficient movement is made possible by the repetition of sensory inputs and the refinement of **motor outputs**. Fitness professionals should be able to recognize what an

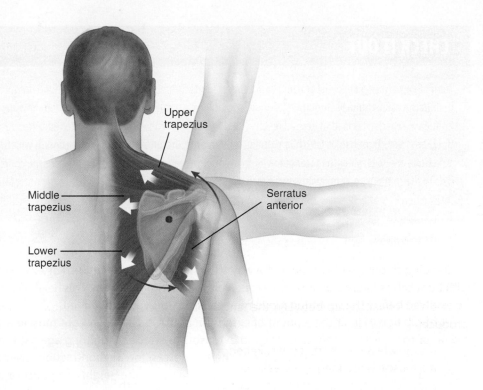

FIGURE 4.24 Force-couple relationship.

exercise should look like and provide cues necessary to elicit a change in a client's form. The change in form is a change in motor recruitment patterns to allow for safer, more efficient, and more effective motor behavior.

Motor behavior is the response of the Human Movement System to internal and external environmental stimuli. The study of motor behavior examines the manner by which the nervous, muscular, and skeletal systems interact to produce skilled movement, using sensory information from internal and external environments. Motor behavior is the collective study of three concepts introduced earlier in this chapter:

◆ Motor control
◆ Motor learning
◆ Motor development

Motor control is the study of posture and movements with the involved structures and mechanisms used by the CNS to assimilate and integrate sensory information with previous experiences. Motor control is concerned with which CNS structures are involved with motor behavior to produce movement. *Motor learning* is the utilization of processes through practice and experience, leading to a relatively permanent change in one's capacity to produce skilled movements (Schmidt & Wrisberg, 2000). Finally, *motor development* is defined as the change in motor behavior over time throughout the lifespan (Gabbard, 2008).

Motor behavior
Motor response to internal and external environmental stimuli.

Flexibility in Human Movement

Optimal functioning of the Human Movement System is largely reliant on flexibility. When flexibility is limited, faulty movement patterns arise and are reinforced while working out. It can be

CHECK IT OUT

Think about a young child just starting to eat finger foods. There is usually much more food on the floor than in the child's mouth! Through repetition, the child can recall that some positions and movements from past experiences lead to desired results (food in mouth), whereas others lead to undesired results (food on floor). This enables the child to make refinements. Motor control is concerned with which CNS structures are involved with motor behavior to produce movement. After enough practice the child begins to learn desired and undesired outcomes of eating finger foods and can modulate the outcomes to satisfaction.

challenging to get clients to move the way they should during exercise. For example, a client with tight calves might lean forward excessively in squatting motions. This flexibility issue must be resolved before the squatting movement can be improved and refined.

Tight hip flexors limit the amount of extension at the hip. When a tight muscle is stretched too far or too quickly it contracts. The hip extensors are not only fighting against the external weight, but also the internal resistance of the hip flexors, forcing contraction. Overactive hip flexors can decrease the amount of weight lifted in a squat, the height of a jump, or the speed of a sprint.

Kinetic Chain Dysfunction

The **kinetic chain** is the combination and interrelation of the actions of the nervous, muscular, and skeletal systems to create movement. The body stacks bone on top of bone and joint on top of joint to create a chain that links structure, movement, and function together to perform daily activities. As some links in the chain move, others must stabilize and support the other parts of the system. If a particular component of the kinetic chain becomes dysfunctional it can result in a chain reaction that may cause dysfunction in other parts of the Human Movement System. For example, if a client walks with his or her feet externally rotated, links all of the way up the kinetic chain will be impacted. Sometimes the area of visible dysfunction presents symptoms of pain in other areas higher up the chain.

Posture is the alignment of all parts of the kinetic chain with the prevailing purpose of countering the constant forces placed on the body by maintaining structural efficiency. Structural efficiency is the structural alignment of each segment—myofascial, neuromuscular, and articular components—of the Human Movement System that allows the body to be aligned and balanced in relation to its center of gravity. **Biotensegrity**, a term coined by Stevin Levin, MD, is a concept that has been introduced to describe how the body maintains its structural integrity (Levin, 1981). Bones are discontinuous compression-resistant beams housed with tension-generating elements such as muscles, tendons, and ligaments; fascia is both a compression and tension element (Swanson, 2013). The structural efficiency of the musculoskeletal system relies on the compression-resistant, tension-generating biotensegrity system (Swanson, 2013).

The importance of the structural integrity and efficiency of the human body is seen when the body is viewed as a whole with interconnected components that rely on optimal **range of motion (ROM)** and means of support. Movement outside optimal ROM and inefficient

Kinetic chain

The combination and interrelation of the actions of the nervous, muscular, and skeletal systems to create movement.

Posture

Position and bearing of the body for alignment and function of the kinetic chain.

Biotensegrity

The examination of how biological structural integrity may occur.

Range of motion (ROM)

The range through which a joint may be freely moved with no resistance or pain.

support can create a chain reaction throughout the Human Movement System with the potential for soft tissue stress, altered sensory input, and decreased motor recruitment. These can initiate stresses and lead to the cumulative injury cycle. The **cumulative injury cycle** is a cycle whereby an injury will induce inflammation, muscle spasm, adhesions, altered neuromuscular control, and muscle imbalance. Muscle imbalance can lead to more inflammation, and the cycle repeats, thus limiting the ability of the neuromuscular system to work efficiently.

Neuromuscular efficiency is the ability of the neuromuscular system to enable all muscles (agonists, antagonists, synergists, and stabilizers) to work synergistically to produce, reduce, and dynamically stabilize the entire kinetic chain. Optimum neuromuscular and structural efficiency leads to optimum length–tension relationships, force-couple relationships, and arthrokinematics. If one component is altered, all components are altered, therefore leading to altered sensorimotor integration, neuromuscular inefficiency, and tissue fatigue and breakdown.

Posture is the visual representation of neuromuscular efficiency or inefficiency. If the nervous system is not operating the way it should, movement is often impacted. If the muscular system is not functioning the way it should, movement is often impacted. If the arthrokinematics of the skeletal system are not functioning properly, movement is impacted. The fitness professional looks at posture, static and dynamic, to see which alignment patterns are altered within the Human Movement System and then implements a corrective strategy to amend the dysfunction. Note that the fitness professional is trying to address *patterns*, not pain. Often, if the movement patterns are addressed, pain may be as well. However, clients with pain management issues should be referred to a licensed practitioner.

Contributors of Kinetic Chain Dysfunction

The three major causes of kinetic chain dysfunction, once injury is removed from the equation, are repetitive movement, suboptimal positioning, and/or frequent lack of movement. All of these can lead to poor posture and potentially repetitive stress injuries. Repetitive movements can lead to pattern overload.

Pattern Overload

Pattern overload is a **repetitive stress injury (RSI)** that happens as a result of repetitious movement patterns that take place in an athletic or conditioning environment. For example, golf training is a dynamic rotational movement pattern that can lead to pattern overload. There tends to be a large range of age and ability among golf participants, and pattern overload can occur early in training. Pattern overload can happen from many small repetitive patterns or from a few impactful movements. Golfer's elbow (medial epicondylitis) is inflammation of the soft tissues at the inside of the elbow because of the stress put on the inside elbow of the dominant (trailing) forearm. It can occur on some individuals' first trip to the driving range, or it can occur after years of playing. The overload may occur earlier for some, whereas others may never be affected. It is best for fitness professionals to develop an understanding of optimal movement, so if/when an altered pattern begins to manifest the fitness professional can cue the client into more optimum positioning.

Culture and Lifestyle

Repetitive motion stresses are by no means limited to the world of sport. Culture plays a role in postural and kinetic chain dysfunction. The daily lives of millions of people include high heels, overloaded backpacks, and asymmetrical loading of the shoulders with bags, purses, and

Cumulative injury cycle

A cycle whereby an injury will induce inflammation, muscle spasm, adhesions, altered neuromuscular control, and muscle imbalances. Muscle imbalance can lead to more inflammation, and the cycle repeats.

TRAINER TIPS

Make sure your clients know that posture does not just relate to how upright they are sitting or standing. Let them know that it also is related to the constant structure of their body and that good posture is important in achieving results.

Pattern overload

Repetitive physical activity that moves through the same patterns of motion, placing the same stresses on the body over time.

Repetitive stress injury (RSI)

Injury due to pattern overload.

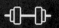
Suboptimal positioning
Less than optimal body positioning that when repeated reinforces poor motor patterns and can lead to abnormal stress and pattern overload.

Repetitive lack of motion
Frequent immobility, which holds the potential for repetitive stress injuries.

Hypomobility
Decrease in normal movement and functionality of a joint, which affects range of motion.

briefcases. Some cultural influences may lead to postural imprints such as increased lumbar lordosis, thoracic kyphosis, and/or a protracted shoulder girdle. Occupation, recreation, and hobbies all play a role in posture and structural alignment.

Occupational positioning can lead to postural misalignment by spending time in "office back," which is a rounded thoracic spine, protracted scapula, internally rotated shoulders, and a forward head position. Hobbies such as gardening, painting, and many others have their own repetitive use issues. Overuse does not have to be repetitive. If a movement is attempted that the body is not prepared to do, it only takes one instance of overstress to lead to injury. The goal is not to scare clients from performing daily activities and hobbies, sports, or their jobs, but rather to provide a means to better prepare for all types of movement.

Suboptimal Positioning

Suboptimal positioning can occur in simple movement patterns such as cycling. Some cyclists adduct their knees as if they are hugging the frame of the bicycle. This increased adduction at the hip and knee can put stress on the medial structures of the knee and transfer this poor activation pattern from the bike to other activities of daily living (ADL). Repeating poor movement reinforces poor motor patterns, and repetitive poor motor patterns can lead to abnormal stress and pattern overload.

Unbalanced Training

Resistance training can lead to postural imbalances because individuals often focus on certain muscle groups over others. Some individuals have an affinity for focusing on chest exercises, but without a balanced approach to resistance training the shoulder girdle alignment will alter. When resistance training is not balanced, the posture will not be either. Too often even fitness professionals focus on the pectoralis major and latissimus dorsi when performing a push–pull routine. These two muscle groups are often incorrectly thought to be opposite in action because they are on opposite sides of the body. However, they have more joint actions in common than in opposition. They tend to lead to a protracted shoulder girdle and internally rotated shoulders when they are the center of upper extremity resistance-training focus.

Repetitive Lack of Motion

Repetitive lack of motion can also lead to repetitive stress. A client may wake up in the morning and sit at the breakfast table, sit in the car on the way to work, sit all day at work, and then be so exhausted upon arriving home that he or she needs to sit down. It is clear from this example that the individual experiences a repetitive lack of movement; it is also perhaps understandable how adaptive shortening, stress, chronic fatigue, altered reciprocal inhibition, altered length–tension relationships, and altered arthrokinematics can occur, eventually leading to the potential for repetitive stress injuries.

Injury

Kinetic chain dysfunction reveals how an injury at one location can lead to dysfunction at other locations throughout the body. People take on postures to function around an injury and to avoid pain at the site of injury. Even after pain and motion restrictions subside and strength returns, the individual may need help in breaking the motor patterns that have developed as a means of working around the impairment.

Immobilizations such a casts, splints, braces, and other means of movement restriction can decrease range of motion and cause tissue shortening. Mobility and strength must be restored at and around the site of **hypomobility**; otherwise, muscles that are too short and tight are functionally paired with muscles that are lengthened and weak. This disrupts the neuromuscular balance in their interdependent relationships, leading to structural inefficiencies. Overuse injuries may also arise as a result of ambulatory means during injury, such as pain involving the wrist, elbow, shoulder, neck, or other areas due to repetitive stress from the use of crutches.

Medical Issues

Medical issues such as stroke, heart attack, and other conditions can lead to altered static and dynamic posture. The fitness professional should only work with these individuals after a physician's clearance, and should only focus on movement, not management of medical signs and symptoms.

Surgeries are another medical event that can lead to kinetic chain dysfunction. Scar tissue is a result of even the best surgical outcomes, yet scar tissue mobility is often overlooked in the rehabilitation paradigm. Functional efficiency following surgery must be restored or muscle imbalance and postural changes will develop.

Scientific Concepts Related to Kinetic Chain Dysfunction

Various concepts are related to kinetic chain dysfunction and are addressed frequently when talking about the science behind imbalances. These terms and concepts build the foundation from which other concepts can be introduced.

Altered Reciprocal Inhibition

Reciprocal inhibition was defined earlier, but a similar concept, *altered reciprocal inhibition*, is also involved in kinetic chain dysfunction. **Altered reciprocal inhibition** is the process by which a short muscle, a tight muscle, and/or myofascial adhesions in the muscle cause decreased neural drive of its functional antagonist. An example is when a tight hip flexor complex decreases the neural drive to the prime hip extensor, the gluteus maximus. The inhibited gluteus maximus muscle would then require other synergist hip extensor muscles, such as the hamstrings, to perform the joint action. This is known a *synergistic dominance*.

Synergistic Dominance

Synergistic dominance is a neuromuscular phenomenon that occurs when synergists take over the function of a weak or inhibited prime mover. Tight hip flexors can inhibit the gluteus maximus, diminishing its ability to extend the hip. The synergists of hip extension, the hamstrings and posterior adductor magnus, become the dominant hip extensors.

The concept of synergistic dominance can be explained with an example. Imagine that the gluteus maximus is the best player on a basketball team. The other muscles on the team are

Altered reciprocal inhibition
Process by which a short muscle, a tight muscle, and/or myofascial adhesions in the muscle cause decreased neural drive of its functional antagonist.

Synergistic dominance
When synergists take over function for a weak or inhibited prime movers.

role players. Unfortunately, the gluteus maximus is not feeling well, but insists on staying in the game. The team really wants to win the game, regardless of the faulty state of their star player. What do the other muscles need to do in order to stay in the competition? They must play harder. If the other players/muscles are playing harder, what will be the result of the added intensity? They will fatigue faster. Because this is not a real basketball game, the muscles cannot be taken out when they get tired, so if this elevated play continues while the muscles are fatigued as they struggle to "stay in the game" they are more likely to get hurt.

Coincidentally, the most injured muscle in the lower body is the hamstring, specifically the biceps femoris. This muscle performs is a synergist to the gluteus maximus for hip extension. When the biceps femoris is synergistically dominant it will perform the job of hip extension that the gluteus maximus should be performing. This will lead to the biceps femoris becoming overwhelmed and overused, leading to muscle strains as a repetitive stress injury.

Areas of Kinetic Chain Dysfunction

The Human Movement System, or kinetic chain, is composed of several major joints where various and excessive movement occurs in the lower extremity and where additional movements occur in the core and upper extremity. The joints where these movements take place are the links in the kinetic chain, and are the areas of focus in identifying optimal movement patterns. The major links/joints in the kinetic chain, which are commonly called the "five kinetic chain checkpoints," are as follows:

- Foot and ankle
- Knee
- Lumbo-pelvic-hip complex (LPHC)
- Shoulder girdle
- Head (cervical spine)

It is important to view the human body as a kinetic chain connected with bones, joints, and soft tissues that have tensional integrity (**tensegrity**). It is impossible for one part of the Human Movement System to be unaffected by the other parts. Think of a young child pulling on her mother's sweater as a relation to how soft tissue can be affected by forces. Most of the damage to the sweater may take place at the point of pull, but the elongation of the material happens throughout the weave of the cloth. Boney structures can be thought of like a building with 20 floors. If the 10th floor is structurally unstable, you would not want to be on any of the floors above or below! The body can heal itself to a degree to continue life and movement. The body can also actively, even subconsciously, compensate to avoid pain or allow for particular desired outcomes.

Muscle imbalances can be caused by a variety of mechanisms, including (Alter, 1996; Gossman, Sahrman, & Rose, 1982):

- Postural stress
- Emotional duress
- Repetitive movement
- Cumulative trauma
- Poor training technique
- Lack of core strength
- Lack of neuromuscular efficiency

Tensegrity

Term coined by Buckminster Fuller that refers to a skeletal structure in which compression and tension are used to give a structure its form, providing stability and efficiency in mass and movement.

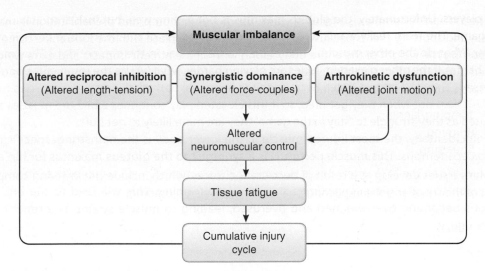

FIGURE 4.25 Muscular imbalance.

Muscle imbalance may be caused by or result in altered reciprocal inhibition, synergistic dominance, arthrokinetic dysfunction, and overall decreased neuromuscular control (**Figure 4.25**).

Foot and Ankle

The foot/ankle complex has many bones and associated joints that support the body during various movements. When issues arise with the foot/ankle complex it can lead to altered mechanics throughout the kinetic chain.

Foot/ankle injuries are among the most common musculoskeletal injuries (Doherty et al., 2014). Common injuries include:

- Plantar fasciitis
- Achilles tendinopathy
- Medial tibial stress syndrome
- Ankle sprains and chronic ankle instability

A common thread in each of these pathologies is a lack of ankle dorsiflexion. This adds particular importance to the implementation of appropriate assessment and movement preparation prior to training. When performing static, transitional, and dynamic movement assessments, the fitness professional is looking for three major faulty joint actions that can be summed up in one word—*pronation*. Pronation of the foot is the sequential combination of dorsiflexion, eversion, and abduction (external rotation) of the foot/ankle complex.

The muscles causing issues are a muscle group called the triceps surae. It is composed of the gastrocnemius (two heads) and soleus (one head) muscles; both muscles join into a tendon commonly known as the Achilles tendon. These muscles are designed to produce regular and repeated plantar flexion on the second-class lever of the ankle to facilitate locomotion. With just that responsibility it can make sense how and why they become so tight, but there are many more complicating factors that may contribute to limited ankle dorsiflexion because of the shortened state of the triceps surae. From footwear, to seated positions, to sleeping under covers, this group adaptively shortens to the forces and positioning placed upon it.

TRAINER TIPS

Make sure you constantly pay attention to the placement of your clients' feet. They are the foundation of the clients' movement.

The foot/ankle complex is a focus of warm-up, movement prep, and prehabilitation in many fitness and sporting events because so many activities take place with the foot/ankle complex supporting the weight of the entire body, along with all the athletic impacts and extra weight added during resistance training. Exercises where the foot/ankle play a dominate role are usually some variation of the following:

◆ Jumping/landing
◆ Running
◆ Squatting

Many issues develop as a result of deceleration forces, which include the lowering component of the squat and the impacting phases of running and jumping.

Knee

The knee is a common site of injury in athletes. Knee injuries and their repair account for more than 50% of injuries among college and high school athletes (Hootman, Dick, & Agel, 2007) (Fernandez, Yard, & Comstock, 2007). In addition, an estimated $2.5 billion is spent annually on knee injuries (Garrick & Requa, 2001). Anatomically, such injuries are so common because the knee is a relatively stable joint stuck directly between two highly mobile joints with very long levers. The ankle is the highly mobile joint below the knee, and the hip is the highly mobile joint above the knee. The long levers are the tibia and femur. It only takes limited range of motion, poor neuromuscular recruitment, and altered arthrokinematics at one of these two joints to cause a potentially devastating injury at the knee. Common knee injuries include:

◆ Patellar tendinopathy (jumper's knee)
◆ Iliotibial band (IT-band) syndrome (runner's knee)
◆ Patellofemoral pain syndrome
◆ Anterior cruciate ligament (ACL) injury (along with injuries to the posterior cruciate [PCL], medial collateral [MCL], and lateral collateral [LCL] ligaments)
◆ Meniscus tears

Common observable movement impairments are pronation distortion syndrome of the lower extremity:

◆ Pronation at the foot/ankle complex: Dorsiflexion, eversion, and external rotation.
◆ Pronation of the knee: Knee flexes and adducts; tibia and femur rotate toward midline.
◆ Pronation of the hips: Flexion, adduction, internal rotation.
◆ Pronation at the hip and/or the foot/ankle: Pronation of the knee; can appear as though the knee is caving in.

Lumbo-Pelvic-Hip Complex

The lumbo-pelvic-hip complex (LPHC) is commonly viewed as the core of the Human Movement System. It is the center of the human body and is directly connected to, influenced by, and has influence on both the upper and lower extremities. This is why LPHC stability is vitally important to injury prevention and sport performance. A properly stabilized core can be properly mobilized.

CAUTION

Some exercises may tend to cause knee pain. The goal of the fitness professional is not necessarily to address this pain, as this is not within the fitness professional's scope of practice. However, by addressing posture and mechanics in form and technique, the fitness professional may help alleviate pain while providing clients with exercise options they once deleted from their repertoire of possibilities.

Injuries associated with LPHC movement compensations are as follows:

◆ Local injuries:
  ● Low back pain
  ● Sacroiliac joint dysfunction
  ● Hamstring, quadriceps, and groin strains
◆ Injuries above the LPHC:
  ● Shoulder and upper extremity injuries
  ● Cervical-thoracic spine
  ● Rib cage dysfunction
◆ Injuries below the LPHC:
  ● Patellar tendonitis
  ● IT-band syndrome
  ● Medial, lateral, or anterior knee pain
  ● Chondromalacia patellae
  ● Plantar fasciitis
  ● Achilles tendonitis
  ● Posterior tibialis tendonitis (shin splints)

The LPHC is an important area to address with almost every movement deficiency presented during assessment and exercise. In almost every movement compensation addressed, the probable underactive muscles include the gluteals of the LPHC.

Shoulder

The shoulder joint, specifically the glenohumeral joint, is a mobile joint because of its unique anatomic features. It is a ball-and-socket joint that compromises stability to allow for greater range of motion. The shoulder joint is a part of the shoulder girdle, which is composed of the scapula, clavicle, and humerus. Much like the LPHC, the shoulder girdle moves in a particular rhythm to allow for increased range of motion. For example, as a client raises his arms overhead, note that the scapula rotates upward. As the arms are brought down, the scapula rotates back downward. When these joints become locked down or limited in their ROM, the glenohumeral joint is often the point of pain.

Common shoulder injuries include:

◆ Rotator cuff strains/tears
◆ Shoulder impingement
◆ Biceps tendinopathy
◆ Shoulder instability

Shoulder impairment can also lead to cervical issues above the shoulders and headaches. Below the shoulder the dysfunction can travel down and possibly lead to low-back pain and dysfunction in the sacroiliac joint. Some of the common muscles clients perform resistance training on, such as the pectorals, anterior deltoids, and latissimus dorsi, are already shortened into upper-extremity postural disorder. This does not mean that these muscles need to stop being trained, rather the movement preparation should have a particular focus on strengthening the underactive muscles, followed by the implementation of an integrated resistance-training program that provides balance between joint actions and the planes of motion.

Cervical Spine

Neck pain is the fourth leading cause of disability, with over 30% of adults worldwide complaining of neck pain at some point in their lives (Goode, Freburger, & Carey, 2010). As with other structures of the body, the cervical spine has an effect on the structures above and below it. The 30 muscles within the neck attach to the cervical spine and shoulder complex. These muscles help with balance and proprioception, stabilization of the head, postural orientation, and whole-body stability. Neck problems can lead to pain and dysfunction through headaches, back pain, and compensations to adjust for posture and balance control. Due to the vital role the neck musculature plays through the control of balance and posture, dysfunction at the cervical spine will lead to dysfunction at several different areas of the body. This can best be illustrated through the pelvo-ocular reflex.

Pelvo-ocular reflex
The neuromotor response of the pelvic girdle and lower extremity that serves to orient the body region in response to head position and visual cues.

The **pelvo-ocular reflex** is the neuromotor response of the pelvic girdle and lower extremity that serves to orient the body region in response to head position and visual cues. As the head moves forward, the pelvis will reflexively rotate anteriorly to readjust one's center of gravity (the pelvo-ocular reflex). This movement can lead to low back pain and movement dysfunction (Cohen, 2015). Poor cervical spine mechanics can lead to neck injuries and other problems, such as:

◆ Neck stiffness
◆ Headaches
◆ Dizziness
◆ TMJ-related symptoms
◆ Cervical strains
◆ Cervical disk lesions

Many people will experience cervical spine dysfunction due to their lifestyle. Oftentimes, such dysfunction is associated with the forward head posture that comes from working at a desk and computer for long periods of time. Others may begin to complain of neck pain if they carry heavy backpacks, purses, and/or children much of the day. Due to the strain these activities place upon the trapezius and levator scapulae muscles, dysfunction, and therefore pain, will be translated to the cervical spine. Those with jobs that require a great deal of overhead work may show signs of cervical spine dysfunction for the same reason. Flexibility exercises for the sternocleidomastoid, levator scapulae, and upper trapezius musculature will become an important part of a training program for those with neck dysfunction and/or pain.

Strengthening the deep cervical flexors, lower trapezius, and cervical-thoracic extensors will also help to alleviate such dysfunction.

Other Systems Related to Human Movement

Although our discussion of the Human Movement System, to this point, has focused largely on the structure, function, and interrelationship of the nervous, muscular, and skeletal systems, other body systems also support individuals during movement. The cardiorespiratory, endocrine, and digestive systems cannot be neglected in the conversation about human movement.

Cardiorespiratory System

The **cardiorespiratory system** is a combination of two closely related systems that interact with each other in order to support energy production for survival, movement, and various types of exercise and performance. The first component of the cardiorespiratory system is the **cardiovascular system**, which consists of the heart, blood vessels, and blood. The other system is the **respiratory system**, which is made up of the trachea, bronchi, alveoli, and lungs. These two systems work together to provide the body with adequate oxygen and nutrients and to remove waste products such as carbon dioxide from the cells in the body (Brooks, Fahey, White, & Baldwin, 2000; Fox, 2006; Hicks, 2000; Murray & Pulcipher, 2001; Vander, Sherman, & Luciano, 2003). Fitness professionals must be familiar with the basics of the anatomy and physiology of the cardiorespiratory system and how it relates to human movement. The intertwining of these two systems is important for fitness professionals beyond health and fitness given its relationship to cardiopulmonary resuscitation (CPR), a skill and certification required to work in the fitness industry.

Cardiovascular System

The cardiovascular system, or simply the circulatory system, is a closed system that circulates blood through a network of blood vessels via the rhythmic pumping action of the heart (Figure 4.26). The pumping of blood through the body is known as *systemic circulation*.

Heart

The heart is a muscular pump roughly the shape and size of a person's closed fist. It is located in the middle region of the thorax called the *mediastinum*, behind the sternum between the sternal attachments of the second through sixth ribs. The heart is obliquely positioned so that the apex (the rounded point), along with nearly two-thirds of the heart's mass, is to the left of the midline of the body, and only one-third to the right of the midline.

The heart must supply blood to the body, as well as to itself. Myocardial cells receive blood from the left and right coronary arteries, which then branch into smaller arteries. Once blood circulates through the network of capillaries it drains back to the inside of the heart for systemic circulation via the coronary veins.

Cardiac muscle is one of three types of muscle in the human body. The others are skeletal muscle and smooth muscle. Cardiac and skeletal muscle are similar in that they contain myofibrils and sarcomeres aligned side-by-side, giving them a striated appearance (Brooks et al., 2000; Fox, 2006; Tortora & Nielsen, 2008; Vander et al., 2003). Unlike skeletal muscle, cardiac

Cardiorespiratory system
System of the body composed of the cardiovascular and respiratory systems.

Cardiovascular system
System of the body composed of the heart, blood, and blood vessels.

Respiratory system
System of the body composed of the lungs and respiratory passages that collect oxygen from the external environment and transport it to the bloodstream.

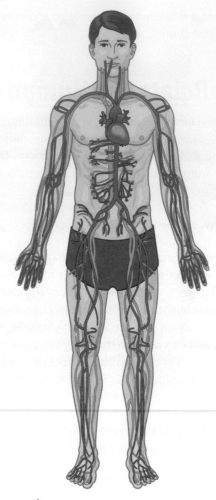

FIGURE 4.26 The cardiovascular system.

Sinoatrial (SA) node

A specialized area of cardiac tissue located in the right atrium of the heart that initiates the electrical impulses that determine the heart rate; often termed the "pacemaker for the heart."

Atrioventricular (AV) node

Small mass of specialized cardiac muscle fibers located on the wall of the right atrium of the heart that receives impulses from the sinoatrial (SA) node and directs them to the walls of the ventricles.

---

muscle is involuntary, meaning that an individual does not have to consciously think about activating the heart for contractions to occur.

Cardiac Muscle Contraction

The average number of times the heart beats per minute is known as the person's heart rate. Average heart rate is 70–80 beats per minute, or bpm (Brooks et al., 2000; Murray & Pulcipher, 2001; Tortora & Nielsen, 2008). Once an impulse enters the heart, the specialized muscle fibers of the heart are connected in such a way that conduction between muscle cells allows the heart to contract as one functional unit. The initiation of the electrical signal happens at the **sinoatrial (SA) node**, which can be thought of as the "pacemaker of the heart." It is located between the top and bottom chambers on the right side of the heart. The signal allows the electrical conduction system of the heart to stimulate the mechanical contraction of the myocardial cells. Because the top chamber must pump before the bottom chamber in order to function, the electrical pathway must enter a delay to offset the contraction timing. This is done by the SA node sending a signal to an internodal pathway called the **atrioventricular (AV) node**. The AV node is a small mass of specialized cardiac muscle fibers located on the wall of the right

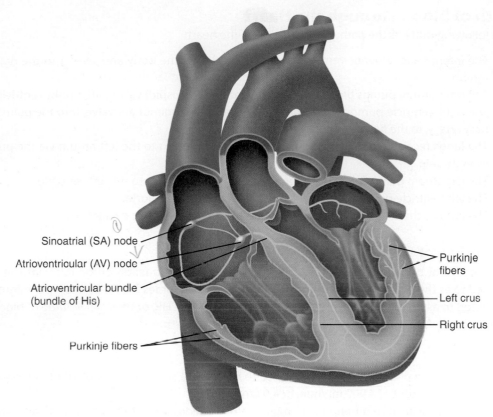

Sinoatrial (SA) node

Atrioventricular (AV) node

Atrioventricular bundle
(bundle of His)

Purkinje fibers

Purkinje fibers

Left crus

Right crus

FIGURE 4.27 Conduction system of the heart.

atrium of the heart that receives impulses from the SA node and directs them to the walls of the ventricles (**Figure 4.27**).

Structure of the Heart

The interior of the heart is divided into four chambers: top and bottom and left and right. The right side of the heart receives blood from the body and sends it to the lungs. The left side of the heart receives blood from the lungs and sends it back out into the body. The top chambers are known as *atria* (plural for *atrium*), and there is a right atrium and a left atrium. The atria receive blood from veins. **Veins** are the blood vessels that transport blood into the heart. The right atrium receives deoxygenated blood from the body. The left atrium receives oxygenated blood back into the heart from the lungs. The atria pump blood down into the same-side **ventricles**, which are larger chambers and are more muscular than the atria. Ventricles are considered the "pumping chambers" of the heart and need more force to push blood farther distances. The left ventricle is particularly muscular because it is tasked with pushing blood out into the systemic circulation, which moves blood throughout the entire body. Think of ventricles as vents, but rather than letting air out of the room they let blood out of the heart. The blood vessels that the ventricles "vent" into are called **arteries**. They are the blood vessels that allow the passage of blood away from the heart.

The chambers of the heart are separated from one another by the **atrioventricular (AV) valves**; major veins and arteries are separated from the chambers by semilunar valves that serve to prevent blockage, backflow, or spillage of blood back into the chambers. *Semilunar* means "half-moon" and the valves are so-named because of the crescent shape of the cusps.

MEMORY TIPS

In architecture, an atrium is an open-roofed hall, so think of the atrium as being the opening on the roof of the heart.

Veins

Vessels that transport blood from the capillaries toward the heart.

Ventricles

The inferior chambers of the heart that receive blood from their corresponding atrium and, in turn, force blood into the arteries.

Arteries

Vessels that transport blood away from the heart.

Atrioventricular (AV) valves

Valves that allow for proper blood flow from the atria to the ventricles.

Path of Blood Through the Heart

The following outlines the path of blood through the heart:

1. The inferior and superior vena cava collect blood from the body and send it to the right atrium.
2. The right atrium pumps blood through the right AV (tricuspid) valve to the right ventricle.
3. The right ventricle pumps out of the heart through the pulmonary valve, into the pulmonary artery, to the lungs.
4. The lungs receive blood from pulmonary artery and return to the left atrium via the pulmonary vein.
5. The left atrium pumps blood through the left AV (mitral) valve to the left ventricle.
6. The left ventricle pumps blood past the aortic valve into the aorta.
7. The aorta is the artery that transports blood toward the systemic circulation.

Function of the Heart

The amount of blood pumped out of the heart with each contraction of the left ventricle is referred to as the heart's **stroke volume (SV)**. The number of times the heart beats per minute is referred to as the **heart rate (HR)**. The SV multiplied by the HR, or the total volume of blood pumped out of the heart per minute, is called the **cardiac output ($\dot{Q}$)**.

$$SV \times HR = \dot{Q}$$

For example, a person with a heart rate of 70 bpm and a stroke volume of 70 mL/beat will have a cardiac output of 4,900 mL/min, or 4.9 L/min.

Monitoring heart rate during exercise gives a good indication of the amount of work the heart is doing at any given time (Brooks et al., 2000; Swain, 2006). Manual HR monitoring is helpful when checking in on a client's workout, but it also used to monitor someone who seems to be sick, pale, clammy, short of breath, or experiencing heart palpitations. **Figure 4.28** illustrates the procedure for manually monitoring a person's heart rate.

Blood Vessels

Blood vessels are hollow tubes that allow for blood to be transported from the heart, throughout the body, and back to the heart, creating a closed circuit (**Figure 4.29**). There are three major types of blood vessels:

- **Arteries**: Carry blood *away* from the heart. As arteries get further away from the heart they become smaller and form small terminal branches called *arterioles*, which end in capillaries.
- **Capillaries**: The **capillaries** are the site of water and gas exchange between blood and tissues.
- **Veins**: Carry blood toward the heart. Other small vessels, called *venules*, collect blood from capillaries. The venules progressively merge with other venules to form veins.

Functions of Blood

Blood supplies the body's organs and cells with oxygen and nutrients to help regulate body temperature, fight infections, and remove waste products. The average adult has 4–6 L of blood in the body, comprising approximately 8% of an individual's body weight. Blood is composed of a liquid portion called plasma (~55% by volume) and formed elements (~45% by volume) comprising red blood cells, white blood cells, and platelets. Formed elements are suspended in the liquid

Stroke volume (SV)

The amount of blood pumped out of the heart with each contraction.

Heart rate (HR)

The rate at which the heart pumps; usually measured in beats per minute (bpm).

Cardiac output ($\dot{Q}$)

Heart rate multiplied by stroke volume; a measure of the overall performance of the heart.

Capillaries

The smallest blood vessels and the site of water and gas exchange between the blood and tissues.

How to Manually Monitor Heart Rate

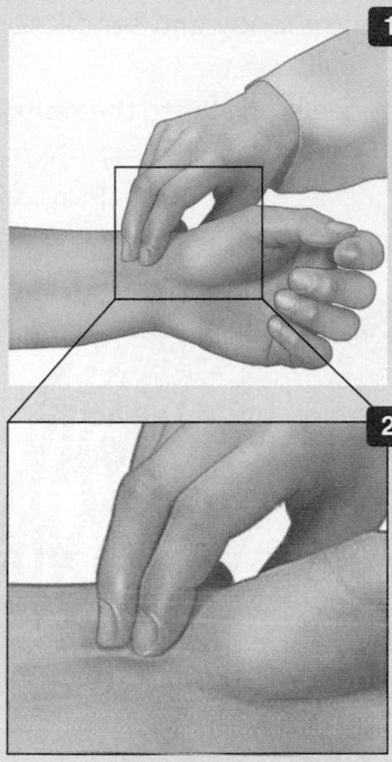

1 Place index and middle fingers around the palm side of the wrist (about one inch from the top of wrist, on the thumb side).

Although some people use the carotid artery in the neck, NASM does not recommend this location for measuring pulse rate. Pressure on this artery reduces blood flow to the brain, which can cause dizziness or an inaccurate measurement.

2 Locate the artery by feeling for a pulse with the index and middle fingers. Apply light pressure to feel the pulse. Do not apply excessive pressure as it may distort results.

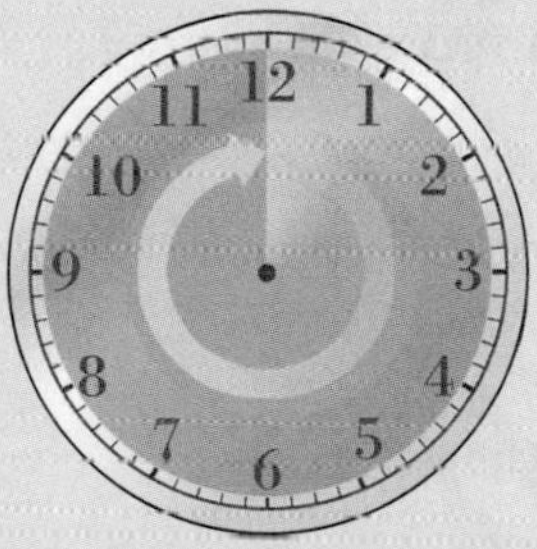

3 When measuring the pulse during rest, count the number of beats in 60 seconds.

There are some factors that may affect resting heart rate, including digestion, mental activity, environmental temperature, biological rhythms, body position, and cardiorespiratory fitness. Because of this, resting heart rate should be measured on waking (or at the very least, after you have had 5 minutes of complete rest).

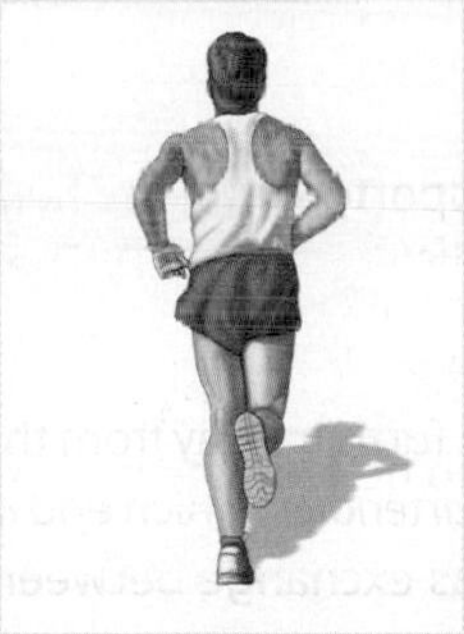

4 When measuring the pulse during exercise, count the number of beats in 6 seconds and add a zero to that number. Adding the zero will provide an estimate of the number of beats in 60 seconds. Or, one can simply multiply the number by 10 and that will provide the health and fitness professional with the same number.

Example: Number of beats in 6 seconds = 17. Adding a zero = 170. This gives a pulse rate of 170 bpm or, 17 x 10 = 170

FIGURE 4.28 How to manually monitor heart rate.

plasma, a watery substance containing nutrients such as glucose, hormones, and clotting agents. The following are the three functions of blood:

◆ Transportation
Blood transports oxygen from the lungs, hormones from the endocrine glands, and nutrients from the gastrointestinal tract to various organs and tissues throughout the body.

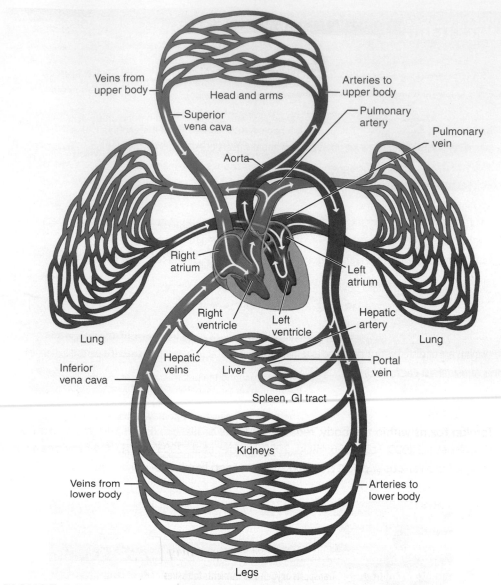

FIGURE 4.29 Blood vessels.

Blood also helps to remove waste products, in addition to helping the body remove heat from internal to external regions of the body.

◆ Regulation
Blood helps regulate body temperature by transferring heat from the internal core out to the appendages. As blood travels close to the skin it gives off heat to the environment or can be cooled depending on external conditions (Brooks et al., 2000; Fox, 2006; Tortora & Nielsen, 2008; Vander et al., 2003). Blood is also essential in regulating the body's pH level (acid–base balance) and in maintaining the water content of cells.

◆ Protection
Blood provides protection from excessive blood loss through its clotting mechanism, which seals off damaged tissue until a scar forms (Fox, 2006; Hicks, 2000; Vander et al., 2003). It also contains specialized immune cells—white blood cells—to fight against

CHECK IT OUT

Fitness professionals will likely work with clients who have a doctor's clearance to exercise after heart disease. The following conditions are a few common heart issues that fitness professionals need to be familiar with to better understand what their clients may have experienced:

Myocardial infarction (heart attack): A heart attack happens when the flow of oxygen-rich blood to a section of heart muscle suddenly becomes blocked and the heart does not get oxygen. If blood flow is not restored quickly, the section of heart muscle begins to die.

Congestive heart failure: A chronic condition where blood does not pump as well as it should, creating congestion within the heart.

Cardiac arrest: A sudden stop in effective blood circulation due to the failure of the heart to contract effectively or at all.

Arrhythmias: An arrhythmia is an abnormal heart rhythm. There are different types of arrhythmias:

- Bradycardia is an abnormally slow heart rate due to faulty SA node signals.
- Tachycardia is an abnormally fast heart rate due to faulty SA node signals.

Fibrillation: Fibrillation is an irregular quivering or spasm of the heart that can lead to cardiac arrest. Many gyms are outfitted with automated external defibrillators (AED) that can be used if a person experiences cardiac arrest due to fibrillation.

foreign toxins within the body, reducing the risk of disease and illness from pathogens (Brooks et al., 2000; Fox, 2006; Hicks, 2000; Vander et al., 2003). **Table 4.4** provides a summary of the various support mechanisms provided by blood.

TABLE 4.4 Support Mechanisms of Blood	
Mechanism	**Function**
Transportation	Transports oxygen and nutrients to tissues
	Transports waste products from tissues
	Transports hormones to organs and tissues
	Carries heat throughout the body
Regulation	Regulates body temperature and acid balance in the body
Protection	Protects the body from excessive bleeding by clotting
	Contains specialized immune cells to help fight disease and sickness

Respiratory System

The respiratory, or pulmonary, system brings oxygen into and removes carbon dioxide from the lungs. This is the function of breathing. The respiratory and cardiovascular systems work

TABLE 4.5 Structures of the Respiratory Pump	
Bones	Sternum
	Ribs
	Vertebrae
Muscles—inspiration	Diaphragm
	External intercostals
	Scalenes
	Sternocleidomastoid
	Pectoralis minor
Muscles—expiration	Internal intercostals
	Abdominals

together to ensure proper cellular function by transporting oxygen from the external environment (outside the body) and transferring it to the bloodstream. They are also responsible for transferring carbon dioxide from the blood to the lungs and eventually transporting it out of the body into the external environment (Brown, 2000; Leech, Ghezzo, Stevens, & Becklake, 1983).

Breathing, or ventilation, is the process of moving air in and out of the body using all components of the respiratory pump (**Table 4.5**). The respiratory pump acts as a mechanism to help pump blood back to the heart during inspiration by decreasing pressure within the thoracic cavity. This causes a drop in pressure in the right atrium of the heart and helps improve venous blood flow back to the heart.

Breathing in is called *inspiration* (or *inhalation*). It is an active process involving several muscles, including the following:

- Diaphragm
- External intercostals
- Scalenes
- Sternocleidomastoid
- Pectoralis major

Sometimes individuals become confused about the function of the diaphragm because when they sing they are told to use their diaphragm. Loudly singing or speaking happens as a result of breathing out, but the diaphragm is a muscle of breathing in, which means it can only passively help with breathing out by relaxing its contraction.

Inspiratory ventilation can be considered either normal or heavy. Normal breathing is quiet and uses the primary muscles of breathing, such as the diaphragm and external intercostals. Heavy breathing is louder and requires the secondary muscles of respiration, such as the scalenes and pectoralis minor.

Breathing out, known as *expiration* (or *exhalation*), can be passive or active. During normal breathing expiratory ventilation is passive, because it results from the relaxation of the contracting inspiratory muscles. During heavy or forced breathing, expiratory ventilation relies on the activity of expiratory muscles to compress the thoracic cavity and force air out (Brown, 2000; Fox, 2006; Hicks, 2000; Sharp, Goldberg, Druz, & Danon, 1975; Tortora & Nielsen, 2008; Vander et al., 2003).

Respiratory Airways

The purpose of ventilation is to move air in and out of the body. There are two categories of respiratory passages: the conducting airways and the respiratory airways.

Conducting airways consists of all the structures that air travels through before entering the respiratory airways (**Table 4.6**). The nasal and oral cavities, mouth, pharynx, larynx, trachea, and bronchioles provide a gathering station for air and oxygen to be directed into the body (**Figure 4.30**), allowing the air to be purified, humidified, and warmed or cooled to match body

TABLE 4.6 Structures of the Respiratory Passages	
Conducting airways	Nasal cavity
	Oral cavity
	Pharynx
	Larynx
	Trachea
	Right and left pulmonary bronchi
	Bronchioles
Respiratory airways	Alveoli
	Alveolar sacs

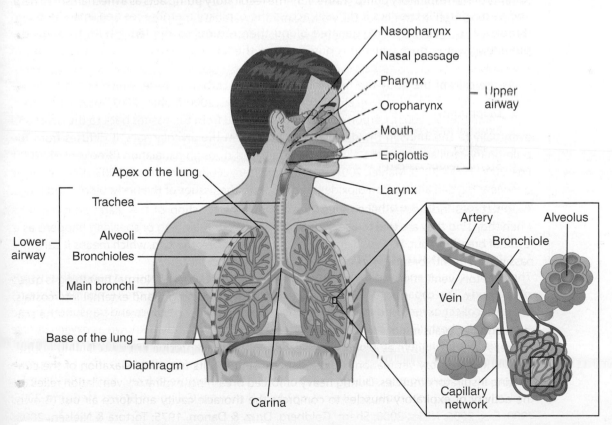

FIGURE 4.30 The Respiratory passages.

temperature (Brooks et al., 2000; Brown, 2000; Fox, 2006; Mahler, 2001; Swain, 2006; Vander et al., 2003).

The respiratory airways collect the channeled air coming from the conduction airways and allow gases such as oxygen and carbon dioxide to be transferred into and out of the blood-stream. At the end of the bronchioles, sit the alveoli, which are made up of alveolar sacs (Figure 4.24). It is in these sacs that gases such as oxygen and carbon dioxide are transported into and out of the bloodstream through a process known as *diffusion* (Brooks et al., 2000; Fox, 2006; Mahler, 2001; Tortora & Nielsen, 2008; Vander et al., 2003). Diffusion is how oxygen gets from the outside environment to the tissues of the body.

Cardiorespiratory System Function

Together, the cardiovascular and respiratory systems make up the cardiorespiratory system. They form a vital support system to provide the Human Movement System with essential el-ements (such as oxygen), while removing waste products that can cause dysfunction in the body.

An essential element to sustain life is oxygen (Brooks et al., 2000). The respiratory sys-tem provides the means to gather oxygen from the environment and transfer it into the body. It is inhaled through the nose and mouth, and conducted through the trachea, and then down through the bronchi, where it eventually reaches the lungs and alveolar sacs (Brooks et al., 2000; Fox, 2006; Hicks, 2000; Mahler, 2001; Tortora & Nielsen, 2008; Vander et al., 2003). Simultaneously, deoxygenated blood is pumped from the right ventricle to the lungs through the pulmonary arteries. Pulmonary capillaries surround the alveolar sacs, and as oxygen fills the sacs it diffuses across the capillary membranes and into the blood (Brooks et al., 2000). The oxygenated blood then returns to the left atrium through the pulmonary veins, from which it is pumped into the left ventricle and out to the tissues of the body.

As the cells of the body use oxygen they produce carbon dioxide, which needs to be re-moved from the body (Brooks et al., 2000; Fox, 2006; Hicks, 2000; Mahler, 2001; Tortora & Nielsen, 2008; Vander et al., 2003). Carbon dioxide is transported from the tissues back to the heart and eventually to the lungs in the deoxygenated blood. In the alveolar sacs, it diffuses from the pulmonary capillaries into the alveoli and is released through exhalation (Brooks et al., 2000; Fox, 2006; Hicks, 2000; Mahler, 2001; Tortora & Nielsen, 2008; Vander et al., 2003). In a simplistic overview, oxygen and carbon dioxide trade places in the tissues of the body, blood, and lungs. As one is coming in, the other is going out.

Oxygen Consumption

The cardiovascular and respiratory systems work together to transport oxygen to the tissues of the body. The capacity to efficiently use oxygen is dependent on the respiratory system's ability to collect oxygen and the cardiovascular system's ability to absorb and transport it to the tissues of the body (Franklin, 2000). The use of oxygen by the body is known as *oxygen uptake* (or *oxygen consumption*; Brooks et al., 2000; Brown, 2000; Fox, 2006; Hicks, 2000; Mahler, 2001; Tortora & Nielsen, 2008; Vander et al., 2003). Resting oxygen consumption ($\dot{V}O_2$) is approxi-mately 3.5 mL of oxygen per kilogram of body weight per minute (3.5 mL $\cdot$ kg^{-1} $\cdot$ min^{-1}), and is typically termed 1 metabolic equivalent, or 1 MET (American College of Sports Medicine, 2005;

Brooks et al., 2000; Franklin, 2000; Hicks, 2000; Leech et al., 1983; Swain, 2006; Timmons, 1994). It is calculated as follows:

$$\dot{V}O_2 = \dot{Q} \times \text{a--}\dot{v}\,O_2 \text{ difference}$$

The equation for oxygen consumption is known as the *Fick equation*. According to the Fick equation, oxygen consumption, $\dot{V}O_2$, is a product of cardiac output, $\dot{Q}$ or ($HR \times S\dot{V}$), multiplied by the arterial-venous difference (difference in the O_2 content between the blood in the arteries and the blood in the veins), a--$\dot{V}O_2$. From the Fick equation, it is easy to see how influential the cardiovascular system is on the body's ability to consume oxygen, and that heart rate plays a major factor in determining $\dot{V}O_2$.

Maximal oxygen consumption ($\dot{V}_{O2max}$) may be the best measure of cardiorespiratory fitness (ACSM, 2005; Brooks et al., 2000; Hicks, 2000; Swain, 2006). $\dot{V}O_{2max}$ is the highest rate of oxygen transport and utilization during maximal exercise (ACSM, 2005; Franklin, 2000; Leech et al., 1983). $\dot{V}O_{2max}$ values can range anywhere from 40–80 mL $\cdot$ kg^{-1} $\cdot$ min^{-1}, or approximately 11–23 METs (ACSM, 2005; Swain, 2006). The only way to determine $\dot{V}O_{2max}$ is to directly measure ventilation, oxygen consumption, and carbon dioxide production during a maximal exercise test. However, because the equipment needed to measure $\dot{V}O_{2max}$ is very expensive and not readily available, the use of a submaximal exercise test to estimate or predict $\dot{V}O_{2max}$ is the preferred method (ACSM, 2005; Guthrie, 2006). Some of the tests that can be used to predict $\dot{V}O_{2max}$ include the Rockport walk test, the step test, and the YMCA bike protocol test (ACSM, 2005; Guthrie, 2006). It is important to note that numerous assumptions are made when predicting versus directly measuring $\dot{V}O_{2max}$, which can lead to over- or underestimates of what an individual's true $\dot{V}O_{2max}$ actually is (ACSM, 2005; Guthrie, 2006).

Abnormal Breathing Patterns

Any difficulty or changes to normal breathing patterns can affect the normal response to exercise (Timmons, 1994). The following are abnormal breathing scenarios associated with stress and anxiety:

- A shallow breathing pattern can result from the predominant use of the secondary respiratory muscles rather than the diaphragm. This breathing pattern can become habitual, causing overuse to the secondary respiratory muscles, such as the scalenes, sternocleidomastoid, levator scapulae, and upper trapezius.
- Increased activity in respiratory muscles and excessive tension may result in headaches, lightheadedness, and dizziness.
- Excessive breathing (short, shallow breaths) can lead to altered carbon dioxide and oxygen levels in the blood, causing feelings of anxiety.
- Inadequate oxygen and retention of metabolic waste within muscles can create fatigued, stiff muscles.
- Inadequate joint motion of the spine and rib cage, as a result of improper breathing, can cause joints to become restricted and stiff.

All of these situations can lead to a decreased functional capacity that may result in headaches, feelings of anxiety, fatigue, and poor sleep patterns, as well as poor circulation.

Endocrine System

The endocrine system is a system of organs known as **glands** that secrete hormones into the bloodstream to regulate a variety of bodily functions, such as mood, growth and development,

Maximal oxygen consumption ($\dot{V}O_{2max}$)
The highest rate of oxygen transport and utilization achieved at maximal physical exertion.

TRAINER TIPS

To prevent nausea and postworkout headaches, watch your clients for abnormal breathing patterns.

CAUTION ⚠

It is not the fitness professional's job to try to diagnose breathing problems. If a client presents any of these scenarios, refer the client immediately to a medical professional for assistance.

Gland
An organ that secretes hormones into the bloodstream to regulate a variety of bodily functions, such as mood, growth and development, tissue function, or metabolism.

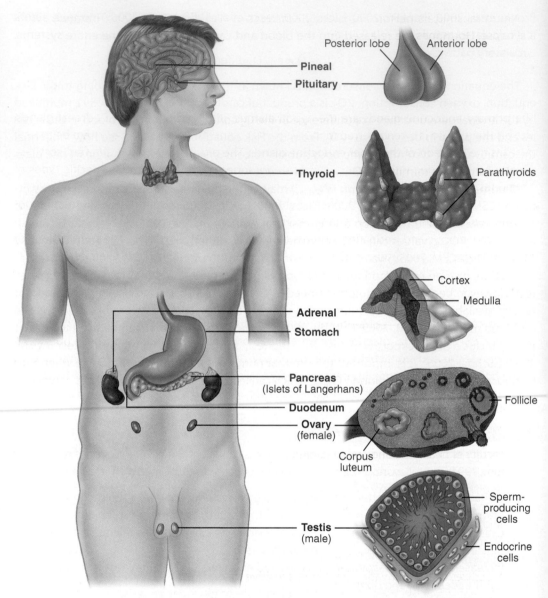

FIGURE 4.31 Endocrine organs.

Hormones

Chemical messengers that enter the bloodstream to attach to target tissues and target organs.

Target cells

Cells that have hormone-specific receptors, ensuring that each hormone will communicate only with specific target cells.

tissue function, and metabolism (**Figure 4.31**). **Hormones** are the chemical messengers that enter the bloodstream to attach to target tissues and target organs. The **target cells** have hormone-specific receptors, ensuring that each hormone will communicate only with specific target cells.

The endocrine system is responsible for regulating multiple bodily functions to stabilize the body's internal environment, much like a thermostat regulates the temperature in a room. Hormones produced by the endocrine system affect virtually all of the body's functions, including, but not limited to, triggering muscle contraction, stimulating protein and fat synthesis, activating enzyme systems, regulating growth and metabolism, and determining how the body will physically and emotionally respond to stress (McArdle, Katch, & Katch, 2010).

Neurotransmitters perform regulatory functions as well, but over a short distance across a synapse. Hormones are released into the blood and carried throughout the entire systemic circulatory pathway.

Endocrine Glands

The primary endocrine glands are the hypothalamus, pituitary, thyroid, and adrenal glands. The pituitary gland is often referred to as the "master gland" of the endocrine system because it controls the function of the other endocrine glands. The pituitary has three different sections, or lobes: the anterior, intermediate, and posterior lobes. Each lobe secretes specific types of hormones.

The pituitary gland and hypothalamus, which are both located in the brain, ultimately control much of the hormonal activity in the body. Together they represent an important link between the nervous and endocrine systems (Tortora & Grabowski, 1996). The purpose of this chapter will be to focus on those glands and hormones directly involved in exercise.

Catecholamines

The two catecholamines—epinephrine (or adrenaline) and norepinephrine—are hormones produced by the adrenal glands, which are situated on top of the kidneys. These hormones help prepare the body for activity; more specifically, they are part of the stress response known as the *fight or flight response*. In preparation for this activity, the hypothalamus (an endocrine gland in the brain) triggers the adrenal glands to secrete more epinephrine. The increase in epinephrine results in specific physiological effects that help to sustain exercise activity (Tortora & Grabowski, 1996; Wilmore & Costill, 2004):

- Increases heart rate and stroke volume.
- Elevates blood glucose levels.
- Redistributes blood to working tissues.
- Catecholamines (CATS) can increase 10 to 20 times resting levels (influenced by intensity and duration).
- Norepinephrine rise > 50% $\dot{V}O_2$max
- Epinephrine rises > 70% VO_2max
- Mobilizes fats by activating hormone-sensitive lipase (HSl).
- Generates glucose via glycogenolysis, glycolysis, or gluconeogenesis.
- Stimulates sweating.
- Promotes vasodilation in needed areas versus vasoconstriction in non-needed areas.

↑increase in epinephrine

Testosterone and Estrogen

Testosterone (TST) is produced in the testes of the male and in small amounts in the ovaries and adrenal glands of the female. Males produce up to 10 times more testosterone than females (McArdle et al., 2010). Testosterone is the hormone that is primarily responsible for the development of male secondary sexual characteristics, such as facial and body hair and greater muscle mass. Estrogen is produced primarily in the ovaries in the female, with small amounts produced in the adrenal glands in males.

For both males and females, however, testosterone plays a fundamental role in the growth and repair of tissue. Increased levels of testosterone are indicative of anabolic (tissue-building) training status.

Cortisol

In contrast to testosterone, cortisol is typically referred to as a catabolic hormone, which means it is associated with the breaking down of tissue. When the body experiences acute stress, such as exercise, cortisol is secreted by the adrenal glands and serves to maintain the energy supply through the breakdown of carbohydrates, fats, and protein. Chronic stress from overtraining, excessive stress, poor sleep, and inadequate nutrition can elevate cortisol levels, leading to unwanted and potentially harmful side effects (McArdle et al., 2010) such as:

- Breakdown of muscle tissue
- Decreased fat utilization
- Increased body composition (specifically abdominal fat)
- Decreased metabolism

[handwritten margin note: excess cortisol]

Growth Hormone

Growth hormone is an anabolic hormone responsible for most of the growth and development that occurs during childhood up until puberty, when the primary sex hormones take over. Growth hormone increases the development of bone and muscle and promotes protein synthesis and fat burning; it also strengthens the immune system. Growth hormone is stimulated by:

- Estrogen
- Testosterone
- Deep sleep
- Hypertrophy training (up to 23 times baseline)
- Max strength training (up to 3 times baseline)

Note that high-intensity interval training (HIIT) has little to no impact on growth hormone production.

Thyroid Hormones

The thyroid gland is located at the base of the neck, just below the thyroid cartilage, which is sometimes called the Adam's apple. This gland releases vital hormones that are primarily responsible for human metabolism, namely triiodothyronine (T3) and thyroxin (T4). Thyroid hormones have been shown to be responsible for:

- Carbohydrate, protein, and fat metabolism
- Basal metabolic rate
- Protein synthesis
- Sensitivity to epinephrine
- Heart rate
- Breathing rate
- Body temperature

[handwritten margin note: thyroid hormones responsible for...]

Effects of Exercise on the Endocrine System

Research has indicated that testosterone and growth hormone levels increase primarily after hypertrophy training and moderately with maximum strength lifts. They are very mildly impacted by low to moderate aerobic exercise or HIIT. The presence of cortisol in the bloodstream is often taken to be indicative of overtraining. This is perhaps a little simplistic, as cortisol is a necessary part of maintaining energy levels during normal exercise activity and may even facilitate recovery and repair during the postexercise period (McArdle et al., 2010). Problems may arise as a result of extremely intense training modalities; additionally, prolonged bouts of endurance training have been found to lower testosterone levels while raising cortisol levels. Under these circumstances, catabolism (breakdown) is likely to outstrip anabolism (build up) and give rise to symptoms of overtraining (McArdle et al., 2010).

Hormones produced by the endocrine system affect virtually all forms of human function and determine how the body physically and emotionally responds to stress. Exercise programming has a significant impact on hormone secretion. Fitness professionals should become familiar with how pertinent hormones respond to exercise to maximize programming strategies and avoid overtraining.

Digestive System

The digestive system is a long tube (~30 feet) called the *alimentary canal*. It performs the vital function of getting nutrients to cells and removing food waste. The term *gastrointestinal (GI) tract* is often used interchangeably with *alimentary canal*, but the GI tract refers specifically to only the stomach and intestines (Patton & Thibodeau, 2015). Food cannot be absorbed into cells without being broken down into small components mechanically and chemically, altered chemically, and then absorbed into the bloodstream and delivered to the cells in the organs and tissues of the body.

Mouth

The process of getting food into the digestive system starts at the mouth with eating, or *ingestion*, and begins the digestion process by mechanically breaking down food through chewing. Accessory organs of the digestive system help begin the process:

- The salivary glands produce saliva to assist with the chemical breakdown of food.
- The tongue has taste receptors and helps with food manipulation.
- Teeth provide the initial and greatest amount of mechanical breakdown of food.

Once food has been chewed to the point of swallowing it is called a *bolus*. When the bolus is swallowed it leaves the mouth and enters the pharynx.

Pharynx and Esophagus

The pharynx is the space between the mouth and both the trachea and esophagus. With swallowing, the opening to the trachea closes so that the bolus can enter the esophagus. The esophagus, or gullet, is about 10 inches long and provides passage of the food bolus to the stomach. The undulating muscular mechanism that causes food to travel down the esophagus is called *peristalsis*.

Stomach

The stomach is a C-shaped muscular pouch that acts as a temporary storage facility and helps break down food both chemically and mechanically. It also serves to absorb water, amino acids and water soluble vitamins for use in the body.

Small Intestine

The small intestine is the longest section of the alimentary tube (about 7–13 feet) that serves as passage from the stomach to the large intestine. It is a twisted, coiled, and muscular tube. It is where the majority of digestion actually takes place. It has three main areas:

- Duodenum (Latin for "12 finger widths")
- Jejunum (Latin for "empty")
- Ileum (Latin for "twisted intestine")

Because the small intestine can only process food in small amounts, the pyloric sphincter serves as the "gatekeeper" between the stomach and small intestine. As food travels through the small intestine and digestion occurs, it is important that only the desired nutrients get into the bloodstream. The billions of bacteria in the GI tract must be prevented from entering the body.

Large Intestine

The large intestine starts where the small intestine ends (ileocecal valve) and ends at the anus. The large intestine is larger than the small intestine in diameter only. The large intestine has several major, visually distinct, regions:

- Ascending colon
- Transverse colon
- Descending colon
- Sigmoid colon

The sigmoid colon is the S-shaped part of the colon once it enters the pelvic girdle. From the sigmoid colon feces enters the rectum and then exits the anal canal through the anus. The large intestine has several jobs, but ultimately its role is to dry out undigested "leftover" food in the intestines and to eliminate it as feces.

It is important for fitness professionals to know the basics of digestive anatomy and how food is broken down and enters the bloodstream to feed the cells, tissues, and organs of the body through the previously discussed circulatory system.

Conclusion

Understanding the Human Movement System is integral to effective performance as a fitness professional. This chapter has provided the essential knowledge related to the Human Movement System, the interactions of the kinetic chain, common areas of kinetic chain dysfunction, and other systems related to human movement. Through application of basic human movement concepts and a deep understanding of the kinetic chain, the fitness professional is better prepared to identify common movement dysfunctions and provide appropriate solutions in supporting client progress.

Case in Review

When talking about the Human Movement System to your friend, you find yourself using your own body to help explain the kinetic chain checkpoints. Similar to the baseline knowledge your friend has of the Human Movement System, you will find that your clients know little about their own body and the interrelationship of the three systems. Simply put, the body's nervous, muscular, and skeletal systems provide us the ability to move in specific ways. When we continue to move in a manner that the body was not designed for, over time signs of poor posture will result. To determine proper posture, five spots on the body called the kinetic chain checkpoints are used to assess alignment. These points include the feet, knees, hips, shoulders, and cervical spine. When they are in alignment, your friend will have proper posture.

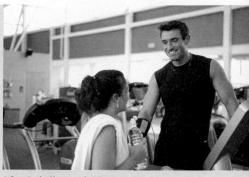
© Sean Locke Photography/Shutterstock

Regardless of the position or exercise someone is performing, you should always check posture by assessing the five kinetic chain checkpoints. Only when aligned will proper form be achieved. When talking with your friend about possible influencers, you ask questions to help identify lifestyle trends with regards to how your friend sits, stands, and moves throughout the day. Some examples of influencers could include your friend's profession, daily activities, hobbies, footwear, and common accessories (bags, purses, briefcases, etc.). The influencers will guide you to the areas that either need to be addressed from a dysfunctional perspective or in increasing one's ability to perform in that specific area.

References

Alexander, B., & Viktor, K. (2010). Proportions of hand segments. *International Journal of Morphology, 28*(3), 755–758.

Alter, M. J. (1996). *Science of flexibility* (2nd ed.). Champaign, IL: Human Kinetics.

American College of Sports Medicine. (2005). *ACSM's resource manual for guidelines for exercise testing and prescription* (5th ed.). Baltimore, MD: Lippincott Williams & Wilkins.

Basmajian, J. (1985). *Muscles alive: Their functions revealed by EMG* (5th ed.). Baltimore, MD: Williams & Wilkins.

Bergmark, A. (1989). Stability of the lumbar spine. A study in mechanical engineering. *Acta Orthopaedica Scandinavica, 230*(suppl), 20–24.

Brooks, G., Fahey, T., & Baldwin, K. (2005). *Exercise physiology: Human bioenergetics and its applications* (4th ed.). New York, NY: McGraw-Hill.

Brooks, G. A., Fahey, T. D., White, T. P., & Baldwin, K. M. (2000). *Exercise physiology: Human bioenergetics and its application* (3rd ed.). New York, NY: McGraw-Hill.

Brown, D. D. (2000). Pulmonary responses to exercise and training. In W. E. Garrett & D. T. Kirkendall (Eds.), *Exercise and sport science* (pp. 117–132). Philadelphia, PA: Lippincott Williams & Wilkins.

Clark, M. A. (2001). *Integrated training for the new millennium*. Thousand Oaks, CA: National Academy of Sports Medicine.

Cohen, S. P. (2015). Epidemiology, diagnosis, and treatment of neck pain. *Mayo Clinic Proceedings, 90*(2), 284–299. doi:http://dx.doi.org/10.1016/j.mayocp.2014.09.008

Crisco, J. J., & Panjabi, M. M. (1991). The intersegmental and multisegmental muscles of the spine: A biomechanical model comparing lateral stabilizing potential. *Spine, 7,* 793–799.

do Rosário, J. L. P., Diógenes, M. S. B., Mattei, R., & Leite, J. R. (2013). Can sadness alter posture? *Journal of Bodywork and Movement Therapies, 17*(3), 328–331.

Doherty, C., Delahunt, E., Caulfield, B., Hertel, J., Ryan, J., & Bleakley, C. (2014). The incidence and prevalence of ankle sprain injury: A systematic review and meta-analysis of prospective epidemiological studies. *Sports Medicine, 44*(1), 123–140.

Fernandez, W. G., Yard, E. E., & Comstock, R. D. (2007). Epidemiology of lower extremity injuries among U.S. high school athletes. *Academic Emergency Medicine, 14*(7), 641–645.

Fox, S. I. (1996). *Human physiology* (5th ed.). Dubuque, IA: Wm C Brown Publishers.

Fox, S. I. (2006). *Human physiology* (9th ed.). New York, NY: McGraw-Hill.

Franklin, B. A. (2000). Cardiovascular responses to exercise and training. In W. E. Garrett & D. T. Kirkendall (Eds.), *Exercise and sport science* (pp. 104–115). Philadelphia, PA: Lippincott Williams & Wilkins.

Gabbard, C. (2008). *Lifelong motor development*. San Francisco, CA: Pearson Benjamin Cummings.

Garrick, J. G., & Requa, R. K. (2001). ACL injuries in men and women—How common are they? In L. Y. Griffin (Ed.), *Prevention of noncontact ACL injuries*. Rosemont, IL: American Academy of Orthopaedic Surgeons.

Goode, A. P., Freburger, J., & Carey, T. (2010). Prevalence, practice patterns, and evidence for chronic neck pain. *Arthritis Care and Research, 62*(11), 1594–1601. doi:10.1002/acr.20270

Gossman, M. R., Sahrman, S. A., & Rose, S. J. (1982). Review of length-associated changes in muscle: Experimental evidence and clinical implications. *Physical Therapy, 62,* 1799–1808.

Gross, J., Fetto, J., & Rosen, E. (1996). *Musculoskeletal examination*. Malden, MA: Blackwell Sciences.

Guthrie, J. (2006). Cardiorespiratory and health-related physical fitness assessments. In American College of Sports Medicine (Ed.), *ACSM's resource manual for guidelines for exercise testing and prescription* (6th ed.; pp. 297–331). Baltimore, MD: Lippincott Williams & Wilkins.

Hall, S. (2014). *Basic biomechanics* (7th ed.). New York, NY: McGraw-Hill Education.

Hamill, J., & Knutzen, J. M. (1995). *Biomechanical basis of human movement*. Baltimore, MD: Williams & Wilkins.

Hamill, J., & Knutzen, J. M. (2003). *Biomechanical basis of human movement* (2nd ed.). Baltimore, MD: Lippincott Williams & Wilkins.

Hamill, J., Knutzen, K., & Derrick, T. (2015). *Biomechanical basis of human movement* (4th ed.). Philadelphia, PA: Lippincott Williams & Wilkins.

Hicks, G. H. (2000). *Cardiopulmonary anatomy and physiology*. Philadelphia, PA: WB Saunders.

Hootman, J. M., Dick, R., & Agel, J. (2007). Epidemiology of collegiate injuries for 15 sports: Summary and recommendations for injury prevention initiatives. *Journal of Athletic Training, 42*(2), 311–319.

Inman, V. T., Ralston, H. J., & Todd, F. (1981). *Human walking*. Baltimore, MD: Williams & Wilkins.

Innes, K. A. (1999). The effect of gait on extremity evaluation. In W. I. Hammer (Ed.), *Functional soft tissue examination and treatment by manual methods* (2nd ed.; pp. 357–368). Gaithersburg, MD: Aspen Publishers.

Knudson, D. (2007). *Fundamentals of biomechanics* (2nd ed.). New York, NY: Springer.

Leech, J. A., Ghezzo, H., Stevens, D., & Becklake, M. R. (1983). Respiratory pressures and function in young adults. *American Review of Respiratory Disease, 128,* 17–23.

Levin, S. M. (1981). The icosahedron as a biologic support system. *Proceedings of the 34th Annual Conference on Engineering in Medicine and Biology, 23,* 404.

Levangie, P., & Norkin, C. (2001). Basic concepts in biomechanics. In *Joint structure and function: A comprehensive analysis* (3rd ed.). Philadelphia, PA: FA Davis.

Luttgens, K., & Hamilton, N. (1997). *Kinesiology: Scientific basis of human motion* (9th ed.). Dubuque, IA: Brown & Benchmark Publishers.

Luttgens, K., & Hamilton, N. (2007). *Kinesiology: Scientific basis of human motion* (11th ed.). New York, NY: McGraw-Hill.

Mahler, D. A. (2001). Respiratory anatomy. In American College of Sports Medicine (Ed.), *ACSM's resource manual for guidelines for exercise testing and prescription* (4th ed.; pp. 74–81). Baltimore, MD: Lippincott Williams & Wilkins.

McArdle, W., Katch, F., & Katch, V. (2010). *Exercise physiology: Nutrition, energy, and human performance* (7th ed.). Philadelphia, PA: Lippincott Williams & Wilkins.

Milner-Brown, A. (2001). *Neuromuscular physiology*. Thousand Oaks, CA: National Academy of Sports Medicine.

Mooney, V. (1997). Sacroiliac joint dysfunction. In A. Vleeming, V. Mooney, T. Dorman, C. Snijders, & R. Stoeckhart (Eds.), *Movement, stability, and low back pain* (pp. 37–52). London, UK: Churchill Livingstone.

Murray, T. D., & Pulcipher, J. M. (2001). Cardiovascular anatomy. In American College of Sports Medicine (Ed.), *ACSM's resource manual for guidelines for exercise testing and prescription* (4th ed.; pp. 65–72). Baltimore, MD: Lippincott Williams & Wilkins.

National Institutes of Health (2015). *Exercise for your bone health*. Available from: http://www.niams.nih.gov/Health_Info/Bone/Bone_Health/Exercise/default.asp

Neumann, D. (2010). *Kinesiology of the musculoskeletal system: Foundations for rehabilitation* (2nd ed.). St. Louis, MO: Mosby/Elsevier.

Nordin, M., Lorenz, T., & Campello, M. (2001). Biomechanics of tendons and ligaments. In M. Nordin & V. H. Frankel (Eds.), *Basic biomechanics of the musculoskeletal system* (3rd ed.; pp. 102–126). Philadelphia, PA: Lippincott Williams & Wilkins.

Norkin, C. C., & Levangie, P. K. (1992). *Joint structure and function: A comprehensive analysis* (2nd ed.). Philadelphia, PA: FA Davis.

Norkin, C. C., & Levangie, P. K. (2000). *Joint structure and function: A comprehensive analysis* (3rd ed.). Philadelphia, PA: FA Davis Company.

Panjabi, M. M. (1992). The stabilizing system of the spine. Part I. Function, dysfunction, adaptation, and enhancement. *Journal of Spinal Disorders & Techniques, 5,* 383–389; discussion 397.

Patton, K., & Thibodeau, G. (2015). *The human body in health and disease* (6th ed.). New York, NY: Elsevier Science Health Science.

Richardson, C., Jull, G., Hodges, P., & Hides, J. (1999). *Therapeutic exercise for spinal segmental stabilization in low back pain*. London, UK: Churchill Livingstone.

Schmidt, R. A., & Lee, T. D. (1999). *Motor control and learning: A behavioral emphasis* (3rd ed.). Champaign, IL: Human Kinetics.

Schmidt, R. A., & Wrisberg, C. A. (2000). *Motor learning and performance* (2nd ed.). Champaign, IL: Human Kinetics.

Sharp, J. T., Goldberg, N. B., Druz, W. S., & Danon, J. (1975). Relative contributions of rib cage and abdomen to breathing in normal subjects. *Journal of Applied Physiology, 39,* 608–619.

Solomonow, M., Baratta, R., Zhou, B. H., Shoji, H., Bose, W., Beck, C., & D'Ambrosia, R. (1987). The synergistic action of the anterior cruciate ligament and thigh muscles in maintaining joint stability. *American Journal of Sports Medicine, 15,* 207–213.

Swain, D. P. (2006). Cardiorespiratory exercise prescription. In American College of Sports Medicine (Ed.), *ACSM's resource manual for guidelines for exercise testing and prescription* (6th ed.; pp. 448–462). Baltimore, MD: Lippincott Williams & Wilkins.

Swanson, R. L., (2013). Biotensegrity: A unifying theory of biological architecture with applications to osteopathic practice, education, and research—a review and analysis. *Journal of the American Osteopathic Association, 113,* 34–52.

Timmons, B. (1994). *Behavioral and psychological approaches to breathing disorders*. New York, NY: Plenum Press; 1994.

Tortora, G. J. (2001). *Principles of human anatomy* (9th ed.). New York, NY: John Wiley & Sons.

Tortora, G. J., & Nielsen, M. (2008). *Principles of human anatomy* (11th ed.). New York, NY: Wiley.

Tortora, G. J., & Grabowski, S. R. (1996). *Principles of anatomy and physiology* (8th ed.). New York, NY: HarperCollins.

Vander, A., Sherman, J., & Luciano, D. (2001). *Human physiology: The mechanisms of body function* (8th ed.). New York, NY: McGraw-Hill.

Vander, A., Sherman, J., & Luciano, D. (2003). *Human physiology: The mechanisms of body function* (9th ed.). New York, NY: McGraw-Hill.

Watkins, J. (1999). *Structure and function of the musculoskeletal system*. Champaign, IL: Human Kinetics.

Wilmore, J. H., & Costill, D. L. (2004). *Physiology of sport and exercise*. Champaign, IL: Human Kinetics.

CHAPTER 5

CLIENT-BASED NUTRITION SCIENCES

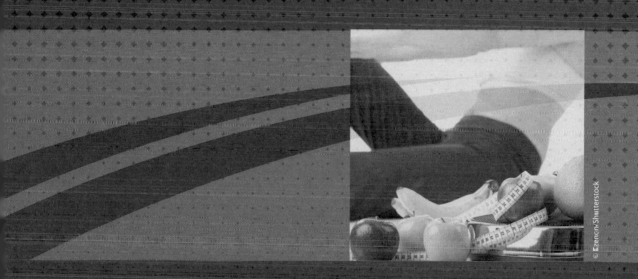
© Ezenen/Shutterstock

OBJECTIVES

After studying this chapter, you will be able to:

1 **Describe** the structure and function of macronutrients.

2 **Describe** the role of water in the function of the body.

3 **Describe** the role macronutrients play in everyday satiation and performance.

4 **Use** scientific laws to explain basic weight loss and weight gain.

5 **Analyze** components on food labels and government nutrition guidelines.

6 **Explain** foundational supplementation concepts.

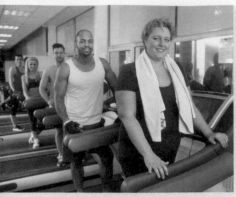

© StockLite/Shutterstock

Case Scenario

Jennifer, a potential client, has expressed in casual conversation her interest in losing weight for an upcoming wedding that she will be attending in 4 months. Although she has not been tracking her daily food intake, Jennifer says that she feels that she eats healthy but that she cannot seem to lose weight, even with the 2-mile walk she takes daily after work. Without offending Jennifer, you ask her how much weight she wants to lose and get a reply of 20 pounds. With the wedding just around the corner, Jennifer wants to get started to ensure she reaches her weight loss goal and provides you with the following information about herself:

- Age: 35

- Weight: 170 pounds

- Height: 5′6″

- Health issues: None

As you continue your conversation with Jennifer, she tells you that she has been told to avoid carbohydrates in order to lose weight, but has done so with no success. With the wedding rapidly approaching, she has begun to research diet and meal plans found on the Internet that guarantee success but involve purchasing a monthly membership.

- What additional information would you need from Jennifer to get a better understanding on how you could possibly help her with her weight loss goal?

- How will you consult, educate, and coach Jennifer on her nutrition needs while remaining within a fitness professional's scope of practice?

Introduction to Fitness-Based Nutrition

CAUTION

In most states only licensed professionals or registered dieticians can legally provide nutritional counseling and dietary prescriptions to consumers.

The science of nutrition originated from the study of nutrient deficiencies, such as scurvy resulting from a deficiency of vitamin C. Nutrition is a young science founded in disciplines such as biochemistry, physiology, psychology, food science, and others. Today, the field has evolved to include other areas, such as disease prevention, weight loss, sociology, and sports nutrition. Nutrition is an evolving and quickly changing science. As new research is conducted, new information provides fresh insights. Public guidelines and recommendations are then changed to reflect this information. However, sometimes new information is misinterpreted by the general public, leading to confusion and misinformation. Therefore, it is important to rely on licensed professionals, such as registered dietitians, to communicate and interpret the science behind the research findings. In most states only licensed or registered dietitians can legally provide nutritional counseling and diet prescription. However, it is critical for fitness professionals to stay current on nutrition research and guidelines throughout their careers by attending conferences and reading publications by reputable organizations. Staying up-to-date on nutrition information is important for engaging in informed discussions with clients—this is the extent of the fitness professional's scope of practice. That being said, it is the intent of this chapter to provide the fitness professional with a foundation in nutrition to better inform discussions with clients and to benefit one's own health and well-being.

A **calorie** is a scientific unit of energy. The calories used to measure food energy are also called **kilocalories**, or kcals. The scientific definition of a kilocalorie is the amount of energy needed to raise the temperature of 1 kilogram of water 1 degree Celsius. In nutrition, when discussing how many calories are in in a particular food or drink, this is referring to how much energy is released by the nutrients in that food once the food has been digested and absorbed. The nutrients that provide calories are called **macronutrients**, and include carbohydrates, fats, and proteins.

Carbohydrates

For the general public, one of the most misunderstood of all the nutrients is carbohydrates. They are eliminated as part of many weight loss programs, blamed for the obesity epidemic, and said to cause diseases like diabetes. The truth is that they supply much-needed energy (4 calories per gram), they spare protein, and they help to maintain blood sugar. Carbohydrates are a diverse class of nutrients, and each specific type has particular health benefits. Therefore, the type of carbohydrate one consumes is important. Whereas sugar in excess can lead to obesity and diabetes, fiber helps to maintain gastrointestinal health and may have a role in preventing colon cancer (Otles & Ozqoz, 2014).

Structure of Carbohydrates

Carbohydrates are made up of carbon and water and are categorized as either simple or complex based on how many carbon/water units they contain. A carbohydrate with more than 10 carbon/water units is a **complex carbohydrate**. Complex carbohydrates include the fiber and starch found in whole grains and vegetables. A carbohydrate with less than 10 carbon/water units is a **simple carbohydrate**. These may be categorized as monosaccharides or disaccharides. Monosaccharides are made up of a single sugar unit and include **glucose** (blood sugar), **fructose** (found in fruit, honey, and some vegetables), and **galactose** (part of lactose). Disaccharides are made up of two sugar units and include **sucrose** (table sugar), **lactose** (sugar in dairy products), and **maltose** (rare in our food supply). See **Table 5.1** for a summary of some food sources of simple and complex carbohydrates.

Function of Carbohydrates

The human body stores a very limited amount of carbohydrates in the liver and the skeletal muscle in the form of **glycogen**. Liver glycogen helps to maintain **blood glucose**, the sugar that is transported in the blood to supply energy to the body, including fueling the brain and other cells in the body that cannot use fat as a fuel. Because these carbohydrate supplies are limited, they must be restored on a regular basis. The liver's glycogen stores can be depleted overnight or during a 90-minute endurance activity. When glycogen stores are depleted, the

Calorie

A scientific unit of energy.

Kilocalorie

A unit of energy equal to 1,000 calories. It is the amount of heat energy required to raise the temperature of a kilogram or liter of water by 1 degree Celsius.

Macronutrients

Nutrients that provide calories.

Complex carbohydrate

A carbohydrate with more than 10 carbon/water units. Includes the fiber and starch found in whole grains and vegetables.

Simple carbohydrate

A carbohydrate with fewer than 10 carbon/water units. Includes glucose, sucrose, lactose, galactose, maltose, and fructose.

Glucose

A simple sugar manufactured by the body from carbohydrates, fat, and (to a lesser extent) protein that serves as the body's main source of fuel.

Fructose

Known as fruit sugar; found in fruits, honey, syrups, and certain vegetables.

Galactose

Combines with glucose in lactose.

Sucrose

Often referred to as table sugar, it is a molecule made up of glucose and fructose.

MEMORY TIPS

You can use the mnemonic "Super Fun and Loud Margie Gets Gum" to remember the simple carbohydrates: **s**ucrose, **f**ructose, **l**actose, **m**altose, **g**lucose, and **g**alactose.

TABLE 5.1 Sources of Complex and Simple Carbohydrates

Carbohydrate Type	Food Sources
Complex	
Starches	Grains, wheat, rice, corn, oats, potatoes, pasta, peas
Fiber	*Soluble:* Nuts, apples, blueberries, oatmeal, beans *Insoluble:* Bran, brown rice, fruit skins
Simple	
Disaccharides	Table sugar (sucrose), milk (lactose), ice cream (lactose), beer (maltose), sweet potatoes (maltose), molasses (maltose)
Monosaccharaides	Glucose, fructose, galactose

Lactose

A sugar present in milk that is composed of glucose and galactose.

Maltose

Sugar produced in the breakdown of starch. Rare in our food supply.

Glycogen

A complex carbohydrate that is stored in the liver and muscle cells. When carbohydrate energy is needed, glycogen is converted into glucose for use by the muscle cells.

Blood glucose

Also referred to as "blood sugar"; the sugar that is transported in the body to supply energy to the body's cells, including fueling the brain and other cells in the body that cannot use fat as a fuel.

High-fructose corn syrup (HFCS)

A sweetener made from cornstarch and converted to fructose in food processing.

liver will break down other substances to maintain blood glucose. Initially it will primarily break down protein. Therefore, one of the primary functions of carbohydrates is to spare protein.

Carbohydrates are an important fuel during exercise. They are an important part of sports nutrition before, during, and following exercise. They are the predominant fuel source during high-intensity activities such as sprinting. As mentioned earlier, carbohydrates are stored in small amounts in the muscle and liver and can be depleted during prolonged, intense exercise lasting longer than 60–90 minutes. The availability of carbohydrates as a fuel for muscle contraction and the central nervous system, especially the brain, makes it critical for optimal exercise performance (Burke, Hawley, Wange, & Jeukendrup, 2011).

High-Fructose Corn Syrup

Part of the controversy surrounding carbohydrates is related to recent evidence that a large portion of carbohydrate intake in the United States comes from simple sugars, especially those used in snack foods and sweetened beverages. One of the primary contributors to this high sugar intake is **high-fructose corn syrup (HFCS)**, which is made from cornstarch and converted to fructose in food processing. It is used in processed foods as a cheap sweetener and is abundant in diets heavy in processed foods. Its prevalence has been linked to the increase in obesity rates, causing many manufacturers to develop HFCS-free foods in response to consumer pressure. Although evidence suggests that any impact consuming products with HFCS in them has on obesity or related diseases is similar to that of consuming sucrose and is more related to the added calories these sugars provide than anything unique about HFCS, many countries have banned it (Johnston et al., 2013). The best way to limit or completely avoid HFCS is to consume a diet high in fruits, vegetables, and other natural foods and to avoid processed foods. Much debate remains as to whether there is a direct link between HFCS and obesity, but the public health messages to consume more fruits and vegetables that have come from the attention to this issue are beneficial regardless (Rippe, 2013).

Recommended Intake of Carbohydrates

Some debate surrounds the recommended intake for carbohydrates. When expressed as a percentage of total calories, it is recommended that adults consume 45–65% of their total calories from carbohydrates, primarily as complex carbohydrates and whole grains (Food and Nutrition

Board of the Institutes of Medicine, 2005). This wide range accounts for the variation in the amount needed based on a person's activity level. Individuals exercising more than 60–90 minutes a day or athletes training twice a day need more carbohydrates than an individual sitting at a desk all day with minimal activity. Carbohydrate intake may also be expressed in grams per kilogram of body weight (weight in pounds/2.2 = weight in kilograms). Inactive individuals only need around 3 grams per kilogram per day, those exercising for more than an hour likely need 4–5 grams per kilogram body weight per day, and athletes who are training intensely may need as much as 8–12 grams per kilogram body weight. These recommendations are based on research on carbohydrate intake and optimal performance in athletes. However, many athletes and fitness enthusiasts reach a healthy weight and optimal performance on different levels of carbohydrate intake. The recommendations provide a place to start, but each individual must find what works best for his or her particular goal (Burke et al., 2011).

Importance of Carbohydrate Type

As mentioned earlier, the type of carbohydrate one consumes has important health implications. Carbohydrates are naturally present in almost all plant foods such as fruits, vegetables, grains, and legumes, and in milk, primarily as complex carbohydrates. The majority of carbohydrates added to processed foods is in the form of simple sugar. It is advised that most, if not all carbohydrates come from complex carbohydrates such as vegetables, grains, pasta, and rice. Eating whole-grain varieties of these foods is optimal and will provide more nutrients and more fiber than consuming highly processed varieties of the same food. For example, brown rice has more nutrients and fiber than white rice, and is therefore the healthier option. All rice starts high in nutrients, but during processing the outer parts of the kernel are removed, leaving the white inner part, which has calories but does not have the same level of nutrients, even when enriched. The same is true of wheat and grains—brown, whole-grain varieties are a healthier choice than the white, highly processed versions. The concept of consuming more nutrients per calorie is called **nutrient density**. It is ideal for everyone to consume most of their foods from very nutrient-dense foods, and it is especially beneficial for those trying to lose weight. See **Table 5.2** for information on the nutrient density of different foods.

Protein

Another macronutrient that provides calories is protein. **Proteins** are long chains of amino acids with nitrogen attached. Recommendations for protein intake and its potential role in weight loss have received much attention in the media. Protein has been promoted as the main nutrient required by the body, and given a reputation as a "cure all," of which you can never have too much. Although crucial to human health, muscular growth, and maintenance of soft tissues, protein alone does not promote optimal health or cure a myriad of weight and health problems as some would like to believe. Protein is, however, an important part of a balanced diet and a vital macronutrient.

Protein Structure

Like carbohydrates and fats, proteins contain carbon, hydrogen, and oxygen, but they differ in that they also contain nitrogen. Proteins are made up of a combination of **amino acids** linked together (**Table 5.3**). **Essential amino acids** are those that cannot be made by the body and

---

TRAINER TIPS

Consuming more whole, natural foods and avoiding processed foods is a simple message with a lot of health-related impact. Following this advice automatically minimizes the consumption of HFCS as well as sodium, saturated fats, trans fats, preservatives, and even extra calories, while increasing consumption of foods high in nutrients.

Nutrient density
The nutrient content of a food relative to its calories.

Protein
Long chains of amino acids linked by peptide bonds. Serve several essential functional roles in the body.

Amino acids
The building blocks of proteins; composed of a central carbon atom, a hydrogen atom, an amino group, a carboxyl group, and an R-group.

Essential amino acids
Amino acids that cannot be produced by the body and must be acquired by food.

TABLE 5.2 Nutrient Density

HIGH NUTRIENT DENSITY (Good)	Nonstarchy vegetables (raw leafy green veggies > solid green veggies > all other nonstarchy vegetables)
	Beans
	Fresh fruits
	Starchy vegetables
	Whole grains
	Raw nuts and seeds
	Fish
	Fat-free dairy
	Poultry
	Eggs
LOW NUTRIENT DENSITY (Not as good)	Red meat
	Full-fat dairy
	Cheese
	Refined grains—crackers, chips, white pasta, etc.
	Oils
	Refined sweets—sugar, baked goods, candy, soda

Green = eat frequently   Yellow = eat keeping portions in mind   Red = eat sparingly

TABLE 5.3 Amino Acids

Essential	Nonessential	Conditionally Essential
Isoleucine	Alanine	Arginine
Leucine	Asparagine	Histidine
Lysine	Aspartic acid	
Methionine	Cysteine	
Phenylalanine	Glutamic acid	
Threonine	Glutamine	
Tryptophan	Glycine	
Valine	Proline	
	Serine	
	Tyrosine	

therefore must be acquired in food. If essential amino acids are not consumed in adequate amounts, the body cannot make the proteins it needs for growth, maintenance, repair, or any of its other functions without breaking down skeletal muscle. **Nonessential amino acids** are also needed by the body, but the body can make them so they do not have to be consumed. In some disease conditions nonessential amino acids cannot be made by the body, and they become **conditionally essential amino acids**.

Functions of Proteins

Protein is best known for its role in muscle growth and repair. However, it also plays a vital role in the development, maintenance, and repair of all tissues in the body. It is involved in fluid balance, blood clotting, enzyme production, acid–base balance, immune function, and hormone regulation, and it serves as a carrier for several nutrients. Protein also supplies energy (4 calories per gram), but providing energy is not its primary function.

Protein also plays a critical role in the function of many cells and enzymes in the body. For example, the cells that line the intestine are replaced about every 3 days. Red blood cells live approximately 4 months, and skin cells are constantly replaced by new skin. All of this requires protein, and if cell turnover is increased by illness or stress, protein needs can increase.

Recommended Protein Intake

The Dietary Reference Intake (DRI) for protein is 0.8 grams per kilogram of body weight per day (USDA, 2010). When expressed as a percentage of total calories, the recommendation is that 10–35% of an individual's daily calories should come from protein. As mentioned earlier, however, there is some debate in the nutrition field with regard to protein intake recommendations. Many researchers suggest that the current recommendations are based on outdated methodology and are too low. They contend that new research has shown that certain groups, such as the elderly and athletes, require more protein than is currently recommended (Wolfe, 2012). Individuals regularly participating in endurance and/or resistance exercise require more protein than sedentary individuals (Phillips & Van Loon, 2011). Recommendations are 1.2–1.4 grams per kilogram body weight for endurance athletes and 1.6–1.7 grams per kilogram body weight for strength athletes. Most athletes naturally consume adequate amounts of protein regardless of recommendations (Jeukendrup & Gleeson, 2010).

Food Sources of Protein

A **complete protein** is one that provides all of the essential amino acids in the amount the body needs and that is also easy to digest and absorb. Typically animal proteins like those found in meats, eggs, and dairy products and the vegetable protein in soy are considered highly digestible complete proteins. Foods that do not contain all of the essential amino acids in the amount needed by the body are called **incomplete proteins**. These include beans, legumes, grains, and vegetables. People who do not eat meat and dairy products can still consume an adequate intake of complete proteins by combining incomplete proteins called **complementary proteins**. An example of this is eating rice and beans; beans are low in the amino acid lysine, but rice is rich in lysine. Putting beans and rice together creates a complete protein (Hewlings & Medeiros, 2011). **Table 5.4** lists some good dietary sources of protein.

Nonessential amino acids
Amino acids that are produced by the body and do not need to be consumed in dietary sources.

Conditionally essential amino acids
Nonessential amino acids that cannot be produced due to disease and as a result must be acquired in dietary sources.

Complete protein
A protein that provides all of the essential amino acids in the amount the body needs and is also easy to digest and absorb; also called a *high-quality protein*.

Incomplete protein
Food that does not contain all of the essential amino acids in the amount needed by the body.

Complementary proteins
Consuming two or more incomplete proteins together to provide needed amino acids.

Lipids

A group of compounds that includes triglycerides (fats and oils), phospholipids, and sterols.

Fatty acid

A chain of carbons linked or bonded together, and the building blocks of fat within the human body.

Triglyceride

The chemical or substrate form in which most fat exists in food as well as in the body.

Phospholipid

Type of lipid in which one fatty acid has been replaced by a phosphate group and one of several nitrogen-containing molecules.

Sterols

A subgroup of the steroids and an important class of organic molecules.

Carboxyl group (–COOH)

A carbon atom joined to a hydroxyl group by a single bond and to an oxygen atom by a double bond.

Methyl group (–CH$_3$)

An alkyl derived from methane that has one carbon atom bonded to three hydrogen atoms.

TABLE 5.4 Complete Protein Food Sources

Whole egg	Yogurt and granola
Milk and milk products	Oatmeal with milk
Meat and poultry	Lentils and bread
Fish	Tortillas with beans or bean burritos
Rice and beans	Macaroni and cheese
Peanut butter on whole-wheat bread	Hummus (chickpeas and sesame paste) with bread
Sunflower seeds and peanuts	Bean soup with whole-grain crackers

Fat

In addition to carbohydrates and proteins, fats also provide energy to the body. Fats are also called **lipids** and are defined as substances that are insoluble in water. Lipids include **fatty acids**, **triglycerides**, **phospholipids**, and **sterols** such as cholesterol. Triglycerides, which contain fatty acids, are found in foods such as meat, butter, and nuts. The fat stored in our bodies is mostly in the form of triglycerides.

Structure of Fat

Like carbohydrates, lipids are composed of carbon, hydrogen, and oxygen, but they contain almost twice as many hydrogen atoms. This is why lipids provide almost twice as much energy as carbohydrates—9 calories per gram, compared to the 4 calories per gram that carbohydrates provide.

Fatty acids are chains of carbon that are linked or bonded together. One end of the fatty acid has a **carboxyl group** (–COOH), which allows the fatty acid to mix with water. The other end has a **methyl group**, represented by –CH$_3$, which does not mix with water but does mix with other fats in the body.

Fats are classified based on their *saturation*. A **saturated fat** consists of a chain of carbons that is saturated with all of the hydrogens it can hold; there are no double bonds. Another prevalent fatty acid in today's food supply is trans-fatty acids. These are the result of hydrogenation (the process of adding hydrogen to unsaturated fatty acids to make them harder at room temperature and increase food shelf-life). Some fatty acids have areas that are not completely saturated with hydrogens, and therefore have double bonds where the hydrogens are missing. These fatty acids are called **unsaturated fatty acids**. A fatty acid with just one missing hydrogen is a *monounsaturated fatty acid*. If there are several spots where hydrogens are missing, it is referred to as a **polyunsaturated fatty acid**. The level of saturation has important health implications, which is why it is important to understand this classification. In addition, it is also important where in the chain the double bonds occur, because the location of the double bonds influence the function of a fatty acid in the body. There are two types of polyunsaturated fatty acids: **omega 3** and **omega 6**. Omega-3 fatty acids have anti-inflammatory affects and help to decrease blood clotting. Omega-6 fatty acids promote blood clotting and cell membrane formation. Maintaining the proper ratio of these two fatty acids

TABLE 5.5 Food Sources and Types of Fats			
Monounsaturated Fats	**Polyunsaturated Fats**	**Saturated Fats**	**Trans-Fats**
Olive oil, canola oil, peanut oil, sesame oil, safflower, avocados, peanuts, almonds, pistachios	Vegetable oils: soy, corn, and sunflower oils Omega-3 fatty acids: herring, mackerel, salmon, sardines, flaxseeds Walnuts	Meat, poultry, lard, butter, cheese, cream, eggs, whole milk Tropical oils: coconut oil, palm, and palm kernel oil Many baked goods	Stick margarine, shortening Fried foods: fried chicken, doughnuts Fast food Many baked goods and pastries

is important in maintaining health. **Table 5.5** lists common food sources for the various types of dietary fats.

A triglyceride is the primary form of fat found in food and in the body. It is composed of a **glycerol** molecule with three fatty acids attached. A phospholipid is very similar to a triglyceride but instead of the third fatty acid it has a phosphate group attached, which allows it to mix with water, as well as blood. The ability of a fat to mix with water is called **emulsification**. In food processing, many manufacturers will add the emulsifier lecithin found in eggs to mix oil and water. Sterols are very different structurally. The best known sterol is cholesterol, but many hormones, including testosterone and estrogen, are also sterols. They play an important role in health but are not needed in the food supply because they are made in the body.

Functions of Fat

Lipids serve many functions in the body, including storing energy, supplying essential fatty acids, absorbing and transporting fat-soluble vitamins, protecting and insulating vital organs, adding satiety and flavor in food, providing cell membrane structure, and serving as a precursor for steroid hormones.

Fats are the major source of energy in the body. The typical adult male of normal weight and body fat has 100,000 calories of stored fat. In comparison, he will only have about 1,500 calories of stored carbohydrate. It is a dense source of calories, supplying more than double the calories of carbohydrates and protein at 9 calories per gram (Hewlings & Medeiros, 2011).

Recommended Intake of Fat

Adults age 19 and older should consume 20–35% of their total calories from fat (Food and Nutrition Board of the Institutes of Medicine, 2005). The types of fats consumed, rather than the total amount of fat, is an important influence on the risk of cardiovascular and other diseases. Animal fats tend to have a higher proportion of saturated fatty acids than plant-based foods (Hewlings & Medeiros, 2011). A strong body of evidence indicates that a higher intake of saturated fats in the diet is associated with increased levels of total blood cholesterol and **low-density lipoprotein (LDL) cholesterol.** LDL is the molecule that carries lipids throughout the body and delivers cholesterol, which can accumulate on artery walls. Higher total and LDL cholesterol are risk factors for heart disease. Therefore, it is recommended that adults consume less than 10% of their total calories from saturated fats, replacing them with polyunsaturated and monounsaturated fats.

Saturated fat
A chain of carbons that is saturated with all of the hydrogens that it can hold; there are no double bonds.

Unsaturated fatty acids
Fatty acids that have areas that are not completely saturated with hydrogens, and therefore have double bonds where the hydrogen is missing.

Polyunsaturated fatty acids
Fatty acids that have several spots where hydrogens are missing.

Omega-3 fatty acids
Fatty acids that have anti-inflammatory effects and help to decrease blood clotting.

Omega-6 fatty acids
Fatty acids that promote blood clotting and cell membrane formation.

Glycerol
A simple polyol (sugar alcohol) compound. It is a colorless, odorless, viscous liquid. The glycerol backbone is central to all lipids known as triglycerides.

TABLE 5.6 Macronutrient Intake Recommendations	
Macronutrient	**Recommended Intake**
Carbohydrate	
General population	45–65% total daily calories OR 3 g/kg body weight per day
Those exercising more than 1 hour per day	4–5 g/kg body weight per day
Athletes or high-intensity exercisers	8–12 g/kg body weight per day
Protein	
General population	0.8 g/kg OR 10–35% total daily calories
Endurance athletes	1.2–1.4 g/kg body weight per day
Strength athletes	1.6–1.7 g/kg body weight per day
Fat	
Total consumption	20–35% total daily calories
Saturated fat	Less than 10% total daily calories

Data from: Food and Nutrition Board of the Institute of Medicine (2005); Jeukendrup & Gleeson, 2010

Food Sources of Fats

Meat, cheese, butter, egg yolks, whole milk, and creamy sauces and soups are all sources of saturated fat. Vegetable oils, such as soybean, corn, and sunflower oils, and fish, especially salmon and cold water fish, as well as flaxseed and walnuts, are good sources of polyunsaturated fatty acids. Olive, canola, peanut, safflower, and sesame oils, as well as nuts and avocados, are good sources of monounsaturated fatty acids.

Table 5.6 provides a summary of the recommended intakes of the three macronutrients.

Vitamins and Minerals

Vitamins and minerals are often referred to as *micronutrients* because they are required in smaller amounts than the macronutrients. This does not mean that they have a less important role in maintaining health. In fact, they are essential to health and vitality because of the important roles they play in every function in the body. For example, even though they do not themselves provide energy, they play a critical role in the body's ability to obtain energy from carbohydrates, fats, and proteins. Iron, for example, plays an important role in transporting oxygen through the blood to the working muscles.

The recommended amounts of essential vitamins and minerals can be obtained through a healthy diet with lots of vegetables, fruits, whole grains, fat-free dairy, and lean meats (Harvard Health, 2015). However, many people feel they are unable to eat healthy every day, and therefore choose to take a multivitamin that will supply 100% of the recommended vitamins and minerals. Multivitamins are fine if taken as a supplement to a healthy diet, but they should not be considered a replacement for a healthy diet. Many components in foods, such as **phytochemicals** and fiber, cannot be substituted by a dietary supplement. Furthermore, taking multivitamins that are greater than 100% of what is recommended and/or using many additional individual vitamin and mineral supplements introduces the risk of **toxicity** and/or

Emulsification

The ability of a fat to mix with water.

Low-density lipoprotein (LDL)

The molecule that carries lipids throughout the body and delivers cholesterol that can accumulate on artery walls.

Phytochemicals

Biologically active compounds found in plants.

Toxicity

The degree to which a substance can cause damage to an organism.

of having too much of one nutrient interfere with the absorption of another. For example, too much niacin can lead to flushing and burning of the skin, and excess iron can lead to cirrhosis of the liver. Although intense physical activity may increase the need for some vitamins, such as vitamins C, B_2, and possibly B_6, A, and E, the increased requirements can be met by consuming a healthy balanced diet that meets an athlete's caloric needs (Jeukendrup & Gleeson, 2010). Fitness professionals should encourage their clients to consume a healthy balanced diet to obtain the necessary vitamins and minerals and not to rely on supplements.

Tables 5.7 and 5.8 provide a brief overview of some of the major functions of important vitamins and minerals and good food sources for each. Fitness professionals can use this information in encouraging clients to obtain the vitamins and minerals they need from a balanced diet.

TABLE 5.7 Major Functions of Vitamins in the Body and Good Food Sources

Vitamin	Role in Body	Good Food Sources
Vitamin A	Essential for proper development and maintenance of eyes and vision. Needed to maintain integrity of skin, digestive tract, and other tissues. Required for proper immune system function. Support of cell differentiation.	Eggs Vitamin A–fortified dairy products Green, leafy vegetables
Beta-carotene (provitamin A)	Antioxidant role. Like other provitamin A carotenoids (alpha-carotene and beta-cryptoxanthin), can be converted to vitamin A in the body.	Sweet potatoes Carrots Pumpkin
Vitamin D	Helps maintain calcium in the blood by increasing calcium absorption in the digestive tract and decreasing calcium loss in urine.	Milk Salmon Tuna
Vitamin E	Antioxidant role. Protects red blood cells, muscles, and other tissues from free-radical damage.	Vegetable oil Wheat germ Nuts
Vitamin K	Necessary for normal blood clotting. Required for strong bones.	Collards and kale Spinach Brussel sprouts
Vitamin C (ascorbic acid)	Antioxidant role. Involved in collagen formation. Aids in iron absorption.	Oranges and other citrus fruits Green peppers Broccoli (cooked)
Thiamin (vitamin B_1)	Coenzyme for several reactions in energy metabolism. Necessary for muscle coordination and proper development and maintenance of central nervous system.	Cereal and grains Pork Nuts and seeds
Riboflavin (vitamin B_2)	Coenzyme for several reactions in energy metabolism.	Milk and yogurt Green, leafy vegetables Eggs
Niacin (vitamin B_3)	Coenzyme for several reactions in energy metabolism. In very large doses, lowers cholesterol. (Note: Large doses should only be taken under physician supervision.)	Peanuts, roasted Tuna Whole grains

(continues)

TABLE 5.7   Major Functions of Vitamins in the Body and Good Food Sources (*cont.*)

Vitamin	Role in Body	Good Food Sources
Vitamin B$_6$ (pyridoxine)	Coenzyme for reactions involved in amino acid processing. Aids in breakdown of carbohydrate stores (glycogen) in muscles and liver.	Fish Beans and peas Spinach and greens Bananas
Folic acid (folacin)	Essential for manufacture of genetic material. Aids in red blood cell formation. Required for cell division.	Asparagus Brussel sprouts Spinach Cantaloupe Whole grains
Vitamin B$_{12}$ (cobalamin)	Essential for proper DNA synthesis and regulation. Helps form red blood cells. Maintains myelin sheath of nerves.	Meat and seafood Milk products Eggs
Pantothenic acid	Coenzyme for reactions involved in energy metabolism.	Abundant in many foods
Biotin	Energy metabolism	Abundant in many foods

Adapted with permission from Hewlings, S. H., & Medeiros, D. M. (2011). *Nutrition: Real people real choices*. Dubuque, IA: Kendall Hunt.

TABLE 5.8   Major Functions of Minerals in the Body and Good Food Sources

Mineral	Role in Body	Food Sources
Calcium	Component of mineral crystals in bone and teeth. Involved in muscle contraction, initiation of heartbeat, blood clotting, and release and function of several hormones and neurotransmitters.	Yogurt Milk Green, leafy vegetables Legumes
Phosphorus	As phosphate, a component of mineral crystals in bone and teeth. Component of high-energy molecules in cells (ATP, CP). Found in cell membranes.	Nuts and seeds Milk Meat
Magnesium	Involved in energy metabolism. Component of many different enzymes.	Nuts Grains Split peas
Iron	Component of heme structure found in hemoglobin, myoglobin, and cytochromes that transports oxygen in blood or stores and handles oxygen in cells. Found in molecules involved in collagen production and energy metabolism. Antioxidant properties.	Meat Prune juice Spinach Fortified cereals
Zinc	Component of numerous enzymes.	Raw oysters Meat Pecans Wheat germ
Copper	Component of several enzymes involved in energy metabolism. Antioxidant activity. Plays role in collagen production and hormone and neurotransmitter production.	Beef liver Oysters Clams (cooked)

TABLE 5.8 Major Functions of Minerals in the Body and Good Food Sources (*cont.*)		
Mineral	**Role in Body**	**Food Sources**
Selenium	Component of antioxidant enzymes. Involved in thyroid hormone function.	Tuna Brown rice Eggs
Iodine	Component in thyroid hormone.	Codfish Iodized salt Shrimp
Fluoride	Involved in strengthening teeth and bones.	Shrimp (canned) Fluoridated water Carrots (cooked)
Chromium	Involved in glucose metabolism.	Broccoli Grape juice Potatoes (mashed)
Sodium	Promotes blood volume balance. Nerve impulse generation. Muscle contraction. Acid–base balance.	Processed foods Table salt Soy sauce Soups
Potassium	Cell membrane balance. Nervous impulse generation. Muscle contraction. Acid–base balance.	Potatoes Bananas Avocado Bran

Adapted with permission from Hewlings, S. H., & Medeiros, D. M. (2011). *Nutrition: Real people real choices*. Dubuque, IA: Kendall Hunt.

If a client suggests she is considering taking vitamin C to prevent a cold, the fitness professional can suggest she consume plenty of fresh fruits and vegetables high in vitamin C, including citrus fruits and broccoli. However, it is not within the fitness professionals' scope of practice to prescribe diets or supplements to their clients.

Additional information on vitamins and minerals can be found on the USDA website at https://fnic.nal.usda.gov/food-composition/vitamins-and-minerals. A list of Dietary Reference Intakes (DRIs) can be located at https://fnic.nal.usda.gov/dietary-guidance/dietary-reference-intakes.

Alcohol

Alcohol provides 7 calories per gram, and therefore contributes to energy intake. When metabolized by the body, alcohol yields energy, but it does not provide vitamins, minerals, or contribute to the body's growth and maintenance. Because alcohol has other properties that can damage health and well-being, it is not classified as a nutrient. Although some cardiovascular health benefits have been associated with moderate intake, particularly of red wines, the negative health outcomes of excessive intake far outweigh the modest suggested benefits. This is mostly because the term *moderation* is "loosely" interpreted. Moderate alcohol consumption is defined as one drink per day for women and up to two drinks per day for men. A drink is defined as one 5-ounce glass of wine, one 12-ounce beer, or one 1-ounce shot of hard liquor. Any health

TRAINER TIPS ⫟⫟⫟

If clients complain they are not losing weight despite sticking to a healthy diet and exercise routine, alcohol may be to blame as a source of extra unneeded calories.

Chemical energy

Energy contained in a molecule that has not yet been released in carbohydrates, fats, and proteins.

Metabolism

All of the chemical reactions that occur in the body that are required for life. It is the process by which nutrients are acquired, transported, used, and disposed of by the body.

Adenosine triphosphate (ATP)

Energy storage and transfer unit within the cells of the body.

Catabolism

A metabolic process that breaks down molecules.

Anabolism

A metabolic process that builds molecules.

benefits associated with alcohol consumption can be obtained by other sources. For example, consuming grape juice, berries, or pomegranates regularly can provide similar health benefits provided by drinking a glass of red wine daily, without the potential negative health consequences (Hewlings & Medeiros, 2011).

Metabolism

A car must have fuel for its engine, a fire must have wood to burn, and the human body must have a constant supply of energy for its movement and maintenance. It may seem that energy is needed only when the body is moving, but the body requires a constant input of energy to maintain basic life activities, such as contraction of the heart and the rise and fall of the lungs.

Although carbohydrates, fats, and proteins all provide calories, they do not provide usable energy simply by their ingestion. After food is ingested and the nutrients are absorbed, several chemical reactions must take place in the body before the food becomes usable energy. The energy in food is **chemical energy**, or energy contained in a molecule that has not yet been released, in carbohydrates, fats, and proteins.

Turning chemical energy into a form the body can use requires a series of chemical reactions called metabolism. **Metabolism** is the sum of biochemical reactions that occur in the cells of the body to obtain usable energy from food in the form of **adenosine triphosphate (ATP)**. The processes of metabolism does more than just break down molecules for energy, or **catabolism**. They can also go in the other direction and build molecules, a process called **anabolism**. The body is in a constant state of breakdown and buildup. If an individual's weight remains relatively stable, then, overall, these pathways are in balance. An example of an anabolic process is the building of muscle through **protein synthesis**. An example of a catabolic process is **glycolysis**, which breaks down glucose to a usable form of energy, or ATP. The body then uses this energy in the muscle contractions required to blink an eye or throw a baseball. These processes are called **metabolic pathways** because they refer to not just one step, but to a series of chemical reactions that either break down or build up compounds in the body. Metabolic processes occur in every cell of the body. An important part of the cell is the **mitochondria**, where most of the energy-producing pathways occur (Hewlings & Medeiros, 2011).

Creation of Usable Forms of Energy

Although carbohydrates, fats, and proteins contain potential energy in the form of chemical energy, the body cannot use it "as is." It must first convert this chemical energy into a usable form, ATP. Vitamins and minerals cannot be broken down to give the body energy, but they play important roles in the pathways used to generate ATP. Before covering the steps molecules stored in carbohydrates, fats, and proteins go through to become usable energy, it is important to recall the **first law of thermodynamics**: energy is neither created nor destroyed, rather it is transferred from one form to another. This is what is occurring in metabolism. Energy, in the form of *electrons*, is transferred from one form to another by the chemical reactions that occur. The ultimate goal of these reactions is to create usable energy for the body. Of course, not all of the potential energy in food consumed is transferred to ATP; some energy is lost as body heat.

Pathways to Energy

The pathway by which ATP is produced depends on the availability of oxygen in the cells. If there is enough oxygen, then **aerobic metabolism** takes place, and large amounts of ATP are produced. If there is not enough oxygen in the cells (e.g., a person is sprinting as hard as possible), then **anaerobic metabolism** occurs, and smaller amounts of ATP are produced. Anaerobic metabolism can occur for only a short time, about 2–3 minutes, before fatigue sets in. The pathway used also depends on the source of potential energy. Any carbohydrates that were consumed are now glucose in the blood and have been delivered to the cells. Similarly, fats are stored as triglycerides, and proteins are contained in the body's tissues.

A third pathway that can generate ATP is the ATP phosphocreatine (ATP-PC) system. Phosphocreatine (a molecule composed of phosphagen and creatine) is stored within the muscles of the human body and can be utilized for short bursts of energy (10–15 seconds) in the absence of oxygen. A phosphagen molecule is transferred from phosphocreatine to an adenosine diphosphate (ADP) molecule to form an ATP molecule for immediate energy use. This system is primarily utilized for activities that require high power or strength, such as sprinting or maximal lifts for low repetitions. Note that this system is activated at the beginning of all physical activities due to its ability to produce energy very rapidly in comparison with the other systems. **Figure 5.1** provides an overview of the energy obtained from the different systems during exercise.

Pathway to Energy: Carbohydrates and Glucose

Once in the cell, glucose is broken down via glycolysis. Glucose will go through many chemical reactions in glycolysis to ultimately become a substance called **pyruvate**. Oxygen is not required for these steps to take place. Throughout this pathway, as glucose changes form, ATP is produced. If enough oxygen is available, once the glucose has become pyruvate, it enters the mitochondria for aerobic metabolism and becomes a substance called **acetyl-CoA**. Many steps in the metabolic pathways can go in either direction, but once pyruvate becomes acetyl-CoA it cannot go back. Now that the pyruvate has become acetyl-CoA it can join with other substances

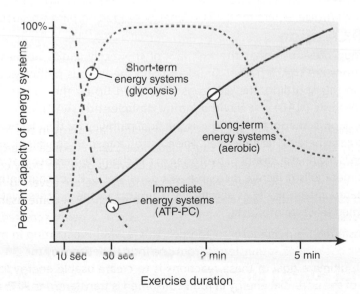

FIGURE 5.1 Energy during exercise.

Protein synthesis

An anabolic process that results in the building of muscle.

Glycolysis

A catabolic process that breaks down glucose to a usable form of energy, ATP.

Metabolic pathway

A series of chemical steps or reactions that either break down or build up compounds in the body.

Mitochondria

Organelle found in the cytoplasm of eukaryotic cells that contains genetic material and enzymes necessary for cell metabolism, converting food to energy.

First law of thermodynamics

Energy can neither be created nor destroyed, only transferred from one form to another.

Aerobic metabolism

Chemical reactions in the body that require the presence of oxygen to extract energy from carbohydrates, fatty acids, and amino acids.

Anaerobic metabolism

Chemical reactions in the body that do not require the presence of oxygen to create energy through the combustion of carbohydrates.

Pyruvate

A byproduct of anaerobic glycolysis that is an intermediate in several metabolic pathways.

Acetyl-CoA

An important molecule in metabolism that is formed as an intermediate in the oxidation of carbohydrates, fats, and proteins. After glucose has become pyruvate, and if there is enough oxygen available, it enters the mitochondria for aerobic metabolism and becomes acetyl-CoA.

Krebs cycle

Central metabolic pathway in all aerobic organisms. The cycle is a series of eight reactions that occur in the mitochondrion. These reactions take a two-carbon molecule (acetate) and completely oxidize it to carbon dioxide.

Tricarboxylic acid (TCA) cycle

Another term for the Krebs cycle. A tricarboxylic acid is an organic carboxylic acid whose chemical structure contains three carboxyl functional groups (−COOH). The best known example of a tricarboxylic acid is citric acid.

Lactate

A byproduct of anaerobic metabolism that occurs when oxygen delivery to the working muscles cannot meet the demands of the tissue.

and start the pathway called the **Krebs cycle** or the **tricarboxylic acid (TCA) cycle.** The Krebs cycle requires oxygen and produces a lot of ATP. If not enough oxygen is available, which occurs when sprinting or when first beginning exercise, a substance called **lactate** is created from the pyruvate. This provides some energy, but not as much as is produced by the Krebs cycle.

Pathway to Energy: Fats and Triglycerides

Fats are stored as triglycerides in the body, and therefore the first step in converting fats to ATP is to break down the triglycerides into fatty acids and glycerol. The glycerol can then be converted to pyruvate or glucose in the liver. The fatty acids are broken down in a pathway called **beta-oxidation** (β-oxidation). In this pathway, enzymes break the carbon chains that make up fatty acids two carbon atoms at a time and convert them to acetyl-CoA, which can then join with other substances and begin the Krebs cycle. The substance that acetyl-CoA joins with is called **oxaloacetate (OAA)**. It is made from carbohydrates, so if carbohydrates are low OAA is also low. Some describe the relationship between fat and carbohydrate metabolism as "fat burns in a carbohydrate flame," meaning that the body needs carbohydrates to burn fats. When carbohydrate supplies are very limited, such as during starvation, uncontrolled diabetes, or while eating a very low carbohydrate diet, fat burning is slowed because OAA is low, and therefore the Krebs cycle is "slower." When this happens, the body forms **ketone bodies**, which can be used as an alternative fuel source, especially for the brain and central nervous system.

Pathway to Energy: Protein and Amino Acids

Under normal circumstances, protein and amino acids are not used to any large extent for energy. However, during starvation or when carbohydrate supplies are limited, amino acids can be used to make ATP. The first step in the breakdown of amino acids is to remove the nitrogen group. This is called **deamination**. Once the nitrogen is removed, the **carbon skeleton** is what remains of the amino acids. The nitrogen is converted to urea and excreted in the urine. Unlike glucose and fatty acids, carbon skeletons can enter the energy-producing pathways at different spots. Depending on which amino acid the carbon skeleton came from, it can enter as pyruvate or acetyl-CoA, or at different places in the Krebs cycle.

Site of ATP Creation

It was mentioned previously that the first law of thermodynamics applies to metabolic reactions. Electrons are transferred or shuttled along the various pathways of metabolism to create ATP. In this shuttling, the electrons are picked up by the carriers **nicotinamide adenine dinucleotide (NAD)** and **flavin adenine dinucleotide (FAD)**, which take the electrons to the **electron transport chain**. This is the final pathway for the electrons and the primary site in the cell where ATP is generated. The electron transport chain is an aerobic process because oxygen is the final acceptor of hydrogen in the chain. Remember that when the body uses anaerobic metabolism, lactate is created as it generates ATP. Consequently, not as much ATP can be created anaerobically as aerobically. Throughout the process, water and carbon dioxide are formed as waste products.

Building and Storing Energy

As has been described, multiple metabolic pathways are used to break down molecules for energy. Remember, however, that the body does not always immediately use the potential energy from food; some of it is used to build or repair tissue or stored for future use. Such pathways, as mentioned previously, are *anabolic*.

Creation of Glucose

Glucose is created in a pathway called **gluconeogenesis**; the term literally means "making new glucose." The body needs a constant supply of glucose to maintain blood glucose levels and to fuel the brain, central nervous system, and red blood cells. During periods of starvation or when carbohydrate stores are depleted, such as on a low-carbohydrate diet or during very long bouts of exercise, the body breaks down other substances to yield glucose. These other substances can be amino acids, lactate, glycerol, or pyruvate.

Glucose Storage

Once enough carbohydrates are consumed to meet the body's immediate energy needs, the remaining glucose is converted to glycogen for storage. Glycogen is stored in the liver and the muscles. Liver glycogen is used to maintain blood glucose levels between meals; muscle glycogen can only be used inside the muscle for energy. Glycogen stores are very limited and can be depleted quickly. If carbohydrates are not consumed, the body will most likely experience what many athletes refer to as "hitting the wall." Basically, the body will run out of energy and have to either stop or slow down.

Fat Storage

Fats are stored mostly in **adipose** (fat) **tissue**; a small amount is stored in the muscles. Fats are produced by a pathway called **lipogenesis**. Because acetyl-CoA is the starting point, anything that can form acetyl-CoA can be converted into fat and stored. This includes fats themselves, carbohydrates, alcohol, and amino acids (yes, protein in excess can be made into fat). Once the acetyl-CoAs are linked, glycerol is added, and they are stored as triglycerides.

Creation of New Proteins

As previously mentioned, proteins are generated through a process called protein synthesis whereby amino acids are linked together. Unlike fats and carbohydrates, proteins do not have a large storage form in the body. However, a small amount of amino acids, called the **amino acid pool**, is stored in the blood and cells. The amino acids used in protein synthesis are drawn from the amino acid pool and various other sources. The body can make nonessential amino acids from the carbon skeletons it gets from pyruvate, essential amino acids, and other compounds. In addition, some amino acids can be obtained from the breakdown of body tissues. Of course, some amino acids, especially essential amino acids, must come from the diet.

Water

When clients complain of feeling fatigued or are unable to complete workouts, the problem may be related to their fluid balance. Although balance among all nutrients is important, water is essential to life and is required in the greatest amount. A person generally cannot survive for more than a few days without consuming some water. Fitness professionals must know the signs of dehydration and closely monitor their clients for any symptoms. The human body is 40–70% water, most of which (70%) is found in muscle tissues. Because men have more muscle tissue than women do, the male body has a greater percent of water by weight. When

---

Beta-oxidation

The breakdown of triglycerides into smaller subunits called free fatty acids (FFAs) to convert FFAs into acetyl-CoA molecules, which are then available to enter the Krebs cycle and ultimately lead to the production of additional ATP.

Oxaloacetate (OAA)

A crystalline organic compound that is a metabolic intermediate in many metabolic processes.

Ketone bodies

Two molecules, acetoacetate and β-hydroxybutyrate, that are synthesized in the liver from acetyl-CoA.

TRAINER TIPS

If clients are seeking to build or maintain muscle, skipping meals or fasting is not recommended because protein is likely to be used to make glucose for energy (in a negative energy–balance environment) rather than utilizing the protein for anabolic means.

MEMORY TIPS

When the body's glycogen stores run low energy levels will drop. Many endurance athletes refer to this fatigue as "hitting the wall" or "bonking."

Deamination

The first step in the breakdown of amino acids; it includes the removal of the nitrogen group.

Carbon skeleton

The skeletal structure of an organic compound; it is the series of atoms bonded together that form the essential structure of the compound.

Nicotinamide adenine dinucleotide (NAD)

A coenzyme found in all living cells that is a carrier in the electron transport chain.

Flavin adenine dinucleotide (FAD)

A redox cofactor, more specifically a prosthetic group, involved in several important metabolic reactions.

Electron transport chain

A series of compounds that transfer electrons from electron donors to electron acceptors, generating ATP in the process.

Gluconeogenesis

Formation of glucose from noncarbohydrate sources, such as amino acids.

Adipose tissue

One of the main types of connective tissue where fat is stored.

Lipogenesis

The metabolic pathway responsible for formation of fat.

comparing a man and a woman who both weigh 150 pounds, the man's body would contain 10% more water. Similarly, an individual person with a greater percent of body weight consisting of muscle will have more water than an individual of the same weight with more body fat. Water is important for controlling body temperature, maintaining the body's acid–base ratio, and regulating blood pressure (Jeukendrup & Gleeson, 2010; McArdle, Katch, & Katch, 2015).

Structure of Water

Water is an inorganic substance, meaning that it does not contain carbon. In contrast, fats, protein, carbohydrates, and vitamins are organic substances that contain carbon. Water consists of two hydrogen **atoms** and one oxygen atom bonded together. This bond is unique, and allows other substances to dissolve in water.

Function of Water

Water serves a number of critical functions in the body. It serves as the medium by which the body transports nutrients (such as the B vitamins), diffuses gases, and rids the body of waste. It lubricates joints, cushions vital organs, and provides structure to the skin and body tissue. It also helps to maintain body temperature via evaporation. As the body sweats and releases water through the skin, the water evaporates to cool the body. Water also helps to stabilize body temperature by absorbing heat generated by exercise and environmental conditions (McArdle et al., 2015).

General Guidelines for Water Intake

The Dietary Reference Intake (DRI) for water is a general recommendation. For women, it is approximately 2.7 liters (91 ounces) of total water from all beverages and foods each day; for men the recommendation is approximately 3.7 liters (125 ounces) per day (Institute of Medicine, 2004). Water needs can be met by drinking water and by consuming foods containing water. For instance, many fruits and vegetables, such as tomatoes, lettuce, watermelon, grapefruit, and cucumbers, are 85–95% water by mass (Hewlings, & Medeiros, 2011). **Table 5.9** provides recommended water intake by gender and by activity.

Water Balance

Hydration status depends on the balance between water loss and water intake. No other nutrient fluctuates within the body as much as water does. Water loss depends on many factors. For example, the temperature and humidity of the environment, the individual's age, the intensity

TABLE 5.9 Recommended Water Intake

Gender or Exercise Status	Recommended Intake
Women	2.7 L (91 oz.) per day
Men	3.7 L (125 oz.) per day
2 hours pre-exercise	14–20 oz.
15 minutes pre-exercise	16 oz., if tolerated
During exercise	4–8 oz. every 15–20 minutes or 16–32 ounces every hour
Postexercise	50 ounces for every kilogram (2.2 pounds) of body weight lost

Data from: *Dietary Reference Intakes*, Institute of Medicine, 2004

and duration of the activity the individual is participating in, and the individual's fitness level can all influence how much water is lost per day. To avoid dehydration, it is very important to balance water intake with water loss. It is important to encourage clients who work or exercise outdoors to pay close attention to their fluid intake, because not consuming enough water can have a negative impact on their workouts in and out of the gym. It is crucial to inform active people that weight loss through water loss, such as jogging while wearing plastic suits, is very dangerous, and can even lead to death.

Water Loss

Overall water balance from input to output is summarized in **Table 5.10**. Because mild daily sweating and the exhalation of air humidified by the lungs generally go unnoticed, these and other minor water losses, such as secretions from the eyes, are often referred to as **insensible water losses**. In addition, mild sweating is often separated from activity-induced sweat, which has a higher mineral content and is visually obvious. Sweat can be a significant route of water loss for athletes and for people who live in warm climates (Hewlings & Medeiros, 2011).

During exercise the body produces a large amount of heat, which must be released in order to keep body temperature in an acceptable range. The body's primary method of doing this is through sweating. As sweat evaporates, it draws off heat and cools the body. In hot-weather exercise, an individual can sweat as much as 30–90 ounces of water per hour. How much one sweats is determined by the type of clothing worn, the intensity of training, gender, and the weather. If the weather is hot and humid, sweat will not evaporate as quickly, making it more difficult to adequately cool the body. In dry climates, by contrast, sweat evaporates very quickly to cool the body—sometimes so quickly individuals do not realize how much fluid they are losing, resulting in dehydration.

Dehydration

Dehydration can affect performance and threaten health, and ultimately even life. A loss of 2–3% of body weight as water (3.0–4.5 pounds for a 150-pound person) can both decrease exercise capacity and increase the risk of death. For the average client, even a small level of dehydration can cause fatigue and make it difficult to put forth the effort needed to get the most out of a workout. Dehydration, which affects the body's ability to cool itself with sweat and leads to overheating, is often compounded with a severe loss of **electrolytes**. This can result in heatstroke. Confusion typically results from dehydration and heatstroke, causing victims to make poor decisions, further worsening their condition. **Table 5.11** lists the signs of dehydration.

TABLE 5.10 Water Balance from Intake and Output

Water Intake		Water Output	
Source	*Intake*	*Source*	*Loss*
Food	600–800 mL	Urine	900–1,200 mL
Beverages	1,000 mL	Mild sweating	400 mL
Metabolic water (from digestion)	200–300 mL	Lungs	300 mL
		Feces	200 mL
Total	**1,800–2,100 mL**	**Total**	**1,800–2,100 mL**

Hewlings & Medeiros, 2011

Amino acid pool
A mixture of amino acids available in the cell derived from dietary sources or the degradation of protein.

Atom
The basic, and smallest, unit of a chemical element.

TRAINER TIPS

Have your clients set a timer on their phone to remind them to drink water.

TRAINER TIPS

It is important to tell clients who are just beginning an exercise program that fluid needs may increase as a result of sweating and that they may need to increase their water intake to stay hydrated.

Insensible water loss
Water lost through mild daily sweating and exhalation of air humidified by the lungs, as well as other minor water losses, such as secretions from the eyes, that generally go unnoticed.

Electrolytes
Minerals in blood and other body fluids that carry an electrical charge.

TABLE 5.11 Signs of Dehydration

Dry mouth	Headache	Rapid heartbeat
Sleepiness or tiredness	Constipation	Rapid breathing
Thirst	Dizziness	Fever
Decreased urine output	Sunken eyes	Delirium
Dry skin	Low blood pressure	Unconsciousness

The best way to avoid dehydration when exercising is to "drink early, drink often." An individual exercising for an extended period of time in the heat should never wait until thirsty to start drinking, because it may be too late by that point. To stay ahead of fluid losses, it is important to begin taking in fluid before the workout begins and then continue to drink fluid periodically throughout the workout. Several fitness-tracking apps are available that people can use to set customized tips and reminders to consume water. **Table 5.12** offers some general guidelines for fluid replacement during exercise.

Monitoring Hydration Status

An objective way to check hydration status, and the easiest method next to monitoring thirst, is assessing urine color and volume. If urine is light in color when the volume and frequency

TABLE 5.12 Guidelines for Fluid Replacement and Exercise

Before Exercise
- Ensure high fluid intake for several days before competition (urine should be pale in color).
- Consume 14–20 ounces (1.75–2.5 cups) of fluid 2 hours before exercise.
- Consume 16 ounces about 15 minutes before exercise, if tolerated.
- Consume water or sports drinks rather than soda or juice.
- Fluid absorption is accelerated with a 6% carbohydrate drink (any popular sports drink).
- Cold water or fluid is more rapidly absorbed.

During Exercise
- Drink 4–8 ounces (0.5–1.0 cup) every 15–20 minutes or 16–32 ounces of fluid every hour.
- If the weather is very hot, more fluid may be required.
- Consuming fluids with 500–700 grams of sodium per 33 ounces of water enhances fluid replacement.
- Drink sports drinks containing 6–8% glucose for exercise lasting longer than 60 minutes.
- Sodas, teas, and juices are not ideal, and may result in the reverse of the desired effect.
- Drinking plain water without electrolytes can also be a problem.
- Take electrolyte pills with water and/or eat food if sports drinks are not favorable.

After Exercise
- Consume 50 ounces of fluid for every kilogram (2.2 pounds) of body weight lost.
- For exercise longer than 1 hour in duration, consuming a drink containing sodium and glucose will promote rapid rehydration.

Data from American College of Sports Medicine. (2009). ACSM position stand: Exercise and fluid replacement. *Medicine and Science in Sports and Exercise, 39*(2), 377–390.

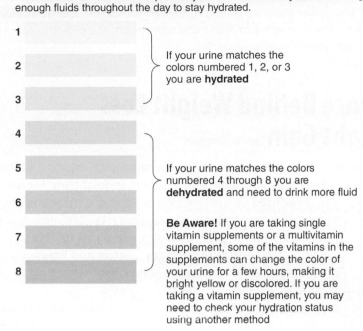

This urine color chart is a simple tool you can to assess if you are drinking enough fluids throughout the day to stay hydrated.

1

2 — If your urine matches the colors numbered 1, 2, or 3 you are **hydrated**

3

4

5 — If your urine matches the colors numbered 4 through 8 you are **dehydrated** and need to drink more fluid

6

7 — **Be Aware!** If you are taking single vitamin supplements or a multivitamin supplement, some of the vitamins in the supplements can change the color of your urine for a few hours, making it bright yellow or discolored. If you are taking a vitamin supplement, you may need to check your hydration status using another method

8

FIGURE 5.2 Urine color chart.

are near normal, then the individual is probably getting enough water. Darker urine indicates a need to drink more water (**Figure 5.2**). Another effective method to monitor fluid loss is to track weight before and after exercise.

Electrolytes

Electrolytes are minerals that include potassium, sodium, calcium, chloride, magnesium, and phosphate. The body needs and uses electrolytes both for their electrical properties and to control fluid balance between the various systems of the body. Electrolytes are lost in sweat. Dehydration and heatstroke are frequently made even worse by electrolyte imbalance. Sodium and potassium are the most important electrolytes depleted in sweat. They must be replaced when significant amounts are lost or the condition of **hyponatremia** (low sodium) and/or **hypokalemia** (low potassium) may result.

Electrolyte replacement is most important in prolonged physical activity, and severe depletion is unlikely to occur in workouts or exercise of less than 2 hours unless an individual begins in a dehydrated or depleted state. Temperature and humidity also affect the rate of electrolyte loss. Therefore, clients who have just started exercising or have just started exercising in a hot environment may be more at risk than those who are used to it. Without extremes of heat, prolonged exercise, or high-intensity workouts, salt losses are usually replenished by normal postexercise dietary intake. Moreover, most Americans eat plenty of salt, and therefore are generally less susceptible to electrolyte depletion from normal exercise (Jeukendrup & Gleeson, 2010).

Sports Drinks

Sports drinks are ideal for individuals who exercise for longer than 60 minutes. Regardless of environmental conditions, sports drinks are generally not necessary for individuals exercising fewer than 60 minutes. Inactive individuals do not need to consume sports drinks, and such drinks can actually be a source of unneeded calories. For those exercising for longer than

Hyponatremia

Loss of significant amounts of sodium, resulting in an increase in the body's water levels.

Hypokalemia

Loss of significant amounts of potassium, resulting in weakness, fatigue, constipation, and muscle cramping.

60 minutes or in an overly hot environment, the ideal drink for fluid replacement is one that tastes good, does not cause stomach discomfort when consumed in large amounts, promotes rapid emptying from the stomach, provides rapid absorption, and provides some energy in the form of carbohydrate for the working muscles.

The Science Behind Weight Loss and Weight Gain

In the field of nutrition, the topic that has perhaps generated the most misinformation, fueled the most myths, and been the topic of many conversations is weight loss. Every aspect of Western culture seems to be influenced by the latest dieting trend: advertisements, infomercials, coffee break conversations, the newest items on popular restaurant menus, and public policy. Although it may seem overwhelming, the attention being given to this topic is somewhat justified. In fact, according to the **Centers for Disease Control and Prevention (CDC)**, more than two-thirds of American adults and one-third of children are overweight or obese (Ogden, Carroll, Kit, & Flegal, 2014; CDC, 2014).

Obesity is a serious public health problem. In addition to being a risk factor for approximately 30 potentially deadly and chronic diseases, including heart disease, stroke, type 2 diabetes, osteoarthritis, and certain cancers, obesity itself is now considered a **chronic disease**. Undoubtedly, either avoidance of weight gain or weight loss are among the reasons most clients seek fitness professionals (Melton, Dali, Katula, & Mustian, 2015). Helping an individual lose weight can be a daunting task. Although a fitness professional can have some control over a client's workouts, the professional's control over the client's eating is minimal. In addition, many approaches for weight loss have been developed. There is not one specific approach that will work for everyone for weight loss. Creating a caloric deficit by consuming less calories and burning more is the best successful method to lose weight regardless of the specific approach taken (Atallah et al., 2014).

Which Diets Work?

In 2013, the weight loss market in North America generated more than $66 billion. Several studies have compared the various weight loss programs to assess their short- and long-term results. The outcomes of these studies are mixed, especially in those looking at weight loss over 12 months or more. However, all long-term results were modest for the various weight loss programs, and one did not emerge that was more effective than the others (Atallah et al., 2014).

Low-carbohydrate diets have become very popular. These types of diets vary in just how low carbohydrate intake should be, but they are developed under similar principles—the main one being that carbohydrates are to blame for weight gain and obesity. Advocates of these diets claim that they are more effective for losing weight and improving diabetes and heart disease than balanced weight loss diets (Noakes, 2013). However, studies comparing low-carbohydrate and balanced weight loss programs consuming the same number of calories found that participants in both groups lost a similar amount of weight over 3–6 months and over 1–2 years of follow up. Researchers suggest that this indicates that the weight loss is a result of a reduction in total calorie intake rather than any manipulation of macronutrient composition (Naude et al., 2011).

In order to lose weight, a calorie deficit must be created; an individual must burn more calories than are consumed. In turn, to maintain weight, a person must burn as many calories

Centers for Disease Control and Prevention (CDC)

Federal agency that conducts and supports activities related to public health.

Chronic disease

A persistent disease lasting 3 months or longer.

as are consumed. To gain weight, more calories must consumed than are burned. Calories in versus calories out is an oversimplified explanation of a complex issue; however, this simple statement holds truth, and summarizes the fact that maintaining weight is really an issue of balance. Any successful weight loss strategy must create a caloric deficit either by decreasing caloric intake or increasing caloric expenditure through exercise and increasing lean body mass (Hall et al., 2011). **Table 5.13** lists the calories expended when engaging in various types of activities.

Whether an individual follows a low-carbohydrate diet, a balanced diet, or any of the other plans available, it is important not to choose a plan that is hard to follow long term or that offers unrealistic outcomes. Fitness professionals cannot, by law in most states, prescribe diets. They can, however, guide clients towards healthy balanced eating that creates a caloric deficit. Fitness professionals can help create that deficit by promoting physical activity to burn calories. In addition, they can guide clients away from extreme weight loss plans or those that promise unrealistic results. Fitness professionals can refer clients who require the prescription of a specific diet to a registered dietitian.

TABLE 5.13 Calories Burned by Various Physical Activities

	Approximate Calories Used (Burned) by a 154-pound Man	
MODERATE Physical Activities	**In 1 hour**	**In 30 minutes**
Hiking	370	185
Light gardening/yard work	330	165
Dancing	330	165
Golf (walking and carrying clubs)	330	165
Bicycling (less than 10 mph)	290	145
Walking (3.5 mph)	280	140
Weight training (general light workout)	220	110
Stretching	180	90
VIGOROUS Physical Activities	**In 1 Hour**	**In 30 Minutes**
Running/jogging (5 mph)	590	295
Bicycling (more than 10 mph)	590	295
Swimming (slow freestyle laps)	510	255
Aerobics	480	240
Walking (4.5 mph)	460	230
Heavy yard work (chopping wood)	440	220
Weight lifting (vigorous effort)	440	220
Basketball (vigorous)	440	220

Reproduced from How Many Calories Does Physical Activity Use (Burn)? U.S. Food and Drug Administration. (2015). Available from: http://www.choosemyplate.gov/physical-activity-calories-burn

CHECK IT OUT

Beware of weight loss plans that:

- Promise dramatic weight loss ("Lose 30 pounds in 30 days!").
- Promise one easy permanent solution.
- Promise permanent weight loss with no effort.
- Say "Studies show that . . .," but provide no references from reputable scientific journals.
- Tell you to eliminate or drastically reduce intake of any one food or food group.
- Promise weight loss with no exercise.
- Encourage consuming fewer than 1,200 calories per day.
- Encourage liquid meals.
- Include pills, creams, or patches.
- Say you can lose weight and eat all you want.
- Suggest the consumption of pills or drinks to "block absorption" of certain foods.
- Encourage you to buy their food or supplements.
- Use the word *miracle*.
- Use testimonials to sell their plan.
- Use dramatic before-and-after photos as selling techniques.
- Provide no maintenance or follow-up plan.
- Do not encourage permanent lifestyle changes.

Adapted from Hewlings, S. H., & Medeiros, D. M. (2011). *Nutrition: Real people real choices*. Dubuque, IA: Kendall Hunt.

The Environment of Eating

When clients are trying to lose weight it is just as important for them to examine *why* they eat as *what* they eat. Food intake is governed not only by internal cues of hunger and satiety, but also by social or emotional forces, not to mention just the pleasure of tasting something delicious. Eating for nonphysiological reasons often occurs in social situations in which food is the medium of social exchange. Holidays, parties, and celebrations surrounding food are a big part of enjoying life (Wagner, Larson, & Wengreen, 2012). One way to control overeating in social situations is to use behavior modification techniques. Eating habits that can contribute to weight gain, such as snacking at work or eating ice cream before bed, also can be managed with behavior modification techniques. Some individuals use food to handle stress, anger, sadness, or loneliness. They look to food as a way to relax or as a reward. Although food meets nutritional needs, it cannot fulfill emotional needs. If a client is using food to cope with emotions and/or stress, advise the client to seek the assistance of a psychologist or other mental health professional for help determining the root of his or her emotional eating and to identify new, healthy coping mechanisms.

Strategies for Better Eating

Decreasing caloric intake can be challenging for some people, but there are some good strategies that can act as a starting point. A good place to start for many individuals is to assess what they drink on a daily basis. Many people are not aware of just how many calories are in many sugar-sweetened beverages and coffee drinks. As many as 1,000 calories a day can be cut just by limiting these beverages and replacing them with water. For example, consider a client who drinks a large sweetened coffee drink in the morning (220 calories), a 16-ounce sports drink at lunch (100 calories), and two light beers with some friends in the evenings (220 calories total). That is 540 calories from beverages in one day! These are **empty calories**, and therefore provide few nutrients.

Another helpful tip is to consume a large green salad at least once a day, being careful not to add high-calorie items like cheese, croutons, and salad dressings. This will help to decrease hunger and provide lots of nutrients without many calories. Research indicates that serving larger portion sizes of low-calorie, high-nutrient foods helps people to feel full longer (Rolls, 2012).

From there, a daily intake of plenty of vegetables, fruits, and whole grains, as well as low fat dairy and lean meats, is the foundation of a healthy diet. People who are trying to lose weight do not have room in their diet for the little extras like sweets and extra portions. In fact, controlling portion size is a critical aspect to successful weight loss.

The following are some general guidelines that fitness professionals can provide to their clients who have weight loss as one of their fitness goals (Hewlings & Medeiros, 2011):

- ◆ *Have regular meals.* In addition to keeping metabolism high, eating small regular meals helps keep caloric intake low. Research shows that restrained eaters—those who suppress hunger to skip meals and starve themselves—frequently end up binging or overeating. This response is a physiological reaction to both hunger and deprivation. Eat three to six meals a day, spaced at fairly regular intervals, about 3 to 4 hours apart.
- ◆ *Eat in a calm, conscious, and relaxed manner.* Chew your food, so you get to taste it. Avoid stress-driven eating by paying more attention to what you are doing—eating—than to what is going on around you. By doing so, you will be more receptive to the internal cues that let you know when you have eaten enough.
- ◆ *Shop with limits.* At the grocery store, make your food purchases wisely. Bring home only foods that will contribute to a healthy diet. Most people tend to overeat certain foods, usually sweets and salty snacks.
- ◆ *Learn to cook.* Satisfying food offers a variety of tastes and textures. When its natural flavor has not been killed by overcooking or overprocessing food does not require as much added fat or sugar to taste good. This food is hard to find in the commercial world. Your best bet is to cook it yourself.
- ◆ *Make cooking easy.* Try to cook when you have time, rather than when you are starved and rushed. Learn a repertoire of quick and easy meals. Prepare foods ahead of time as much as possible, and keep a good supply of basic ingredients in the pantry.
- ◆ *Don't clean your plate.* There are two ways to waste extra food: throw it out or eat it. If you feel guilty about throwing food out, save it for tomorrow's lunch or compost it.
- ◆ *When you cook, go for it.* Cook as if you are cooking for several people and then portion the food out before you eat. Put all but the one portion you are eating into freezer-safe containers and refrigerate or freeze. You have just eliminated the excuse that you have no time to cook a healthy meal, as you will have several available throughout the week.
- ◆ *Don't wait until you are famished to eat.* You will tend to overeat if you wait until you are so hungry you will eat anything.
- ◆ *When you attend a party or event bring a healthy dish or salad.* If you bring a healthy option, you will have something healthy to eat when you are there. It might be a good

Empty calories
Calories that provide little or no nutrients.

idea to eat a healthy snack before you go so that you are not hungry when faced with the abundant buffet table.

♦ *Plan.* If you know you tend to get really hungry at 3:00 PM and end up heading for the candy to satisfy your hunger, eat a small healthy snack at 2:30 PM to prevent that hunger.

♦ *Mix your meals.* Eating carbohydrates, fats, and proteins together will help keep you fuller longer and will provide a balance of nutrients.

♦ *Don't eat out of a pot or serving dish; fix your plate.* People are more likely to overeat and not even be aware that they are doing so if they don't fix a set portion size on their plate.

♦ *Don't read or watch TV while eating.* You will tend to be distracted and may overeat as a result.

♦ *Eat slowly.* It takes time for the brain to get the signal that you are full. If you eat too fast, by the time you feel full you will end up being stuffed.

♦ *Have a plan for dining out.* Order sauces on the side and cut portions in half right from the start, putting half the dish in a "to go" container before you start eating. Order extra steamed vegetables instead of higher calorie sides like macaroni and cheese or french fries.

Food Labels and Government Nutrition Guidelines

So, what is a healthy diet? A very basic definition is that a healthy diet is a plan of eating that incorporates balance, variety, and moderation while meeting individual nutritional needs and goals while balancing energy intake to maintain a healthy weight. It is important to note that nutritional needs change over the life span. In addition, nutritional needs differ for athletes and for those who are sick, pregnant, or taking certain medications.

Another factor to consider when meal planning is the nutrient density of the foods being consumed. As discussed earlier, nutrient density refers to the nutrient content of a food relative to its calories. For example, when comparing 200 calories from a sugar candy with a 200-calorie banana it may seem like they are the same, since both provide the same calories. Although both foods provide 200 calories, the banana provides several nutrients, including important vitamins and minerals, whereas the candy is essentially just sugar. The candy represents empty calories; therefore, the healthier choice would be the banana.

These basic concepts can be incorporated into a healthy eating plan in a number of ways. Health and fitness professionals can refer to government guidelines to provide clients with additional information with regards to their meal planning strategy. As part of its role in improving the health of all Americans, the U.S. government has developed guidelines such as the Dietary Guidelines, the Daily Recommended Intakes, and MyPlate, as well as laws governing what must appear on food labels. These are all meant to work together and to provide guidelines to be individualized into a variety of eating plans. These can be great places to which you can refer your clients.

The Dietary Guidelines for Americans

The Dietary Guidelines for Americans has been published jointly every 5 years since 1980 by the U.S. Department of Health and Human Services (HHS) and the U.S. Department of Agriculture (USDA). The latest guidelines were released in 2015. They summarize science-based advice to promote health through diet and physical activity and to reduce risk for major diseases such as heart disease and stroke. The recommendations reflect the knowledge that the major causes of death and disease in the United States are related to an unhealthy diet, a sedentary lifestyle, and obesity. The overall purpose is to encourage most Americans to eat fewer calories, be more active, and make healthier food choices. The latest guidelines can be found at: http://health .gov/dietaryguidelines/.

The nutrition label found on food can be used to implement these guidelines on a daily basis. The Dietary Guidelines are intended to be general, and therefore do not provide information on the specific requirements of each nutrient. For example, the Dietary Guidelines say "Consume more of certain foods and nutrients such as fruits, vegetables, whole grains, fat-free and low-fat dairy products, and seafood" rather than providing specific recommendations for nutrients like calcium. The requirements for each nutrient are listed in **dietary standards**. Dietary standards provide recommended intakes for specific nutrients. They can be used to plan diets for individuals and groups.

The Dietary Reference Intakes

The **Dietary Reference Intakes (DRIs)** are reference values used to plan and assess nutrient intakes of healthy individuals. The DRIs include four nutrient-based reference values: **Recommended Dietary Allowance (RDA)**, **Adequate Intake (AI)**, **Estimated Average Requirement (EAR)**, and **Tolerable Upper Intake Level (UL)**. The DRIs are established for healthy individuals, and do not apply to those with chronic or acute disease, who need extra nutrients, or who are recovering from a diagnosed deficiency. For example, a person who smokes may require more than the RDA of vitamin C. DRIs can be used to plan menus for individuals, and institutions, such as hospitals and school cafeterias, use the DRIs to ensure that they provide adequate nutrition and not too much of any one nutrient or too many calories.

As noted earlier, an individual can use the DRIs to assess their diet. For example, several online tools as well as smartphone apps are available that people can use to compare their food intake with each of the recommendations. Such tools often provide assessments indicating the percentage consumed of the recommended intake of vitamin C, iron, calcium, and so on.

Energy and Macronutrient Requirements

People often ask, "How many calories should I eat?" One general recommendation is the **Estimated Energy Requirement (EER)**. It is based on formulas designed to include individual characteristics such as age, gender, height, weight, and level of physical activity. The tools used to assess DRIs will also calculate the user's calorie needs based on a set of formulas.

Because macronutrients contribute to calories consumed, it is important to provide guidelines for how much each macronutrient should contribute to overall caloric intake. The recommendations for carbohydrates, fats, and proteins have been discussed in previous sections and are provided under the **Acceptable Macronutrient Distribution Range (AMDR)**. The AMDR is a recommended range of macronutrient requirements based on a person's total daily calorie needs and the balance of nutrients that are associated with a decreased risk of chronic disease:

- Protein: 10–35% of total daily calories
- Fat: 20–35% of total daily calories
- Carbohydrates: 45–65% of total daily calories

Dietary standards
Recommended intakes for specific nutrients.

Dietary Reference Intakes (DRIs)
A general term for a set of reference values used to plan and assess nutrient intakes of healthy individuals.

Recommended Dietary Allowance (RDA)
Estimated amount of a nutrient per day considered necessary for good health.

Adequate Intake (AI)
Estimated amount of a nutrient per day consumed by people assumed to be maintaining adequate nutrition.

Estimated Average Requirement (EAR)
Estimated amount of a nutrient per day at which the needs of 50% of the population will be met.

Tolerable Upper Intake Level (UL)
Highest level of a nutrient per day that is unlikely to pose a risk of adverse health effects.

Estimated Energy Requirement (EER)
General recommendation for calorie intake based on formulas designed to include individual characteristics such as age, gender, height, weight, and level of physical activity.

There is some debate surrounding these numbers; however, these numbers provide a guide and a place to start that can be adjusted to meet individual goals and needs. Recall that an endurance athlete would need to eat more carbohydrates than an inactive person.

MyPlate

MyPlate has evolved from the original food pyramid. It is a planning and assessment tool that individuals can use to incorporate the recommendations into daily meal choices. The MyPlate website can be found at www.choosemyplate.gov/. It provides useful meal planning and healthy eating tools and promotes physical activity. It is a great place to refer clients to in order to encourage them to assess their nutrition and calorie intake on their own. If they require detailed assistance with the information they receive, the fitness professional can refer them to a registered dietitian.

Food Labels

Food labels are another tool for meal planning. They can help individuals make healthy food choices by listing information about the nutrient content of a food and how it fits into an overall healthy diet. The "overall diet" that the nutrient content of a specific food is compared to is called the **daily value**. It is like the DRI but is just one value for each nutrient, because the label is not big enough to show values for different ages and genders. It is based on a 2,000- and a 2,500-calorie diet. Several changes will be made to food labels, starting in 2016. The Food and Drug Administration (FDA) provides a website that describes these changes and goes through each section of the food label. It is an excellent tool to which you can refer clients.

Foundations of Supplementation Concepts

Dietary supplements are a huge part of our culture for both health and athletic performance, whether in an attempt to get the most out of each workout or to enhance that competitive edge in events. When supplements are used to benefit athletic performance or exercise they are called **ergogenic aids**. Although supplements can offer a way to fill in the gaps of a healthy diet and exercise program, many faulty claims have been made, and there is confusion about the role of supplements in health and sport performance. The internet, magazines, and television are heavy with advertisements for products that claim to have the answer for those who want to gain muscle, improve athletic performance, lose weight, obtain more energy, and more. With so many claims and promises, it is no surprise that marketing data has shown a dramatic increase in sales of supplements in the United States, with sales totaling more than $13 billion in 2013 (Euromonitor, 2015). Approximately 65% of Americans use dietary supplements (Dickinson & MacKay, 2014). Because of their popularity, it is safe to assume that fitness professionals are often approached by their clients for advice on the latest supplement.

It is important to recognize that not all supplements provide false claims; in fact several have been shown to provide health and performance benefits when taken correctly. The difficult part is differentiating the beneficial ones from those that are harmful, and those that simply fail to do what they claim. In addition, as the supplementation industry continues to grow, the scientific research into its claims grows as well. Therefore, fitness professionals need to remain

Acceptable Macronutrient Distribution Range (AMDR)
Recommendations for intake of carbohydrates, fats, and proteins.

Daily value
Guide to nutrients found within one serving of food.

Ergogenic aids
Supplements used to benefit athletic performance or exercise.

up-to-date on the latest information. The following are some good resources to keep up with the latest information on supplements:

- Dietary Supplement Fact Sheets from the National Institute of Health, Office of Dietary Supplements: https://ods.od.nih.gov/factsheets/list-all/
- Food and Drug Administration: www.fda.gov/Food/DietarySupplements/default.htm
- National Center for Complementary and Integrative Health: https://nccih.nih.gov/health/supplements
- Council for Responsible Nutrition: www.crnusa.org
- International Society for Sports Nutrition: www.jissn.com/series/ISSNPosP

What Is a Dietary Supplement?

The **Dietary Supplement Health and Education Act of 1994 (DSHEA)** was enacted by Congress following public debate concerning the importance of dietary supplements in promoting health, the need for consumers to have access to current and accurate information about supplements, and controversy over the FDA's regulatory approach to this product category. According to the DSHEA, a supplement is (www.fda.gov/Food/DietarySupplements/Using DietarySupplements/ucm480069.htm#what_is):

- A product intended to supplement the diet that contains one or more of the following dietary ingredients: a vitamin; a mineral; an herb or other botanical; an amino acid; a dietary substance used to supplement the diet by increasing the total daily intake; or a concentrate, metabolite, constituent, extract, or combination of these ingredients.
- Intended for ingestion in pill, capsule, tablet, or liquid form.
- Not represented for use as a conventional food or as the sole item of a meal or diet.
- Labeled as a dietary supplement.

In defining a supplement, it is also important to understand how the supplement industry is regulated. Since the passing of the DSHEA in 1994, the FDA regulates dietary supplements under a different set of regulations from those covering "conventional" foods and drugs (prescription and over the counter). Under the DSHEA, the supplement manufacturer, not the FDA, must ensure that a dietary supplement is safe before it is marketed (FDA, 2016). According to the FDA:

> Unlike drug products that must be proven safe and effective for their intended use before marketing, there are no provisions in the law for the FDA to 'approve' dietary supplements for safety or effectiveness before they reach the consumer. Under DSHEA, once the product is marketed, the FDA has the responsibility for showing that a dietary supplement is 'unsafe,' before it can take action to restrict the product's use or removal from the marketplace.

The important thing to remember is that the FDA does not get involved until *after* the product has been on the market. In other words, the FDA does *postmarketing surveillance* of supplements, but does not ensure their safety or effectiveness. The agency may restrict a substance only if it poses a "significant and unreasonable risk" after it is being sold and used. The FDA handles consumer complaints of unsafe products, improper or illegal labeling claims, and package inserts.

Before Taking a Supplement

Many supplements can be safely consumed without adverse effects on the health of the individual if consumed correctly. Unfortunately, there are not strict regulatory standards that are applied

Dietary Supplement Health and Education Act of 1994 (DSHEA)
Act that defines and regulates dietary supplements. Enacted by Congress following public debate concerning the role of dietary supplements in promoting health.

TRAINER TIPS

Oftentimes clients will support a supplement, claiming it is FDA approved. It is important for the trainer to explain to the client what that means and provide some standards on decision making with regard to supplement use.

to dietary supplements. With the growing popularity of supplements and the growth of their advertising, many clients will ask fitness professionals for guidance when they are considering utilizing supplements in their nutritional program. The fitness professional should not provide guidance or advice in regards to the consumption of supplements by their clients. Without a complete understanding of their medical history and medication usage, as well as potential side effects and negative drug interactions with supplements, it can be understood that the fitness professional should direct their client to their medical professional for discussions on supplementation usage. Some other tips that a fitness professional can follow for supplement discussions with clients are:

◆ Think about the overall nutritional needs. Supplements are called supplements as they are intended to supplement an overall healthy nutritional intake that may be lacking in a few key areas. The individual should be aware of potential toxicity risks if taking in too much of a certain nutrient. A full nutritional profile and understanding should be reviewed before any supplementation recommendations are made.

◆ A licensed professional should always be referred to before making supplementation decisions. It is important to understand the potential deficiencies within one's diets, what risks there are for potential toxic dosage, as well as any issues that may occur because of medication and/or medical conditions. A full understanding of these interactions along with the medical history of the individual needs to be considered before making any educated recommendations for supplements.

◆ Be skeptical of claims that are made by companies. If the supplement is advertised with claims that are too good to be true, they should be researched to ensure that they truly do provide the desired effect safely. This will require an understanding of the research that is cited by the claims, as well as understanding of who funded that particular research. This should include learning a deep understanding of fraudulent claims. Many supplement companies will use marketing and advertising concepts in order to reach the consumer. Understanding these concepts and evaluating supplement claims with a level of skepticism will ultimately protect the consumer from spending money on substances that may be ineffective and/or harmful to their health.

Supplement Types

There are various types of supplements with supporting rationales for their use. The most common supplements clients inquire about are addressed here, along with discussion that can be helpful when talking to clients.

Protein Supplements

Protein supplements are one of the most commonly used and talked about ergogenic aids by active individuals. Protein supplements are frequently consumed by athletes and active people to achieve greater gains in muscle mass and strength and improve physical performance. They are often marketed as providing superior muscle-building properties to the protein provided in food. Although these supplements provide a convenient source of protein after a workout, or when a protein-rich meal is needed on the run, they are not superior to protein-rich foods, such as egg whites, in stimulating muscle growth (Pasiakos, McLellan, & Lieberman, 2015). Research supports that individuals engaged in regular exercise training require more dietary protein than sedentary individuals. Protein intakes of 1.4–2.0 grams per kilogram of body weight per day for physically active individuals is not only safe, but also may improve the adaptations to exercise training (Campbell et al., 2007).

A variety of different types of protein supplements are available. **Whey proteins** and **casein** constitute the two major protein groups of cow's milk. Milk protein is 80% casein and

Whey protein

A mixture of globular proteins isolated from whey, the liquid material created as a byproduct of cheese production.

Casein

Protein commonly found in mammalian milk.

20% whey protein. Whey is a byproduct of cheese making. In its raw form whey consists of fat, lactose, and other substances. Supplement manufacturers take this raw form and process it to produce **whey protein concentrate (WPC)** and **whey protein isolate (WPI)**. Whey is considered a fast protein because the body absorbs it quickly. Casein is a slow protein and takes longer to absorb. Because of this, most supplements contain whey protein. A few different types of whey proteins are marketed. Whey protein concentrates are rich in whey proteins and also contain fat and lactose. Whey protein isolates are low in fat and lactose. Although whey proteins are a good source of protein, they are not superior to other forms.

While protein supplements contain all of the amino acids, typically both essential and nonessential, some supplements contain one or a few of the individual amino acids rather than a complete protein like whey. **Arginine** is a conditionally essential amino acid; normally the body can synthesize sufficient amounts to meet its needs. Arginine is involved in protein synthesis and the formation of several compounds in the body. Dietary supplements containing arginine have been marketed with the purpose of increasing vasodilation, thereby elevating blood flow to the exercising muscle and enhancing the metabolic response to exercise. Current research indicates that arginine does promote vasodilation. Although it is most beneficial to people who have heart disease, are recovering from trauma, or have a compromised immune function, it is used by many body builders and fitness enthusiasts to increase blood flow to the working muscle. Doses of 3–18 grams per day seem well tolerated, whereas doses in excess of 30 grams per day have been shown to produce negative side effects such as low blood pressure and rapid heart rate (Alvares et al., 2011). It does not appear to be effective for enhancing lean body mass in healthy individuals. More research needs to be done before a definitive statement on the benefits of arginine can be made (Paddon-Jones, Borsheim, & Wolfe, 2004).

Branched-Chain Amino Acids

The **branched-chain amino acids (BCAAs)**—leucine, isoleucine, and valine—are essential. They differ from the other amino acids because they can be used for energy directly in the muscle, without having to go to the liver to be broken down during exercise. It has been suggested that ingesting them before and/or during long-duration activity may help delay fatigue, but studies have not strongly supported this theory. However, the BCAAs, especially leucine, may play a critical role in recovery from exercise by preventing muscle breakdown. Other studies have shown that BCAA supplementation improves immune system function after exercise to exhaustion. It has been suggested that young adults consuming a moderate-protein diet on a daily basis (1.4 grams per kilogram body weight) consume 20–25 grams of high-quality protein, providing 2.5–3.0 grams of leucine after exercise enhances recovery; older adults engaged in resistance training and consuming a moderate-protein diet consume 35–40 grams of high-quality, fast-digesting protein (like whey protein) following resistance training to maximize muscle growth and recovery (Guimarães-Ferreira et al., 2014).

Caffeine

Caffeine is one of the most widely used drugs in the world. In some supplements it is listed as guarana or kola nut. It can be found in coffee, tea, chocolate, soft drinks, some pain relievers, some cold medicines, and many weight-loss pills. It has long been known that moderate to high caffeine doses (5–13 grams per kilogram body weight) ingested approximately 1 hour before and during exercise increases endurance exercise performance. Research has also shown that caffeine is ergogenic in some short-term high-intensity exercise and sport situations. Lower caffeine doses (≤ 3 grams per kilogram body weight, or approximately 200 milligrams) taken before exercise also increase athletic performance, and low and very low doses of caffeine taken late in prolonged exercise also show a benefit. The response to caffeine intake can vary from person to person, therefore

Whey protein concentrate (WPC)

Dietary supplement obtained by removal of sufficient nonprotein constituents from pasteurized whey.

Whey protein isolate (WPI)

Dietary supplement obtained by separating components from milk.

Arginine

Conditionally essential amino acid that the body can normally synthesize in sufficient amounts; however, in some disorders the body cannot make enough, and it becomes essential.

Branched-chain amino acids (BCAAs)

Essential amino acids, including leucine, isoleucine, and valine, that can be used for energy directly in the muscle and do not have to go to the liver to be broken down during exercise.

TABLE 5.14 Caffeine Content of Foods and Beverages

Food/Beverage	Serving Size	Caffeine Content, mg
Coffee		
Brewed	250 mL	100–150
Drip	250 mL	125–175
Instant	250 mL	50–70
Espresso	1 shot	50–110
Tea		
Green (medium)	250 mL	25–40
Black (medium)	250 mL	40–60
Cola drinks	355 mL	35–50
Energy drinks	250 mL	80–150
Chocolate		
Dark	50 mg	20–40
Milk	50 mg	8–16

The values are a range and some products could be outside the range provided as a function of brewing time and other factors. For example, an analysis of 97 espresso shots taken from retail stores in Australia showed a range of 24–214 mg/shot.
Data from Tarnopolsky, M. A. (2010). Caffeine and creatine use in sport. *Annals of Nutrition and Metabolism, 57*(Suppl 2), 1–8. Epub 2011 Feb 22.

it is important to determine whether the ingestion of 200 milligrams of caffeine before and/or during training and competitions is beneficial on an individual basis (Spriet, 2014). People who consume it on a daily basis can become adapted and may have to use more caffeine to achieve the same effect. **Table 5.14** provides the caffeine content of a number of foods and beverages.

Caffeine has some side effects. Individuals who do not regularly consume it can experience gastrointestinal distress, nervousness, rapid heart rate, headaches, and increased blood pressure (Hewlings & Medeiros, 2011).

Creatine

Creatine is made in the body and can be consumed in the diet, mostly from meat and fish. It is part of creatine phosphate, the key component of the immediate energy system used primarily during sporting events lasting 10 seconds or less (such as track sprints). Higher intakes of creatine seem to result in higher levels of creatine phosphate in the muscle cells, thus making more energy available for very high-intensity activity such as strength training and sprinting. Research has shown that creatine supplementation results in small (1–2%) increased gains in strength or speed when combined with appropriate training (Tarnopolsky, 2010). Most studies have also reported an acute increase in fat-free mass after 5–7 days of creatine supplementation (Tarnopolsky, 2010). The effect is greater in men than women, and the effect in men is approximately 1.5 kilograms. This increase in fat-free mass is due to an increase in water; however, in combination with resistance-exercise training, the increase in fat-free mass can be related to an increase in muscle mass. It is important to note that not everyone responds to creatine supplementation the

Creatine
Compound made in the body but that can also be consumed in the diet, mostly from meat and fish. Involved in the supply of energy for muscular contraction.

same. Response depends on the frequency and type of training and on the levels produced and present in the body when supplementation begins. Vegetarians and others who do not consume much creatine naturally appear to achieve a greater response from supplementation. Absolutely no result exists without training, and creatine does not benefit aerobic conditioning. Many individuals who have taken it complain of side effects, including headaches, abdominal cramps, and muscle cramps. On the other hand, creatine supplementation in common dosages results in urinary concentrations 90 times greater than normal (Tarnopolsky, 2010). This suggests it could damage the kidneys if used long term. As always, follow the dosing outlined with the product and carefully consider taking creatine on an individual basis (Tarnopolsky, 2010).

HMB (beta-hydroxy beta-methylbutyrate)

HMB (beta-hydroxy beta-methylbutyrate) is a product of the breakdown of the essential amino acid leucine. HMB supplementation is claimed to exert positive effects both in healthy (i.e., increasing sport performance as well as reducing exercise-related muscle damage) and pathological (i.e., preserving and increasing muscle mass) conditions, perhaps by reducing protein breakdown and enhancing protein synthesis (Zanchi et al., 2010). It is synthesized naturally in humans and is also available in some foods, such as citrus fruits and catfish. Whether HMB has a necessary physiological function or is merely a product of leucine breakdown remains unclear. Most studies support the effectiveness of HMB in preventing exercise-related muscle damage in healthy trained and untrained individuals as well as muscle loss during chronic eases (Molfino et al., 2013; Wilson et al., 2013). Up to 3 grams (38 grams per kilogram body weight per day) of HMB taken for 2 weeks has been found to improve strength and **fat-free mass (FFM)** and reduce muscle damage in a dose-dependent manner, whereas higher doses, such as 6 grams, have shown no additional benefits. The 3 gram (or 38 grams per kilogram body weight per day) dose may be an optimal dosage, especially if taken right before or right after the workout. No adverse side effects have been reported; however, too few well-controlled studies have been conducted to conclude that it is safe at doses above the recommended 3 grams (Molfino, Gioia, Rossi-Fanelli, & Muscaritoli, 2013; Wilson et al., 2013).

Prohormones and Anabolic Steroids

In 2014 the U.S. government passed the Anabolic Steroid Control Act to expand the list of substances from previous versions of the act to include many prohormones. These substances are now considered Class 3 narcotics, and it is a felony to make, distribute, or possess them. Therefore, any "supplement" claiming to raise hormone levels is either illegal or making false claims.

HMB (beta-hydroxy beta-methylbutyrate)
A metabolite of the essential amino acid leucine that is synthesized in the human body. Used as a supplement to increase muscle mass and decrease muscle breakdown.

Fat-free mass (FFM)
Total body mass, without the fat. It is the lean or nonfat components of the body.

Conclusion

Our understanding of human nutrition is constantly evolving. As new research is conducted, new information provides further insight. Often, public guidelines and recommendations are changed to reflect this new science. This fluctuating information is often misinterpreted by the general public and can lead to confusion and misinformation. Therefore, it is important to rely on licensed professionals such as registered dietitians and scientists to communicate and interpret the science. It is critical to stay current throughout one's career by attending conferences and reading publications, such as this one, by reputable organizations. Staying up-to-date on current information is important to inform discussions with clients. This is the extent of the scope of practice for the fitness professional. In most states only licensed or registered dietitians can legally provide nutritional counseling and diet prescription.

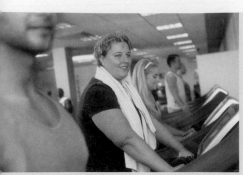

© StockLite/Shutterstock

Case in Review

Jennifer has approached you with the goal of losing 20 pounds over a 4-month period and wants to know how she can leverage a meal plan to help her do so. Before you begin to look deeper into Jennifer's lifestyle, it is important to set clear expectations on what you can and cannot help Jennifer with on her quest to lose weight. As a fitness professional, be transparent in the services and education you can provide to your client in regards to nutrition guidance. Although there are no concerning health issues evident with Jennifer, it is important to let her know that as a fitness professional you have the ability to educate her about nutrition, but only with regards to providing guidance and you cannot prescribe specific meal plans.

When talking with Jennifer about her weight loss goal, operate within the scope of practice; asking her to list the details of her daily diet, her current understanding of nutrition, and any additional activities she engages in aside from her daily walks. Compiling such information will help you get an idea of what Jennifer already knows as well as highlight opportunities that can be used to further educate her about the food she ingests. While probing Jennifer, it is important to be sensitive to her lifestyle to help facilitate trust that is required to obtain honest answers.

Although you are not a registered dietician, you have the ability to educate Jennifer on how our bodies use various types of nutrients and how integrating certain foods will help with reaching her goal. Throughout the consultation, you provide guidance on healthy eating for weight loss without giving specific recommendations.

References

Alvares, T. S., Meirelles, C. M., Bhambhani, Y. N., Pascjoalin, V. M., & Gomes, P. S. (2011). L-Arginine as a potential ergogenic aid in healthy subjects. *Sports Medicine, 41*(3), 233–248.

American College of Sports Medicine. (2009). ACSM position stand: Exercise and fluid replacement. *Medicine and Science in Sports and Exercise, 39*(2), 377–390.

Atallah, R., Fillion, K. B., Wakil, S. M., Genest, J., Joseph, L., Poirier, P., Rinfret, S., Schiffrin, E. L., & Eisenberg, M. J. (2014). Long-term effects of 4 popular diets on weight loss and cardiovascular risk factors: A systematic review of randomized control trials. *Circulation. Cardiovascular Quality and Outcomes, 76*, 815–827.

Burke, L. M., Hawley, J. A., Wonge, S. H. S., & Jeukendrup, A. E. (2011). Carbohydrates for training and competition, *Journal of Sports Sciences, 29*(S1), S17–S27.

Campbell, B., Kreider, R. B., Ziegenfuss, T., La Bounty, P., Roberts, M., Burke, D., . . . Antonio, J. (2007). International Society of Sports Nutrition position stand: Protein and exercise. *Journal of the International Society of Sports Nutrition, 4*, 8.

Centers for Disease Control, (2014). Obesity and Overweight. Retrieved on 5/3/2016. http://www.cdc.gov/nchs/fastats/obesity-overweight.htm

Dickinson, A., & MacKay, D. (2014). Health habits and other characteristics of dietary supplement users: A review. *Nutrition Journal, 13*, 14.

Euromonitor. (2015). Vitamins and dietary supplements in the US. Available from: http://www.euromonitor.com/vitamins-and-dietary-supplements-in-the-us/report

Food and Drug Administration. (2016). *Questions and answers on dietary supplements.* Available from http://www.fda.gov/Food/DietarySupplements/UsingDietarySupplements/ucm480069.htm#what_is

Guimaraes-Ferreira, L., Cholewa, J. M., Naimo, M. A., Zhi, X. I., Magagnin, D., de Sa, R. B., . . . Zanchi, N. E. (2014). Synergistic effects of resistance training and protein intake: Practical aspects. *Nutrition, 30*(10), 1097–1103.

Hall, K. D., Sacks, G., Chandramochan, D., Chow, C. C., Wang, Y. C., Gortmaker, S. L., & Swinburn, B. A. (2011). Quantification of the effect of the energy imbalance on body weight. *Lancet, 378*, 826–837.

Harvard Health. (2015). Making sense of vitamins and minerals: Choosing the foods and nutrients you need to stay healthy. Available from: http://www.health.harvard.edu/heart-health/vitamins-and-minerals-choosing-the-nutrients-you-need-to-stay-healthy

Hewlings, S. H., & Medeiros, D. M. (2011). *Nutrition: Real people real choices.* Dubuque, IA: Kendall Hunt.

Institute of Medicine, Food and Nutrition Board. (2004). *Dietary reference intakes: Water, potassium, sodium, chloride, and sulfate.* Washington, D.C.: National Academies Press.

Institute of Medicine, Food and Nutrition Board. (2005). *Dietary reference intakes for energy, carbohydrate, fiber, fat, fatty acids, cholesterol, protein, and amino acids.* Washington, D.C.: National Academies Press.

Jeukendrup, A., & Gleeson, M. (2010). *Sports nutrition: An introduction to energy production and performance.* Champaign, IL: Human Kinetics.

Johnston, R. D., Stephenson, M. C., Crossland, H., Cordon, S. M., Palcidi, E., Cox, E. F., . . . Macdonald, I. A. (2013). No difference between high-fructose and high-glucose diets on liver triacylglycerol or biochemistry in healthy overweight men. *Gastroenterology, 145*(5), 1016–1025.

McArdle, W. D., Katch, F. I., & Katch, V. L. (2015). *Exercise physiology: Nutrition, energy, and human performance* (8th ed.). Baltimore, MD: Wolters Kluwer Health.

Melton, D., Dali, T. K., Katula, J. A., & Mustian, K. M. (2015). Women's perspectives of personal trainers: A qualitative study. *Sport Journal, 14*(1), 1–18.

Molfino, A., Gioia, G., Rossi-Fanelli, F., & Muscaritoli, M. (2013) Beta-hydroxy-beta-methylbutyrate supplementation in health and disease: A systematic review of randomized trials. *Amino Acids, 45*(6), 1273–1292.

Naude, C. E., Schoones, A., Senekal, M., Young, T., Garner, P., & Volmik, J. (2014). Low carbohydrate versus isoenergetic balanced diets for reducing weight and cardiovascular risk. A systematic review and meta-analysis. *PLoS One, 9*(7), e100652.

Noakes, T. D. (2013). Low-carbohydrate and high fat intake can manage obesity and associated conditions. Occasional survey. *South African Medical Journal, 103*, 826–830.

Ogden, C. L., Carroll, M. D., Kit, B. K., & Flegal, K. M. (2014). Prevalence of childhood and adult obesity in the United States, 2011–2012. *JAMA, 311*(8), 806–814.

Otles, S., & Ozqoz S. (2014). Health effects of dietary fiber. *Acta Scientiarum Polonorum. Technologia Alimentaria, 13*(2), 191–202.

Paddon-Jones, D., Borsheim, E., & Wolfe, R. R. (2004). Potential ergogenic effects of arginine and creatine supplementation. *Journal of Nutrition, 134*(10 Suppl), 2888S–2894S.

Pasiakos, S. M., McLellan, T. M., & Lieberman, H. R. (2015). The effects of protein supplements on muscle mass, strength, and aerobic and anaerobic power in healthy adults: A systematic review. *Sports Medicine, 45*(1), 111–131.

Phillips, S. M., & Van Loon, L. J. C. (2011). Dietary protein for athletes: From requirements to optimum adaptation. *Journal of Sports Sciences, 29*(Suppl. 1), S29–S38.

Rippe, J. M. (2013). The metabolic and endocrine response and health implications of consuming sugar-sweetened beverages: Findings from recent randomized controlled studies. *Advances in Nutrition, 4*(6), 677–686.

Rolls, B. J. (2012). Dietary strategies for weight management. *Nestle Nutrition Institute Workshop Series, 73*, 37–48.

Spriet, L. L. (2014). Exercise and sports performance with low doses of caffeine. *Sports Medicine, 44*(Suppl 2), S175–S184.

Tarnopolsky, M. A. (2010). Caffeine and creatine use in sport. *Annals of Nutrition and Metabolism, 57*(Suppl 2), 1–8. Epub 2011 Feb 22.

U.S. Department of Agriculture and U.S. Department of Health and Human Services (USDA). (2010). *Dietary Guidelines for Americans 2010* (7th ed.). Washington, D.C.: U.S. Government Printing Office.

Wagner, D. R., Larson, J. N., & Wengreen, H. (2012). Weight and body composition change over a six-week holiday period. *Eating and Weight Disorders, 17*(1), e54–56.

Wilson, J. M., Fitschen, P. J., Campbell, B., Wilson, G. J., Zanchi, N., Taylor, L., . . . Antonio, J. (2013). International Society of Sports Nutrition Position Stand: beta-hydroxy-beta-methylbutyrate (HMB). *Journal of the International Society of Sports Nutrition, 10,* 6.

Wolfe, R. R. (2012). The role of dietary protein in optimizing muscle mass, function and health outcomes in older individuals, *British Journal of Nutrition, 108*(Suppl. 2), S88–S93.

Zanchi, N. E., Gerlinger-Romero, F., Guimarães-Ferreira, L., de Siqueira Filho, M. A., Felitti, V., Lira, F. S., . . . Lancha, A. H. Jr. (2010). HMB supplementation: Clinical and athletic performance-related effects and mechanisms of action. *Amino Acids, 40,* 1015–1025.

CHAPTER 6

CONCEPTS OF INTEGRATED TRAINING

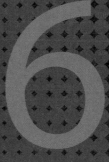

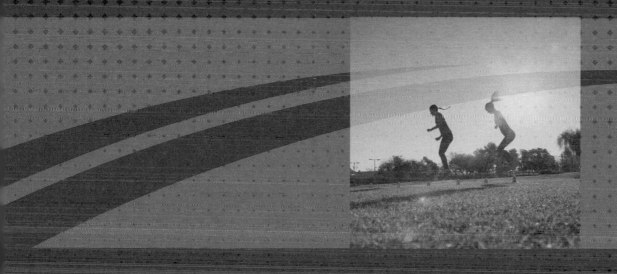

OBJECTIVES

After studying this chapter, you will be able to:

1. **Define** the principles of integrated training.

2. **Describe** the components, scientific rationale, and supporting evidence for integrated training.

3. **Explain** how the basic and applied sciences work together in an integrated approach.

4. **Apply** basic science to the development of an integrated training program.

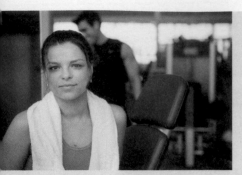

© Sean Locke Photography/Shutterstock

Case Scenario

You have become quite knowledgeable about the Human Movement System and biomechanics, and are now easily able to explain and dissect your daily movements. Your friend, who you have been working out with over the past few months, has complained to you on numerous occasions that she experiences frequent neck and lower back pain. Your friend is clearly committed and routinely joins you when coming to the gym—predominately running on the treadmill and frequenting an indoor spinning class that is regularly offered—but she has still been experiencing pain. She believed that exercise would help to alleviate her pain, and you have started to notice her frustration that it has not.

You have learned that she works in an office cubicle the majority of the week. How would you explain to her what integrated training is, and how it could help to minimize the neck and lower back pain she is experiencing? Keep in mind that your friend is relatively new to exercising on a regular basis and believes that hard work and results are directly proportionate.

How would you explain and incorporate the following components of integrated training to help her minimize her neck and lower back pain?

- Core training

- Balance training

- Reactive training

- Speed, agility, and quickness (SAQ) drills

- Resistance training

Introduction to Integrated Training

The previous chapters in this book have described the Human Movement System, biomechanics, and the nutrition necessary to set the stage for supporting client results. This chapter will continue to connect those topics by relating them to the scientific rationale for integrated training. This is the foundation for successful program design. To begin, it is important to understand the history and definition of *integrated training*.

The original personal trainers were bodybuilders, helping clients who wanted to achieve large, well-defined musculature for either competing on stage or simply improving personal appearance. Traditional bodybuilding exercise programs focus specifically on developing muscle strength and **hypertrophy** using single-joint or single-muscle exercises. Traditional selection and sequencing of exercises evolved from the bodybuilding community to a focus on the

Hypertrophy

Enlargement of skeletal muscle fibers in response to overcoming force from high volumes of tension.

methodology of isolation. These programs used isolation exercises and were structured around specific muscles or muscle groups that create movement at a particular joint. Most exercise machines focus on this type of muscle action in a single plane of motion.

However, fitness professionals began to notice a need for programs that addressed a person's functional and structural capacity. Activities of daily living and structural changes caused by emerging technologies and conveniences have led to the need for these types of programs. **Function** is an important component of an individual's everyday performance. It is defined as integrated, multiplanar movement that involves acceleration, stabilization, and deceleration. Integrated training arose out of the need for programs that involved a more well-rounded approach that met an individual's everyday needs to maintain function. Given that this is a three-dimensional and multiplanar world, with varying external demands and environments, training programs needed to evolve similarly. Programs had to shift from a one-size-fits-all model to a more diverse programming schematic that considered a person's goals, needs, environment, and abilities in a safe and systematic fashion. This led to the rise of the concept of integrated training.

Function
Integrated, multiplanar movement that involves acceleration, stabilization, and deceleration.

Components of Integrated Training

Integrated training is a comprehensive training approach that combines all the components necessary to help any client achieve optimum performance. The integrated training concept incorporates all forms of exercise as part of a progressive system. Integrated training includes all elements of effective movement: flexibility; cardiorespiratory; core; balance; reactive; speed, agility, and quickness (SAQ); and resistance training. Integrated training is built upon the primary training principles, thus ensuring that individuals achieve their goals in a safe and effective manner. These principles include the general adaptation syndrome, the principle of specificity, the principle of overload, and the principle of variation.

Integrated training
A comprehensive training approach that combines all the components necessary to help a client achieve optimum performance.

General Adaptation Syndrome

The **general adaptation syndrome (GAS)** provides an overview of how the Human Movement System adapts to the demands imposed by physical activity (**Table 6.1**). Exercise places a physical stress on the body. Every exercise stress applied results in specific biochemical, neurological, and mechanical adaptations in the body. A new exercise stimulus creates a response until the

General adaptation syndrome (GAS)
(1) How the kinetic chain responds and adapts to imposed demands. (2) How the body responds and adapts to stress.

TABLE 6.1 The General Adaptation Syndrome

Stage	Reaction
Alarm reaction	Initial reaction to stressor, such as increased oxygen and blood supply to the necessary areas of the body.
Resistance development	Increased functional capacity to adapt to stressor, such as increasing motor unit recruitment.
Exhaustion	A prolonged intolerable stressor produces fatigue and leads to a breakdown in the system or injury.

Alarm phase

The first stage of the GAS; the initial phase of response to a new stimuli within the Human Movement System.

Adaptation phase

The second stage of the GAS in which physiological changes take place in order to meet the demands of the newly imposed stress.

Intermuscular coordination

The ability of the neuromuscular system to allow all muscles to work together with proper activation and timing.

Exhaustion phase

The third stage of GAS in which stress continues beyond the body's ability to adapt, leading to potential physiological and structural breakdown.

Overtraining syndrome (OTS)

Excessive frequency, volume, or intensity of training, resulting in fatigue; also caused by a lack of proper rest and recovery.

MEMORY TIPS

Think of the alarm phase as an alarm clock. The alarm phase wakes your body up and alerts the kinetic chain to a new stimulus, much as an alarm clock wakes you up and alerts you to a new day.

body has adapted to the stimulus. Three specific phases of how the body adapts to an exercise stimulus have been identified (Selye, 1976):

1. **Alarm phase**: The alarm phase, which is also referred to as the *shock phase*, is the initial response to the imposed demands of exercise, lasting approximately 2–3 weeks. This is when the initial neuromuscular adaptations of the body (e.g., strength, coordination) occur. During this phase, most of the strength gains will be due to neuromuscular adaptations, not actual structural changes within the Human Movement System. An individual in this phase may feel fatigued, weak, or sore as his or her body adapts to the demands of exercise. These symptoms are temporary and will resolve as physical activity continues.

2. **Adaptation phase**: In the adaptation, or resistance, phase, the body adapts to the applied stimuli by changing structures within the human body and their physiological function. For example, during this phase individual muscle fibers experience an increase in thickness and improved motor unit synchronization, both of which can help increase the net magnitude of force production. This phase is characterized by progressive improvements in strength due to more efficient neural recruitment of the involved muscle fibers, increased muscle volume, and more efficient **intermuscular coordination**. This phase can last approximately 4–12 weeks after the introduction of the training stress.

3. **Exhaustion phase**: In this phase, the body can no longer tolerate the physiological stresses and imposed demands of the applied training stimulus. Once an individual has reached the exhaustion phase, further adaptations may halt, and the risk of overtraining greatly increases. **Overtraining syndrome (OTS)**, sometimes described as being "under-recovered," can affect various parts of the kinetic chain. OTS can lead to a host of physiological problems, including recurring illness, loss of sleep, moodiness, decreased physical performance, and overuse injuries. Applying appropriate rest periods between training sessions decreases the risk of OTS (Selye, 1976).

The GAS establishes the rationale for changing the **acute variables** on a regular basis. As the kinetic chain adapts to a specific type of exercise, it may cease to experience the intended adaptations, making it necessary to change the acute variables to ensure that the body continues to experience the desired changes.

Principle of Specificity

Changes to the kinetic chain do not occur without a preceding stimulus. The concept that the Human Movement System will adapt and change in response to the specific types of exercises applied is known as the principle of specificity. Also referred to as the **specific adaptation to imposed demands (SAID) principle**, it states that the type of exercise stimulus placed on the body will determine the expected physiological outcome. Each system of the body (e.g., neural, endocrine, muscular, skeletal) will respond and adapt to the specific physical demands applied through a progressively challenging exercise program. This principle implies that what an individual trains for is the specific outcome he or she will get. If a client wants to run a marathon, the focus of the program should be on endurance. If an older client wants to work on balance to better avoid falls, the focus of the program should be on incorporating stabilization training strategies. In both examples, the programming is unique to the needs of the client, while also incorporating all the components of integrated training. The fitness professional must have a good understanding of the client's activities and goals so that he or she can create a program that will meet the mechanical, neuromuscular, and metabolic demands associated with the client's goals (Barnett, Ross, Schmidt, & Todd, 1973).

Mechanical Specificity

Mechanical specificity refers to the weight and movements placed on the body. Daily and activity-specific movement patterns and forces need to be fully acknowledged in order to develop a program that will meet the mechanical needs of the client. For example, to develop endurance in the legs, lighter weights would be used with a high number of **repetitions**. Similarly, transverse plane movements to mimic the swing of a golf club or baseball bat would be incorporated into a sport-specific training program. The client's goals and physical capabilities will dictate the mechanical specificity of the training protocol (Tan, 1999; Kraemer & Ratamess, 2000).

Neuromuscular Specificity

Neuromuscular specificity refers to the specific exercises using different speeds and movement patterns that are performed to increase neuromuscular efficiency. For every movement, a set recruitment pattern of muscular tissue must be produced by the nervous system. This controls the coordination and speed of specific muscle fibers to meet the performance demands required by the specific activity. For example, to develop higher levels of power, high-velocity exercises are used to develop the ability to contract the muscle fibers as quickly as possible. If stability is a goal, training in environments that are unstable, yet controllable, helps the nervous system develop better control of finite muscle contractions to maintain balance (Gabriel, Kamen, & Frost, 2006; Hakkinen, 1994; McEvoy & Newton, 1998).

Metabolic Specificity

Metabolic specificity refers to the energy demand placed on the body. When training for endurance events, it is important for the body to efficiently utilize the aerobic energy system. If the individual is participating in shorter but more intense bouts of activity, the programming should emphasize the anaerobic energy pathway. Because of this, the cardiorespiratory training programs for a marathon runner and a sprinter will be vastly different (Harmer et al., 2000; Parra, Cadefau, Rodas, Amigo, & Cusso, 2000).

Overload Principle

The **overload principle** states that in order to create physiological changes, an exercise stimulus must be applied at an intensity greater than the system is accustomed to receiving. This increased stimulus results in the system adapting to the increased demands, and providing a desired change. When the body is not overloaded, it ceases to change. The body will reach a level of **homeostasis** when presented with the same recurring stimuli. This principle is the foundation for the GAS. In order for adaptation to occur, the program needs to challenge the Human Movement System safely and effectively. Adjusting the acute variables will provide the added stimulus needed in order to overload the system and push it out of homeostasis. This is why fitness professionals change a workout routine after a certain number of sessions (de Hoyo et al., 2015; Ramírez-Campillo et al., 2015; Tous-Fajardo, Gonzalo-Skok, Arjol-Serrano, & Tesch, 2015). The fitness professional needs to be able to balance the overload principle with the GAS in order to avoid overtraining. Smart programming with integrated training will

---

Acute variables
The components that specify how each exercise is to be performed.

Specific adaptation to imposed demands (SAID) principle
States that the type of exercise stimulus placed on the body will determine the expected physiological outcome.

Mechanical specificity
(1) The specific muscular requirements using different weights and movements that are performed to increase strength or endurance in certain body parts. (2) The weights and movements placed on the body.

Repetition
One complete movement of a single exercise.

Neuromuscular specificity
The specific muscular contractions using different speeds and patterns that are performed to increase neuromuscular efficiency.

Metabolic specificity
Energy demand placed on the body.

Overload principle
States that in order to create physiological changes an exercise stimulus must be applied at an intensity greater than the body is accustomed to receiving.

Homeostasis

The ability or tendency of an organism or a cell to maintain internal equilibrium by adjusting its physiological processes.

Principle of variation

Rationale for challenging the kinetic chain with a wide variety of exercises and stimuli.

Set

A group of consecutive repetitions.

provide the rest necessary to avoid overtraining, while still maximizing the overload principle to achieve the client's goals.

Principle of Variation

The **principle of variation** is an important rationale for challenging the kinetic chain with a wide variety of exercises. According to the GAS, the Human Movement System will experience adaption to an exercise stimulus after approximately 8–12 weeks. An integrated program constantly adjusts the acute variables. The variables are adjusted to meet a specific goal during a planned period of training. By making a long-term programming plan, the principle of variation can be maximized to achieve the desired goals. Variation can also keep a person from reaching the exhaustion phase, while also maximizing the overload principle. By applying these principles in unison when developing a program, the fitness professional can develop a program that helps the client to reach his or her highest level of individual performance.

Rationale to Support Integrated Training

Integrated training is a comprehensive way to ensure a client's safety and health by using an organized, systematic approach to developing a training program. Each component of an integrated training program is selected based on the varying needs of today's fitness client. Research suggests that musculoskeletal pain is more common now than it was 40 years ago (Harkness, Macfarlane, Silman, & McBeth, 2005). Many causes of movement dysfunction are related to everyday life (e.g., work, movement patterns, inactivity). Also, the less conditioned the musculoskeletal system is, the higher the risk of injury becomes (Barr, Griggs, & Cadby, 2005). That being said, an exercise program needs to address all of the components of health-related physical fitness. Vital components of a safe and effective exercise program are the use of specific exercises to train essential areas of the body, such as the stabilizing muscles of the hips, trunk, and neck, and to use a proper progression of acute variables (e.g., **sets**, repetitions, and rest periods).

Low Back Pain

Low back pain is a primary cause of musculoskeletal degeneration in the adult population (**Figure 6.1**), affecting approximately 80% of all adults (Cassidy, Carroll, & Cote, 1998; Walker, Muller, & Grant, 2004). Research has shown that low back pain is common among workers in enclosed workspaces, such as offices, as well as those engaged in manual labor. Low back pain is also seen in people who often sit for long periods of time, typically more than 3 hours (Omokhodion, 2002; Omokhodion & Sanya, 2003; Volinn, 1997).

Knee Injuries

An estimated 80,000–100,000 anterior cruciate ligament (ACL) injuries occur each year in the United States (**Figure 6.2**). Approximately 70% of these are noncontact injuries (Griffin et al., 2000). ACL injuries have a strong correlation with the development of arthritis in the affected

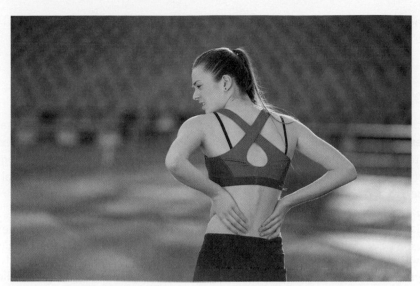

FIGURE 6.1 Low back pain.
© Andrey Orletsky/Shutterstock

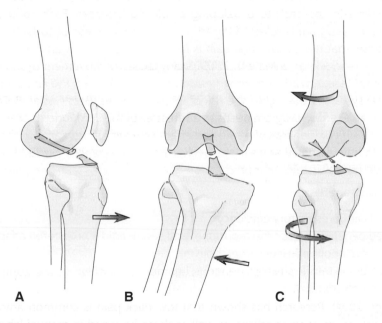

A   B   C

FIGURE 6.2 ACL tear.

knee (Hill et al., 2005). Most ACL injuries occur in people 15–25 years of age (Griffin et al., 2000). This comes as no surprise, considering the lack of activity and increased obesity occurring in this age group, in part due to an abundance of automation and technology, combined with a lack of mandatory physical education in schools (Zack et al., 2004). Fortunately, research suggests that enhancing neuromuscular stabilization may alleviate the high incidence of noncontact injuries (**Figure 6.3**; Mandelbaum et al., 2005).

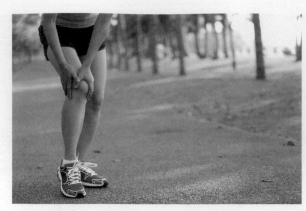

FIGURE 6.3 Noncontact knee injury.
© lzf/Shutterstock

With more people living sedentary lifestyles, while at the same time living longer, today's average client is often not ready to begin physical activity at the same level a typical client could 30 years ago (Centers for Disease Control and Prevention, 2004; Haskell et al., 2007). Therefore, today's training programs cannot stay the same as those used in the past. The new mindset in the fitness industry is on creating programs that address functional capacity as part of a safe program designed specifically for each individual. In other words, training programs must consider an individual's goals, needs, and abilities in a safe and systematic fashion. This is best achieved by introducing an integrated approach to program design.

Integrated Training and the OPT Model

The Optimum Performance Training (OPT) model was conceptualized as a training program for a society that has more structural imbalances and susceptibility to injury than ever before. It is a process of programming that systematically progresses any client to any goal. The OPT model is built on a foundation of principles that allows any client to achieve peak levels of physiological, physical, and performance adaptations:

Physiological benefits:

- Improved cardiorespiratory efficiency.
- Enhanced beneficial endocrine (hormone) and serum lipid (cholesterol) adaptations.
- Increased metabolic efficiency (metabolism).
- Increased tissue tensile strength (tendons, ligaments, muscles).
- Increased bone density.

Physical benefits:

- Decreased body fat.
- Increased lean muscle mass.

Performance benefits:

- Improved flexibility.
- Better balance.
- Enhanced endurance.
- Improved speed, agility, and quickness.
- Greater strength.
- More power.

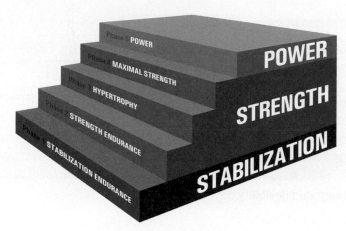

FIGURE 6.4 The OPT model.

The OPT model is a comprehensive approach to training that combines flexibility, cardiorespiratory, core, balance, reactive, SAQ, and total body resistance training for each level and phase of programming (Figure 6.4). In fact, given an individual's state of health, integrated training that focuses on incorporating each of these aspects may help reduce the risk of injury, increase neuromuscular efficiency, stabilize dynamic joints, and improve speed and reaction times. Research has demonstrated increased performance and fitness measures using this integrated approach (Clemson et al., 2012; Distefano et al., 2013; Ratamess et al., 2007). We will review each of the components of an integrated training program and their benefits in more detail.

Integrated Flexibility Training

Flexibility is defined as the normal extensibility of all soft tissue that allows for optimal range of motion of a joint. Structural changes due to decreased activity and pattern overload can create muscle imbalances and poor soft tissue extensibility around joints (i.e., poor flexibility), which can decrease performance and increase the risk of injury (Amako, Oda, Masuoka, Yokoi, & Campisi, 2003; Hartig & Henderson, 1999; Kay & Blazevich, 2012; Knapik, Bauman, Jones, Harris, & Vaughan, 1991; Witvrouw, Danneels, Asselman, D'Have, & Cambier, 2003). The integrated flexibility continuum incorporates different forms of flexibility (i.e., myofascial release and static, active, and dynamic stretching) at different programming levels of the OPT model based on the person's goals, capabilities, and structural limitations (Figure 6.5).

Integrated flexibility is performed to correct muscle imbalances, increase joint range of motion, decrease muscle soreness, relieve joint stress, improve muscle extensibility, and maintain the functional length of all muscles. These factors increase neuromuscular efficiency and enhance overall function. If an individual does not have the proper extensibility and neuromuscular control around a joint, exercise performance will be limited. For example, if a person's pectoralis major is too tight, the shoulder's range of motion is limited, creating internal rotation of the humerus and lengthening the posterior deltoids and mid/lower trapezius. Over time this limitation in shoulder extensibility, and decreased function of the posterior muscles, will decrease stabilization at the shoulder and eventually lead to injury. Research has indicated that flexibility training may decrease the occurrences of low back pain, joint pain, and overuse injuries (Gadjoski, 2001; Hartig & Henderson, 1999; Pope, Herbert, & Kirwan, 2002).

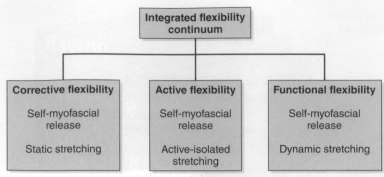

FIGURE 6.5 Integrated flexibility continuum.

Flexibility Improvement

In order to achieve ideal extensibility, the integrated flexibility continuum identifies how muscle physiology plays a role in stretching techniques. Muscles, tendons, ligaments, and joint capsules contain small sensory receptors called *mechanoreceptors* that send messages from the source to the nervous system to detect any distortion in soft tissues, such as stretch, touch, and pressure. Two important mechanoreceptors involved in flexibility are muscle spindles (**Figure 6.6**) and the Golgi tendon organs (**Figure 6.7**). Muscle spindles are sensitive to the change of length of a muscle, whereas Golgi tendon organs are sensitive to changes in the tension of the muscles.

These mechanoreceptors are integral in regaining muscle extensibility. Prolonged tension in a muscle creates an inhibitory action called **autogenic inhibition**. When stretching a muscle, the muscle spindles are initially stimulated to help protect the muscle from stretching too far, causing the muscle to contract. This can be experienced by the feeling of initial "tightness" when initiating the stretch. As the stretch is held, more tension is created, stimulating the Golgi tendon organ, which then overrides the muscle spindles, causing the muscle to relax. At this

Autogenic inhibition

The process by which neural impulses that sense tension are greater than the impulses that cause muscles to contract, providing an inhibitory effect to the muscle.

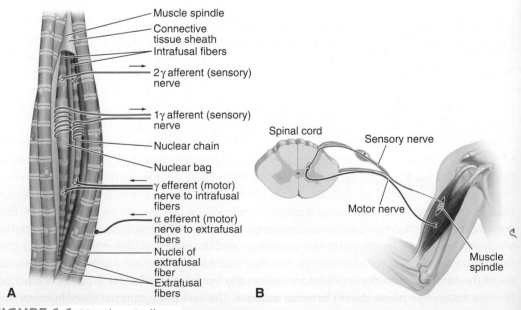

FIGURE 6.6 Muscle spindles.

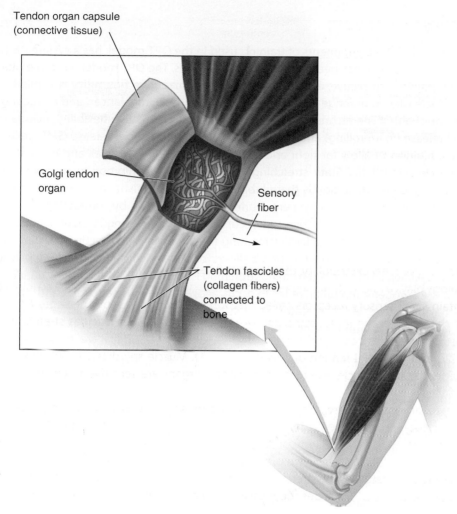

FIGURE 6.7 Golgi tendon organs.

point, the "tightness" first experienced when engaging in the stretch decreases, allowing the joint to be placed in a new position to further stretch the muscle. Over time, this can lead to permanent changes in the muscle and the associated tissues (e.g., fascia, tendon), resulting in tissues that are more extensible and ultimately leading to a greater range of motion. Because autogenic inhibition is activated through the development of tension, it becomes important that stretches are held for a specific period of time (20–60 seconds) so that enough tension is created to stimulate this reflex (Chaitow, 1997; Etnyre & Abraham, 1986).

Multiplanar Extensibility

Muscles work in all three planes of motion. To help maximize tissue extensibility in all three planes of motion, it becomes important to stretch a muscle in all three planes of motion. Stretching in only one plane could lead to compensation, and the potential for further imbalances. For example, for the latissimus dorsi to have optimal multiplanar extensibility it must be extensible in the sagittal plane during shoulder flexion, the frontal plane during shoulder abduction, and the transverse plane during external rotation. This will allow optimal glenohumeral and scapula-thoracic movement, decreasing the risk of synergistic dominance around those joints.

Flexibility Continuum

Flexibility, like all of the components of training used in the OPT model, has a systematic progression based on the client's needs, goals, and capabilities. The OPT model has three phases of flexibility training: corrective, active, and functional. **Corrective flexibility** is applied with the goal of increasing joint range of motion, improving muscle imbalances, and correcting altered joint mechanics. The techniques used when applying corrective flexibility include self-myofascial release (foam-rolling) and static stretching. Self-myofascial release (SMR) relies on autogenic inhibition to allow for tight and/or overactive muscles to relax and elongate, improving muscle extensibility. Static stretching utilizes reciprocal inhibition to improve muscle extensibility. Reciprocal inhibition is the inhibition of an antagonistic muscle while the agonist contracts to allow for joint movement. During static stretching, by contracting the antagonist, further decreases in neural drive can occur to the muscle being stretched, enhancing the stretch. For example, when statically stretching the hip flexors, contracting the gluteals to further decrease neural drive to the hip flexors allows for greater lengthening of the hip flexors. As mentioned earlier, a key element to static stretching is to hold the stretch for 20–60 seconds to allow for the autogenic inhibition reflex to occur, allowing the muscle to relax and stretch.

Active flexibility uses **active-isolated stretching**, allowing for an agonist and its synergist muscles to move a limb through a full range of motion while the antagonists are being stretched. For example, an active supine hamstring stretch is performed by extending the knee through the contraction of the quadriceps, while relaxing the hamstrings for the stretch. The stretch is held for 2–5 seconds at the end range of motion, and then relaxed. This would be repeated for the specified number of repetitions.

Functional flexibility utilizes **dynamic stretching**. Dynamic stretching requires multiplanar extensibility with optimal neuromuscular control though a full range of motion. Examples of dynamic stretches include bodyweight squats or walking lunges with medicine ball rotation. Dynamic stretches should be reserved for those who have progressed to a higher level of the OPT model. These individuals should have developed good neuromuscular control and reduced their muscle imbalances.

Integrated Cardiorespiratory Training

Of the various components that comprise a client's total physical fitness program, cardiorespiratory training is probably the most misunderstood and underrated. Clients often fail to understand why cardiorespiratory training is so important to their total training program. In order to understand how to perform cardiorespiratory training in the most effective and efficient way, the fitness professional must understand the client's overall goals.

The following are the most common goals of cardiorespiratory training:

◆ To improve health by reducing cardiovascular risk factors (e.g., unhealthy body composition, poor blood lipid profile, high blood pressure).
◆ To assist in weight management.
◆ To improve performance in work, life, and sports.
◆ To reduce mental anxiety.

Cardiorespiratory training is more than just training the aerobic energy system. In order to meet the goals outlined above, the aerobic energy system *and* the anaerobic energy system

---

Corrective flexibility

Flexibility training that is applied with the goal of improving muscle imbalances and correcting altered joint mechanics.

Active-isolated stretching

Flexibility exercises in which agonists move a limb through a full range of motion, allowing the antagonists to stretch.

Dynamic stretching

Multiplanar extensibility with optimal neuromuscular control through a full range of motion.

TRAINER TIPS

Clients who are not used to stretching may feel greater tightness when you have them stretch their muscles before an exercise or workout. Assure them that this tightness will soon subside during the stretch.

must both be trained. This is especially true for clients who constantly switch between their aerobic and anaerobic energy systems, maximizing performance and minimizing fatigue (e.g., soccer players during a match). This type of conditioning is referred to as *interval training*.

Methods for Prescribing Exercise Intensity

In order to properly program for cardiorespiratory training, the fitness professional must be able to prescribe specific intensities for the client to perform at. Fitness professionals have several different ways to prescribe intensity for cardiorespiratory work.

Peak $\dot{V}O_2$ Method

The traditional gold standard for cardiorespiratory fitness is $\dot{V}O_{2max}$, the maximal volume of oxygen (in liters) per kilogram body weight utilized per minute. In other words, $\dot{V}O_{2max}$ is the maximal amount of oxygen that an individual can use during intense exercise. Once $\dot{V}O_{2max}$ is determined, a common method to establish exercise training intensity is to have clients exercise at a percentage of their $\dot{V}O_{2max}$. However, accurately measuring $\dot{V}O_{2max}$ is often impractical for fitness professionals, because it requires clients to perform cardiorespiratory exercise at maximal effort. This requires a great deal of personal motivation from the client. Sophisticated equipment is also required to monitor the client's ventilation response (oxygen consumed and carbon dioxide expired). Therefore, submaximal tests to estimate $\dot{V}O_{2max}$, are utilized for cardiorespiratory programming.

$\dot{V}O_{2max}$
The highest rate of oxygen transport and utilization achieved at maximal physical exertion.

Maximal Heart Rate Method

For years, a person's maximal heart rate (HR_{max}) was determined through the use of the age-related heart rate formula of (220 − Age). Despite the acceptance of this formula, research spanning more than two decades revealed a large error inherent in the estimation of HR_{max} of around 7–11 beats per minute (Visich, 2003). Consequently, the formula $HR_{max} = 220 − Age$ has little scientific merit for use in exercise physiology and related fields. It is for this reason that the regression formula of 208 − (0.7 × Age) has been adopted, because it has been shown that this method of determining HR_{max} is much more closely related to age compared to the 220 − Age formula (Tanaka, Monahan, & Seals, 2001). This equation is very simple to use, and can be easily implemented as a general starting point for measuring cardiorespiratory training intensity. However, fitness professionals should keep in mind that this, or any other simple formula, is not a definitive HR_{max} value.

Heart Rate Reserve (HRR) Method

The **heart rate reserve (HRR) method**, also known as the Karvonen method, is a method of establishing training intensity based on the difference between a client's predicted maximal heart rate and his or her resting heart rate. Because heart rate and oxygen uptake are linearly related during dynamic exercise, selecting a predetermined training or target heart rate (THR) based on a given percentage of oxygen consumption is the most common and universally accepted method of establishing exercise training intensity. The HRR method is defined as:

Heart rate reserve (HRR) method
A method of establishing training intensity based on the difference between a client's predicted maximal heart rate and his or her resting heart rate.

$$THR = [(HR_{max} − HR_{rest}) \times \text{Desired intensity}] + HR_{rest}$$

6	No exertion at all
7	Extremely light
8	
9	Very light
10	
11	Light
12	
13	Somewhat hard
14	
15	Hard (heavy)
16	
17	Very hard
18	
19	Extremely hard
20	Maximal exertion

FIGURE 6.8 Rating of perceived exertion (Borg scale).

Rating of Perceived Exertion Method

A subjective **rating of perceived exertion (RPE)** is a technique used to express or validate how hard a client feels he or she is working during exercise. When using the RPE method, a person is subjectively rating the perceived difficulty of exercise. It is based on the physical sensations a person experiences during physical activity, including increased heart rate, respiration rate, and sweating and muscle fatigue. The client's subjective rating should be reported based on the overall feelings of effort, including an overall sense of fatigue and not just isolated areas of the body (e.g., tired legs during treadmill testing). Although the RPE scale is a subjective measure, if clients report their exertion ratings accurately it does provide a fairly good estimate of the actual heart rate during physical activity. Moderately-intense activity is equal to "somewhat hard" (12–14) on the 6–20 Borg scale (**Figure 6.8**).

Talk Test

The talk test is an informal method used to gauge exercise training intensity. The belief has always been that if clients reach a point at which they are not able to carry on a simple conversation during exercise because they are breathing too hard, then they are probably exercising at too high of an intensity. A number of studies have reported a correlation between the talk test, $\dot{V}O_2$, the **ventilatory threshold (T_{vent})**, and heart rate during both cycle ergometer and treadmill exercise (Foster et al., 2008; Persinger, Foster, Gibson, Fater, & Porcari, 2004). Thus, it appears that the talk test can help fitness professionals and clients monitor proper exercise intensity without having to rely on measuring heart rate or $\dot{V}O_{2max}$. A summary of the methods for prescribing exercise intensity is provided in **Table 6.2**.

Rating of perceived exertion (RPE)

A technique used to express or validate how hard a client feels he or she is working during exercise.

Ventilatory threshold (T_{vent})

The point during graded exercise at which ventilation increases disproportionately to oxygen uptake, signifying a switch from predominately aerobic energy production to anaerobic energy production.

CHECK IT OUT

Consider the following example of a 25-year-old client with a desired training intensity of 85% of his heart rate maximum. If this 25-year-old client has a resting heart rate of 40 bpm (which is considered very good), then the formulas would be solved as follows:

Age-Related Heart Rate

$$220 - 25 = 195\ HR_{max}$$
$$195 \times 85\% = 165.75$$

Thus, 166 bpm is the client's target heart rate.

Regression Formula

$$208 - (0.7 \times 25) = 190.5\ HR_{max}$$
$$190.5 \times 85\% = 161.925$$

Thus, 162 bpm is the client's target heart rate.

Heart Rate Reserve

$$220 - 25 = 195\ HR_{max}$$
$$195 - 40 - 155$$
$$155 \times 85\% = 132$$
$$132 + 40 = 172\ bpm$$

Thus, 172 beats per minute is the client's target heart rate.

TABLE 6.2 Methods for Prescribing Exercise Intensity

Method	Formula
Peak $\dot{V}o_2$	Target $\dot{V}o_2 = \dot{V}o_{2max} \times$ intensity desired
Peak heart rate (HR)	Target HR (THR) = $HR_{max} \times \%$ intensity desired
Heart rate reserve (HRR)	Target heart rate (THR) = $[(HR_{max} - HR_{rest}) \times \%$ intensity desired$] + HR_{rest}$
Ratings of perceived exertion (RPE)	6- to 20-point scale
Talk test	The ability to speak during activity can identify exercise intensity and ventilatory threshold

TRAINER TIPS

Before prescribing specific exercise intensities for clients, ensure that they have had the foundational health assessments and that they are healthy enough for high-intensity training.

Benefits of Interval Training and Zone Training

If the goal is to bring positive physical changes to a client's cardiorespiratory system, then overloading is necessary. An increased workload will cause fatigue and, with the proper recovery, eventually yield cardiorespiratory improvements. If the workloads are of the right elevated

Anaerobic threshold

The point during high-intensity activity when the body can no longer meet its demand for oxygen and anaerobic metabolism predominates; also called the *lactate threshold*.

Interval training

Training that alternates between intense exertion and periods of rest or lighter exertion.

Resting heart rate (RHR)

The number of contractions of the heart occurring in 1 minute while the body is at rest.

magnitude (i.e., slightly more than the body is currently used to), then adaptation occurs. It is important to note that the overload happens during the exercise, whereas the adaptations occur during recovery. Recovery is, therefore, a vital part of any client's program.

In order to overload the cardiorespiratory system and achieve the desired adaptations, zone training may be employed. Three zones are applied to zone training. Zone 1 consists of an individual maintaining a training heart rate of approximately 65–75% of his or her HR_{max}. This zone is referred to as the recovery, or cardio base, zone. Clients who stay in this zone without variation will initially improve their volume of oxygen consumption, but will quickly plateau. When this occurs weight loss slows or sometimes stops. If Zone 1 intensity is maintained, the only solution to end the plateau is to keep increasing the length of time exercising.

Zone 2 is close to a person's **anaerobic threshold** at 76–85% of HR_{max}. In this zone, the body can no longer produce enough energy for the working muscles with just the aerobic energy system. The higher the intensity the body can train at while remaining aerobic, the greater the number of calories burned from fat. Thus, one of the main goals of cardiorespiratory training is to increase the anaerobic threshold. This can be effective for fat reduction. However, as with Zone 1, if a participant continues to only train in this zone, then plateaus will occur. To improve fitness level or increase metabolism, the client must overload the body. This leads to Zone 3 training.

A true high-intensity workout would be considered reaching 90% of HR_{max}, which may require several short sprints. Zone 3 will be getting close to peak exertion levels. A client may exercise in Zone 3 for 30–60 seconds and then recover in Zones 1 or 2 before repeating (i.e., **interval training**). For most individuals, exercising in Zone 3 once per week is enough to obtain the benefits of this level of higher intensity without overtraining.

Preventing Overtraining During Zone Training

The fitness professional can use a client's **resting heart rate (RHR)** to determine if the client is being overtrained. For 5 days, the fitness professional will have the client record his or her true RHR (i.e., heart rate upon waking in the morning), and then calculate the average RHR for that time period. When taking a pulse in the fitness setting, the client's heart rate should be no more than 8 bpm higher than the RHR. If the client's heart rate is more than 8 bpm higher than the average morning pulse, it is advised that the client reduce the training load for the day.

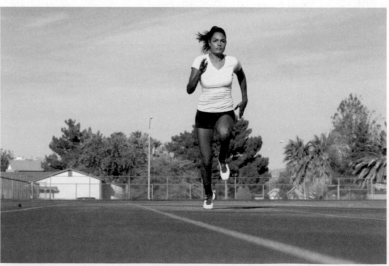

© LifetimeStock/Shutterstock

CHECK IT OUT

Another useful test to check for overtraining is to instruct the client to lie flat on the floor for several minutes and rest. The fitness professional should take the client's heart rate and then instruct the client to stand up. The client's heart rate after standing up should not increase by more than 10 bpm. If there is an increase of more than 10 bpm upon standing, it is advised that the client take that day off from training. Refrain from this test if a client should not lie down due to medical conditions.

CAUTION

Be sure to keep an eye out for obvious signs of overtraining in each client, including:

- Inability to reach target training zones.
- Inadequate sleep at night.
- Chronically elevated resting heart rate.
- Increased number of injuries.
- More frequent illness.
- Persistent muscle soreness.
- Chronic fatigue.

Integrated Core Training

Core training is the foundation of optimal movement. It is where movement begins and ends. Without adequate neuromuscular control, stabilization, strength, and power in the core musculature, clients cannot optimally harness the strength and power of their prime movers. Integrated core training is a systematic and progressive approach to develop muscular balance, neuromuscular efficiency, endurance, strength, and power in the core.

Structure and Function of the Core

Anatomically, the core is synonymous to what is termed the *lumbo-pelvic-hip complex* (LPHC). (Figure 6.9). This is the area of the body that lies between the inferior portion of the chest and the inferior portion of the gluteals. It consists of both passive and active structures, including bones, connective tissues (e.g., ligaments, fascia), and muscles; all must work together in an integrated fashion to ensure optimal function and movement. The core works to absorb and transfer forces to and from the upper and lower extremities. The muscles of the core also help to stabilize the lumbar spine, pelvis, and hips, protecting these regions from excessive stress and injury.

Activating the Core

The best method to activate the muscles of the core has been widely debated. The two activation methods most frequently utilized are the drawing-in maneuver and abdominal bracing.

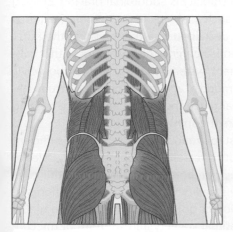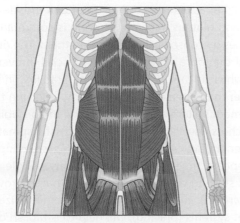

FIGURE 6.9 Lumbo-pelvic-hip complex.

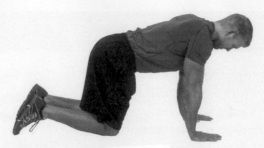

FIGURE 6.10 Quadruped with abdominal bracing.

Although each technique emphasizes the activation of one core system over the other (stabilization vs. movement system), both are crucial in ensuring optimal core stability and strength.

The Drawing-In Maneuver

The drawing-in maneuver was first introduced through research that looked at the role the transverse abdominus played in spinal stabilization and low back pain (Hodges & Richardson, 1996, 1997a, 1997b; Hodges, Richardson, & Jull, 1996). It was found that people who suffered from low back pain displayed a delay in activity of the transverse abdominus and lumbar multifidi associated with quick movements of the extremities (Hodges & Richardson, 1996). The research also showed that independent contraction of the transverse abdominus might contribute to stiffness of the sacroiliac joint (Hodges & Richardson, 1997a, 1997b). Further evidence pointed to increased stability when performing an intentional contraction of the abdominal muscles using the drawing-in maneuver (Hodges et al., 1996).

The maneuver is performed by drawing the navel back toward the spine without spinal flexion; this is similar to pulling the stomach in when trying to button a pair of tight jeans. The premise behind the drawing-in maneuver is that it contracts the transverse abdominus bilaterally to form a corset, which is thought to increase the segmental stability of the lumbar spine (Hodges & Richardson, 1997b). The maneuver also helps to activate the inner unit of the core, creating stability (Aroski, Valta, Airaksinen, & Kankaanpaa, 2001).

Abdominal Bracing

The second technique to activate the core for optimal stability is abdominal bracing. Bracing is referred to as a cocontraction of outer unit muscles, such as the rectus abdominus, external obliques, and gluteus maximus. Bracing is commonly described as a tightening of the outer unit muscles by consciously contracting them. The premise behind this technique is that contraction of the more superficial core muscles (movement system) will improve lumbo-pelvic stiffness, which, in turn, will lead to spinal stability. This mode of activation focuses on trunk stability rather than intersegmental stability, asserting that given the proper endurance training the movement system muscles will also work to stabilize the spine (McGill, 2001).

Researchers have concluded that successful spinal stabilization depends on both sufficient tension-generating capacity and nervous system input to recruit the appropriate muscles at the appropriate times (McGill, 2001). Many people lack neuromuscular control of the core. Therefore, starting clients with exercises that improve stability via the local stabilization system (drawing-in), and then progressing to the utilization of both the stabilization and global movement systems (bracing), will help to establish optimal stability and strength of the core (**Table 6.3**).

TRAINER TIPS

Clients can learn the drawing-in maneuver by performing the "cat" exercise from the quadruped position (Figure 6.10).

TRAINER TIPS

Clients can learn proper abdominal bracing techniques through exercises such as the low or high prone iso-abs (Figure 6.11) and floor bridge (Figure 6.12).

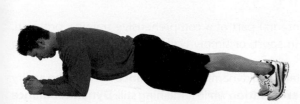

FIGURE 6.11 Prone iso-abs.

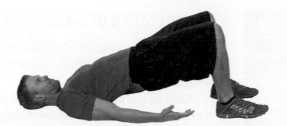

FIGURE 6.12 Floor bridge.

TABLE 6.3 Global and Local Musculature Subsystems

Local Stabilization System	Global Stabilization System	Global Stabilization System (cont.)
Transversus abdominis	Quadratus lumborum	Latissimus dorsi
Internal oblique	Psoas major	Hip flexors
Lumbar multifidus	External oblique	Hamstring complex
Pelvic floor muscles	Portions of internal oblique	Quadriceps
Diaphragm	Rectus abdominis	
	Gluteus medius	
	Adductor complex • Adductor magnus • Adductor longus • Adductor brevis • Gracilis • Pectineus	

CHECK IT OUT

Care should be taken when performing abdominal bracing. The technique can increase intra-abdominal pressure if the client holds his or her breath while bracing. This is the Valsalva maneuver. The intra-abdominal pressure can increase the blood pressure and potentially cause the client to pass out. The client should be coached to continue breathing during all exercise.

Integrated Balance Training

Integrated balance training is a systematic and progressive training process designed to develop neuromuscular efficiency. Balance training simulates **proprioceptively enriched environments** (i.e., unstable, yet controlled), teaching the body how to recruit the right muscle, at the right time, with the right amount of force. This leads to increased inter- and **intramuscular coordination**, which will result in greater force production and injury prevention.

TRAINER TIPS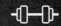

Proprioceptively enriched environments can be created by having clients close one or both eyes, balance on one leg, use a foam pad or inflatable disc, or exercise in sand.

Proprioceptively enriched environments
Unstable, yet controllable environments.

Intramuscular coordination
The ability of the neuromuscular system to allow optimal levels of motor unit recruitment and synchronization within a muscle.

Balance

Ability to maintain the body's center of gravity within its base of support.

Static balance

Ability to maintain equilibrium in place with no external forces.

Perturbation

A disturbance of equilibrium; shaking.

Dynamic balance

Ability to maintain equilibrium through the intended path of motion when external forces are present.

Sensorimotor control

A complex interaction involving the muscular system, PNS, and CNS to obtain balance or postural control.

Postural stability

Ability to prepare, maintain, anticipate, and restore stability of the entire Human Movement System.

Importance of Balance Training

Balance training has quickly become an integral part of a comprehensive training program. Whether running, climbing, participating in sport, or simply walking, **balance** is required to execute the desired task.

Balance can be divided into two forms: static and dynamic. **Static balance** refers to the ability to maintain a static equilibrium through a **perturbation** while remaining still. **Dynamic balance** refers to the ability to maintain the intended path of motion following an external perturbation, or force placed on the moving body. Every individual requires both forms of balance, regardless of the activity they are participating in. Although it may appear that athletes would require greater balance and postural control based on the demands of their sport, every client faces the challenge of keeping balance to perform activities of daily living, such as playing with children or walking through their home. Therefore, it is important to incorporate balance training into every client's program as an integrated part of a comprehensive training regimen.

Balance is influenced by age, inactivity, and injury. For example, as age increases, the ability to balance, or maintain postural control, decreases. The very task of maneuvering stairs can create a significant risk of injury for older adults, who may lack the ability to decelerate and control their center of gravity, potentially resulting in a fall. Injury has been shown to decrease an individual's ability to balance as well. Research has shown that sensory input to the central nervous system (CNS) is altered after ankle sprains and ligamentous injuries to the knee, as well as when experiencing lower back pain (Hodges & Richardson, 1996; Ross & Guskiewicz, 2004; Solomonow, Barratta, & Zhou, 1987). These changes within the kinetic chain create imbalances, such as altered length–tension relationships, altered force-couple relationships, and altered joint motion. Consequently, this can lead to decreased neuromuscular efficiency, resulting in diminished balance and postural stability (Liebenson, 1996; Olsen, Myklebust, Engebretsen, Holme, & Bahr, 2005; Sahrmann, 1997). The cycle of injury is perpetuated by a lack of joint (postural) stabilization. Inefficient balance can create a pattern of overload and stress throughout the kinetic chain due to faulty movement patterns and compensations. Research has supported the use of balance in not only reconditioning clients following injury, but using balance training as a preventative measure to increase postural stability and reduce the risk of injury (Hewett, Lindenfeld, Riccobene, & Noyes, 1999; Olsen et al., 2005; Wedderkopp, Kaltoft, Holm, & Froberg, 2003).

Science of Balance

The human body goes through a dynamic process of controlling its center of mass upon a continually changing base of support. Balance is a necessity because the body's base of support shifts with every step. To obtain balance, or postural control, the body uses a complex interaction among the muscular system, peripheral nervous system (PNS), and CNS. This process is referred to as **sensorimotor control**. It is a dynamic process of constant review, feedback, and modification based on the integration of sensory information, motor commands, and resultant movements (Lephart, Riemann, & Fu, 2000; Peterka, 2002; Riemann & Lephart, 2002). In addition, sensorimotor control is designed to prepare, maintain, anticipate, and restore the stability of the entire Human Movement System (**postural stability**), including each segment of the Human Movement System (**joint stability**; Lephart et al., 2000; Peterka, 2002; Reimann & Lephart, 2002).

The body controls posture through a series of complex processes that involve visual, vestibular, and proprioceptive inputs from the Human Movement System (Lephart et al., 2000;

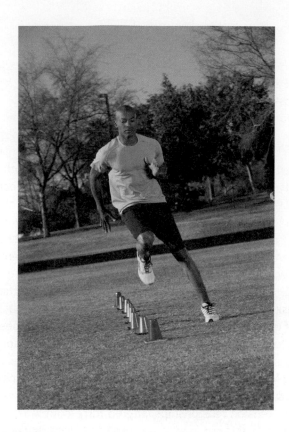

Reimann & Lephart, 2002). Maintaining postural equilibrium requires sensory detection of motion, **sensorimotor integration**, and the execution of appropriate musculoskeletal responses (Lephart et al., 2000; Peterka, 2002; Reimann & Lephart, 2002). All of this can be challenged during balance training, which, in turn, can help to improve dynamic postural stability.

Integrated Reactive Training

Reactive training, including plyometric training, enhances the **rate of force production** (i.e., the speed at which motor units are activated), which is regulated by the CNS. Reactive training teaches the body how to react, adapt, and respond quickly to the demands placed upon it. Integrated reactive training teaches the body how to respond at realistic speeds to changes in the environment that will be encountered during functional activities. By overloading the CNS, reactive training enhances neuromuscular efficiency and the rate of force production and stimulates the proprioceptive mechanisms and elastic properties of the Human Movement System.

Success in most functional activities, ranging from sport to everyday movement patterns, depends on the speed at which an individual can create force. For example, the basketball player who can produce the most power to jump will have an advantage rebounding the ball. In everyday situations, the ability to generate force quickly (such as jumping out of the way of a fellow pedestrian) is necessary in avoiding potentially dangerous situations. Reactive training represents an important component of function in both athletes and general population clients. Reactive training works to improve motor learning and neuromuscular efficiency by requiring the neuromuscular system to increase the rate of force production, **motor unit recruitment**, and **firing frequency**, and to enhance **motor unit synchronization**.

Joint stability
Ability to prepare, maintain, anticipate, and restore stability at each joint.

Sensorimotor integration
The ability of the nervous system to gather and interpret information to anticipate and execute the proper motor response.

Reactive training
Exercises that use quick, powerful movements involving an eccentric contraction immediately followed by an explosive concentric contraction.

Rate of force production
Ability of muscles to exert maximal force output in a minimal amount of time.

Motor unit recruitment
The activation of motor units in a successive manner to produce more strength.

Firing frequency
The number of activation signals sent to a single motor unit in 1 second.

Motor unit synchronization
The simultaneous recruitment of multiple motor units resulting in more muscle tissue contracting at the same time.

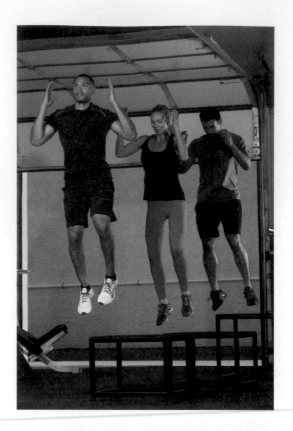

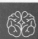
Incorporating reactive training into an integrated training program can help increase power and decrease reaction times.

Science Behind Reactive Training

Reactive training focuses on developing quick, powerful movements involving an eccentric contraction, followed immediately by an explosive concentric contraction. This is accomplished through the stretch–shortening cycle, also known as the **integrated performance paradigm** (Figure 6.13). In theory, a muscle that is loaded (eccentrically), stabilized (isometrically), and then unloaded (concentrically) will contract more forcefully. All movement patterns that occur during functional activities involve a series of repetitive stretch–shortening cycles.

The neuromuscular system must react quickly and efficiently following an eccentric muscle action in order to produce a concentric contraction and impart the necessary force and acceleration in the appropriate direction. The ultimate goal of reactive training is to increase the reaction time of the muscle action spectrum. The body will only move within the range of speed that the nervous system has been programmed to allow (Little & Williams, 2005; Young, McDowell, & Scarlett, 2001). Reactive training works to improve neuromuscular efficiency and the range of speed set by the nervous system.

The integrated performance paradigm has three phases. They include the eccentric (loading) phase, the **amortization phase**, and the concentric (unloading) phase. The first phase of a reactive movement, the loading phase, increases muscle spindle activity by prestretching the muscle prior to activation. Using the vertical jump as an example, the dip down immediately before the jump would be the eccentric, or loading, phase. The second phase is the amortization, or transitional, phase. This phase involves dynamic stabilization and takes place between the end of the eccentric contraction and the initiation of the concentric contraction.

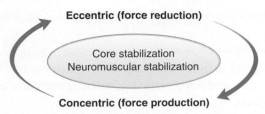

Eccentric (force reduction)

Core stabilization
Neuromuscular stabilization

Concentric (force production)

FIGURE 6.13 Integrated performance paradigm.

The amount of time in this phase is inversely related to performance: the shorter the amount of time, the more powerful the response; the longer the delay, the less power generated. Therefore, the amortization phase should be quick for optimum power generation. Reactive training works to quicken the amount of time the muscles spend in the amortization phase. The last phase is the concentric, or unloading, phase. This phase occurs immediately after the amortization phase and involves a concentric contraction. Returning to the example of the vertical jump, the upward jump would be considered the concentric phase.

Importance of Reactive Training

Reactive training is important because it develops a quick and powerful neuromuscular response, allowing for safe movement at functionally applicable speeds. This is particularly important for the performance of activities of daily living. People do not move at specified tempos under controlled conditions when performing everyday activities. By utilizing an integrated and progressive reactive training program, the individual will be better equipped to move at these speeds efficiently, effectively, and with reduced injury potential.

Three mechanisms have been proposed as to how reactive training enhances performance:

- Enhanced muscle spindle activity.
- Desensitization of the Golgi tendon organ.
- Enhanced neuromuscular efficiency.

Enhanced Muscle Spindle Activity

The Human Movement System will only move within a set speed, regardless of how strong a muscle is. Muscle spindle activation will cause a muscle to contract. Muscle spindles are excited via the fast loading of muscle through eccentric muscular contractions. Reactive training focuses on a fast eccentric muscle load to capitalize on the energy produced for a more powerful concentric muscle contraction. Simply put, increased muscle spindle activity can help to contract the muscle faster and improve reactive capabilities.

Desensitization of the Golgi Tendon Organ

A muscle can accept more tension without the inhibitor effects of the Golgi tendon organ. This is what is meant by desensitizing the Golgi tendon organ. It increases the stimulation threshold for muscular inhibition. This allows greater force to be produced, due to a greater load being applied to the musculoskeletal system.

Enhanced Neuromuscular Efficiency

Reactive training helps to promote increased neuromuscular control over agonists and synergists, making the nervous system more reflexive. These neural adaptations increase neuromuscular efficiency regardless of the muscle's size, resulting in more efficient movement and control.

These three attributes allow for the nervous system to optimize power output during the stretch–shortening cycle. Beyond power, reactive training has been shown to provide other benefits, such as increased jumping ability, running economy, and rate of force development and injury prevention.

Speed, Agility, and Quickness (SAQ) Training

Performance training incorporates speed, agility, and quickness (SAQ) training to prepare athletes for the demands of their sport. Many athletes play sports that require all three attributes; therefore, their training regimens should provide a combination of these training elements. However, even the typical client can utilize and benefit from SAQ training to improve their daily functioning and overall conditioning. The ability to generate speed, change direction quickly, and adjust to environmental demands can ensure that the average person stays injury-free. This type of training can also add a component of "fun" to their routine while helping to burn calories.

Science of Speed

Speed, commonly associated with sprinting, is defined as the straight-ahead pace of an individual. An individual's speed is determined by **stride rate** and **stride length**, combined with the force being applied to the ground (Mero, Komi, & Gregor, 1992). Research has shown that to increase sprint speed a specific training regimen of speed drills is beneficial (Little & Williams, 2005; Young et al., 2001). In addition, research has also found that integrated training, using both strength and speed training, is more beneficial than resistance training alone in increasing performance (Kotzamanidis et al, 2005).

Speed
The straight-ahead velocity of an individual.

Stride rate
The number of strides taken in a given amount of time (or distance).

Stride length
The distance covered with each stride.

TRAINER TIPS

Minimize your client's risk for injury by implementing SAQ training. Although the client might feel as though you are conditioning him or her for sports performance, SAQ training is a great way to burn calories while adding variety to the client's training.

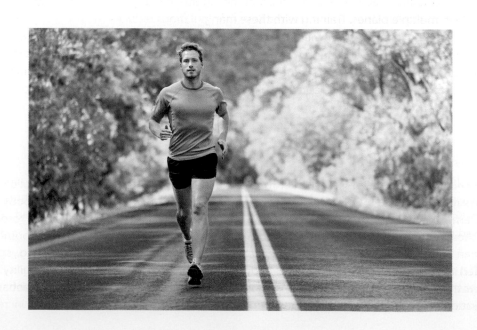

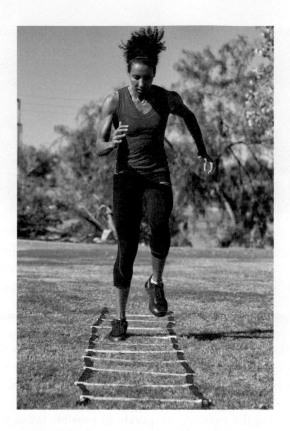

Science of Agility

Agility requires high levels of neuromuscular efficiency to maintain an individual's center of gravity over a changing base of support while changing direction at various speeds. Agility differs from speed in a few ways. Whereas speed focuses on uniplanar movement with a constant forward acceleration, agility requires constant management of acceleration, deceleration, and stability in multiple planes. Training with these manipulations reduces the risk of injury by enhancing the body's ability to effectively control eccentric forces in all planes of motion. Several research studies support the finding that incorporating various SAQ drills into a training program can reduce the incidence of injury to the lower extremity while improving performance (Hewett et al., 1999; Olsen et al., 2005).

Agility
The ability to maintain center of gravity over a changing base of support while changing direction at various speeds.

Science of Quickness

Quickness involves the ability to react to a stimulus without hesitation during functional or sports-related activities. Components of quickness include a change in head, trunk, body, leg, foot, arm, and/or hand position in the fastest possible time. In training for quickness, research has shown that progressive training methods work best to enhance performance (Bloomfield, Polman, O'Donoghue, & McNaughten, 2007). Shifting from planned or known cues (e.g., speed ladder) to unknown variable cues (e.g., auditory or visual commands) during an agility drill allows the athlete to properly progress without overloading the nervous system, and enhances activation strategies for running and cutting (Bloomfield et al., 2007).

Quickness
The ability to react to a stimulus with an appropriate muscular response without hesitation.

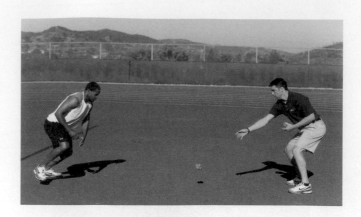

Importance of SAQ Training

SAQ training is commonly associated with athletes and athletic performance. Some individuals may not see the importance of SAQ training as it applies to the general population and functional movements. In order to realize the importance of SAQ training for everyone, it must be noted that the goal of progressive SAQ training is to develop these adaptations to be performed at speeds that are functional and applicable. The focus of this training should be on performing the exercises correctly and increasing the speed of the correct performance over time, rather than on performing the exercises as quickly as possible (as suggested by the terms). This will help to develop the desired adaptations of speed, agility, and quickness. It is important for individuals to maintain these functional assets, because agility is required for walking on different surfaces, around objects, and in unpredictable circumstances, such as a crowded grocery store. The same can be said for quickness. At times it is important for an individual to show quickness through a reaction to a given stimulus. Getting out of the way of a moving object, moving out of harm's way, or moving to save a falling individual or object all require a level of quick reaction to an outside stimulus. Sometimes this will require the production of a linear speed. Speed, agility, and quickness are all intimately connected to provide the capacity to respond quickly to outside stimuli in a varied environment as fast as possible and in a safe and efficient manner.

Integrated Resistance Training

Resistance training has been shown to create numerous health and movement benefits, and it has become an integral part of disease and injury prevention. Although resistance training has its roots in physical change (e.g., strength, hypertrophy, fat loss), the health benefits have reached beyond traditional uses to various ages and levels of ability. The broad scope of resistance training uses has brought forth the desire to understand different programming schemes to meet the needs of different individuals performing this activity. Resistance training programming is highly utilized in the OPT model, and comes with four major adaptations: stabilization endurance, strength, hypertrophy, and power. In order to fully understand how these different components of integrated training work together to reach adaptation, an understanding of the science of muscle contraction is needed.

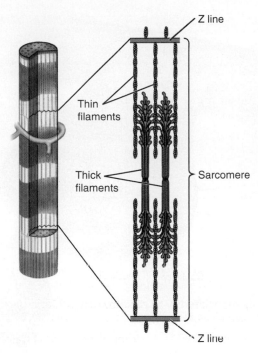

Z line

Thin filaments

Thick filaments

Sarcomere

Z line

FIGURE 6.14 Sarcomere.

Muscle Fibers and Their Contractile Elements

Muscle fibers are encased by a plasma membrane known as the sarcolemma. Each muscle fiber contains cellular components, including plasma called sarcoplasm (which contains glycogen, fats, minerals, and oxygen-binding myoglobin), nuclei, and mitochondria (which transform energy from food into energy for the cell). Unlike other cells, muscle fibers also have structures called myofibrils. Myofibrils contain myofilaments that are the actual contractile components of muscle tissue. These myofilaments are known as actin (thin, stringlike filaments) and myosin (thick filaments). The actin (thin) and myosin (thick) filaments form a number of repeating sections within a myofibril. Each section is referred to as a sarcomere (**Figure 6.14**). A sarcomere is the functional unit of the muscle, much like the neuron is the functional unit of the nervous system. The sarcomere lies in the space between two Z lines. Each Z line denotes another sarcomere along the myofibril. Two protein structures that are also important to muscle contraction are tropomyosin and troponin. Tropomyosin is located on the actin filament and blocks myosin binding sites also located on the actin filament, keeping myosin from attaching to actin when the muscle is in a relaxed state. Troponin, which is also located on the actin filament, plays a role in muscle contraction by providing binding sites for both calcium and tropomyosin when a muscle needs to contract.

Neural Activation

Skeletal muscles (**Figure 6.15**) will not contract unless they are stimulated to do so by motor neurons. Neural activation is the communication link between the nervous system and the muscular system (**Figure 6.16**). Motor neurons originating from the CNS communicate with

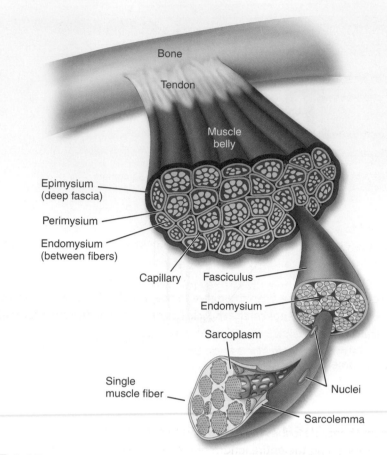

FIGURE 6.15 Structure of the skeletal muscle.

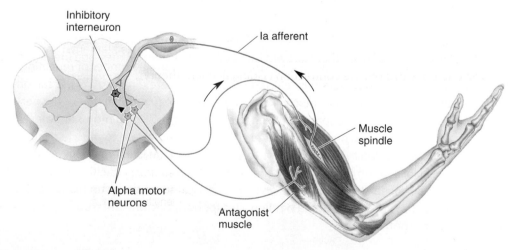

FIGURE 6.16 Neural activation.

Motor unit

One motor neuron and the muscle fibers it connects (innervates) with.

muscle fibers through a specialized synapse called the neuromuscular junction. One motor neuron and the muscle fibers it connects (innervates) with is known as a **motor unit**. The point at which the motor neuron meets an individual muscle fiber is called the neuromuscular junction (nerve to muscle). This junction is actually a small gap between the nerve and muscle fiber

CHECK IT OUT

Motor units will fire independently of each other in order to contract the same muscles or different muscles. An adaptation that must occur in order to develop strength is the coordination of these motor units to fire at specific times in relation to each other to develop the proper force. As more specific muscle fibers fire in a synchronized fashion, force can be developed to focus on a specific movement in overcoming a specific resistance. Motor unit synchronization is a neuromuscular adaptation that needs to take place in order to develop maximal levels of force and strength.

and is often referred to as a synapse. Electrical impulses (also known as action potentials) are transported from the CNS down the axon of the neuron. When the impulse reaches the end of the axon (axon terminal), chemicals called neurotransmitters are released. Neurotransmitters are chemical messengers that cross the synapse between the neuron and muscle fiber, transporting the electrical impulse from the nerve to the muscle. Once neurotransmitters are released, they link with receptor sites on the muscle fiber specifically designed for their attachment. The neurotransmitter used by the neuromuscular system is acetylcholine (ACh). Once attached, ACh stimulates the muscle fibers to go through a series of steps that initiates muscle contractions.

Sliding Filament Theory

The sliding filament theory describes how thick and thin filaments within the sarcomere slide past one another, shortening the entire length of the sarcomere, thus shortening muscle and producing force (**Figure 6.17**).

Excitation–Contraction Coupling: Putting It All Together

Excitation–contraction coupling is the process of neural stimulation creating a muscle contraction. It involves a series of steps that start with the initiation of a neural message (neural activation) and end up with a muscle contraction (sliding filament theory).

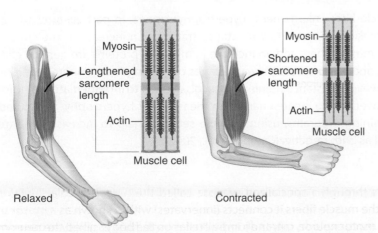

FIGURE 6.17 Sliding filament theory.

Endurance/Stabilization

Training for endurance is not limited to athletes engaging in endurance activities, but is central to overall programming schemes to improve stabilization. Creating muscular endurance is critical to helping the body increase core and joint stabilization. Without this, one cannot effectively build muscle size, strength, and power. Stabilization endurance training focuses on the recruitment of tissues in the body responsible for postural stability (primarily type I muscle fibers). Type I muscle fibers are slow to fatigue, and are important for long-term contractions required for postural control and stabilization. These muscle fibers are emphasized in training for stabilization endurance. Research has shown that resistance training protocols with higher repetition ranges and lower loads demonstrate a greater propensity for improving measures of local endurance (Campos et al., 2002).

Strength

Strength is the ability of the neuromuscular system to provide internal tension and exert force against external resistance. Strength gains can occur rapidly in beginning clients and can increase with a structured, progressive resistance training program. Often, client goals require an increase in strength, whether for sport or recreation.

Maximal strength is the most force a muscle can produce in a single, voluntary effort, regardless of the speed. For a muscle to increase strength, more motor units must be recruited. Using heavier loads increases the demand and recruitment of more muscle fibers. Therefore, neuromuscular considerations must be made prior to training for strength. Strength is built upon the foundation of stabilization, requiring the muscles, tendons, and ligaments to be prepared for the load that is required to increase strength beyond the initial stages of training in beginning clients. Strength training matches the characteristics of type II muscle fibers, which are larger in size, quick to produce maximal tension, and fatigue more quickly than type I muscle fibers. Due to their characteristics, the acute variables have to be manipulated to get the most out of muscle physiology. According to research, the majority of strength increases will occur during the first 12 weeks of resistance training (Hass, Garzarella, De Hoyos, & Pollock, 2000; Marx et al., 2001).

Hypertrophy

Skeletal muscle fiber enlargement (hypertrophy) occurs, in part, as a response to increased volumes of tension as created by resistance training. An increase in the cross-sectional area of individual muscle fibers and an increase in myofibril proteins are general characteristics of hypertrophy, and can begin in the early stages of training in beginners, regardless of exercise intensity. However, resistance training protocols use low to intermediate repetition ranges with progressive overload to create changes in measures of hypertrophy. Structured, progressive resistance training programs, using multiple sets, will help to increase hypertrophy in older adults as well as both genders (Campos et al., 2002).

Power

The ability to react, explode, cut, and jump all relies on the body's ability to generate the greatest possible force in the shortest amount of time. **Power** is defined as the neuromuscular system's

---

Strength

Ability of the neuromuscular system to provide internal tension and exert force against external resistance.

Maximal strength

The maximum force a muscle can produce in a single voluntary effort, regardless of the rate of force production.

Power

The ability to produce a large amount of force in a short amount of time.

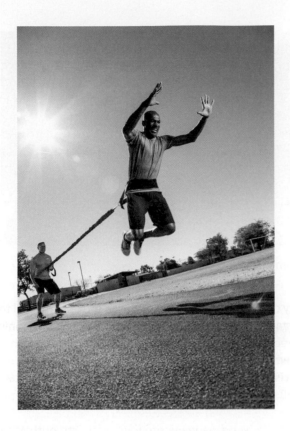

ability to increase the rate of force production (i.e., the speed at which the motor units are activated). Power is built upon the foundation of stabilization and strength, because it requires neuromuscular efficiency (as gained through stabilization training) and increased motor unit activation (as gained through strength training). The adaptation of power uses stabilization and strength adaptations, and applies them at more realistic speeds and forces. Power can be enhanced through an increase in force or an increase in velocity. The higher the force (heavier load), the slower the movement, and vice-versa: the lower the force (lighter load), the faster the movement. To maximize this type of training, both heavy and light loads must be moved as fast as possible to create the adaptation of power (Ebben & Watts, 1998; Hoffman et al., 2005).

Resistance Training Systems

Many resistance training systems are currently is use. Some of the most common resistance training systems used in the health and fitness industry include the single-set system, the circuit training system, the multiple-set system, the peripheral heart-action system, the pyramid system, the tri-set system, the superset system, and the split-routine system.

Single-Set System

In the single-set system, the individual performs one set of each exercise. The single-set system is one of the oldest training methods, and is still quite popular with many fitness professionals and strength coaches because of the proposed safety of the system (Hass et al., 2000).

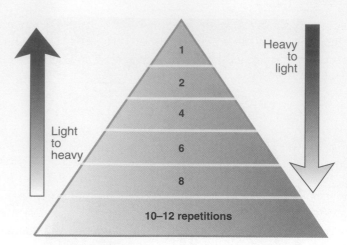

FIGURE 6.18 Pyramid set.

Multiple-Set System

The multiple-set system of training consists of two or three warm-up sets of increasing resistance, followed by several sets of the same resistance. This resistance training system has been popular since the 1940s.

Pyramid System (Light-to-Heavy/Heavy-to-Light System)

In the light-to-heavy system, the individual performs 10–12 repetitions with a light load. Resistance is then increased for each set while the repetitions are decreased, until the individual can only perform one to two repetitions, usually in four to six sets. The heavy-to-light system works in the opposite direction. The individual begins with a heavy load for one to two repetitions and then decreases the load and increases the repetitions for four to six sets (**Figure 6.18**).

Superset System

The superset system has evolved into two distinct but similar types of programs. One form of super-setting uses several sets of two exercises for antagonistic muscles. For example, an individual may perform a bench press immediately followed by cable rows (chest/back). The second type of super-setting uses one set of several exercises in rapid succession for the same muscle group or body part. For example, an individual may perform a dumbbell incline press, a ball push-up, and a cable chest press all in succession (chest superset).

Circuit training
A series of exercises performed in order to ensure a full-body resistance training session combined with cardiorespiratory exercise.

Circuit-Training System

Circuit training programs consist of a series of exercises that an individual performs one after the other, with minimal rest. For example, an individual may perform a stability ball dumbbell chest press, stability ball dumbbell row, dumbbell front lunge and press, cable curls standing on a foam pad, triceps pushdowns on a balance plate, and single-leg squat touchdowns on a half foam roll. These exercises should be performed immediately one after another. Circuit training is a great training system for those with limited time and for those who want to alter body composition.

Peripheral Heart-Action System

The peripheral heart-action system is a variation of circuit training. The training session is divided into two to four sequences, all of which contain four to six different exercises alternating between upper body and lower body exercises. For example, after performing the first sequence the individual rests for 30–45 seconds, and then performs the second sequence, and so on. This system is very beneficial for incorporating an integrated, multidimensional program and for altering body composition.

Tri-Set System

The tri-set system is similar to the peripheral heart-action system in that it incorporates groups of exercises. As the name implies, it consists of groups of three exercises for the same body part. Individuals perform the exercises with little or no rest between each exercise, typically performing two to four sets of each exercise. For example, an individual may perform a dumbbell shoulder press, a cable triceps pushdown, and then a ball dumbbell triceps extension.

Split-Routine System

Many bodybuilders and mass-dominant athletes (e.g., football) use the split-routine system. Bodybuilders must perform many exercises for the same body part to bring about optimum muscular hypertrophy. A typical split routine consists of training chest/shoulders/triceps on Monday and Thursday and back/biceps/legs on Tuesday and Friday. This enables the individual to achieve the desired volume of training in a reasonable period of time.

Conclusion

Today, fitness professionals must take a holistic approach in designing and implementing training programs. Today's clients are moving less, but living longer. This requires programming that addresses all aspects of human movement to ensure that peak performance is achieved. This can be accomplished through the use of integrated training, which incorporates flexibility, cardiorespiratory, core, balance, reactive, SAQ, and resistance training into one comprehensive routine. However, as with all programs, a system must be in place to progress clients in a safe and effective manner. This is achieved by utilizing the OPT model to progressively design and implement integrated training in an individualized manner, leading to a more confident fitness professional and clients safely achieving their goals. Knowing the terminology and principles behind integrated training ensures that the fitness professional understands the scientific rationale underlying this type of training, which is essential for effective client support and the fitness professional's long-term success.

TRAINER TIPS

The peripheral heart-action system is a good system to use with clients with cardiovascular disease, because alternating between upper and lower body exercises helps to increase blood flow to the extremities.

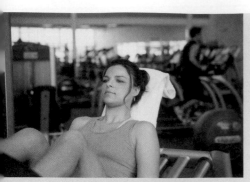

© Sean Locke Photography/Shutterstock

Case in Review

Your friend has been complaining to you about ongoing neck and lower back pain, and has been feeling discouraged because she thought regular exercise would help alleviate her pain. Because your friend hasn't achieved the results she was hoping for, she has expressed to you that she is losing her motivation to exercise, and has come to you for advice due to your knowledge of biomechanics. You begin by explaining the importance of integrated training and how it can be used to minimize the pain she is experiencing. You advise her that integrated training is the incorporation of all aspects of fitness into a single program and explain the importance of total body training in order to address the pain she is experiencing, as well as reduce the possibility for injury in the future.

To further expound on how you could incorporate integrated training into her workout, you explain how combining aspects of core, balance, reactive, SAQ, and resistance training will help minimize the pain she experiences from extended periods in the seated position at work:

- **Integrated core training.** Core training is important to prevent neck and lower back pain, because the core serves as the stabilization system for the spine. Most of the weight of the body will fall on the spine to support the torso. This puts a great deal of stress on the musculature supporting the spine, including the core. If these muscles are weak, the strain placed on them will inevitably lead to pain and potential injury due to the overloading of untrained musculature in these areas. By incorporating core exercises through the different phases of the OPT model, the local musculature will become more efficient in its daily functional capacity.

- **Integrated balance training.** By further challenging the stabilization (local) musculature system, balance training can help to prevent lower back and neck pain by improving the body's ability to balance itself in a changing environment. Integrating balance training into a workout will develop the neuromuscular system in a way that will help to stabilize and protect the spine through the coordinated firing of the trunk muscles.

- **Integrated reactive training.** Reactive training is important for the prevention of lower back and neck issues, because it trains the body to absorb and produce external forces. If the body is able to better absorb forces placed upon it, then this inherently decreases the risk for injury. Training for proper landing mechanics or force production through the core will allow the body to better protect the spine when high levels of power are required to either accelerate or decelerate a force.

- **Integrated SAQ training.** SAQ training can help to decrease potential back and neck issues by training the body to maintain good posture at functionally applicable speeds. By maintaining the proper biomechanics throughout the associated movements, the body will not be placed in compromising positions that could lead to potential injury. The core will remain stable and balanced regardless of the quick movements and changes of direction that may be required due to outside stimulus.

- **Integrated resistance training.** Resistance training can be utilized to develop overall strength and stability of the musculature that supports and stabilizes the spine. By integrating a systematic resistance training progression into a program, the individual will be able to better protect the spine during functional activities. The supporting musculature will then not have to be recruited to assist in activities they are not intended for due to a lack of prime mover strength. Think of lifting a heavy box off the floor: if the gluteal muscles are not firing or not strong enough, the erector spinae will be recruited to help. However, this muscle is not designed to perform this task and may become injured in the process.

After your thorough explanation, your friend now has a clear understanding of the importance and benefits of an integrated approach to training that utilizes various components to meet her individual needs.

References

Amako, M., Oda, T., Masuoka, K., Yokoi, H., & Campisi, P. (2003). Effect of static stretching on prevention of injuries for military recruits. *Military Medicine, 168*(6), 442–446.

Aroski, J. P., Valta, T., Airaksinen, O., & Kankaanpaa, M. (2001). Back and abdominal muscle function during stabilization exercises. *Archives of Physical Medicine and Rehabilitation, 82*(8), 1089–1098.

Barnett, M. L., Ross, D., Schmidt, R. A., & Todd, B. (1973). Motor skills learning and the specificity of training principle. *Research Quarterly, 44*(4), 440–447.

Barr, K. P., Griggs, M., & Cadby, T. (2005). Lumbar stabilization: Core concepts and current literature, part 1. *American Journal of Physiological Medical Rehabilitation, 84*(6), 473–480.

Bloomfield, J., Polman, R., O'Donoghue, P., & McNaughton, L. (2007). Effective speed and agility conditioning methodology for random intermittent dynamic type sports. *Journal of Strength and Conditioning Research, 21*(4), 1093–1100.

Campos, G., Luecke, T. J., Wendeln, H. K., Toma, K., Hagerman, F. C., Murray, T. F., . . . Staron, R. S. (2002). Muscular adaptations to three different resistance training regimens: Specificity of repetition maximum training zones. *European Journal of Applied Physiology, 88*(1–2), 50–60.

Cassidy, J. D., Carroll, L. F., & Cote, P. (1998). The Saskatchewan Health and Back Pain Survey. The prevalence of low back pain and related disability in Saskatchewan adults. *Spine, 23*(17), 1860–1866.

Centers for Disease Control and Prevention (CDC). (2004). Summary health statistics for U.S. adults: National Health Interview Survey, 2002. *Vital Health Statistics, 10*(222), 1–151.

Chaitow, L. (1997). *Muscle energy techniques.* New York, NY: Churchill Livingstone.

Clemson, L., Fiatarone Singh, M. A., Bundy, A., Cumming, R. G., Manollaras, K., O'Laughlin, P., & Black, D. (2012). Integration of balance and strength training into daily life activity to reduce rate of falls in older people (the LiFE study): Randomised parallel trial. *BMJ, 345,* e4547.

de Hoyo, M., Pozzo, M., Sañudo, B., Carrasco, L., Gonzalo-Skok, O., Domínguez-Cobo, S., & Morán-Camacho, E. (2015). Effects of a 10-week in-season eccentric-overload training program on muscle-injury prevention and performance in junior elite soccer players. *International Journal of Sports Physiology and Performance, 10*(1), 46–52.

Distefano, L. J., Distefano, M. J., Frank, B. S., Clark, M. A., & Padua, D. A. (2013). Comparison of integrated and isolated training on performance measures and neuromuscular control. *Journal of Strength and Conditioning Research, 27*(4), 1083–1090.

Ebben, W. P., & Watts, P. B. (1998). A review of combined weight training and plyometric training modes: Complex training. *Strength and Conditioning, 20*(5), 18–27.

Etnyre, B. R., & Abraham, L. D. (1986). Gains in range of ankle dorsiflexion using three popular stretching techniques. *American Journal of Physiological Medicine, 65,* 189–196.

Foster, C., Porcari, J. P., Anderson, J., Paulson, M., Smaczny, D., Webber, H., . . . Udermann, B. (2008). The talk test as a marker of exercise training intensity. *Journal of Cardiopulmonary Rehabilitation and Prevention, 28*(1), 24–30.

Gabriel, D. A., Kamen, G., & Frost, G. (2006). Neural adaptations to resistive exercise: Mechanisms and recommendations for training practices. *Sports Medicine, 36*(2), 133–149.

Gadjosik, R. (2001). Passive extensibility of skeletal muscle: Review of the literature with clinical implications. *Clinical Biomechanics, 16,* 87–101.

Griffin, L. Y., Agel, J., Albohm, M. F., Arendt, E. A., Dick, R. W., Garrett, W. E., . . . Wojtys, E. M. (2000). Noncontact anterior cruciate ligament injuries: Risk factors and prevention strategies. *Journal of American Academic Orthopedic Surgery, 8*(3), 141–150.

Hakkinen, K. (1994). Neuromuscular adaptation during strength training, aging, detraining and immobilization. *Critical Review of Physical Medicine, 6,* 161–198.

Harkness, E. F., Macfarlane, G. J., Silman, A. J., & McBeth, J. (2005). Is musculoskeletal pain more common now than 40 years ago? Two population-based cross-sectional studies. *Rheumatology (Oxford), 44*(7), 890–895.

Harmer, A. R., McKenna, M. J., Sutton, J. R., Snow, R. J., Ruell, P. A., Booth, J., . . . Eager, D. M. (2000). Skeletal muscle metabolic and ionic adaptations during intense exercise following sprint training in humans. *Journal of Applied Physiology, 89*(5), 1793–1803.

Hartig, D. E., & Henderson, J. M. (1999). Increasing hamstring flexibility decreases lower extremity overuse injuries in military basic trainees. *American Journal of Medicine, 27*(2), 173–176.

Haskell, W. L., Lee, I. M., Pate, R. R., Powell, K. E., Blair, S. N., Franklin, B. A., . . . Bauman, A. (2007). Physical activity and public health: Updated recommendations for adults from the American College of Sports Medicine and the American Heart Association. *Medicine and Science in Sports and Exercise, 39*(8), 1423–1434.

Hass, C. J., Garzarella, L., De Hoyos, D., & Pollock, M. L. (2000). Single versus multiple sets in long-term recreational weight lifters. *Medicine and Science in Sports and Exercise, 32*(1), 235–242.

Hewett, T. E., Lindenfeld, T. N., Riccobene, J. V., & Noyes, F. R. (1999). The effect of neuromuscular training on the incidence of knee injury in female athletes: A prospective study. *American Journal of Sports Medicine, 27*(6), 699–706.

Hill, C. L., Seo, G. S., Gale, D., Totterman, S., Gale, M. E., & Felson, D. T. (2005). Cruciate ligament integrity in osteoarthritis of the knee. *Arthritis Rheumatology, 52*(3), 794–799.

Hodges, P. W., & Richardson, C. A. (1996). Inefficient muscular stabilization of the lumbar spine associated with low back pain. *Spine, 21*(22), 2640–2650.

Hodges, P. W., & Richardson, C. A. (1997a). Contraction of the abdominal muscles associated with movement of the lower limb. *Physical Therapy, 77,* 132–142.

Hodges, P. W., & Richardson, C. A. (1997b). Feedforward contraction of transversus abdominis is not influenced by the direction of arm movement. *Experimental Brain Research, 114,* 362–370.

Hodges, P. W., Richardson, C. A., & Jull, G. (1996). Evaluation of the relationship between laboratory and clinical tests of transverse abdominus function. *Physiotherapy Research International, 1,* 30–40.

Hoffman, J. R., Ratamess, N. A., Cooper, J. J., Kang, J., Chilakis, A., & Faigenbaum, A. D. (2005). Comparison of loaded and unloaded jump squat training on strength/power performance in college football players. *Journal of Strength and Conditioning Research, 19*(4), 810–815.

Kay, A. D., & Blazevich, A. J. (2012). Effect of acute static stretch on maximal muscle performance: A systematic review. *Medicine and Science in Sports and Exercise, 44*(1), 154–164.

Knapik, J. J., Bauman, C. L., Jones, B. H., Harris, J. M., & Vaughan, L. (1991). Preseason strength and flexibility imbalances associated with athletic injuries in female collegiate athletes. *American Journal of Sports Medicine, 19*(1), 76–81.

Kotzamanidis, C., Chatzopoulos, D., Michailidis, C., Papaiakovou, G., & Patikas, D. (2005). The effect of a combined high-intensity strength and speed training program on the running and jumping ability of soccer players. *Journal of Strength and Conditioning Research, 19*(2), 369–375.

Kraemer, B. J., & Ratamess, N. A. (2000). Physiology of resistance training. *Orthopedic Physical Therapy Clinics of North America, 9*(4), 467–513.

Lephart, S. M., Riemann, B. L., & Fu, F. H. (2000). Introduction to the sensorimotor system. In: S. M. Lephart & F. H. Fu (Eds.), *Proprioception and neuromuscular control in joint stability* (pp. 37–51). Champaign, IL: Human Kinetics.

Liebenson, C. (1996). Integrating rehabilitations into chiropractic practice (blending active and passive care). In: *Rehabilitation of the spine: A practitioner's manual* (pp. 165–191). Baltimore: Williams & Wilkins.

Little, T., & Williams, A. G. (2005). Specificity of acceleration, maximum speed, and agility in professional soccer players. *Journal of Strength and Conditioning, 19*(1), 76–78.

Mandelbaum, B. R., Silbers, H. J., Watanabe, D. S., Knarr, J. F., Thomas, S. D., Griffin, L. Y., . . . Garrett, W., Jr. (2005). Effectiveness of a neuromuscular and proprioceptive training program in preventing anterior cruciate ligament injuries in female athletes: 2-year follow-up. *American Journal of Sports Medicine, 33*(7), 1003–1010.

Marx, J. O., Ratamess, N. A., Nindl, B. C., Gotshalk, L. A., Volek, J. S., Dohi, K., . . . Kraemer, W. J. (2001). Low-volume circuit versus high-volume periodized resistance training in women. *Medicine and Science in Sports and Exercise, 33*(4), 635–643.

McEvoy, K. P., & Newton, R. U. (1998). Baseball throwing speed and base running speed: The effects of ballistic resistance training. *Journal of Strength and Conditioning Research, 12*(4), 216–221.

McGill, S. M. (2001). Low-back stability: From formal description to issues for performance and rehabilitation. *Exercise and Sport Sciences Review, 29*(1), 26–31.

Mero, A., Komi, P. V., & Gregor, R. J. (1992). Biomechanics of sprint running. *Sports Medicine, 13*(6), 376–392.

Olsen, O. E., Myklebust, G., Engebretsen, L., Holme, I., & Bahr, R. (2005). Exercises to prevent lower limb injuries in youth sports: Cluster randomised controlled trial. *BMJ, 330*(7489), 449.

Omokhodion, F. O. (2002). Low back pain in a rural community in South West Nigeria. *West African Journal of Medicine, 21*(2), 87–90.

Omokhodion, F. O., & Sanya, A. O. (2003). Risk factors for low back pain among office workers in Ibadan, Southwest Nigeria. *Occupational Medicine (London), 53*(4), 287–289.

Parra, J., Cadefau, J. A., Rodas, G., Amigo, N., & Cusso, R. (2000). The distribution of rest periods affects performance and adaptations of energy metabolism induced by high-intensity training in human muscle. *Acta Physiologica Scandanavia, 169*, 157–165.

Persinger, R., Foster, C., Gibson, M., Fater, D. C., & Porcari, J. P. (2004). Consistency of the talk test for exercise prescription. *Medical Science Sports Exercise, 36*(9), 1632–1636.

Peterka, R. J. (2002). Sensorimotor integration in human postural control. *Journal of Neurophysiology, 88*(3), 1097–1118.

Pope, R. P., Herbert, R. D., & Kirwan, J. D. (2002). Effects of ankle dorsiflexion range and preexercise calf muscle stretching on injury risk in Army recruits. *Australian Journal of Physiotherapy, 44*, 165–177.

Ramírez-Campillo, R., Henríquez-Olguín, C., Burgos, C., Andrade, D. C., Zapata, D., Martínez, C., . . . Izquierdo, M. (2015). Effect of progressive volume-based overload during plyometric training on explosive and endurance performance in young soccer players. *Journal of Strength and Conditioning Research, 29*(7), 1884–1893.

Ratamess, N. A., Kraemer, W. J., Volek, J. S., French, D. N., Rubin, M. R., Gómez, A. L., . . . Maresh, C. M. (2007). The effects of ten weeks of resistance and combined plyometric/sprint training with the Meridian Elyte athletic shoe on muscular performance in women. *Journal of Strength and Conditioning Research*, *21*(3), 882–887.

Riemann, B. L, & Lephart, S. M. (2002). The sensorimotor system, part I: The physiologic basis of functional joint stability. *Journal of Athletic Training*, *37*(1), 71–79.

Ross, S. E., & Guskiewicz, K. M. (2004). Examination of static and dynamic postural stability in individuals with functionally stable and unstable ankles. *Clinical Journal of Sport Medicine*, *14*(6), 332–338.

Sahrmann, S. (1997). Diagnosis and treatment of muscle imbalances and musculoskeletal pain syndrome. Continuing Education Course, St. Louis. Available from: https://www.neseminars.com/more-info.asp?product=235

Selye, H. (1976). *The stress of life.* New York, NY: McGraw-Hill.

Solomonow, M., Barratta, R., & Zhou, B. H. (1987). The synergistic action of the ACL and thigh muscles in maintaining joint stability. *American Journal of Sports Medicine*, *15*, 207–213.

Tan, B. (1999). Manipulating resistance training program variables to optimize maximum strength in men: A review. *Journal of Strength and Conditioning Research*, *13*(3), 289–304.

Tanaka, H., Monahan, K. D., & Seals, D. R. (2001). Age-predicted maximal heart rate revisited. *Journal of the American College of Cardiology*, *37*(1), 153–156.

Tous-Fajardo, J., Gonzalo-Skok, O., Arjol-Serrano, J. L., & Tesch, P. (2015). Change of direction speed in soccer players is enhanced by functional inertial eccentric overload and vibration training. *International Journal of Sports Physiology and Performance*, *11*(1), 66–73.

Visich, P. S. (2003). Graded exercise testing. In: J. K. Ehrman, P. M. Gordon, P. S. Visich, & S. J. Keteyan (Eds.), *Clinical exercise physiology* (pp. 79–101). Champaign, IL: Human Kinetics.

Volinn, E. (1997). The epidemiology of low back pain in the rest of the world. A review of surveys in low- and middle-income countries. *Spine*, *22*(15), 1747–1754.

Walker, B. F., Muller, R., & Grant, W. D. (2004). Low back pain in Australian adults: Prevalence and associated disability. *Journal of Manipulative and Physiological Therapy*, *27*(4), 238–244.

Wedderkopp, N., Kaltoft, M., Holm, R., & Froberg, K. (2003). Comparison of two intervention programmes in young female players in European handball—with and without ankle disc. *Scandinavian Journal of Medicine and Science in Sports*, *13*(6), 371–375.

Witvrouw, E., Danneels, L., Asselman, P., D'Have, T., & Cambier, D. (2003). Muscle flexibility as a risk factor for developing muscle injuries in male professional soccer players. A prospective study. *American Journal of Sports Medicine*, *31*(1), 41–46.

Young, W. B., McDowell, M. H., & Scarlett, B. J. (2001). Specificity of sprint and agility training methods. *Journal of Strength and Conditioning Research*, *15*(3), 315–319.

Zack, M. M., Moriarty, D. G., Stroup, D. F., Ford, E. S., & Moddad, A. H. (2004). Worsening trends in adult health-related quality of life and self-related health—United States, 1993–2001. *Public Health Report*, *119*(5), 493–505.

CHAPTER 7

NAVIGATING THE PROFESSIONAL FITNESS ENVIRONMENT

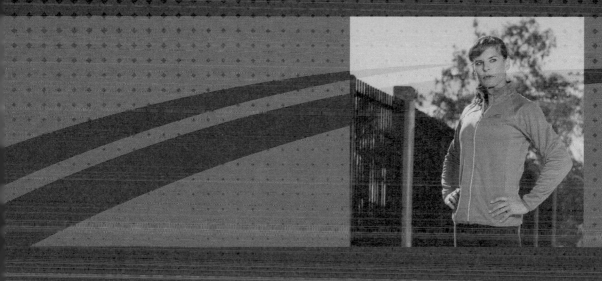

OBJECTIVES

After studying this chapter, you will be able to:

1   **Summarize** the major fitness facility types employing fitness professionals.

2   **Differentiate** the departmental roles at major fitness facility types.

3   **Compare** the employment requirements of an independent fitness professional to those of working for a fitness facility.

4   **Explain** strategies used to obtain employment as a fitness professional at the different fitness facility types.

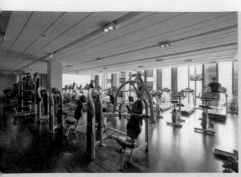
© zhu difeng/Shutterstock

Case Scenario

You are a few weeks away from taking the exam required to obtain your NASM Certified Personal Trainer certification and are starting to think about different locations in your area to apply to for employment. Just recently, a large national club opened near the small group training facility you have been a member of for the past 2 years. Also, while driving to a friend's house you noticed advertising for a small boutique club operating out of a large commercial building. You begin to consider your ideal working environment and to identify the types of clients you would prefer to work with. You have come up with the following questions you need to answer before making a decision as to which fitness facility would be the best fit with your abilities and personality as a fitness professional:

- What key characteristics do you find most beneficial with regard to each type of gym, and how do they align with your career as a fitness professional?

- What are the clientele differences between the facility types, and how will that play a role in your decision to choose which facility to apply to?

- What are some possible considerations with regards to working at fitness facilities of various types?

Introduction to Navigating the Fitness Environment

Demographics

Statistical data relating to the population and the particular groups in it.

Psychographics

The study of personality, values, opinions, attitudes, interests, and lifestyles.

All fitness facilities are unique, and certain functions and reporting structures will differ from one to another. However, the function an employee supports often dictates the general department he or she will work in. In some situations, such as large-scale national chain clubs and high-end and boutique facilities, other niche departments may exist. These niche areas may include court sports (e.g., tennis, racquetball, basketball), aquatics, rock-climbing walls, cafés, and day spas. All of these may have their own managerial departments and specialized employees. Fitness professionals should learn about the services their club or potential employer provides for members, because this will give them insight into the primary goal or focus of that facility, as well as a deeper understanding of ways to later promote their services within the organization. Factors to evaluate include the key characteristics, common clientele, and the organizational setting of each environment.

Professionals should also take the time to understand the **demographics** and **psychographics** associated with a facility, and identify any populations that are being

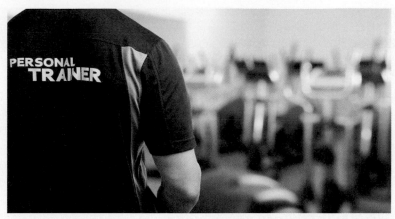

© ruigsantos/Shutterstock

underserved or overlooked. Psychographic profiles of the population can be useful in determining what factors may influence a person's purchasing decisions. Furthermore, if a club is mature and stable, with existing professionals who are comfortably booked, then the new fitness professional may need to identify an underserved niche market within the existing member base to establish his or her own clientele.

Fitness center employees function in a variety of roles and responsibilities. Employees at medium to small facilities will often have multiple roles and functions. As the facility grows in size, employees begin to take on more specialized roles, dividing the organization into more specific departments. Common departments at a typical large-scale facility are fitness (i.e., personal trainers, group fitness instructors), sales, front desk and **operations** (including maintenance), general management, and specialty departments (e.g., sports, aquatics, café, child care, spa).

Whereas a working knowledge of the Human Movement System and the concepts of integrated training are essential for employment in the fitness industry, it is also important to understand the various fitness environments that are available. Each setting has different operational and employment requirements the fitness professional must consider prior to selecting the option that best meets his or her individual personality and needs.

Operations

Activities involved in the day-to-day functions of a business that do not directly generate revenue.

Large-Scale Facilities and National Chains

Large-scale facilities and national chains are branded fitness facilities that typically have multiple locations, are very large in size, and, through marketing efforts, often become the reference point in many consumers' minds. They account for the majority of revenue generated in the fitness industry and are the largest employers of fitness professionals (Bixlar, 2014). These centers often have multiple membership options, and offer additional specialty services, such as child care, court sports, aquatics, and cafés. From a potential member perspective, this facility option is often appealing because it has a recognizable brand, is established in the industry, provides a product that is easy to understand, is often open long hours, and has many quality programming options. In this environment, the company supplies the marketing materials to attract members and has a dedicated sales team to promote products and services, allowing fitness professionals to focus on instruction and building a client base.

CHECK IT OUT

Key characteristics of large-scale facilities and national chains:

- Large marketing and advertising budgets to help establish or reinforce their brand name.
- Expanded selection of commercial-grade cardio and resistance machines, free weights, group fitness rooms, and open training areas.
- Often have specialty facilities, such as court sports, aquatics, a café, child care, and a spa.
- Large locker rooms and shower facilities, often with a sauna or steam room.
- Fitness professionals employed directly by the company as members of a larger team.
- Large preexisting membership base.
- Comprehensive new hire onboarding programs and training.
- Use of proprietary company systems and technology solutions for both back-office business purposes and member–trainer interactions.
- High level of departmental structure.
- High focus on sales and client retention.

Common Clientele

The common clientele of large-scale facilities will often be representative of the population that lives or works in the general neighborhood of the facility. These clubs often attract financially conservative consumers who value established and proven programs, as well as the familiarity, consistency, and reliability commonly associated with a large brand name. With so many offerings, not every member will have the desire or the means to participate in personal training. Rather, they will use the facility for à la carte access to fitness equipment, group classes that come standard with their membership, or use of the courts and swimming pool. Families are often drawn to these facilities due to the access to child care and the availability of multiple fitness activities for all ages.

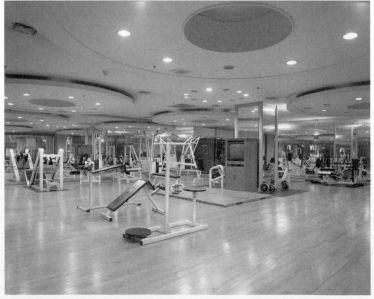

© wizdata/Shutterstock

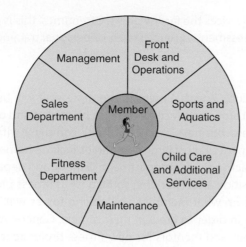

Large Scale Fitness Facility

Organizational Setting

In most situations, these facilities will have new trainer onboarding programs so a new professional may learn the company's culture and standard operating procedures, and shadow other more experienced professionals. The next step will generally involve taking new members through complimentary assessments and performing other activities inside the facility. These activities will help the new fitness professional build a lead base by working the floor and possibly assisting at the front desk. New fitness professionals should initially expect very little control over their scheduled hours, because the schedule will vary based on the facility's needs and the seniority of the existing staff.

Fitness Department

In most large-scale facilities, the fitness department encompasses not only personal training, but also group fitness instruction. Within these centers the fitness department serves a vital role as both a member-retention tool as well as a **top-line** revenue driver. In addition to providing the direct services of personal training and group fitness instruction, professionals will often be responsible for selling the fee based services that they provide. Most large fitness facilities will set weekly, monthly, or quarterly sales targets for fitness professionals, or targets around another **driver of sales**, such as the number of sessions scheduled and serviced. Fitness professionals may also be responsible for instructing free personal training sessions or group training classes, because they are often offered as an incentive to new members by the sales department. This provides the fitness professional an early opportunity to prospect and begin building a client base. These opportunities should be utilized to begin building relationships with potential clients.

Sales Department

Sales department employees will perform various activities to increase member acquisition and revenue generation through both prospecting and follow-up interaction with current members. In most situations they will be compensated with a base pay, either hourly or salary, and then earn a commission on the products or services that they sell. Whereas sales employees may not be certified fitness professionals, they need to have a strong knowledge of health and fitness in order to efficiently interact with prospects and provide facility tours to drive revenue. Once a new member joins, it is the sales department's responsibility to introduce them to

Top-line
A company's overall sales or revenues, before any discounts or returns.

Driver of sales
Activities that create opportunities for future sales.

the additional fee-based services the facility offers. Oftentimes, this is done through the use of complimentary fitness assessments, group classes, or personal training sessions.

Management

The larger the club, and company that owns it, the more staff will be needed for back-office tasks and administration. Large-scale facilities tend to be owned and operated by corporations and use the same standard business practices of any company with numerous employees. Roles within the management of most large companies include human resources, accounting, and managerial staff for each individual department. General and departmental managers may have moved into their position after spending some time as fitness professionals. This will give them a good perspective on what members are looking for, as well as best practices fitness professionals can employ in order to grow in their careers. General managers can be used as professional career coaches and mentors for new fitness professionals looking to forge their own career path.

Front Desk and Operations

Front desk employees are often the first impression of the facility to a new member or prospect. They will typically screen calls, greet visitors on arrival, and process payments for memberships and **ancillary revenue** items (e.g., snacks and drinks, club merchandise). Though they typically provide services that do not directly generate substantial amounts of revenue for the club, they serve vital functions that are aimed at member retention and allow other departments in the facility to operate more efficiently. Front desk employees will provide the first, and perhaps only, interaction with a club member during a visit. Being helpful and upbeat during the first interactions with potential new members can be the difference between them signing up or not. Front desk employees are also the staff who will oftentimes know the names of members and welcome them each time they come into the facility. Because of this, their level of customer service can define the visit the member has at the club that day.

Sports and Aquatics

Many large clubs will have sports and athletics facilities available to members in addition to standard fitness equipment and exercise space. These offerings may be included with a membership or in some cases be available for an additional fee. These can include, but are not limited to, basketball courts, indoor running tracks, racquetball courts, rock-climbing walls, tennis complexes, and swimming pools. With these different activities comes the need for other specialized employees, such as referees, tennis professionals, and lifeguards.

Child Care and Additional Services

The primary role of child care attendants is to monitor, entertain, and ensure the safety of members' or prospects' children while they are working out. In addition to providing activities, toys, and games for children to play with while their parents are working out, larger facilities are beginning to incorporate youth fitness into this area. This is also typically the department that will organize youth events, specialty groups (e.g., martial arts lessons), and youth sports leagues.

Large clubs also tend to have additional services available to members that go above and beyond the fitness realm. Many are beginning to include in-house cafés, offering coffee shop–style service with healthy food and juice bars. Some even offer classes on nutrition and cooking. Full-service spas are also common among the larger national chain facilities, providing massage therapy, hair stylist, skin care, and nail salon services for members.

Ancillary revenue
Revenue beyond the sale of memberships and services generated by the direct sale of products to customers.

CHECK IT OUT

The average size of the facility varies based on the type of fitness center:

- Large-scale national chains: 20,000+ square feet
- Medium-sized fitness centers: 8,000–20,000 square feet
- Small group training facilities: 1,000–8,000 square feet
- Boutique and high-end facilities: 4,000–20,000+ square feet

Maintenance

The maintenance and janitorial crews often have the least direct interaction with members and clients. However, if the equipment in a facility is often out of service or if the facility is consistently unclean, member retention will become increasingly difficult. It is thus the job of the maintenance staff to ensure that the club stays clean and that the equipment is always in optimal working condition. Whereas medium to small facilities may split these duties up among the training and front desk staff, large-scale national clubs have the resources to employ full-time crews dedicated to the upkeep of the facility and maintenance of the equipment.

Medium-Sized Fitness Centers

Medium-sized fitness centers may be smaller facilities operated by the same corporations that run the large-scale clubs. These smaller satellite facilities may be located in less densely populated areas and may have slightly altered service offerings than their larger sister clubs. In other cases, medium-sized clubs may be independently owned franchises. These tend to be **turn-key** business solutions where an owner will invest in the startup costs and the company selling the franchise will assist with finding a location, supplying the equipment, and providing base-level operations training. It is then up to the owner to run the facility as his or her own business, while paying royalties back to the parent company to maintain rights to use the brand and business model. Medium-sized clubs can also be independently owned facilities, which are not franchises, or they may be part of a growing small business with multiple locations in an area or city.

Most of these facilities will offer commercial-grade strength and cardio equipment, technology solutions to connect fitness professionals and clients, and have similar **profit centers** as the large-scale facilities. On the other hand, these clubs may provide fewer additional amenities, choosing to focus on members who are looking to complete a workout in the most efficient way possible. Because of this, medium-sized facilities will usually not have court sports or swimming pools; however, they frequently will provide 24-hour access and come with much lower membership costs than the large-scale clubs. Personal training and group exercise services will also vary from club to club, with some employing them in-house, similar to a large-scale facility, and others developing contract relationships with independent fitness professionals for use of the space and equipment. These services are typically per-session fee based, as the club membership offerings tend to be simple, primarily revolving around access to the facility.

Turn-key
A complete product or service that is ready for immediate use.

Profit center
A part of an organization with assignable revenues and costs, and hence ascertainable profitability.

CHECK IT OUT

Key chracteristics of medium-sized facilities and national chains:

- Large workout space with commercial-grade equipment.
- Offer exercise convenience and simplicity for members.
- Offer personal training and group fitness classes as additional purchased services.
- Use technology to easily connect with members.
- Lower membership costs, with less complex membership options.
- Shower/changing/locker rooms and snack bar services.
- Fewer specialized facilities (e.g., café, aquatics, court sports).
- Often located in less-densely populated suburban areas.
- More local community involvement and outreach.
- Can be supported by national brands or be unique local businesses.
- Often run as a small businesses.
- Primary revenue source comes from membership acquisition and retention.
- Often have no dedicated sales or marketing teams.
- More shared operational responsibility for employees.

Common Clientele

Similar to the large-scale facilities, medium-sized facilities will mostly appeal to the fiscally conservative client who is attracted to this model by the simple membership options and low cost. For various reasons, these individuals will find benefit in a smaller club with fewer amenities. These facilities may also develop an atmosphere to attract a specific type of client or niche group in the community. These members may not be interested in additional activities or programming options, focusing instead on the ability to workout. These individuals may select the medium-sized facility based on the equipment available as well as when the peak hours are at the particular location. With potentially less space available, it may be more important for these members to have access to the desired equipment, and to visit the club at times they know the equipment will be available. Clientele may also select a facility based on a specific class offered or staff member they prefer. Facilities of this nature tend to appeal to teenage athletes, college students, working professionals, and senior clients who are seeking to increase their physical fitness, but who do not prioritize the need for the extra amenities of a large-scale facility membership.

Organizational Setting

Fitness professionals working in medium-sized facilities often find similar working conditions as their colleagues in large-scale locations. The essence of working at a franchise location is the turn-key systems that allow owners to operate with the same basic programs and services as large-scale facilities do. Fitness professionals in these facilities may enjoy greater flexibility with their daily schedule, but there will probably be less on-the-job training and support in developing a client base. The organizational structure is less complex as well, typically divided by management, the fitness team, and operations employees. Some medium-sized fitness centers will

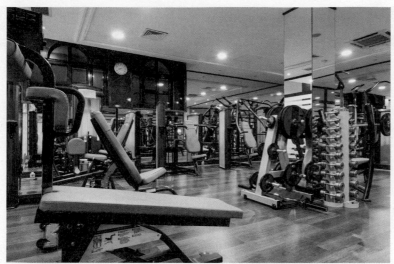

© Marko Poplasen/Shutterstock

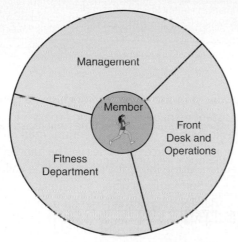

Medium Sized Fitness Facility

have the budget for more specialized employees, such as cleaning crews or dedicated sales-people; however, the fitness professional needs to be prepared for cross-functional operational duties to ensure the club members receive the expected level of service they are looking for.

Fitness Department

As with large gyms, the fitness department will mainly encompass personal training and group instruction services. Also, relative to the size of the club, the vast majority of the sales activities will be conducted by the fitness staff. This may include giving tours or presentations or going out in to the community to assist with local marketing events to drive membership. Without a dedicated sales staff, and with a smaller membership base to draw from, more responsibility on building a full client base may fall upon the fitness professional. This will require more dedication to individual promotion and lead-generation efforts. With smaller departments, the fitness professional may also take part in cleaning and maintenance operations, as well as working the floor to ensure a clean and safe environment for the members. These activities provide an opportunity for the fitness professional to interact with members and become a visible part of the facility's community.

CHECK IT OUT

Equipment malfunctions can happen at any time, with both new and used equipment. As a best practice, fitness professionals should be familiar with the safe operation of every piece of equipment in the facility, as well as understand where and how to report an equipment malfunction when one is discovered. Maintenance logs should be kept for all equipment and updated any time service is needed or performed. The following should always be checked for functionality prior to placing a client on a piece of equipment:

- Treadmill belts.
- Elliptical and stationary bike pedals and tracks.
- Belts, chains, or brake-supplied resistance on bikes and rowers.
- Handles and seats on bikes rowers and resistance machines.
- Electrical displays and cords on all powered equipment.
- Cables and pins on resistance machines

Implementing a regular preventive maintenance program can extend the life and usage of most major equipment, and decrease the chance of injury to a member or client. Thus, fitness professionals should seek an active role in understanding and participating in the equipment maintenance program at their facility.

Management

Management will typically consist of the owner or franchisee, a general manager, and a few (depending on club size) assistant managers overseeing fitness and operations activities. With fewer resources, general tasks such as materials ordering, marketing, accounting, business development, payroll, and human resources activities will be handled by the general manager and other employees as needed. These individuals may also be called upon to provide training or class instruction services during times when training staff is unavailable for scheduled appointments. Due to the understanding of the fitness industry required for these positions, a successful fitness professional may be able move their career to general management of a fitness facility.

Front Desk and Operations

The front desk employees at medium-sized facilities are usually fitness enthusiasts who are not yet certified as fitness professionals. Job tasks usually include answering phones, giving tours to prospects, signing up new walk-in members, and taking payments for fees and snack bar items. These employees may also be responsible for cleaning the gym and performing simple maintenance tasks that do not require specialized repair skills. In situations where in-house staff are unable to make repairs, professional repair services can be contracted from outside vendors. Also, it is not uncommon for external janitorial services to be contracted by these facilities.

Small Group Training Facilities

Small group training facilities are typically smaller in size and do not normally contain the large selection of commercial fitness machines a medium-sized or large-scale facility does. Small group facilities may rely upon smaller pieces of equipment, such as kettlebells, suspension trainers, sandbags, battling ropes, and plyo boxes to meet the training needs of their members.

CHECK IT OUT

Key characteristics of small group training facilities:

- Catering to niche fitness solutions.
- Numerous creative avenues of personal training and group training classes.
- Mostly independent-owner operated, with some franchise brands.
- Small number of employees with shared operational, administrative, and sales responsibilities.
- High level of community involvement and grassroots marketing.
- May be specialized, requiring new-hire training in facility-specific methods.

These facilities will often occupy a standard storefront and are often focused on niche market activities such as athletic performance enhancement, "boot camps", circuit-style group training, and other assorted group training modalities. Because of this, these facilities will have far less walk-in traffic and rely more heavily on local marketing and referrals to grow the business. The small size also limits the availability of changing and shower facilities. Whereas many are independently owned and operated by fitness professionals, the number of franchises operating in this sector is growing. The membership model for these facilities can be implemented differently than others in the industry. This type of gym primarily operates with clients working directly with fitness professionals, in scheduled one-on-one or group training sessions, with little to no "open gym" access for patrons. The membership model of these facilities is often driven by how many classes or sessions a member attends in a given time period, typically by week or month. The facility may also offer a per session price that can be bundled for a larger number of sessions at a discounted rate. This allows for freedom of scheduling and access to classes for the clientele. Members are not always committed to the same classes at the same times every week, but have the freedom to choose different classes based on their personal schedule and preferences. The smaller size of the business generally means that fewer employees are needed. This leads to a larger sharing of responsibilities, while the majority of staff are all fitness professionals.

Common Clientele

The type of client who chooses a small group training facility is generally a person who enjoys being in a group setting and views working out as a social experience. Some facilities will even host non-workout-related gatherings, giving members the opportunity to interact with each other and build a community-based culture in which members are encouraged to hold each other accountable. Further, the idea of a professionally designed workout led by a coach or trainer, for a fraction of the cost of an individual training session, often appeals to young professionals and those focused on value. Small group clientele also tend to be highly dedicated to their niche training.

Organizational Setting

Because of the diversity of the target markets each company is attempting to serve, facilities will vary significantly within this market segment. Fitness professionals may find it more

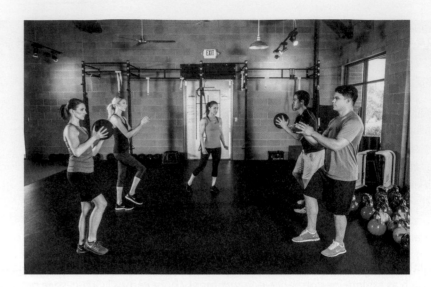

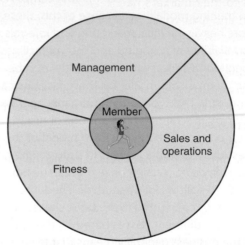

Small Group Training Fitness Facility

challenging to be hired in these types of facilities, because the owners or managers often seek out fitness professionals who may have specialized training or experience working within the facility's niche training brand. Additionally, turnover in these types of facilities is often low. Thus, unless the company is adding more classes or expanding in locations, there are typically fewer job openings, because one fitness professional can lead multiple classes per day. Fitness professionals should also anticipate that these types of facilities will require them to attend or shadow a number of classes in order to learn the programming and instruction methods unique to the company's position within the market.

Management

Most managerial, administrative, and human resources tasks are handled by the owner or general manager in small group training facilities. High levels of entrepreneurial skill, business acumen, and dedication are required for success in this category of facility. Managers in these facilities need to not only have great depth of knowledge in fitness, but they must also be skilled in the area of business operations. Seeking out extra education surrounding entrepreneurial skills may be a vital component of running a successful small group training facility.

Fitness, Sales, and Operations

In small group facilities, running the gym is a team effort. Fitness professionals will also be the sales and operations staff. When not directly instructing classes or personal training sessions, employees will assist the owner or manager with manning the front desk, selling nutrition products and snacks, and cleaning the facility and equipment. Fitness professionals are also the sales and marketing team in a small group training facility. They are responsible for client retention as well as for boosting the business's reputation through word-of-mouth and local outreach in their communities.

Boutique and High-End Facilities

Boutique and high-end facilities range in size and scope. Boutique facilities are often in the form of high-end studios that focus on attracting and serving a niche segment of the market. Similar to small group training facilities, these studios are specialized in a specific form of training or area that appeals to their market's needs. What differentiates them, however, is their generally upscale design and luxury feel. Along with that comes an equally upscale cost of membership and service fees. Boutique studios vary in size but are generally small, sometimes located in office buildings, near business districts, or in affluent suburbs. The larger high-end facilities may only have one location, or they may have a few branches in larger metropolitan markets. Oftentimes, they are also offered as part of larger members-only golf or tennis clubs. These facilities may provide multiple specialized service offerings similar to the large-scale national chain clubs, which may even be unique to the individual facility. These clubs and studios focus on providing high-end amenities, equipment, and fitness professionals. Exclusivity and privacy are also highly marketed, with clubs often restricting the number of available memberships and maintaining a waitlist for acceptance.

CHECK IT OUT

Key characteristics of boutique and high-end facilities:

- Offer a luxury fitness experience, ranging from small boutique studios to large resort-style clubs.
- Focused on exclusivity and privacy.
- Emphasis on exceptional customer service.
- Contain the best equipment, facilities, and fitness professionals.
- Resort/spa-style design and feel.
- More expensive than standard fitness facilities.
- Generally located near business centers or in affluent suburbs.
- Higher demand for training services.
- Fitness professionals often earn higher per-session rates for services.
- More difficult to build a deep client base, due to less foot traffic and club exclusivity.
- Difficult point of entry for new inexperienced fitness professionals without having specialized skills few others can provide.

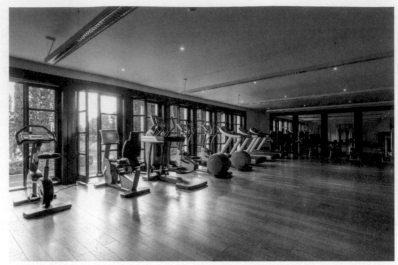

© Marko Poplasen/Shutterstock

Common Clientele

Patrons of these facilities are generally from highly affluent backgrounds, and are willing to invest more than the average fitness consumer for a resort-style experience. In the large-scale facilities, they expect everything from spa amenities and luxury locker rooms to top-of-the-line equipment, concierge service, and the best personal trainers and group fitness instructors available. The members are often there because they value the undivided attention and the privacy they receive. For boutique studios, the customer is attracted to the private facility's luxury look and feel, and services they cannot receive anywhere else.

Organizational Setting

The members of boutique and high-end facilities pay a premium for the goods and services they consume. In paying these higher prices, these members may expect more specialized skill sets and experience from their fitness professionals. This expectation may drive management to seek out specialized and highly experienced professionals who they can promote to members. Respective to size, organizational structure and job tasks will be similar, if not the same, as the standard versions of small group training studios and large-scale national chains. In a private studio setting, professionals should anticipate to have only one or two managers who are highly involved in every aspect of the facility.

CHECK IT OUT

A fitness professional at a country club should consider creating tennis- or golf-specific programs for avid players. Another programing option is providing summer group training programs for their regular clients' children.

Getting Hired

Fitness professionals applying for a position with a company should spend adequate time researching the facility, its demographics, and its target market. It is recommended to research as many locations of interest as possible, because the more jobs that are applied for, the greater the success a new fitness professional will have of getting hired. Typically, larger companies with more robust human resources departments will have standardized online job postings and offer the option of submitting resumes and applications online. Because smaller companies will tend to not have that level of onboarding support, face-to-face interaction to discover and apply for jobs is still crucial in a market with such a vast range of employer opportunities. Interviewing etiquette and resume writing are also highly important skills that cannot be overlooked. And while many similarities do exist with finding employment in any market, each type of fitness facility will present its own unique challenges.

Applying to Large-Scale Facilities

Large-scale facilities will have standardized hiring practices. Many of these facilities will require that all applications and resumes be submitted through an online portal (typically found through a careers page on the gym's website) to streamline the application process. These jobs are often cross promoted through job search websites, and can be easily discovered by searching online for openings in the desired geographic area. A candidate may be expected to complete an online questionnaire and application as well. Once the application process has been completed online, it is also best to submit an application or resume in person at the facility. This ensures direct contact with the hiring management, which can increase the chances of being considered for the position. It is best to visit during non-peak hours and to respect the management's time. A short 3- to 5-minute introduction and conversation is adequate to communicate commitment and desire from the applicant.

Applying to Medium-Sized and Small Facilities

When the facility is a franchise location or a smaller facility operated by a large corporate entity, the application process will often be online and mimic that of a large facility. With growing availability of technology, smaller independent companies will also post available positions online through job search websites. In the event that there is not an online application process in place, applicants should visit the facility and ask to speak with the personal training director or fitness manager about current openings and the hiring process. Candidates should utilize that time to submit an application (if the facility is hiring) and their resume, and briefly describe their qualifications and why they are interested in working at the facility. If the job was applied for online, as with large facilities, it is best to always follow up in person to submit a resume as well.

CHECK IT OUT

NASM has its own online job board, where certified fitness professionals can post their resumes for discovery by employers looking specifically for NASM Certified Personal Trainers! Potential employers can also list open positions for NASM certified fitness professionals to search out as well. Head on over to the NASM website to check it out!

Resume Writing

When developing a resume, job seekers should follow some basic ground rules and suggestions to ensure that they are viewed in the best light by potential employers. The resume should be concise and, if possible, limited to one page. The applicant's name, phone number, and email address should be displayed centered in the header, with the content below following a standard bulleted outline format. The major headings should reflect formal education and certifications attained, past work experience, and special skills and achievements that could directly relate to a career in the fitness industry.

The highest level of formal education earned should be listed first, followed by industry certifications and specializations. The bulk of the resume should be filled with past work experience. If experience has not been gained directly in an environment similar to the job being applied to, the candidate should elaborate on how skills gained in other experiences could be related to a position as a fitness professional. If an applicant has multiple years of experience building and managing a business in a different industry, that valuable knowledge could directly relate to the necessary tasks of acquiring and retaining personal training clients. Previous job titles and start and end dates of the positions should be listed, and it is best to include the name of previous supervisors. When describing past work experience, always use brief phrasing, action verbs, and quantifiable accomplishments. For example, "during my time with the company, I helped manage a four-person team to complete many projects" could be rephrased as "managed a four-person team to successful completion of essential-outcome projects." This type of phrasing adds power to the experience and will help to capture the attention of the hiring manager, who may have numerous resumes to look through.

The special skills and achievements section is for the applicant to highlight accomplishments that may not be directly covered in experience or formal education. This would include additional skills, pertinent awards earned, personal accomplishments, and any affiliations with professional organizations that relate to the job being applied for. For example, a fitness professional may list additional skills of proficiency using software that relates to personal training, as well as CPR/AED and first aid certifications and professional courses or seminars attended. See **Figure 7.1** for an example of this commonly used resume format.

Interviewing

The interview process will vary from facility to facility; however, the applicant should be honest and straightforward about the information provided. The interview process is an opportunity for the potential employer to gather more information about the candidate, as much as it is an opportunity for the candidate to gather information about the potential employer. Both the candidate and employer should feel that the position is a good fit. It is likely that behavioral-based questions, requiring a candidate to recall a specific time in which he or she performed an activity, will be asked. Examples of this could be, "describe a time when you had to overcome a conflict with a coworker" or "tell me about your greatest workplace achievement, as well as a time when you had to overcome a failure." Candidates should be able to demonstrate how the actions taken, and the outcomes achieved, in these situations would translate to the potential position. They should also be prepared with questions about the position, work environment, opportunity for advancement, continued training, and onboarding process to demonstrate they have researched the information that is available about the position. Candidates should also ask about next steps that should be taken to continue the employment screening process. During the interview, potential employers will not only question the candidate, but they will

---

Full Name

Phone Number – Email Address

Education/Professional Certification(s)

Highest Education Level Degree Name (e.g., Bachelor's Degree, Master's Degree)
(Graduation Date)
School Name – City and State School is Located

Next Highest Education Level Degree Name (if applicable) *(Graduation Date)*
School Name – City and State School is Located

Certification Name – Certifying Company Name *(Date Earned)*
Additional Certification Name (if applicable) – Certifying Company Name *(Date Earned)*

Experience

Current/Most Recent Company Name (Date Range of Employment)
Job Title – *Supervisor:* **Supervisor Name**, Supervisor Title – City and State Job is/was Located
- Concise bullet point of job responsibility with action verbs.
- Concise bullet point of job responsibility with action verbs.

Previous Company Name (Date Range of Employment)
Job Title – *Supervisor:* **Supervisor Name**, Supervisor Title – City and State Job was Located
- Concise bullet point of job responsibility with action verbs.
- Concise bullet point of job responsibility with action verbs.

Previous Company Name (Date Range of Employment)
Job Title – *Supervisor:* **Supervisor Name**, Supervisor Title – City and State Job was Located
- Concise bullet point of job responsibility with action verbs.
- Concise bullet point of job responsibility with action verbs.

Accomplishments and Additional Skills

- Bullet point of additional skills, awards, accomplishments, or professional affiliation.
- Bullet point of additional skills, awards, accomplishments, or professional affiliations.

FIGURE 7.1 Sample resume.

also observe a candidate's behavior to assess the level of professionalism displayed. Thus, interviewees should be conscious of their speech, body language, and appearance when in front of the hiring manager. This starts with dressing professionally and ensuring that high levels of personal hygiene are maintained. Although the workplace is a gym, fitness professionals should dress and present themselves no differently than if they were applying for a formal office job. The following are key factors to consider during an interview:

- Arrive early. Consider traffic around the time of the interview, and plan accordingly.
- Dress in professional attire.
- Bring multiple copies of the resume printed on high-quality paper.
- Have a positive demeanor, smile, and make eye contact.
- Nod and react accordingly to display active listening through body language.
- Have questions prepared and take notes.
- Use professional language.

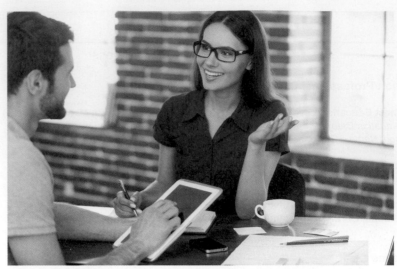

© g-stockstudio/Shutterstock

- ◆ Avoid sloppy or defensive body language, such as crossing arms and legs, slouching, or eye rolling.
- ◆ Avoid "hot button" topics such as religion and politics.

The education, experience, and skills listed on the resume is what earned the interview. When an interview is earned, the hiring manager is already confident enough in those criteria that he or she wants to meet with the applicant, so the time during the interview is more about determining if the individual's personality and demeanor is a good fit with the company's culture. That said, the most important aspects of an interview are to stay calm, confident, prepared, and professional.

Independent Fitness Professionals

Independent fitness professionals work for themselves and develop their own service offerings, prices, and programs. The independent fitness professional must be a true entrepreneur, running every aspect of the business. This means they bear the responsibilities of marketing and advertising, selling products and services, delivering those services and training clients, and managing revenue. Being an independent fitness professional offers the most freedom and flexibility, but it carries with it the greatest amount of responsibility.

CHECK IT OUT

Key chracteristics of operating as an independent fitness professional:

- Freedom of being one's own boss.
- Flexibility of when and where to work with clients.
- Ability to develop unique, custom, and creative programming.
- Must control all aspects of marketing, sales, service, and billing.
- No employment benefits, such as 401k or subsidized health insurance.
- Need to maintain and transport equipment.
- Tax and business licenses and liability insurance are required.

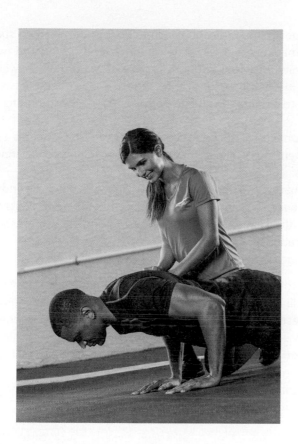

Common Clientele

People seek out the services of independent personal trainers for many different reasons. Some may not want to join a gym or would like to train within the comforts of their own home. Others may be self-conscious and do not want to work out in front of other people. Additionally, some may seek out a niche style of training that only a particular fitness professional offers. It is important for fitness professionals to understand the demographics of the area they would like to serve when they are looking to begin an independent training service. Understanding the common desires and goals of those who may be interested in an independent fitness professional will help the entrepreneur understand how he or she can fit into the market area and develop a business to suit the needs of the individuals in that location.

Organizational Setting

The working environment varies based on the style of training and instruction offered. Regardless of which direction is taken, it will be necessary to purchase basic marketing materials, as well as to maintain liability insurance. Further, fitness professionals considering an independent business should educate themselves on federal and local tax regulations prior to establishing prices or investing in fitness equipment. Independent professionals can work in a number of environments, and often do so across various locations. They can provide creative group classes or personal training sessions outdoors in public spaces, or through facilities that may either require an access fee or potentially a contract relationship. They can also train out of their homes or directly in clients' homes.

If working outdoors, the professional should consider factors such as the average temperature and climate in the area, safety during early morning and twilight hours, access to restrooms, proximity to shelter in the event of a storm or rain, as well as availability and proximity of parking in relation to the area the service will be offered. Also, local municipalities should be consulted to obtain the required permits needed for commercial activity in a public space.

The traveling in-home training option can be lucrative, given that it is a personalized service delivered in the convenience of the client's home. Professionals considering this option should weigh factors such as:

How much and what type of equipment they will need to purchase and regularly transport.

- Travel times between locations, which will affect the volume of clients able to be scheduled.
- Safety issues with regards to meeting and performing assessments with first-time clients.
- Space considerations.
- Liability coverage for both the professional and client.

The working environment for fitness professionals who elect to pay rent or contract with a facility or studio will vary based on each studio's culture and management. The fitness professional should investigate the facility's policies as they relate to priority of equipment and presence of regularly employed trainers and instructors, as well as policies that govern the acquisition of new clients from the facility. Regardless of the option chosen, independent professionals will need to acquire business and tax licenses, set up ways to bill clients and collect fees, maintain a business plan to track finances and forecast opportunities for growth, and develop a marketing plan to successfully promote the business.

Conclusion

Understanding the various work environments provides the fitness professional the knowledge he or she needs to determine what will most likely be the best fit for employment. From large-scale national brands and all-inclusive clubs to small studios and independent businesses, options are available for all personality types and training styles. Visiting locations and making connections with those already employed in the field will provide new perspectives and information, allowing for a more thorough grasp of the real-life experience for fitness professionals.

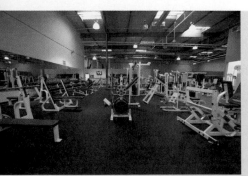
© bikeriderlondon/Shutterstock

Case in Review

You continue to look further into the employment opportunities available in your area that will best fit your career path after becoming a NASM Certified Personal Trainer. Based on your research, you have identified three gyms as potential employment prospects. You have created a table that includes a few characteristics, common clientele, and possible considerations for each gym type to gain further insight as to which one would best align to your professional goals as a fitness professional.

Facility Comparison

Facility Type	Notable Key Characteristics	Common Clientele	Considerations
The new, large-scale national club	• Established brand • Sizable selection of exercise equipment • Large membership base • Departmentally separated • Onboarding programs	• Financially conservative individuals • Families • Those seeking numerous options and amenities	• Little control over scheduled hours • Focus on sales • Will have to build reputation
Your small group training facility	• High level of community involvement • Flexible work hours • Specialized offerings and program designs	• Younger, price conscious audience that likes to socialize and compete with one another	• Self-marketing • Responsible for own clientele pipeline • Additional cross-functional responsibilities
The small boutique club	• Higher price point • Luxury feel • Numerous additional amenity offerings available • Specialized program design offerings	• Affluent populations • Willing to pay for the best equipment and trainers	• Possible membership caps • May be more difficult to build client base due to club exclusivity

Reference

Bixlar, B. (2014). What investors need to know before jumping into the fitness industry. *Franchise Chatter*. Retrieved January 20, from Available at: www.franchisechatter.com/2014/01/20/franchise-chatter-guide-what-investors-need-to-know-before-jumping-into-the-fitness-industry/

CHAPTER 8

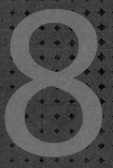

CLIENT ACQUISITION AND CONSULTATIONS

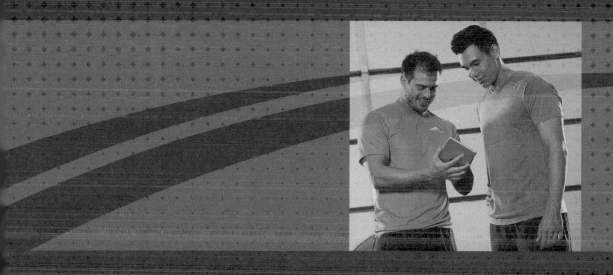

OBJECTIVES

After studying this chapter, you will be able to:

1. **Identify** different prospecting strategies used to reach and acquire potential clients.

2. **Describe** consultation strategies and assessments essential for the client acquisition process.

3. **Employ** rapport-building techniques to establish trust and credibility.

4. **Develop** sales presentation strategies to overcome common client objections.

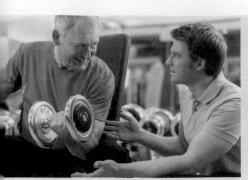

© Kzenon/Shutterstock

Case Scenario

You have accepted a job as a personal trainer at the new fitness facility that just opened down the street from your house. Accepting a personal training position at a large-scale national chain has kicked off your career path of becoming a fitness professional. Over the past 2 weeks, you have become familiar with the different departments within the gym and how they will help you succeed in your new role. While acclimating yourself to the operations of each department, you have been shadowing seasoned personal trainers as they search for new clients and build relationships with the frequent members of the gym.

After becoming accustomed to your new working environment, your manager has given you the green light to begin working with clients on your own. As you begin to work the floor, you quickly realize the need to create strategies, which will enable you to begin feeding your client pipeline. You have identified three key areas you feel are imperative to building your clientele: prospecting activities, client consultation, and making the sale.

Now that you are no longer shadowing other personal trainers, you will first need to create a plan that will help to maximize your success in acquiring and retaining clients. Based on what you have witnessed over the past 2 weeks in the gym, and what you have learned about client acquisition and consultation, you have included the following in your plan:

- *Prospecting activities*: Where will you find new clients?

- *Client* acquisition *and consultation*: How will you establish rapport, credibility, and trust with your potential clients? What types of assessments will you require the client to have and/or complete prior to getting started, and why? What will your next steps be once you have successfully acquired a new client?

- *Making the* sale: What will you present to gain buy-in and commitment? What are some common objections to making a sale you need to be aware of, and how do you plan to overcome them?

Introduction to Client Acquisition and Consultations

Some of the most successful fitness professionals credit their success to not only their knowledge and ability in helping clients achieve fitness-related results, but equally to their ability to market their business and sell their services. Successful fitness professionals must place a large

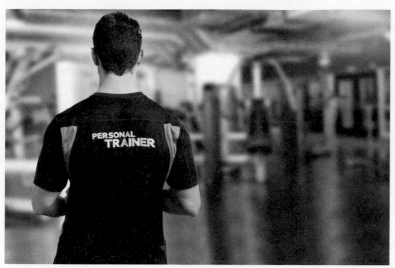

© ruigsantos/Shutterstock

amount of time and energy into sales and marketing in order to accumulate the necessary number of clients needed to maintain their desired income level. Most fitness professionals enter the fitness industry due to their own passion for fitness, as well as their aspiration to help others achieve their fitness goals. A challenge many fitness professionals often face early in their careers is improving their sales and marketing skills to match both their passion for fitness as well as their desire to help others. Fitness professionals who are not successful in marketing themselves in order to create **leads**, and who fail to convert leads into actual clients, may never be able to put their skills into action. Fitness professionals should expect to have to generate a significant portion of their own clientele, regardless of the type of environment they work in. This will require that the professional invest time in **prospecting** activities both inside and outside of the environment they work in. The goal of prospecting is often to drive prospective clients into a trial program or some type of an assessment appointment, in which the fitness professional is then able to present options for personal training services.

One thing is certain, however, and that is the fact that clubs and gyms of all sizes continue to have difficulty finding, and retaining, high-quality fitness professionals due to a general lack of understanding of the sales process. Clubs do not just need fitness professionals who are certified, they need ones who are ready and able to build a book of business. Too many fitness professionals believe that just because they are certified that clients will automatically appear. Many trainers also do not want to have to pressure clients, and will only sell when the opportunity naturally presents itself. However, the most successful professionals are the ones who treat their client list like a business, proactively focusing on marketing their services and recruiting new clients. Three basic things should always be focused on together: *service*, *science*, and *sales*. Earning an accredited certification demonstrates a fitness professional is invested in knowing the science, while a steadfast passion for fitness and helping others will always lead to the best service for clients. However, it is only with a solid understanding of the sales process that a fitness professional can unlock the potential for a prosperous career in the fitness industry.

The client acquisition process begins with the initial meeting and building **rapport**. It will then typically transition from a prospect's expression of interest in the service to scheduling and attending an assessment session. During the assessment, the professional has another opportunity to build rapport, earn trust, and demonstrate credibility and knowledge. Numerous tools are available for transitioning a lead to a client, retaining the client, and eventually earning referrals from the client that can be applied to increase the fitness professional's success.

Leads

Individuals who have shown a certain level of interest in personal training services.

Prospecting

Activities designed to search for potential customers or clients.

Rapport

The aspect of a relationship characterized by similarity, agreement, or congruity.

Prospective Clients and Marketing

In addition to training their clients, fitness professionals will need to allot adequate time to participate in the sales process. New professionals may be surprised by the sales process, and, in turn, may have developed a stigma around having a "sales quota." A goal or quota should not be feared. Sales goals are easily broken down into actionable tasks fitness professionals can track on a day-to-day basis. The three major sources of clients are **point of sale**, **new business**, and **re-signs**. Point-of-sale clients are those who have purchased personal training services of their own volition, whether individually or in a package, at the same time they enrolled as a member at a fitness facility. New business clients, sometimes referred to as *self-generated business*, are those clients who have enrolled in personal training via any number of prospecting activities a fitness professional may have performed inside or outside the fitness facility. Re-signs are clients that choose to purchase additional training services near the end of their training program, and often represent the largest portion of a fitness professional's revenue stream. The level of involvement that fitness professionals are expected to have in the sales process will vary from location to location. In all cases though, it is an important task to develop personal goals for client acquisition and to revisit those goals frequently to determine whether they are being met.

Creating a Plan

Understanding how to build a client book, and possessing the insight to project future needs as they relate to new client acquisition, will allow the fitness professional to dedicate adequate time to complete essential prospecting tasks. Personal training department managers will often give fitness professionals revenue goals. New trainers may start with low targets to reflect their number of clients and, as their client base grows, management will then assign higher revenue goals, as it is expected that fitness professionals will retain the majority of their paying clients while continuing to prospect for new leads. Having a prospecting strategy, and dedicating a certain amount of time to prospecting each day, will give the fitness professional the best opportunity to generate the necessary leads needed to obtain a full client base. Initially, fitness professionals may need to spend most of their time in prospecting activities, because they will not have a full client load at the beginning of their career. As they begin to have success turning leads into actual clients, there will be a shift toward spending more of their time training and less of their time prospecting.

A number of **forecasting** techniques are available to fitness professionals. In large-scale facilities, department managers often will assign fitness professionals a business plan to complete at the end of the month to project what their next month's sessions, service, and revenue generation will most likely look like. In order to estimate new business, the fitness professional can look at the total number of hours he or she anticipates spending to train paid clients per week versus the total number of hours available. Using the total number of hours available, the fitness professional can then work with the manager to estimate the number of new-member fitness assessments or other new business opportunities that he or she will realistically need to fill the remaining time. This will differ for each fitness professional based on the type of facility, the individual's personality, and the hours that are available. The fitness professional should then look to past performance, or facility-specific data, to gain insight as to the *show percentage* (i.e., percent of those booked for assessments who actually appear for their complimentary service) and the *closing percentage* (i.e., percent of those who attend an assessment who end up purchasing a paid service) to estimate the number of new clients he or she could earn that month, and thus the amount of revenue that could be generated from new business.

Point-of-sale client

A client who has purchased a personal training package or program at the time that he or she enrolled in a membership program.

New business

A new client who has purchased personal training services as a result of the fitness professional's prospecting activities.

Re-sign

An existing client who has elected to continue training and purchases additional personal training services or commits contractually to training for a longer period of time.

Forecasting

Process whereby trainers and/or managers apply specific percentages based on previous performance to predict future sales or other measurable outcomes, such as sessions serviced.

CHECK IT OUT

Consider the following basic business plan scenario: A fitness professional has a target to book open hours with 25 assessment opportunities. He suspects that 60% of all appointments booked will show up for the assessment. Because new professionals sometimes have lower closing averages when they first get started, he expects to have a closing average of 20%. Of the 25 prospects that are booked, 15 show up for their appointment. Of those, three actually purchase a paid service. As this cycle repeats each week, the number of fitness assessments booked will decrease, because he has to make time to prepare for and train these new clients.

Face-to-Face Prospecting

The ability to prospect for leads is essential to building a successful fitness career. It is critical to have the mindset that fitness professionals are on perpetual job interviews when they are in the facility in which they work. Even in public fitness professionals may find opportunities to create leads for their business, because one never knows where the next client may come from. For some, the idea of prospecting may be intimidating. The notion that a fitness professional will have to go out onto the workout floor, or even outside within their communities, and speak to people about a service they are selling can cause feelings of discomfort. First and foremost, fitness professionals should have confidence in their unique ability to transform their clients' lives in a positive manner. In many situations, they will not only help their clients achieve a positive health-related objective, but along the way will help their clients build confidence, self-esteem, and a sense of accomplishment that leads them to empower others to do the same. However, not a single client can receive those benefits unless the fitness professional is able to actively promote and sell the services he or she is offering. A fitness professional's skills and knowledge are almost always in demand, so the challenge for many new professionals comes with communicating that there is a fee for their services. Although many struggle with this, the pressure can be alleviated by gaining exposure to a larger number of prospective clients. Simply put, the more people a fitness professional approaches and interacts with regarding the services he or she provides, the more people there will be that sign up as clients.

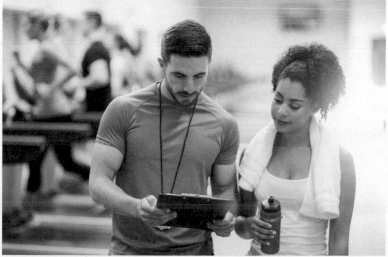

© wavebreakmedia/Shutterstock

For a new fitness professional, actively working the fitness center floor is a great way to begin. Being available to offer suggestions, instruct proper technique on an exercise, or provide new member orientations gives a fitness professional the ability to become the go-to person at the fitness center. Influential members should also be actively recruited into a fitness professional's network. These are the members that are often eager to try new services, so they can go back to their peer group, report experiences, and make recommendations. The ability to be one of the first to try a new product or service reaffirms their position as the opinion leader within their group, and thus they will actively seek out new programs. Opinion leaders are often easily identifiable, because they will generally serve as the messenger to and from their group. The opinion leader will also likely be the person to voice problems, concerns, or unhappiness on behalf of other members to management or a trainer at a fitness facility. In most cases, fitness professionals can seek out the opinion leaders, build rapport by asking about their experience in the facility with different programs, and then seek out a way to improve upon those experiences prior to offering a product or service. Then, the fitness professional can offer the person a complimentary opportunity to try out a new service, presented as an opportunity to earn the person's valuable feedback. This process may not lead to direct business with the individual; however, a positive experience will be reported back to the opinion leader's peer group and in turn increase receptiveness and interest in the new program or service.

A common mistake fitness professionals make is not being proactively involved with the membership. Often, as soon as a session is finished with a client, the fitness professional either leaves the fitness center or retires to a break room to regroup before the next session. Although it is important for fitness professionals to take time for themselves, whenever they are not on the floor interacting with members potential opportunities to prospect are lost. In addition, the fitness professional needs to appear welcoming to the membership. Some individuals may find fitness professionals intimidating, and find it difficult to approach them. Having an inviting appearance by smiling, making eye contact, and being the first to engage in conversation will help put apprehensive gym-goers at ease.

CHECK IT OUT

Focusing on the positives, rather than pointing out any potentially negative attributes, will prevent members or potential clients from being placed in an uncomfortable situation, while simultaneously showing them that the fitness professional respects them as a person and is interested in their overall well-being. If a fitness professional initiates a conversation with a negative comment, it will probably put the member on the defensive. This will not get the relationship off on the right track, no matter how noble the fitness professional's intentions are. The following are some examples of what to say and what not to say.

Appropriate	Inappropriate
"Hello, I hope I am not interrupting your workout, my name is _____. I noticed you doing your last exercise, and I was wondering if it would be alright if I showed you a different variation of the exercise."	"Hello, I need to show you a different exercise. The one you are doing is not right for you."
"Hello, if I can be of any assistance to you today during your workout please do not hesitate to ask as I am the fitness professional on duty today."	"Hello, I am one of the fitness professionals here and I believe you may need my help."

Spectator Prospects

Some clients may seek out services from fitness professionals without being prospected. Sometimes these clients may come in the form of referrals from satisfied clients. They may also have observed personal training sessions from a distance in the fitness center, and the competence exhibited impressed the member enough to approach that particular fitness professional. Thus, a major goal should always be to provide excellent customer service. Fitness professionals can demonstrate excellent customer service by being an educational and motivational resource for any person they come into contact with, while being genuinely interested in helping them to pursue and accomplish their health and fitness goals. Everything fitness professionals say and do is observed within the facility. How sincere they appear when they are approached by members, how much interest they show with their own clients, as well as how gracious they are, may all be a part of how someone decides to trust their health and fitness goals to them in the future. The gym environment is like working in a fish bowl, even when fitness professionals first enter the work environment.

Additional Prospecting Activities

In addition to interacting with members inside the facility, it is essential to have a digital presence in today's marketplace. A core outlet of that digital presence is social media. It is important to understand, however, that whatever is placed on social media will give current and potential clients an opportunity to make judgments—both positive and negative—about the fitness professional, so it is essential to always think critically before posting. Offering educational and motivational information on the common social media platforms is an excellent ways to build a following, while allowing the fitness professional to stay in contact, market, and prospect with a large number of potential clients all at once. This will also give prospective members opportunities to interact with a fitness professional in an environment which may feel more comfortable to them at first. Note that communication of company-sponsored promotions via social media should only be done through channels already set up under the company name. Fitness professionals can then share links from the company site or event page to their personal pages. A fitness professional who works in a facility does not necessarily need his or her own website, because it may create a mixed message for current customers of the facility who make up the core market the fitness professional is trying to offer services to.

Another great possible source of clients is to actively prospect new members by sending them a welcome email, therein offering a free new member orientation or even a personal training session. The use of a personal email address should be avoided, as all business communication should be tied to an email address provided by the employer. If that is something an employer does not provide it is best to set up a new professional email address, effectively separating personal and professional personas. It is also important to seek approval from management prior to beginning this communication with customers. Other possible suggestions for digital prospecting would be to produce and promote a fitness podcast to provide fitness-related information to current and potential clients, or to reach out to online publications to write articles for fitness blogs. Both of these will increase the fitness professional's visibility and popularity, providing a platform to showcase his or her knowledge and expertise.

Beyond "working the floor" and digital prospecting, a number of other activities can be completed to assist in building an active clientele. Company-sponsored events, as well as programs that promote training services to the member base, should be fully explored and participated in. These are valuable opportunities to interact with members who are already somewhat interested in utilizing fitness services. Such events range from manning a promotional table to participating in organized events such as 5K runs or family open houses.

Those wishing to increase their number of leads could also benefit by offering a periodic raffle, in which members have an opportunity to win a set number of sessions. This raffle should be located inside of the facility in a high-traffic area, such as the front desk. The prize needs to be valuable enough to draw interest, without giving too much of the fitness professional's time away for free. For example, offering the same free session promotions that are typically given to new members upon enrollment will serve this purpose nicely. The main benefit, however, is that every submission to the raffle, regardless of whether they win, is a new interested lead to prospect to. To solidify this, the raffle card should request participants to include their name, phone number, email address, and mailing address.

Promotional signage is another great way to get the word out, and should also be strategically placed within the facility. For example, promotional posters for a new youth training program should be placed near the child care room, or perhaps by the court sports and aquatics facilities (if available) that younger audiences utilize more. Conversely, posters for a strongman training program would be better placed near the free-weights area to increase visibility of the program to the target group.

At the end of the day, it is all about increasing exposure to clients. Regardless of what fitness environment a professional is working in, these activities and strategies can be deployed to increase visibility of the fitness professional's services to interested individuals. Of all the different ways to get the word out, it is most important to be creative, unique, and relevant to the population being targeted. That means taking advantage of every avenue available, both old and new, to create as many new leads as possible.

Professional Networking

A fitness professional should work to build a professional referral network. Networking is the process of meeting and interacting with the various stakeholders that serve the same or similar communities or target markets. Networking is a long-term time investment that, given consistent attention, will open opportunities for fitness professionals and business owners. Within the facility, the fitness professional should identify a number of key stakeholders to seek out and interact with in order to develop a foundation for a long-term relationship. Key stakeholders often include department managers, group fitness instructors, and other successful fitness professionals.

The first goal of networking is to establish a meaningful relationship in the hopes that it will eventually lead to business opportunities. In order to build a relationship with other like-minded professionals, fitness professionals will have to show the value of their services to those they would like to include in their referral network. Individuals generally hesitate to refer a client of theirs to someone else if they have not personally experienced the service. For this reason it would benefit those seeking professional relationships to offer complementary assessments and initial sessions to other health and wellness professionals. This way their competencies and skill set can be fully demonstrated, allowing the other professional the ability to experience the professionalism their clients will be treated with. If this is handled properly, it can become a great source of referrals.

External networking events are held in a variety of different venues and opportunities are often limitless. Common networking opportunities include Chamber of Commerce meetings, local charitable events, public speaking engagements, local school events and presentations, onsite corporate wellness days, and even simply meeting local business owners and managers at their workplace. Some business owners and fitness professionals feel that these events are a waste of time, because they are not always easily able to sell or present their services on

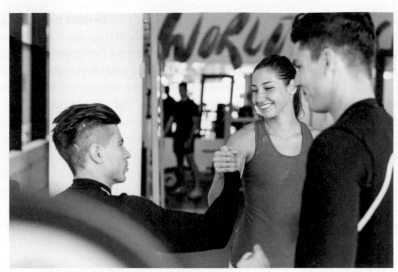

© Andor Bujdoso/Shutterstock

the spot. However, when viewed from a long-term perspective, interacting and participating at these functions often opens doors for fitness professionals to participate in events as "experts" and address the target market directly. With the high demand that exists for access to the knowledge fitness professionals have, networking is key to long-term success within the industry.

Cross-Departmental Interaction and Promotion

Cross-promotion opportunities allow departments or businesses to promote their specific products and services directly to another department's or business's customer base. Cross promotion can be an incredibly powerful tool for fitness professionals who are working as an employee within a fitness facility or as an independent fitness professional with their own business. Cross-promotion activities are often most effective when both parties have something to gain, or at least understand the significance of the role the benefitting department plays in the company's underlying objective as a whole. In many situations, cross-promotion activities are designed for departments to work together in order to fully explain the facility's service offerings. This will often be built into processes inside of the facility. For example, in large facilities the sales department may, as a standard process, encourage prospective members who are on a trial membership to participate in group fitness classes or small group training. In this situation the sales department is likely to gain a sale if the prospective member has a good experience in a popular class. The instructor then benefits by increasing the class size, which may eventually lead to the formation of additional classes.

Prior to establishing cross-promotions with other departments and employees, the fitness professional must, in a similar fashion as training a new client, develop rapport. It may be automatically assumed that employees who work at the same facility all have the same goals, but this is not always the case. Each employee may not have the same understanding of the roles other departments respectively play in a member's life, or knowledge of the other employees' compensation plans. Fitness professionals should inquire about the employees' experience in the facility, such as what aspects they like, what they would change, what their experience has been with various departments, and what ideas they may have for how departments could work together to improve the facility and member experience.

Fitness professionals are often able to build rapport with employees in other departments by utilizing similar body language and communication skills as they would with a potential client. Smiling, making eye contact, introducing themselves, and explaining what role they will be playing in the club, all suggest openness and will make a great first impression. Fitness professionals should also understand that they will often be in a position to offer complimentary or heavily discounted programs to employees; however, this should not be the only focus of interdepartmental communication. Fitness professionals should seek to fully understand what the other employees do, as well as their perceived level of importance. Consistency and reciprocity are key characteristics or behaviors that should be exercised to maintain and develop rapport and trust over a long period of time. Trainers should utilize friendly interactions, and make an effort to periodically check in with those they do not regularly interact with to maintain relationships. Simple comments that let other employees know that they are making a difference are almost always welcomed and will go a long way in helping develop a positive reputation.

The fitness professional can effectively partner with, participate in, and leverage the functions of other departments to grow his or her clientele in a number of different ways. Fitness professionals should understand that the best way to leverage any other department is to understand how that department works, what the primary motivations are for that department's employees, and openly work with employees of that department to assist their efforts as well. Simply stated, a fitness professional should be willing to help promote other departments' objectives in return, and communicate how the cross promotion will ultimately further the objective of the company and benefit all of the stakeholders involved.

Interaction with, and participation in, the new member acquisition process is a common, but sometimes underutilized, strategy in which fitness professionals can quickly grow their clientele. A new fitness professional who takes an interest in the sales department, and offers to assist with presenting or explaining personal training services, stands a good chance of gaining new clients. If the sales team does not understand the training program, they will not be in a good position to communicate the benefits to new members, thus decreasing the number of new clients available to the fitness professional. Fitness professionals can utilize a number of strategies to make this process easier for the sales department employee, which should lead to more new members purchasing personal training services:

◆ Explain the complimentary assessment program to the sales department employee, and how the program benefits new members and the sales department.
◆ Take the sales department employee through the complimentary assessment, so he or she has firsthand knowledge and experience with the program.
◆ Explain the fee-based services the fitness professional provides, and how participation may benefit members and the sales department.
◆ Take the employee through a complimentary training session, so that he or she can refer to the experience when promoting or discussing personal training services with prospective members.
◆ Offer to assist in explaining the personal training services directly to prospective members.
◆ Ask the sales department to assist in promoting an educational topic or seminar to members they enroll as well as to prospective members.
◆ Offer to assist with tours of the facility or demonstrate exercises for prospective members.

Furthermore, if the facility offers a group exercise program, this may be an additional source of potential clients for a fitness professional to market personal training services to. These instructors tend to have tremendous rapport with the members who are loyal to their classes, so building a relationship with the instructor may be mutually beneficial. The fitness professional

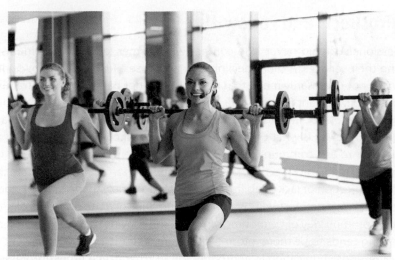

© Syda Productions/Shutterstock

can help market the group instructor's classes to his or her clients and the general membership base and, in turn, the group exercise instructor can help market the fitness professional. Another way to capitalize on this relationship would be to teach a complimentary course (e.g., introduction to foam-rolling and flexibility) marketed directly to the active attendees of the various group fitness classes. This adds value to the membership while also providing the fitness professional the opportunity to show his or her level of expertise on a topic the members may not fully understand. Also, the opportunity to volunteer as an assistant to a group fitness instructor can be utilized by fitness professionals from time to time. The professional can move around the room to correct form and bring to light any movement compensations students may have while the primary instructor focuses on leading the group, therefore demonstrating how personal training services could further enhance the individuals' overall fitness programs.

In addition to promoting, selling, and servicing personal training programs, fitness professionals will often have opportunities to increase their income through the promotion of various additional products and services. Facilities often have business deals to promote specific products, and thus may have a compensation plan that rewards these actions. Some of the more common sources of additional revenue streams include:

- Software-based nutritional coaching
- Healthy snacks, drinks, and dietary supplements
- Fitness accessories and implements
- Spa and massage services
- Online or distance coaching services

Professionals will have the opportunity to regularly interact with the front desk, child care center, and group fitness employees for any number of reasons. However, each department can be leveraged to create mutually beneficial relationships. Essentially, every employee in the facility has the ability to either endorse the training program and the fitness professional or not. Although it is not always within the fitness professional's control to positively influence or manage employees who are less than receptive, the lack of an endorsement should never be from a lack of awareness of the personal training program and its potential benefits. Professionals should seek to first work closely with those who have the greatest contact and direct influence with the members, and then over time look to create awareness in departments that have less member interaction.

Former Prospects and Follow-Ups

Fitness professionals should never lose contact with former leads or individuals who have stopped using their services. A client declining to purchase a fitness program during the first interaction does not necessarily mean that he or she will not have interest in training services at a later date. It is important for the fitness professional to obtain a prospect's contact information in order to allow for future interaction and notification of promotions. In addition, an important question to ask is what their preferred method of communication is. It is better to establish this prior to any communications being sent. Potential communication options are email, phone, social media, and texting. The reason this is important is to eliminate the possibility for miscommunication or lack of ability to connect in a timely manner, and to demonstrate that the client's level of comfort will be a priority moving forward. For example, texting has become a very common way of communicating, but this may not be the preferred method for everyone. Texting tends to be more informal in nature, and the prospective client may prefer handling business communication in another manner. Whenever a fitness professional meets a new prospective client, an email should be sent within 24 hours in order to acknowledge the client and communicate that his or her time and conversation were much appreciated.

Organizing the names and contact information of leads is crucial to a successful prospecting plan. Many facilities offer lead-tracking software or spreadsheets, and the fitness professional should always take advantage of these tools. They allow for proper management of the leads gained and tracking of when each individual was last contacted. As more and more contact information is gathered, utilization of these systems is critical, because there will be numerous leads to contact every day at different points of the follow-up cycle. This ensures that no one lead is contacted too often or too little. It is important to maintain a set call or email schedule for leads that have been collected.

A typical schedule, after the initial 24-hour message has been sent, is a "30-60-90" timeline; that is, direct follow-ups should be made at 30 days, 60 days, and 90 days, with the form of contact being slightly different from the previous one. The 30-day follow-up should be very similar to the 24-hour message, but it should be more personal in nature, acknowledging the interaction that was made and reintroducing the lead to who the professional is, where they train out of, as well as offering help and service without directly pushing a sale. A good approach would be to say, "If there is anything I can do, or if there are any questions I can answer, to assist in reaching your fitness goals, please don't hesitate to contact me!" The fitness professional should always make sure to reference company and individual professional social media outlets as well so the lead can follow and interact more frequently than the monthly email contact.

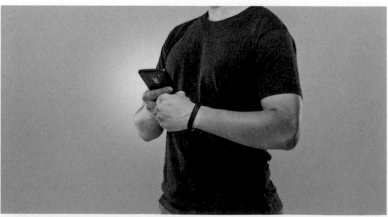

© leungchopan/Shutterstock

Now that the fitness professional is fully introduced to the prospect and remembered, the 60-day follow-up will be more inclusive, listing current promotions at the facility, highlighting any events going on, providing the pricing structure for services, and potentially offering a free session. When sending emails, it is also smart to include fitness tips and other educational information; this will add value to the messages so they do not just seem like advertisements. Once the 90-day mark is hit, the rigor of the contact should be stepped back slightly. Use these emails and calls to simply check in, reintroduce yourself, notify the lead of current events the gym may be holding, as well as continue to provide fitness tips and references to the respective social media outlets. These can even be simple friendly reminders that they are missed and are always welcome to return to the gym, because it may just be the motivation someone needs at that exact time to begin the process of exercising again.

Social media can be another way a fitness professional can maintain contact with former prospects or former clients. If a fitness professional takes the extra time to establish a credible online presence via his or her own website, blog, or social media, this can keep former and prospective clients conscious of the value the fitness professional has to offer on a more consistent basis and will continue to have the fitness professional in mind when the time is right to buy in. Taking the time to send a simple well-timed personal message through social media can go a long way in showing that the fitness professional has a genuine interest in the individual. Additionally, the fitness professional should step back from the digital world and handwrite a personal message on a card and mail it to the client or prospective client. This extra effort can be highly meaningful to a client, as it is easy to send an electronic message, but a handwritten note shows a more personal touch and displays the level of service the lead or client can expect when working with that particular fitness professional.

Re-Signing Clients

Once a steady clientele has been established, re-signs are typically the largest portion of trainer-generated revenue. Fitness professionals should make a list of all clients who have 12–15 sessions or fewer remaining in their package, depending on training frequency per week, then, based on the number of sessions completed weekly, project the date that the client will be nearly out of sessions. If the client has indicated that he or she will continue to train at

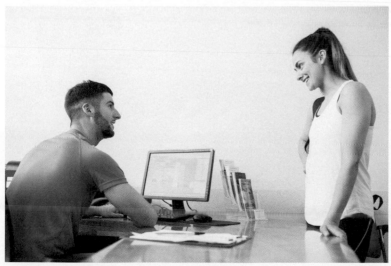

© wavebreakmedia/Shutterstock

the current frequency, the fitness professional should discover how long the client intends to continue the services for. Then, the fitness professional should set follow-ups with the clients to review progress, develop new long-term plans, and present opportunities to continue the purchase of services to further build a lasting relationship.

In the event the client has not yet indicated whether he or she plans to re-sign or not, the same basic prospecting techniques used on new leads should also be applied to re-signing current clients. A large portion of this activity will be through delivering results, creating the desire for the client to keep progressing more and more through the Optimum Performance Training (OPT) model. Continued professionalism, relationship building, and demonstration of value through follow-up contacts will solidify the fitness professional's role in a client's life, leading to long-term buy in and repeat business. Promotional re-sign offers are an effective tool to utilize. For example, offering current clients a free session with the purchase of a set package adds considerable value for the conservative spender (e.g., one free session for every four purchased). Further, increasing the number of re-signs will, in turn, lead to more word-of-mouth referrals from current clients, creating a domino effect of naturally occurring prospecting activity. Eventually, the goal of a robust client list that keeps the fitness professional actively booked will be attained, lowering the necessity for additional prospecting and sales activity, and allowing the fitness professional to focus more exclusively on his or her passion for helping others.

Promoting the Independent Professional

Independent trainers and business owners often must look for external businesses rather than internal departments to establish cross-promotions with. Independent trainers must work as their own marketing department while also performing the sales and operations roles. Whereas the techniques involved with prospecting will be similar for any fitness professional, those who are independent are additionally responsible for identifying and selecting their target markets, creating a product that can serve this market differently or better than an existing product or service, creating a message that accurately communicates this to the market, and finally getting that message out to the market.

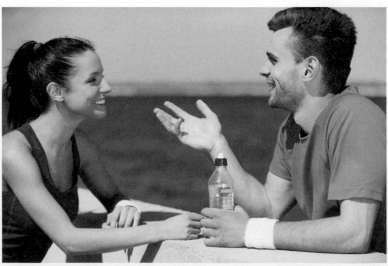

© g-stockstudio/Shutterstock

Creating and establishing a network of businesses that serve a similar market is essential to continually drive leads and new customers to the independent fitness professional. These types of businesses will often serve similar market segments with different service options. They are not competitors, but rather businesses that offer **complementary goods and services**. These businesses may include:

- Massage therapists
- Supplement and nutrition product distributers
- Sports programs and coaches
- Allied health professionals, such as occupational therapists, physical therapists, and physicians
- Small group training facilities
- Healthy restaurants or grocery stores
- Other outlets that promote healthy lifestyles and activities

Leveraging and working with businesses that serve a similar target market can often help independent trainers enhance their reputation in the community, grow their business, and possibly establish discounts for themselves and their clientele. Fitness professionals looking to establish cross promotions with external businesses should seek out businesses that have a good reputation within the community, that promote a complementary product and healthy lifestyle, and that have products which will not cannibalize or act in direct competition with the services the fitness professional offers. When target markets align, the purchase of one complementary good or service will usually increase demand for another.

Whereas fitness professionals employed by a company will normally not have to perform their own external marketing and advertising, independent professionals hold the responsibility of promoting their business themselves. Channels for promotion typically include print media (e.g., magazines, newspapers), radio, television, signage, direct postal mail, and online advertising (e.g., website ads, paid search engine promotion, and paid social media promotion). Each medium offers a way for independent fitness professionals to get their message across to their target market. Most new fitness professionals will find a combination of print and internet advertising to be highly effective. No matter what media outlet is chosen, it is always necessary to pay attention to the cornerstone marketing aspects of *product*, *price*, *placement*, and *promotion* (**Table 8.1**). Many resources and services exist to assist small business owners in marketing their services, and it is best to research all promotional avenues in-depth before deciding which one will work best with regard to both functionality and cost.

> **Complementary goods and services**
> Goods and services that are similar and share a beneficial relationship with another product or service offering, but are not viewed by the consumer as an alternative or direct competition.

TABLE 8.1 The Four Ps of Marketing: Product, Price, Placement, and Promotion

- **Product:** What is being sold.
- **Price:** The monetary value charged for the product, in addition to any costs associated with attaining the product (time, switching costs, assembly, etc.).
- **Placement:** Where the product can be found or accessed, and where in the market it is placed (i.e., high end, mid-market, low cost).
- **Promotion:** Any type of messaging used to get information about the product, price, or placement out to stakeholders, such as consumers, providers, retailers, and/or distributers.

Client Acquisition

Once a fitness professional has turned an interested individual into a lead through prospecting activities and has set an initial consultation meeting, that lead must then be converted into an actual client. Primarily, this is done using techniques to build rapport, trust, and credibility. Additionally, fitness professionals will often use the process of formal consultations with the prospective client to further enhance trust and commitment with regard to the personal training services being provided. Quite often these formal consultations will be complimentary and used as a sales tool to provide quality one-on-one time with the client, thereby giving the fitness professional center stage to prove his or her value, demonstrate his or her expertise, and potentially sign a new client.

Building Rapport

Building rapport with perspective clients is a vital component in building a successful career as a fitness professional. Rapport is the aspect of a relationship characterized by similarity, agreement, or congruity. When meeting an individual for the first time, the fitness professional will have to quickly build rapport to make the prospective client as comfortable as possible. The importance behind establishing rapport quickly is to address any fears or concerns the prospect will need to overcome in order to commit to an exercise program. When potential clients feel comfortable and identify with the fitness professional, they will feel more at ease knowing there is someone who can help them achieve their goals safely and effectively.

CHECK IT OUT

The following are examples of positive body language:

- Hold a relaxed posture, with a straight back.
- Arms should hang comfortably at the sides. Standing with arms crossed is a sign an individual is closed off to the conversation.
- Maintain eye contact, but avoid staring.
- Speak calmly and confidently.

During a first meeting, it is important that fitness professionals make eye contact, introduce themselves by name, and ask the individual for his or her name. They should smile, shake hands, and use positive body language. It is vital that the fitness professional understand how to demonstrate positive body language, because a large part of communication is nonverbal. This will set the stage for the fitness professional to begin building a positive relationship with the prospective client.

Rapport is easier to establish when common ground is found between individuals. In order to find common ground quickly, fitness professionals should have a basic framework of questions they can ask a potential client early on in order to successfully initiate and carry on a conversation. The following examples of conversation-building techniques can be adapted as a framework toward helping a fitness professional build rapport with prospective clients during an initial meeting (Carnegie, 1981):

- *Ask them their name*. This way the client can be addressed by name, which makes the conversation more personal.
- *Find out where they are from*. This can be a talking point in regards to providing background for future conversations. The fitness professional may be familiar with that area or can ask questions about the area in order to show interest in that person as an individual.
- *Ask where they live now*. This allows the fitness professional to find out how long the client has lived in that particular area, as well as opening opportunities to find common ground.
- *Ask about their family*. Most people enjoy talking about their family. This can create opportunities to find rapport in regards to each other's family structure or provide information that can be brought up in future conversations, such as "How are your children doing?"
- *Ask what they do for a living*. This is important in regards to what might be revealed as a part of their particular movement compensations, as well as creating opportunities for the fitness professional to connect with clients over an aspect of life they take part in each and every day.
- *Ask what their hobbies are*. It is possible that a client's hobby could be of particular interest to the fitness professional. However, finding out what they like to do in their free time and/or what they are passionate about will provide the fitness professional opportunities to connect with them in an area that they feel extremely comfortable with.
- *Ask where they see themselves in the future*. This will help to build rapport, because the fitness professional will eventually play an integral role in helping the client achieve his or her future goals.

These questions can be part of a simple framework of conversation starters, allowing for the opportunity to find common ground with a potential client and make a connection. During this type of conversation building, fitness professionals may find something they have in common with prospective clients. They may be from the same home town, share a similar hobby, or have something in common with the prospective client's family situation. Finding a similarity with a prospective client creates common ground, allows for a more relaxed conversation, and provides an anchor the fitness professional can use in future conversations. This way the conversation will become more fluid in nature, allowing the client to feel comfortable rather than as if he or she is being interrogated. As the fitness professional becomes more comfortable communicating with prospective clients, the framework will either become automatic, or the fitness professional will develop a style of communication that flows naturally for him or her. By establishing a framework early in their career, fitness professionals can quickly develop the skills needed to interact with prospective clients.

It is not only important to build rapport during an initial formal session, but on a more casual basis as well. Oftentimes, fitness professionals will have opportunities to meet an individual over much shorter interactions, such as greeting a member as he or she walks into the fitness center. During these encounters, it is important for the fitness professional to learn and use the member's name and to ask a simple question such as, "How has your program been progressing?" This opens the door for the fitness professional to look interested in providing great customer service, as well as allowing the potential client the ability to talk about his or her progress (or lack thereof). Another way a fitness professional can initiate and create rapport is to anticipate a member's needs. For instance, if a member constantly requests a television on a certain channel or frequently purchases the same beverage after each workout, the fitness professional could greet the member by saying, "I already have the television on your favorite channel" or "I'll have your [drink of choice] ready for you when you are finished." These gestures not only show an attention to detail, but they also demonstrate an extremely high level of customer service, solidifying a fitness professional's value to a client.

Barriers to Establishing Rapport

Due to the high importance and value building rapport has for a fitness professional, it is important to gain an understanding of some of the negative behaviors that can become barriers to establishing it. The following are some potential barriers to establishing rapport:

- *Not being an active listener.* Active listening is a communication technique that requires listeners to repeat what they hear to the individual, paraphrased in their own words. This confirms what was heard and ensures understanding by both parties. An example of proper active listening would be for the fitness professional to conclude a conversation with a prospective client by saying, "So if I understand you correctly, your fitness goal would be to lose 20 pounds over the next 6 months." If active listening is not employed during conversations, there is a greater risk that there may be a misunderstanding of some key details between the client and the fitness professional. This technique not only allows for any possible misinterpretations to be cleared up right away, it also shows that the fitness professional is truly engaged in what the client is saying (**Figure 8.1**).
- *Interrupting too often.* As a conversation develops, it is best to allow the potential client to do the majority of the talking. Fitness professionals may feel the need to interject during a conversation to talk about what they feel they can offer, or what they feel is important to the topic being discussed. This communication style may come across as rude, or that the fitness professional is more interested in making a sale than truly listening to what is important to the client. This can be avoided by asking to comment once the client is finished speaking rather than interjecting in a conversation, which will help clients feel that they can fully and safely express themselves.

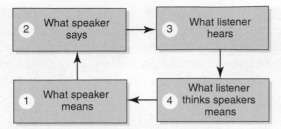

FIGURE 8.1 Verbal communication.

◆ *Being disinterested*. Beginning a structured exercise program can be very intimidating, as well as a significant financial investment many individuals. For these very reasons, it is important that the fitness professional deliver an exceptional level of customer service and focus on the client. Staying focused on the client during the entire session is vital in demonstrating professionalism. When with a client, fitness professionals should not become distracted by a cell phone, talk with other people, talk too much about them selves, or discuss topics that are irrelevant to the fitness experience. In addition, when instructing any exercise, the topic of conversation should stay on any and all teaching cues that are pertinent to that exercise. Conversational discussions should be reserved for rest periods, warm-ups, and cool-downs. Business in the fitness industry will always be customer dependent, so it is imperative that each client or potential customer has 100% of the fitness professional's attention, 100% of the time.

Characteristics of Professionalism

More often than not, a fitness facility is not regarded as a "professional place," making it easy to consider gyms and fitness facilities as being more relaxed and requiring less of the professional edge. However, the act of professionalism is extremely important in the fitness industry, precisely because the environment and context of the surroundings suggest otherwise. Fitness professionals should practice standards of professionalism anywhere and everywhere they go, because working in a club setting implies that they are constantly under evaluation and critique from those around them. How fitness professionals portray themselves does not extend only to the clients in front of them, but also to the hundreds of members able to silently watch their every move. Professionalism is what people see, hear, and experience. It is a level of higher standards that dictates how the fitness professional is treated and regarded by others. Regardless of the surroundings, demonstrating professionalism will warrant respect, courtesy, and admiration from clients and prospective customers.

A lack of professionalism can lead to a cycle of half-hearted business practices. The value of the product and facility and the client's confidence in the fitness professional will begin to decrease, leading to a loss of customers. To ensure that this does not happen, it is important to maintain a professional attitude at the workplace, outside of the workplace, and when conducting business via email or social media. Perception is always a key factor in business. For fitness professionals, even those with the most extensive knowledge, skills, or physically fit appearance, being professional extends beyond spoken words or one's demeanor. Being professional is constant action. Just as in the corporate workplace, "being professional" involves the following:

◆ Always be at least 5 minutes early.
◆ Wear appropriate and professional attire.
◆ Never lose sight of the goal.
◆ Maintain focus on the client.
◆ Seek to inspire others.

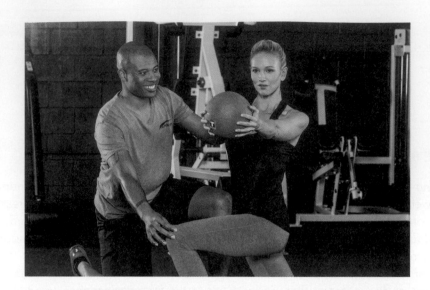

It is generally understood that one should always be on time for meetings, consultations, and sessions. However, in an appointment-based situation "on time" is considered late. The fitness professional should be prepared, ready, and waiting when the client arrives. Practicing good punctuality is not only professional, but it represents preparation, organization, and respect for the client. The modern fitness professional should also dress in a professional manner. Proper attire will usually include well-fitted athletic pants (i.e., not too baggy or too tight), a collared shirt, and clean shoes. Oftentimes, the facility of employment will have guidelines as to what should be worn on the workout floor, or even provide custom uniforms for the staff. Appearance is the first factor a member takes into consideration before any other communication is exchanged. Proper attire brandishes professionalism, organization, and confidence, all of which are preferred by a client when entrusting a fitness professional with his or her goals.

Trust is not given; it is earned. Some individuals who tend to be trustworthy at the beginning of a relationship may eventually lose trust with someone based on certain behaviors. Others will only give trust as it is earned. In either situation, it is important that the relationship be established in a trusting manner, because it is always difficult to earn someone's trust back once it has been lost. The following behaviors will allow the fitness professional to earn and keep the trust of his or her clients:

- *Dependability*. Whether it is starting and ending sessions on time, providing additional educational material as promised, or following up with all communications in a reasonable time frame, dependability is essential to building and maintaining a trusting relationship.
- *Integrity*. Fitness professionals should strive to follow through on what they say and handle themselves in a professional manner at all times. Integrity is generally judged by the accuracy of an individual's words and actions. If fitness professionals are consistent with their actions, words, and behaviors, they should be able to show a high level of integrity to potential as well as current clients.
- *Empathy*. Empathy is awareness, understanding, and sensitivity of the thoughts, emotions, and experiences of another individual without personally having gone through the same thing. Fitness professionals will spend a significant portion of their time with people who may have struggled, or are still struggling, with major health issues. Even though fitness professionals may not have experienced the situations themselves, it is important to always express empathy and caring in all client interactions.

CHECK IT OUT

Fitness professionals who have been fortunate enough to never face any significant health issues will need to avoid using comments such as the following:

- "I can imagine."
- "I understand where you are coming from."
- "I understand how you feel."

    A better way to validate the client's feelings would be to use the following phrases:

- "I am sure that what you are dealing with is difficult."
- "Thank you for sharing your experience with me, I have an idea on how we can work on that."

This line of communication shows clients, or potential clients, that the fitness professional has empathy for their situation and is there to help them with any fitness challenge they are facing.

It is important for the fitness professional to first establish and then maintain credibility. Early on, credibility is established by the fitness professional's ability to build rapport, which helps to turn a potential client into an actual client. Once the professional relationship is established, credibility can be gained by the results clients see from their exercise programs, the professional nature in which they are treated, and the sincere interest their fitness professional shows for them as individuals. It is important to remember that credibility can also be lost if the fitness professional does not always act in a professional manner. The following are ways in which the fitness professional can consistently maintain credibility:

- *Be honest and consistent.* Fitness professionals need to understand that their clients or potential clients are their customers, and that they are the ones that make their business successful. Whether a client has been told to expect a call at a certain time, an exercise program to be designed and ready to take with them after their next session, or simply for their appointment to start at a specific time, honoring any promises that have been made must be a priority for a fitness professional.
- *Be a role model.* Clients look to fitness professionals for more than just their fitness education. They are viewed as a source of motivation and inspiration. Fitness professionals who do not practice what they preach can be looked at as hypocrites, and can lose credibility due to their lack of effort in the very area they are trying to get their clients to make changes in.

Regardless of the size or scope of the position within the center, all fitness professionals should recognize that polite, effective communication and a professional attitude are the cornerstone attributes for the successful establishment of trust and credibility.

Formal Consultations

An important role of a fitness professional is having the ability to correctly perform different assessments, evaluate the results, and then implement an appropriate exercise routine based on those results. In addition to these responsibilities, fitness professionals will need to know how to educate their clients on the importance of any assessment they chose to perform and how it directly relates to that individual's particular goals. This is a crucial step in continuing to establish trust and credibility with a client. Considering that most consultation appointments are complimentary, and used as a tool to convince potential clients to sign up for a paid training package, it becomes even more important to use that time to not only build rapport, but to demonstrate high levels of expertise and professionalism. The formal consultation is the time to truly evaluate what can be done for a client and, in turn, to present that message in a way that communicates the importance of purchasing a fitness professional's services.

The assessments used in a formal consultation also serve as the starting point for how to keep clients as safe as possible while exercising, because fitness professionals interact with individuals of all health and fitness levels. Their job, however, is not to provide medical advice to their clients, but rather to simply understand and explain how common medical conditions can be potentially improved with an integrated training program. It is important to remember that prior to starting any fitness regimen the fitness professional should review the client's medical history and, in light of any persistent issues, ensure that the client has received medical clearance. In addition, a client's lifestyle should also be discussed. Cues based on working conditions, daily activates, and hobbies will provide vital information in determining the starting point for each individual.

Subjective assessment

Assessment used to obtain information about a client's personal history, as well as his or her occupation, lifestyle, and medical background.

The PAR-Q

Subjective assessment provides feedback regarding the client's personal history, such as occupation, lifestyle, and medical background. Note that the information gained during a subjective assessment is not directly measurable and is dependent on what the client is willing to disclose. To make the process of uncovering this vital information easier, the Physical Activity Readiness Questionnaire (PAR-Q) is a standard subjective assessment tool that is readily accessible to fitness professionals (**Figure 8.2**). The obvious purpose of the PAR-Q is to assess prospective clients' readiness to increase their physical activity. Fitness professionals use the PAR-Q to screen clients for possible medical conditions and to ensure that medical clearance from a physician is not required. The fitness professional will also want to gather information on the client's general lifestyle, medical history, and daily movement patterns (**Figure 8.3**). Any and all subjective information that is obtained during the initial consultation should be discussed in detail, especially with regards to how an appropriate exercise program has the potential for positive changes in a particular area. Fitness professionals need to remember that they are simply screening individuals to determine if they are ready to initiate an exercise program, not providing medical advice.

When discussing the client's PAR-Q, lifestyle, and medical history, the fitness professional should only offer information that is important and relevant to the client, and not educate simply for the sake of demonstrating knowledge. The fitness professionals must be able to assess what information is of value to the prospect based on of his or her responses to the questions in the PAR-Q, as well the client's body language or nonverbal cues. The overall aim is to look for good eye contact, engaging conversation, and reciprocation of attention by the client. If the client does not seem involved, change topics to another subject that may be more appealing. At the end of the PAR-Q discussion, the fitness professional should not only have a good understanding of the client's medical history, but also his or her lifestyle, interests, typical workday, and any additional, more personal, information the professional can directly relate to the client with and continue to build trust and rapport.

Questions		
1. Has your doctor ever said that you have a heart condition and that you should only perform physical activity recommended by a doctor?	☐ Yes	☐ No
2. Do you feel pain in your chest when you perform physical activity?	☐ Yes	☐ No
3. In the past month, have you had chest pain when you are not performing any physical activity?	☐ Yes	☐ No
4. Do you lose your balance because of dizziness or do you ever lose consciousness?	☐ Yes	☐ No
5. Do you have a bone or joint problem that could be made worse by a change in your physical activity?	☐ Yes	☐ No
6. Is your doctor currently prescribing any medication for your blood pressure or for a heart condition?	☐ Yes	☐ No
7. Do you know of any other reason why you should not engage in physical activity?	☐ Yes	☐ No

If you have answered "Yes" to one or more of the above questions, consult your physician before engaging in physical activity. Tell your physician which questions you answered "Yes" to. After a medical evaluation, seek advice from your physician on what type of activity is suitable for your current condition.

FIGURE 8.2 The PAR-Q.

Questions		
1. What is your current occupation?	☐ Yes	☐ No
2. Does your occupation require extended periods of sitting?	☐ Yes	☐ No
3. Does your occupation require extended periods of repetitive movements? (If yes, please explain.)	☐ Yes	☐ No
4. Does your occupation require you to wear shoes with a heel (dress shoes)?	☐ Yes	☐ No
5. Does your occupation cause you anxiety (mental stress)?	☐ Yes	☐ No
6. Do you partake in any recreational activities (golf, tennis, skiing, etc.)? (If yes, please explain.)	☐ Yes	☐ No
7. Do you have any hobbies (reading, gardening, working on cars, etc.)? (If yes, please explain.)	☐ Yes	☐ No

FIGURE 8.3 Sample lifestyle and medical history questionnaire.

Objective Assessments

Objective assessments include observations that can be directly measured and quantified by the fitness professional. Unlike subjective assessments, objective assessments are generally performed in order to maintain accurate and repeatable measurements for an individual. This data can then be revisited periodically and reassessed to determine an individual's progress toward certain health and fitness goals. A fitness professional should be able to correctly perform measurements of pulse, blood pressure, and body composition. The information gained from body composition assessments will enable the calculation of a client's body fat percentage.

Pulse

A person's **pulse** is created by blood moving or pulsating through the arteries each time the heart contracts. Each time the heart contracts, or beats, one wave of blood flow can be felt by placing one or two fingers on an artery. Arteries contract and relax rhythmically from the force the blood creates as it circulates, coinciding with the contraction and relaxation of the heart as it pumps blood throughout the body. Therefore, the pulse rate is also known as the heart rate.

A person's pulse can be found in two primary ways. The first method is the **carotid pulse** (Figure 8.4). The carotid pulse is found by lightly placing two fingers on the neck, just to the side of the larynx, roughly 1 inch below the chin. The second method is the **radial pulse** (Figure 8.5). This is the preferred method for the fitness professional to use with clients, because individuals may often be uncomfortable with someone pressing on their neck. The radial pulse can be found by having the client turn his or her hand palm up and then placing two fingers roughly 2 inches below the wrist on the lateral (thumb) side of the arm, generally in line with the first and middle finger of the client's hand. Regardless of the method used, the touch should be gentle, because excessive pressure can lead to inaccurate measurements, as well as discomfort

Objective assessments

Assessments that address observations that can be directly measured and quantified by the fitness professional.

Pulse

The force created by blood moving or pulsating through the arteries each time the heart contracts.

Carotid pulse

Pulse obtained from the carotid artery of the neck.

Radial pulse

Pulse obtained on the forearm, just below the wrist.

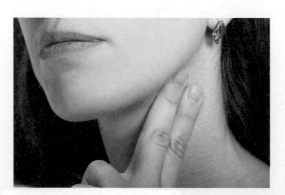

FIGURE 8.4 Carotid pulse.
© Ilya Andriyanov/Shutterstock

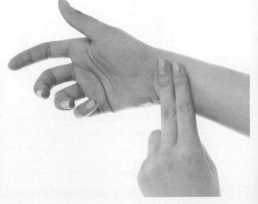

FIGURE 8.5 Radial pulse.
© stockCe/Shutterstock

for the client. Once identified, the pulse is counted for 10 seconds. That number is then multiplied by 6 to determine the beats per minute (bpm).

Blood Pressure

Blood pressure is the pressure of circulating blood against the walls of the blood vessels after blood is ejected from the heart. A blood pressure measurement is composed of two numbers. The first number (the top number) is the **systolic pressure**, and it represents the pressure within the arterial system after the heart contracts. The second number (or bottom number) is called the **diastolic pressure**, and it represents the pressure within the arterial system when the heart is resting and filling with blood. An example of a blood pressure is 120/80 (said "120 over 80"). In this example, 120 is the systolic number and 80 is the diastolic number. Blood pressure measurements always consist of both readings. An acceptable systolic blood pressure measurement for health is less than 120 millimeters of mercury, or mm Hg, and an acceptable diastolic blood pressure is less than 80 mm Hg (American Heart Association, 2014).

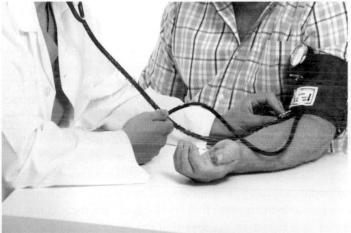

© kurhan/Shutterstock

Blood pressure

The pressure of circulating blood against the walls of the blood vessels after blood is ejected from the heart.

Systolic pressure

The top number of a blood pressure measurement that represents the pressure within the arterial system after the heart contracts.

Diastolic pressure

The bottom number of a blood pressure measurement that represents the pressure within the arterial system when the heart is resting and filling with blood.

Body composition

The relative percentage of body weight that is fat versus fat-free tissue.

Body Composition

Measurements of **body composition** are important for evaluating the general health of a client, as well as tracking goals of both weight loss and muscle gain. Assessments include waist-to-hip ratio, circumference and skinfold measurements, underwater weighing, and bioelectrical impedance. Body composition refers to the relative percentage of body weight that is fat versus fat-free tissue. It is most commonly reported as *percent body fat*. Fat-free mass can be defined as body weight without stored fat, and includes muscles, bones, water, connective tissues, and organs. Fat mass includes both essential fat (crucial for normal body functioning) and nonessential fat (storage fat, or adipose tissue).

Body composition assessments offer a number of benefits for both the fitness professional and the client. Body composition assessments can be used to:

- Identify a client's health risk for excessively high or low levels of body fat.
- Promote the client's understanding of body fat.
- Monitor changes in body composition.
- Enable estimation of a healthy body weight.
- Assist in exercise program design.
- Provide motivation.
- Identify risks associated with chronic diseases.
- Assess the effectiveness of nutrition and exercise choices.

Currently, acceptable percent body fat standards for all ages have not been established, because most body composition studies have been performed with young adults. However, those studies that have been conducted indicate that men typically have 10–20% body fat and women have 20–30%. Based on that research, current body fat targets are 15% for men and 25% for women (Going & Davis, 2001).

Measuring Body Fat

Three methods are available to determine a person's body fat: underwater weighing, bioelectrical impedance, and skinfold measurements. Underwater weighing, which is also referred to as hydrostatic weighing, is the most accurate method to measure body fat, and is commonly used in exercise physiology laboratories. It is based on the concept that fat-free mass is denser than body fat and will sink, while fatty tissue is less dense than water, so only the fat-free mass will register during the specialized weighing. A person's underwater weight is then compared to weight taken on a normal scale to determine an accurate measurement of percent body fat. This method requires large pieces of equipment and advanced levels of training.

Bioelectrical impedance is more commonly used by fitness professionals. With this method, the person holds a portable instrument that conducts an electrical current through the body to estimate body fat. It is based on the idea that tissues that are high in water will conduct electrical currents with less resistance than those with little water, such as adipose tissue. This

CHECK IT OUT

The following formulas can be used to calculate fat mass and lean body mass:

Body fat % × Scale weight = Fat mass
Scale weight − Fat mass = Lean body mass

method of testing body composition can be quick, but it may fluctuate based on the person's hydration level.

Skinfold measurement is the method most often used to determine percent body fat in the fitness setting. With the skinfold method, a caliper is used to obtain an indirect measurement of the thickness of subcutaneous (under skin but on top of muscle) adipose tissue. The idea behind skinfold measurement is that the amount of fat present in the subcutaneous regions of the body is proportional to overall body fat content. Fitness professionals should train with an individual skilled in taking skinfold measurements before performing such measurements with their clients. In addition, the following recommendations apply to obtaining skinfold measurements:

- Take a minimum of two measurements at each site.
- Open the jaws of caliper before removing it from the measurement site.
- Be meticulous when locating anatomic landmarks.
- Do not measure immediately after exercise.
- Instruct the clients ahead of time regarding the test protocol.
- Avoid performing skinfold measurements on extremely obese clients.

The NASM uses the Durnin formula (sometimes called the Durnin-Womersley formula) to calculate percent body fat (Durnin & Womersley, 1974). This formula was chosen because of its simple four-site upper body measurement process. The Durnin formula's four sites of skinfold measurement are as follows:

1. *Biceps*: A vertical fold on the front of the arm over the biceps muscle, halfway between the shoulder and the elbow (**Figure 8.6**).
2. *Triceps*: A vertical fold on the back of the upper arm, with the arm relaxed and held freely at the side. A measurement should also be taken halfway between the shoulder and the elbow (**Figure 8.7**).

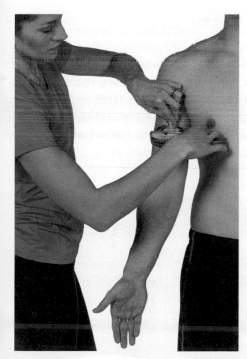

FIGURE 8.6 Biceps skinfold measurement.

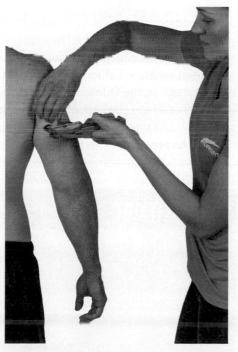

FIGURE 8.7 Triceps skinfold measurement.

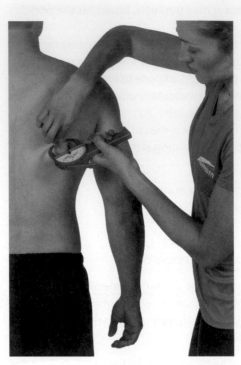

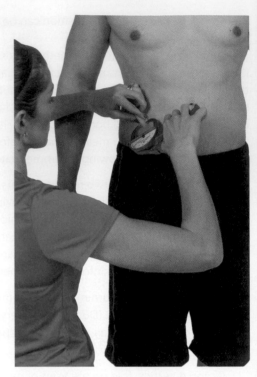

FIGURE 8.8 Subscapular skinfold measurement.

FIGURE 8.9 Iliac crest skinfold measurement.

3. *Subscapular*: A 45-degree angle fold 1–2 centimeters below the inferior angle of the scapula (**Figure 8.8**).
4. *Iliac crest*: A 45-degree angle fold, taken just above the iliac crest and medial to the axillary line (**Figure 8.9**).

All skinfold measurements should be taken on the right side of the body. After the four sites have been measured, the measurements of the four sites are added together. This number is then located on the Durnin-Womersley body fat percentage calculation table based on the client's sex and age (**Table 8.2**). For example, the percent body fat of a 40-year-old female client with a skinfold total of 40 is 28.14% (or rounded down to 28%). Refer to **Table 8.3** for healthy body fat recommendations for active adults.

CHECK IT OUT

The following is an example of a conversation of how a fitness professional might discuss the client's body fat percentage in relation to specific health or fitness goals: "I calculated your body fat percentage, which is an assessment of what part of your body is considered fat mass. We are looking to have a number around 27. Your percentage currently is 31, which indicates you are at a higher risk for certain diseases. However, I am confident that we can bring that number down through dedication to an exercise program."

TABLE 8.2 Durnin-Womersley Percent Body Fat

Sum of Folds	Men					Women				
	<19	20–29	30–39	40–49	>50	<19	20–29	30–39	40–49	>50
5	−7.23	−7.61	−1.70	−5.28	−6.87	−2.69	−3.97	0.77	3.91	4.84
10	0.41	0.04	5.05	3.30	2.63	5.72	4.88	8.72	11.71	13.10
15	5.00	4.64	9.09	8.47	8.38	10.78	10.22	13.50	16.40	18.07
20	8.32	7.96	12.00	12.22	12.55	14.44	14.08	16.95	19.78	21.67
25	10.92	10.57	14.29	15.16	15.84	17.33	17.13	19.66	22.44	24.49
30	13.07	12.73	16.17	17.60	18.56	19.71	19.64	21.90	24.64	26.83
35	14.91	14.56	17.77	19.68	20.88	21.74	21.79	23.81	26.51	28.82
40	16.51	16.17	19.17	21.49	22.92	23.51	23.67	25.48	28.14	30.56
45	17.93	17.59	20.41	23.11	24.72	25.09	25.34	26.96	29.59	32.10
50	19.21	18.87	21.53	24.56	26.35	26.51	26.84	28.30	30.90	33.49
55	20.37	20.04	22.54	25.88	27.83	27.80	28.21	29.51	32.09	34.75
60	21.44	21.11	23.47	27.09	29.20	28.98	29.46	30.62	33.17	35.91
65	22.42	22.09	24.33	28.22	30.45	30.08	30.62	31.65	34.18	36.99
70	23.34	23.01	25.13	29.26	31.63	31.10	31.70	32.60	35.11	37.98
75	24.20	23.87	25.87	30.23	32.72	32.05	32.71	33.49	35.99	38.91
80	25.00	24.67	26.57	31.15	33.75	32.94	33.66	34.33	36.81	39.79
85	25.76	25.43	27.23	32.01	34.72	33.78	34.55	35.12	37.58	40.61
90	26.47	26.15	27.85	32.83	35.64	34.58	35.40	35.87	38.31	41.39
95	27.15	26.83	28.44	33.61	36.52	35.34	36.20	36.58	39.00	42.13
100	27.80	27.48	29.00	34.34	37.35	36.06	36.97	37.25	39.66	42.84
105	28.42	28.09	29.54	35.05	38.14	36.74	37.69	37.90	40.29	43.51
110	29.00	28.68	30.05	35.72	38.90	37.40	38.39	38.51	40.89	44.15
115	29.57	29.25	30.54	36.37	39.63	38.03	39.06	39.10	41.47	44.76
120	30.11	29.79	31.01	36.99	40.33	38.63	39.70	39.66	42.02	45.36
125	30.63	30.31	31.46	37.58	41.00	39.21	40.32	40.21	42.55	45.92
130	31.13	30.82	31.89	38.15	41.65	39.77	40.91	40.73	43.06	46.47
135	31.62	31.30	32.31	38.71	42.27	40.31	41.48	41.24	43.56	47.00

(continued)

TABLE 8.2 Durnin-Womersley Percent Body Fat (*continued*)

Sum of Folds	Men					Women				
	<19	20–29	30–39	40–49	>50	<19	20–29	30–39	40–49	>50
140	32.08	31.77	32.71	39.24	42.87	40.83	42.04	41.72	44.03	47.51
145	32.53	32.22	33.11	39.76	43.46	41.34	42.57	42.19	44.49	48.00
150	32.97	32.66	33.48	40.26	44.02	41.82	43.09	42.65	44.94	48.47
155	33.39	33.08	33.85	40.74	44.57	42.29	43.59	43.09	45.37	48.93
160	33.80	33.49	34.20	41.21	45.10	42.75	44.08	43.52	45.79	49.38
165	34.20	33.89	34.55	41.67	45.62	43.20	44.55	43.94	46.20	49.82
170	34.59	34.28	34.88	42.11	46.12	43.63	45.01	44.34	46.59	50.24
175	34.97	34.66	35.21	42.54	46.61	44.05	45.46	44.73	46.97	50.65
180	35.33	35.02	35.53	42.96	47.08	44.46	45.89	45.12	47.35	51.05
185	35.69	35.38	35.83	43.37	47.54	44.86	46.32	45.49	47.71	51.44
190	36.04	35.73	36.13	43.77	48.00	45.25	46.73	45.85	48.07	51.82
195	36.38	36.07	36.43	44.16	48.44	45.63	47.14	46.21	48.41	52.19
200	36.71	36.40	36.71	44.54	48.87	46.00	47.53	46.55	48.75	52.55

TABLE 8.3 Percent Fat Recommendations for Active Men and Women

Men	Not Recommended	Low	Mid	Upper
Young adult	<5	5	10	15
Middle adult	<7	7	11	18
Elderly	<9	9	12	18
Women				
Young adult	<16	16	23	28
Middle adult	<20	20	27	33
Elderly	<20	20	27	33

Circumference Measurements

A circumference is a measure of the girth of a body segment (e.g., arm, thigh, waist). Circumference methods are affected by both fat and muscle, and therefore do not provide accurate estimates of body composition in the general population. However, the following are some of the benefits of circumference measurements:

◆ Can be used on obese clients
◆ Good for comparisons and progressions

- ◆ Good for assessing fat pattern and distribution
- ◆ Inexpensive to perform
- ◆ Easy to record
- ◆ Little room for technician error

Circumference measurements can also be a source of feedback with clients who have the goal of altering body composition because they are designed to assess changes in the girth of body. The most important factor to consider when taking circumference measurements is consistency. When taking measurements, the tape measure must be kept taut and level around the area that is being measured. The following are seven sites commonly used to obtain circumference measurements:

1. *Neck*: Measure across the larnyx (**Figure 8.10**).
2. *Chest*: Measure across the nipple line (**Figure 8.11**).
3. *Waist*: Measure at the narrowest point of the waist, below the rib cage and just above the top of the illiac crest. If there is no apparent narrowing of the waist, measure at the navel (**Figure 8.12**).
4. *Hips*: With feet together, measure the circumference at the widest portion of the buttocks (**Figure 8.13**).
5. *Thighs*: Measure 10 inches above the top of the patella for standardization (**Figure 8.14**).
6. *Calves*: At the maximal circumference between the ankle and the knee, measure the calves (**Figure 8.15**).
7. *Biceps*: At the maximal circumference of the biceps, measure with arm extended, palm facing forward (**Figure 8.16**).

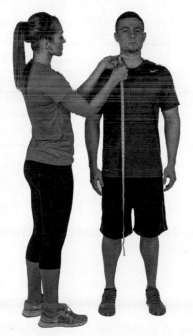

FIGURE 8.10 Neck circumference measurement.

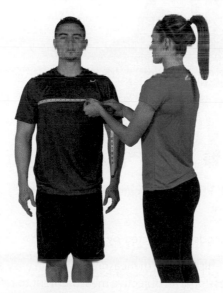

FIGURE 8.11 Chest circumference measurement.

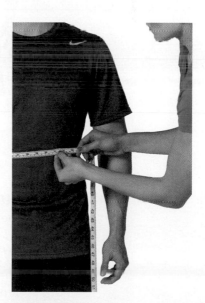

FIGURE 8.12 Waist circumference measurement.

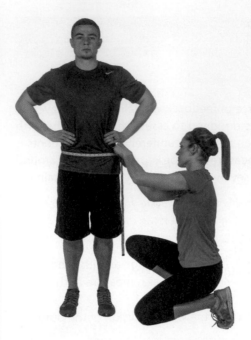

FIGURE 8.13 Hips circumference measurement.

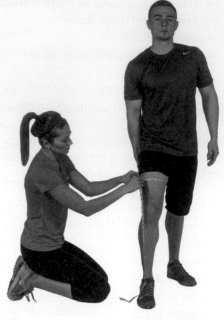

FIGURE 8.14 Thigh circumference measurement

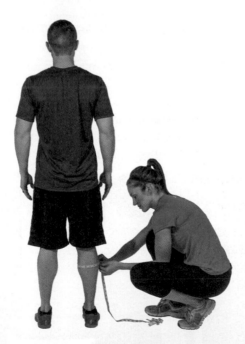

FIGURE 8.15 Calves circumference measurement.

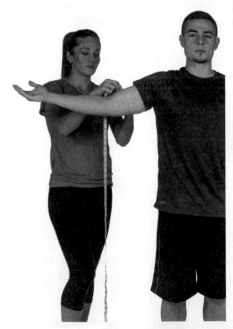

FIGURE 8.16 Biceps circumference measurement.

Waist-to-Hip Measurements

The waist-to-hip ratio girth measurement is an easy assessment to perform and will provide the fitness professional an objective measurement to refer back to as the client progresses with the exercise program. This is an important measurement to obtain because researchers have determined that correlations exist between many chronic diseases and fat stored in the midsection (American College of Sports Medicine, 2010).

The following is an example of a conversation of how a fitness professional might discuss the client's waist-to-hip ratio in relation to specific health or fitness goals: "You have already indicated that losing weight and improving your overall health is your number one priority. For those reasons it is important to find your waist-to-hip ratio. This assessment is a simple way to help determine your overall health, as well as providing us a way to track the progress you will make with the program I design for you."

To perform the assessment, the fitness professional will measure the waist and hip circumferences and then divide the waist measurement by the hip measurement. For example, if a client's waist measures 30 inches, and his or her hips measure 40 inches, dividing 30 by 40 provides a waist-to-hip ratio of 0.75. A ratio greater than 0.80 for women and greater than 0.95 for men is an indicator for disease risk (WHO, 2008; Heyward & Wagner, 2004).

Body Mass Index

Body mass index (BMI) is a rough assessment based on the concept that a person's weight should be proportional to his or her height. An elevated BMI has been linked with increased risk of disease, especially if associated with a large waist circumference (Poirier et al., 2006). Although this assessment is not designed to assess body fat, BMI is a quick and easy method for determining whether a client's weight is appropriate for his or her height. It is important to remember that the BMI measurement does not take into account muscle mass versus body fat. Individuals who weigh the same but have drastically different body fat measurements will still have the same BMI. For example, a man who is 6 feet tall and weighs 200 pounds with a body fat of 7% will have a BMI of 27.1, as will a man who is 6 feet tall and 200 pounds with a body fat percentage of 18%. For this reason, BMI may not always be the best measurement of overall health. BMI is calculated by either dividing the weight in kilograms by the square of the height in meters, or by dividing body weight in pounds by the square of height in inches and multiplying by 703:

$$BMI - Weight (kg)/Height (m^2)$$

$$BMI = [Weight (lbs)/Height (in^2)] \times 703$$

The lowest risk for disease lies within a BMI range of 22–24.9 (**Table 8.4**). Research has indicated that the risk for disease increases with a BMI of 25 or greater. Even though research has proven that the risk of premature death and illness increases with a high BMI score, individuals who are underweight are also at risk (Jakicic et al., 2001; Stevens, 1998).

Body mass index (BMI)
A rough assessment metric based on the concept that a person's weight should be proportional to his or her height.

The following is an example of a conversation of how a fitness professional might discuss the client's BMI in relation to specific health or fitness goals: "I calculated your body mass index, which is a rough assessment of your health based on your weight versus your height. We are looking to have a number below 25, which would be an indication of good health. Your BMI currently is 27.5, which indicates you are at a higher risk for certain diseases. As you have already told me your goal is to become healthier, upon completion of the program I have designed for you I am confident you will see a drop in your BMI, and will feel much healthier."

TABLE 8.4 Body Mass Index Classification		
BMI	**Disease Risk**	**Classification**
<18.5	Increased	Underweight
18.6–21.99	Low	Acceptable
22.0–24.99	Very low	Acceptable
25.0–29.99	Increased	Overweight
30–34.99	High	Obese
35.0–39.99	Very high	Obesity II
>40	Extremely high	Obesity III

The Sales Presentation and Overcoming Objections

The fitness professional can provide information on different personal training packages to potential clients in a number of different ways. Each prospect will have different expectations, fears, and possible objections the fitness professional may need to overcome in order to demonstrate his or her value. The objections that fitness professionals will hear from potential clients will vary. The fitness professional needs to be prepared to discuss how the services offered are more important than the objections the client provides. In general, people will find the time and the money for the things that they find most important to them. Knowing this, a fitness professional needs to try and discover what the potential client considers to be the most important aspect of working out. Asking open-ended questions that require more than a one-word response is vital to this discovery process. The following are important **open-ended questions** to ask during the subjective portion of the assessment:

Open-ended question

A question that cannot be answered with a simple "yes" or "no." It gives the person answering the scope to provide more detailed information.

◆ *Why do you want to begin working out?* The fitness professional should ask this question because it may provide the key point as to why a potential client is exploring working out or hiring a fitness professional to begin with. If the fitness professional discovers the potential prospect's key reason for wanting to exercise, this can then be used as the anchor in presenting the personal training options that best fit the potential client's needs.

◆ *What are your fitness and health goals?* This is an important question because the fitness professional needs to know what the potential client's particular goals are. The more clearly the client can define what his or her fitness goals look like, the easier it will be for the fitness professional to use this as a motivational strategy in the future.

When engaging in the information-gathering process, the fitness professional will need to be able to distinguish between needs and wants. *Needs* are logical explanations for potentially using the services of a fitness professional in an attempt to accomplish certain goals; these are usually more direct in nature. People tend to act immediately on needs without any consideration, so very little emotional impact is involved. *Wants* represent an emotional explanation for seeking out services, and often focus more on aesthetics and perceptions. Prospective clients who are undecided as to whether they wish to purchase services will generally be most influenced by emotions. The goal of the fitness professional is to determine the emotional attachment of the client, and then speak to them on that level.

Follow-up questions are important to clarify what the client's true goals and intentions are. The more specific the answer a potential client provides, the better understanding the fitness professional will have as to what the key emotional triggers may be. The fitness professional has to stay focused on that fact if buy-in is to be achieved with a potential client. Following this process will allow the fitness professional to focus in on what is most important to clients, making the sales process specific on an emotional level to them. Knowing this key bit of information will also aid the fitness professional later on when goal setting and motivational strategies become important.

Once a prospect's strongest motivation has been determined, it is vital that the fitness professional demonstrate that the training services he or she offers will help the potential client accomplish the specific fitness goals. If the fitness professional has been able to build rapport and show the prospect the importance of the findings of the objective assessments, it should feel like more of an educational process than a sales process. Few people would say they like to be sold an item, as much as they would like to be educated on the features of a product.

Sales Presentation

People seek the services of fitness professionals for many different reasons. Fitness professionals have a responsibility to explain and demonstrate the value they will bring to their clients if and when services are purchased. If this value is not conveyed to a prospect, then it is unlikely that the prospect will be converted into an actual client. Being able to show value early in the relationship will be a major determinant of whether a prospect becomes a client or not. Fitness professionals should emphasize the following in any of their presentations or marketing pieces with regards to the value they provide to clients:

- Their education and advanced training
- Their ability to hold their clients accountable
- Their ability to motivate their client to achieve results

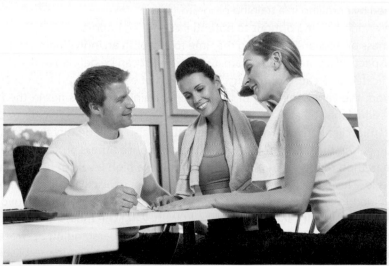

The fitness professional should make sure to touch on the education and advanced training that he or she has earned during the sales presentation to demonstrate that the potential client will be in good hands. In addition, providing this information demonstrates to the prospect the level of commitment that the fitness professional has to making sure that he or she knows the most recent and scientifically valid information available. The prospect may have already tried other programs unsuccessfully, and may have questions regarding why the program failed. The prospect may also have questions regarding the latest fitness trends. When the fitness professional explains his or her education it will be easier for the prospect to ask questions.

Fitness professionals also play a valuable role with regard to the client's motivation, and it is important to not overlook this key point when presenting to prospects. Many people have the desire to get in better physical shape; however, the task may seem overwhelming and they may never find the proper motivation to initiate, and stick with, an exercise program. Fitness professionals should ask prospective clients how they like to be motivated, as well as how they do not like to be motivated. Motivation for one client could be an encouraging word during a workout, whereas for another client it may be more direct and intense. It is important for prospects to understand that if they use the services of a fitness professional, they will be appropriately motivated in the way that works best for them. When fitness professionals not only demonstrate knowledge, but also an ability to dynamically motivate, the prospect will realize multiple levels of value gained by enrolling in a training program.

When presenting training options to potential clients, an important step that is often overlooked by fitness professionals is taking the time to establish an individual's commitment level to different aspects of a potential program. **Commitment** can be defined as the state or quality of being dedicated to a cause or activity. The benefit of establishing the prospect's commitment level from the very beginning of the personal training process lies in the fact that the fitness professional may be able to determine if there are possible roadblocks to overcome to keep the potential client on track with a program. It will also help identify the areas that should be focused on during the sales presentation. For example, if a fitness professional has expertise in training marathon runners, but a potential client has a high level of commitment to losing weight and a low level of commitment to increasing cardiovascular performance, the latter would be avoided in achieving buy-in no matter how much the professional would want to highlight his or her specialty. It is important to identify what the most important goals are for each potential client. This knowledge not only establishes understanding between the potential client and the fitness professional, it can become an anchor point in establishing commitment from a potential client.

Commitment

The state or quality of being dedicated to a cause or activity.

CHECK IT OUT

Jan can only make it to the gym 3 days per week, and she has committed to learning portions of her program so she can workout at home on the days she cannot make it to the fitness center. She is able to commit to a 10-week program. Her program can be designed so she completes her cardiovascular, core, and balance work at home, because these portions of her program will require little to no equipment. If she does these portions of her weekly routine at home she will be able to focus her time in the fitness center on her resistance training program, ensuring that she will complete everything she needs to do to obtain her particular goals. This also allows her to feel a sense of freedom, and that she is not totally dependent on a fitness professional. The key point for Jan is that she would like a fitness professional to spend time early in her personal training program educating her on proper form and technique and on how the home exercises should be completed and progressed.

In this situation, Jan would purchase 10 sessions and use them over a 5- to 10-week period. Her initial appointment after an assessment has been completed would be to teach her the exercises she can perform at home. She would then train with the fitness professional once or twice a week.

Always keeping the clients' goals in mind enables fitness professionals to connect with their clients and demonstrate that they understand what is most important to them. Then, the findings of the assessments can be used to demonstrate how the exercise program, to be designed specifically for them, will create the pathway to achieve their ultimate fitness goals. When it is time to present actual prices to potential clients, the fitness professional should have, at a minimum, completed the following steps:

◆ Identified the client's most important fitness goals.
◆ Completed subjective assessments (i.e., PAR-Q, lifestyle, medical history) and a variety of objective assessments.
◆ Discussed the findings from the assessments.
◆ Established a realistic time frame in which the potential client's fitness goal could be obtained using the different phases of the OPT model.

Determining Price

When a fitness professional is presenting the price for services to potential clients, it is critical that the presentation be based off of the client's goals, the findings of any assessments that have been performed, as well as realistic timelines based on exercise science. When a client has a particular goal, and the appropriate time frame needed to accomplish this goal has been mapped out by the fitness professional, the initial cost of the program has then been established by the potential client rather than the fitness professional. Using integrated program design determines the length and frequency of a potential client's exercise program, thus placing the fitness professional in an educational role while lessening the overall need to sell. From here, the only thing left to determine is how many times per week the client would like to be, or is capable of being, at the gym, and how long he or she can commit to working out for while in attendance. From there, a program can be constructed and presented to the prospect.

Commonly, fitness professionals will try to get potential clients to purchase the biggest personal training package possible, and when faced with objections from the potential clients the only option is to continually offer smaller and smaller packages until the appropriate financial comfort level is reached. However, by using integrated program design as the framework, the fitness professional allows the client to determine the starting point of the training package based on the steps needed to achieve his or her goals. The length of the program and frequency of workouts are based on science, rather than just simple randomness. If the fitness professional faces an objection from the initial price of the program, it can be then shifted to finding options for the client to perform portions of the workout on his or her own, while being guided in less frequent sessions by the fitness professional. The amount of sessions would decrease from what was originally quoted, but the framework of the initial program never changes.

Overcoming Objections to Gain Commitment

Fitness professionals will frequently be faced with objections from potential clients in regard to why they may not be able to utilize personal training services. The fitness professional should be prepared to listen to the client's potential objections, and then politely find ways to present alternatives in order to overcome the objections. Some of the most common objections fitness professionals face are potential clients stating that they cannot afford personal training or that they do not have the time to commit to an exercise program. Other common causes for objection are needing approval from a spouse or other social pressures that may lead to a lack of commitment to a new exercise program, but in the end it will always come down to time and money. Fitness professionals need to be prepared to face these objections, and have a focus on how to turn them into actual sales.

Individuals will find both the time and the money for things that they deem most important to them. To overcome a financial objection, for example, a fitness professional could incorporate strategies to evaluate a client's spending habits on unhealthy items such as coffee beverages, soda, and alcohol, as well as eating meals out frequently. The professional can then relate consumption of these items to how they will, in their own right, create a barrier to achieving fitness goals. If the client stops for a coffee beverage every day before heading to work, the fitness professional can calculate the total calories the individual will consume, as well as how much money is being spent on a weekly or monthly basis, and paint a very strong picture of how the habit is both costly and unhealthy; clearly demonstrating how the money would be better spent on a fitness program. Fitness professionals can show potential clients that in making healthier choices they can find more disposable income than they may have originally thought possible.

Techniques for Overcoming Objections

When faced with an objection, it is important for the fitness professional to listen completely to the objection and allow the client to feel that he or she is being heard. The potential client should not feel that he or she is facing a pressure sales situation. After hearing the objection from the client, four steps can be respectfully initiated in order to increase the chances of showing the potential client the value of the fitness professional's services. The four steps are to validate, isolate, remind, and resolve:

- ◆ *Step 1: Validate.* Validating a person's objection is necessary in order to show that his or her thoughts are understood, and that the fitness professional is not dismissing what is causing the person to initially feel unable to commit to personal training at this point.
- ◆ *Step 2: Isolate.* The fitness professional needs to focus solely on the objection that the individual has presented. Once the objection has been isolated, the fitness professional can focus on finding a solution that the individual may not have thought of.

◆ *Step 3: Remind.* Reminding the person of the main reason that he or she initiated the search to find a fitness and/or personal training program can help to refocus the potential client on the overall importance of reaching his or her goals.

◆ *Step 4: Resolve.* Showing the individual that there is a plan to meet his or her particular goals will make the prospective client believe that the goal can be accomplished, and that the time, effort, and money he or she will need to commit will ultimately be worth it.

Note that these steps should be followed in sequence when attempting to overcome objections from potential clients.

The following are examples of overcoming different objections using the validate, isolate, remind, and resolve method for overcoming objections.

Scenario 1: No Longer Able to Afford Training

Fitness professionals frequently have to deal with objections based on financial concerns. In this scenario, a current client, Mrs. Smith, approaches the fitness professional and states, "I can no longer afford to train with you." The fitness professional can either allow her to simply state that she can no longer afford personal training services, or he or she could try and overcome the client's objection in the following manner:

◆ *Step 1: Validate her feelings about the objection.* "Mrs. Smith, I completely understand that you believe that the 10-week program, as I have initially designed it, would be too much of a financial commitment for you at this point."

◆ *Step 2: Isolate the main concern creating the objection.* "Mrs. Smith, just so I can be clear, is it the length of the 10-week program or simply the cost that is the main issue for you?"

◆ *Step 3: Remind her of why she initially decided it was important to achieve her fitness goal.* "Mrs. Smith, you informed me that you need to lose 20 pounds over the next 10 weeks due to a health concern, and that you are extremely committed to that end. This 10-week program is truly a safe and effective way to get you to your ultimate goal."

◆ *Step 4: Resolve her concerns by providing an alternative solution that she may feel comfortable with.* "Mrs. Smith, I understand if you train with me three times per week over 10 weeks, the cost of 30 sessions will be more than you feel comfortable spending at this time. An alternative would be to train with me one time per week, so I can help you learn your exercise program, monitor your progress, and ensure that you progress to your goal over the next 10 weeks. Does this sound like a good alternative?"

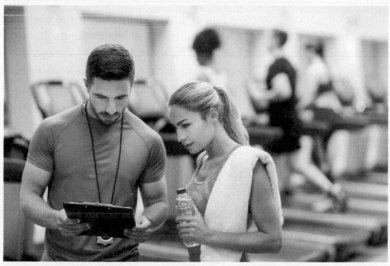

© wavebreakmedia/Shutterstock

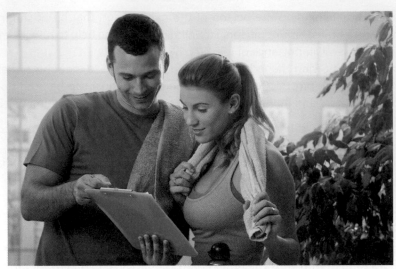

© StockLite/Shutterstock

Scenario 2: Spousal Pressure

Another objection a fitness professional may face is that a client's spouse may not feel the use of a fitness professional is warranted. Here, during a complimentary consultation appointment, a potential client, Kristy, says, "After speaking with my spouse, I feel I do not need to pursue a personal training program at this time." The fitness professional could attempt to overcome this objection in the following manner:

- *Step 1: Validate the individual's feelings about the objection.* "Kristy, I understand your husband feels that you may not need to use personal training at this time. I am sorry to hear that."
- *Step 2: Isolate the main concern creating the objection.* "If you don't mind me asking, is it the cost of personal training, or is it that he feels you should be able to do the program on your own?"
- *Step 3: Remind her of why she initially decided it was important to achieve her fitness goal.* "Kristy, when we initially began your program you indicated that it was extremely important for you to increase your strength and endurance for a 5K race you are running in a few months."
- *Step 4: Resolve her concerns by providing an alternative solution that she may feel comfortable with.* "Working out on your own is beneficial to achieve your goals, but you will make even greater strides with the direction of a fitness professional. We could create a schedule that will allow us to meet less frequently, where I will provide you with the direction to complete your workouts on your own. This way you are more independent and your program will cost less, but we can still keep you on track."

Scenario 3: Lack of Time

Not having time is another common objection professionals will face quite often. In this situation, a client, Paul, approaches his fitness professional and says, "Unfortunately, I seem to no longer have time to work out." The fitness professional could attempt to overcome this objection in the following manner:

- *Step 1: Validate his feelings about the objection.* "Paul, if I am hearing you correctly, you feel you no longer have time to work out, is this correct?"

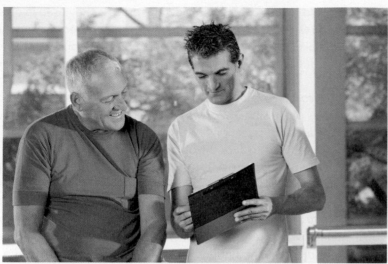

© Robert Kneschke/Shutterstock

- *Step 2: Isolate the main concern creating the objection.* "Paul, is it that you don't want to work out, or is it that just you feel your current program is taking too much of your time?"
- *Step 3: Remind him of why he initially decided it was important to achieve his fitness goal.* "At the beginning of your exercise program you indicated the most important goal you had was to be able to play with your two children again, and how you currently feel that you cannot keep up with them."
- *Step 4: Resolve his concerns by providing an alternative solution that he may feel comfortable with.* "Would you feel better if I was able to recreate your fitness program around your new schedule? That way you can find some extra time as well as maintain your fitness program."

These steps can allow a fitness professional to face and overcome objections potential clients may have when deciding if personal training is right for them and their particular situation. In the face of objection, the most important factor is the ability to redirect the potential client's train of thought back to his or her wants, thus increasing the emotional desire to buy in. Following a blueprint in order to overcome objections will keep the fitness professional on the right track, rather than just simply trying figure out if the individual will purchase any number of sessions. This technique also takes a tremendous amount of pressure off both the potential client and the fitness professional. Early in their careers many fitness professionals feel uncomfortable selling their services. What fitness professionals can easily control, however, is to not to set up additional obstacles themselves that they will then need to overcome. Oftentimes, fitness professionals will interact with potential clients, taking the steps to offer free advice, perform assessments, and even help design exercise programs, but they then stop short of completing the necessary steps to gain clients by failing to present paid personal training options to them. The following are potential internal barriers to successfully presenting a sale:

- *Fear of rejection.* If the fear of rejection is holding a fitness professional back from presenting personal training options to potential clients, a failure to convert a sale should be viewed not as a personal rejection, but simply a failed presentation that can be reviewed and learned from. When fitness professionals remove viewing any rejection as a personal rejection, they should be better able to review the process they used in order to build a better skill set for presenting and closing a sale. Viewing a failed presentation as a personal failure may make it harder to present the next time an opportunity presents itself, thus creating a self-fulfilling prophecy of the inability to present and convert leads into clients.

◆ *Not working to overcome a prospect's objection.* When a prospect has an objection, far too often the fitness professional accepts the objection and fails to try and overcome it. It could be from a fear of rejection, but it could also simply be that the fitness professional was not prepared to face an objection and was not ready to respond accordingly with alternative options. A fitness professional should always be prepared to validate, isolate, remind, and resolve an objection for any common scenario that may present itself.

◆ *Not knowing when to present personal training options to a prospect.* Every time a fitness professional interacts with a prospect he or she should focus on finding an opportunity to present the personal training options. Whenever a prospect discusses a goal, needs help with an exercise, or asks a fitness-related question, an opportunity is created for the fitness professional to present services to that individual. Fitness professionals should focus on the fact that they lose every sale that they do not ask for.

◆ *Not demonstrating enough value to the prospect.* It is important that fitness professionals find the most important reason as to why the potential client has explored initiating an exercise program. Once the *why* has been discovered, the formal consultation should be used as an anchor to solidify the value of a personal training program in the potential client's mind. From there, fitness professionals need to demonstrate how the exercise programs they will design will take potential clients to exactly where they desire to be. When these steps are not completed in detail, or skipped completely, the value the fitness professional has becomes diminished, decreasing the chance of converting a prospect into a client.

The more comfortable fitness professionals are in following these steps the more they will see their sales increase. Very few fitness professionals will be comfortable with this process at the beginning of their career, so it is important for them to practice these techniques, just as they would any other particular skill they were trying to become more efficient in. A great way to improve skills in overcoming objections is to role-play with a friend or family member. This way the validate, isolate, remind, and resolve method will become ingrained and automatic.

Conclusion

The fitness professional has the information needed to assess the needs of the clients he or she acquires. However, it is equally important to be able to locate new clients and retain them in order to be truly successful in any professional fitness setting. As a lack of sales knowledge is one of the main barriers to many fitness facilities' inability to hire and retain quality fitness professionals, those who have sales skills as well as knowledge about, and passion for, fitness will have the edge needed for a successful career in the fitness industry. Building trust and rapport through professionalism, dedicated service, and objective consultations, combined with a thorough understanding of exercise science and integrated program design, will allow the fitness professional to demonstrate the highest levels of value to clients.

Case in Review

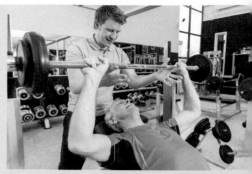

© Kzenon/Shutterstock

It has been roughly 1 week since you shadowed another personal trainer in the gym you have been recently hired by. Eager to begin working with clients, you felt that it is necessary to create a plan that will help maximize your ability to convert potential gym members into future clients. Within your plan, you have begun to list specific insights gained from your shadowing experience.

- *Prospecting activities*: Most new prospects will come from new memberships, free assessments, working the floor, and promoting yourself through social media and other follow-up interactions (e.g., calling and emailing leads).

- *Client acquisition and consultation*: Rapport, credibility, and trust often take time and patience. Finding ways to relate with clients through similar interests can help. You have listed the following starting points to help build relationships with your clients:

  - Find out where they are from.

  - Ask where they live now.

  - Ask about their family.

  - Ask what they do for a living.

  - Ask what their hobbies are.

  - Ask where they see themselves in the future.

- *Use the PAR-Q to assess the clients' readiness to begin various levels of physical activity.* Using a PAR-Q can help surface any medical conditions that may exist, as well as provide insight into the client's general lifestyle and underlying reasons for seeking a fitness professional.

- *During the on-boarding process you will conduct, at a minimum, body fat, circumference, and pulse assessments.* These formal assessments will demonstrate expertise and credibility, bring to light more information on the client's current health and fitness status, as well as provide an excellent base for future assessment comparison and progress tracking.

- *Making the sale:* Present the packages and offerings of the facility while discussing how your NASM CPT education differentiates you from other trainers. Clients will often object to buy-in due to time and/or money. Because of this, it will be important to further understand ways your prospect can free up time and financial restraints, and how to best communicate those messages when presenting your training packages.

References

American College of Sports Medicine. (2010). *ACSM's guidelines for exercise testing and prescription* (8th ed.). Philadelphia, PA: Lippincott Williams & Wilkins.

American Heart Association. (2014). Understanding and measuring high blood pressure. Available at: www.heart.org/HEARTORG/Conditions/HighBloodPressure/AboutHighBloodPressure/Understanding-Blood-Pressure-Readings_UCM_301764_Article.jsp#.VvFxP-bDpEE

Carnegie, D. (1981). *How to win friends and influence people* [Paraphrased from Part 2: Six ways to make people like you.] . New York, NY: Simon and Schuster.

Durnin, J. V. G. A., & Womersley, J. (1974). Body fat assessed from total body density and its estimation from skinfold thickness measurements on 481 men and women aged 16–72 years. *British Journal of Nutrition, 32*, 77–97.

Going, S., & Davis, R. (2001). Body composition. In J. L. Roitman (Ed.), *ACSM's resource manual for guidelines for exercise testing and prescription* (4th ed., p. 396). Philadelphia, PA: Lippincott Williams & Wilkins.

Heyward, V. H., & Wagner, D.R. (2004). Applied body composition assessment (2nd ed.). Champaign, IL: Human Kinetics.

Jakicic, J. M., Clark, K., Coleman, E., Donnelly, J. E., Foreyt, J., Melanson, E., . . . Volpe, S. L. (2001). American College of Sports Medicine Position Stand: Appropriate intervention strategies for weight loss and prevention for weight regain in adults. *Medicine and Science in Sports and Exercise, 113 (6)*, 898–918.

Poirier, P., Giles, T. D., Bray, G. A., Hong, Y., Stern, J. S., Xavier Pi-Sunyer, F., Eckel, R. H. (2006). Obesity and cardiovascular disease: pathophysiology, evaluation, and effect of weight loss: An update of the 1997 American Heart Association Scientific Statement on Obesity and Heart Disease from the Obesity Committee of the Council on Nutrition, Physical Activity, and Metabolism. *Circulation, 113*(6):898-918.

Stevens, J. (1998). The effect of age on the association between body mass index and mortality. *New England Journal of Medicine, 338*, 1–7.

World Health Organization. (2008). *Waist circumference and waist-hip ratio*. (Report of a WHO Expert Consultation). Geneva, Switzerland: World Health Organization.

CHAPTER 9

EXECUTING FORMAL FITNESS ASSESSMENTS

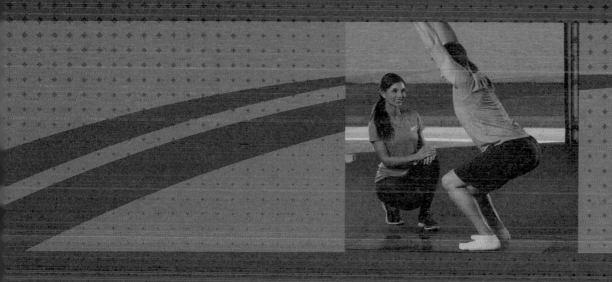

OBJECTIVES

After studying this chapter, you will be able to:

1. **Explain** the scientific components associated with postural, movement, and performance assessments.

2. **Conduct** and interpret basic postural assessments.

3. **Conduct** and interpret basic movement assessments.

4. **Translate** assessment results into a robust goal plan for the client.

5. **Apply** modifications to assessments based on specific populations.

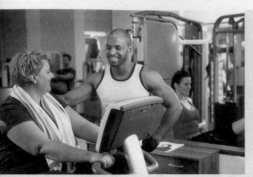

© StockLite/Shutterstock

Case Scenario

You have just signed up your first client, Jennifer, and have reviewed and conducted many of the foundational assessments that fall within the scope of practice of a certified personal trainer. You measured her blood pressure and heart rate, and also gathered information on her medical history. Additionally, she has filled out a lifestyle questionnaire and the PAR-Q for your review. The assessments did not produce any results that would require you to refer Jennifer to a physician, registered dietician, chiropractor, or other healthcare professional.

She is eager to begin her training regimen and has asked you what she should do to begin. To capitalize on her motivation, you schedule a meeting with her to discuss and conduct the necessary movement assessments that are required before you can design a program that fits her specific needs. As you begin your assessments of the human movement system, she looks confused as to why you need even more information before starting a training program.

- How would you educate Jennifer about the need for human movement system assessments?

- How would you explain that these assessments are critical to the development of a training program, regardless of her goals?

- What specific assessments of the human movement system would you conduct on Jennifer, and what would you be looking for with each one?

Introduction to the Scientific Components of Assessments

Designing an individualized, systematic fitness assessment can only be accomplished by having an understanding of the client's goals, needs, and abilities. This entails knowing what a client wants and needs to gain from a training program and how capable (structurally and functionally) he or she is of performing the required tasks within a training program. The information necessary to create the right program for a specific individual (or group of individuals) comes through a proper fitness assessment. This chapter will focus on the components of fitness assessments. It will highlight the importance of postural assessments (both static and dynamic), performance assessments, and how the information obtained from them will enable fitness professionals to design individualized programs for their clients.

The Importance of Posture

Proper postural alignment makes room for optimal neuromuscular efficiency, which helps produce effective and safe movement. Good posture ensures that the muscles of the body are aligned at the proper length–tension relationships necessary for efficient functioning of force-couples. This allows for ideal arthrokinimatics, and effective absorption and distribution of forces throughout the kinetic chain; alleviating excess stress on joints. In other words, proper posture keeps muscles at their ideal lengths so that joint motion happens the way it should. Proper posture is essential in maximizing strength and power gains (Newmann, 2010; Powers, Ward, Fredericson, Guillet, & Shellock, 2003; Sahrmann, 1992, 2002).

The ideal alignment of the musculoskeletal system is known as structural efficiency, and it allows posture to be balanced in relation to the body's center of gravity, so an individual can maintain his or her balance over a constantly changing base of support during movement. For example, consider a block-stacking game. When playing a block-stacking game, the structure is most efficient when the blocks are stacked on top of one another in proper alignment. As blocks are removed, the structure progressively becomes less and less efficient, making it more difficult to control. Eventually, the structure collapses. The same thing can happen to the body. The more out of alignment it becomes over time, the greater the possibility of it breaking down (i.e., injury). **Functional efficiency** is the ability of the neuromuscular system to perform functional tasks with the least amount of energy, decreasing stress on the body's structure. Functional efficiency is a result of *structural efficiency*, or optimal posture.

Functional efficiency
The ability of the neuromuscular system to perform functional tasks with the least amount of energy, decreasing stress on the body's structure.

Muscle Imbalances and Injury

When assessing posture, fitness professionals are evaluating clients for muscle imbalances. This lack of control is also known as **altered neuromuscular efficiency**. In general, when muscle imbalances are present, a certain muscle (or muscles) associated with a joint (or joints) may be in a shortened state while other muscles are in a lengthened state, affecting the position of the joint. It has been shown that muscles in a shortened state also tend to be more "hyperactive," whereas those in a lengthened state tend to be more inhibited (Janda, 1983). This is a result of a phenomenon known as *altered reciprocal inhibition*, which can lead to *synergistic dominance*. Joint movement requires a combination of muscle synergies and *force-couples*. When muscle imbalances are present, the activation sequence is altered, leading to an altered force-couple relationship. This altered force-couple relationship will affect the arthrokinematics of the joints, creating **altered arthrokinematics**. Over time, this can lead to injury via the cumulative injury cycle.

Altered neuromuscular efficiency
Occurs when the kinetic chain is not performing optimally to control the body in all three planes of motion.

Cumulative Injury Cycle

The cumulative injury cycle is the cycle our body goes through to heal an injury. This process begins when tissue is traumatized (e.g., through exercise, movement compensation, etc.) and inflammation occurs at the site of the trauma. This elicits increased muscle tension (or spasm) as a protective mechanism. Fibrotic adhesions (or knots) develop in the soft tissue to further decrease trauma to the region. Over time, these adhesions can decrease the extensibility of the muscle fibers, resulting in further altered neuromuscular control and muscle imbalances (Sahrmann, 2002). If this process is not addressed (through the use of corrective exercise techniques), further imbalances and compensation can occur, leading to injury.

Altered arthrokinematics
Altered joint motion caused by altered length–tension relationships and force-couple relationships that affects the joints and causes poor movement efficiency.

Relative flexibility

The human movement system's way of finding the path of least resistance during movement.

Relative Flexibility

Muscle imbalances can also lead to the development of **relative flexibility**, which is the human movement system's way of finding the path of least resistance during movement (Sahrmann, 2002). A common example of relative flexibility is when an individual with poor ankle dorsiflexion tries to squat. As the individual lowers into the squat, he will have a smaller range of motion due to the relative dorsiflexion. Once this range of motion is reached, additional range of motion through altered arthrokinematics will occur. The altered arthrokinematics are displayed through the feet turning out or raising of the heels. The knees may also move in or out to allow for an even greater range of motion. These movement compensations can lead to further imbalances, which can also initiate (or be a result of) the cumulative injury cycle.

Pre-assessment Information

Before performing a postural assessment, the fitness professional should learn more about the client during a pre-exercise interview. This interview can be helpful in identifying potential structural issues that will need to be addressed. The fitness professional should obtain more information from the client with regard to the following:

- *Occupation*: Collecting information about a client's occupation helps the fitness professional determine common movement patterns that occur during the course of an average day. Collecting this kind of information helps the fitness professional to recognize important clues about the client's musculoskeletal structure and function, potential health and physical limitations, and restrictions that could affect the safety and efficacy of an exercise program.
- *Extended periods of sitting*: If clients are sitting for long periods throughout the day, their hips are also flexed for prolonged periods of time, which, in turn, can lead to tight hip flexors (rectus femoris, tensor fasciae latae, iliopsoas) and postural imbalances within the human movement system. Moreover, if clients are sitting for prolonged periods of time, especially in front of a computer, there is a tendency for the shoulders and head to fatigue under the constant effect of gravity, which again can lead to postural imbalances, including rounding of the shoulders and a forward head.
- *Repetitive movements*: Repetitive movement is a persistent motion that can cause musculoskeletal injury and dysfunction. Repetitive movements can create pattern overload on muscles and joints, which may lead to tissue trauma and eventually kinetic chain dysfunction, especially in jobs that require a lot of overhead work or awkward positions such as construction or painting (Van der Windt et al., 2000). Working with the arms overhead for long periods may lead to shoulder and neck soreness that may be the result of tightness in the latissimus dorsi and weakness in the rotator cuff. This imbalance does not allow for proper shoulder motion or stabilization during activity.
- *Dress shoes*: Wearing shoes with high heels puts the foot/ankle complex in a plantar-flexed position for extended periods. This can lead to tightness in the gastrocnemius, soleus, and Achilles tendon, causing postural imbalance such as decreased dorsiflexion and overpronation at the foot and ankle complex; resulting in flattening of the arch of the foot (Kim, Lim, & Yoon, 2013). They can also contribute to knee and low back pain (Silva, De Sigueira, & da Silva, 2013).
- *Past injuries*: All past and recent injuries should be recorded and discussed in sufficient enough detail to be able to make decisions about whether exercise is recommended or a

medical referral is necessary. Previous history of musculoskeletal injury is a strong predictor of future musculoskeletal injury during physical activity (Kucera, Marshall, Kirkendall, Marchak, & Garrett, 2004). The effect of injuries on the functioning of the human movement system is well documented, especially with regard to the following injuries:

- *Ankle sprains*: Ankle sprains have been shown to decrease neural control to the gluteus medius and gluteus maximus muscles. This, in turn, can lead to poor control of the lower extremities during many functional activities, which can eventually lead to injury (Bullock-Saxton, 1994; Terada, Pietrosimone, & Gribble, 2014).

- *Knee injuries involving ligaments*: Knee injury can cause a decrease in neural control to the muscles that stabilize the patella (kneecap), leading to further injury. Knee injuries that are not the result of contact (noncontact injuries) are often the result of ankle or hip dysfunction, such as the result of an ankle sprain. The knee is caught between the ankle and the hip. If the ankle or hip joint begins to function improperly, this results in altered movement and force distribution of the knee. Over time, this can lead to further injury (Fredericson et al., 2000; Ireland, Willson, Ballantyne, & Davis, 2003; Nyland, Smith, Beickman, Armsey, & Caborn, 2002; Powers, 2003).

- *Low back injuries*: Low back injuries can cause decreased neural control to the stabilizing muscles of the core, resulting in poor stabilization of the spine. This can lead to dysfunction in the upper and lower extremities (Bullock-Saxton, Janda, & Bullock, 1993; Hodges & Richardson, 1996, 1997; Hodges, Richardson, & Jull, 1996).

- *Shoulder injuries*: Shoulder injuries cause altered neural control of the rotator cuff muscles, which can lead to instability of the shoulder joint during functional activities (Kedgley, MacKenzie, Ferriera, Johnson, & Faber, 2007; Yanagawa et al., 2008; Yasojima et al., 2008).

- *Other injuries*: Injuries that result from human movement system imbalances include repetitive hamstring strains, groin strains, patellar tendonitis (jumper's knee), plantar fasciitis (pain in the heel and bottom of the foot), posterior tibialis tendonitis (shin splints), biceps tendonitis (shoulder pain), and headaches.

◆ *Past surgeries*: Surgical procedures create trauma for the body and may have similar effects on the functioning of the human movement system and safety and efficacy of exercise as those of injuries. Surgery will cause pain and inflammation that can alter neural control to the affected muscles and joints if not rehabilitated properly (Graven Nielsen & Mense, 2001; Mense & Simons, 2001).

◆ *Recreation*: Recreation, in the context of assessment, refers to a client's physical activities outside of the work environment, also referred to as *leisure time*. By finding out what recreational activities a client performs, the fitness professional can better design an exercise program to fit the needs of the client. For example, many clients like to golf, ski, play tennis, or perform a variety of other sporting activities in their spare time, and proper exercise training must be incorporated to ensure that clients are trained in a manner that optimizes the efficiency of the human movement system without predisposing it to injury. Knowing this information will also provide direction on the appropriate performance assessments that would be applicable if the client's goal is to also enhance performance.

Asking questions that address these areas can help the fitness professional begin to paint the picture of the client's potential needs before performing any postural assessments. In addition, the responses to these questions can make it easier for the fitness professional to focus on specific areas when performing postural and performance assessments.

TRAINER TIPS ⫞—⫞

The preassessment should be considered an important information-gathering opportunity. The trainer should take this opportunity to ask as many questions as possible to gather all of the information needed for successful assessments and program design.

Postural Assessments

Posture is often viewed as being static. However, posture is constantly changing to meet the demands placed on the kinetic chain. Thus, both static and dynamic posture assessments should be performed. The observation process should search for any movement distortions that may lead to injury. With the limited time that most fitness professionals have for observation, incorporating a systematic assessment sequence is essential.

Static Postural Assessment

Recall that static posture could be considered the starting point from which an individual moves. It provides the foundation or the platform from which the extremities function. An individual's static posture provides a snapshot of the body's alignment, and may in fact provide warning of potential problems that could arise in an exercise program. A client's static posture can inform the fitness professional about the client's lifestyle and provide red flags about a client's potential movement limitations. Is the client slumped over with her shoulders rounded? Does his head jut forward or low back arch excessively? All of these poor postural positions indicate that the body is not in proper alignment. If the body is not in proper alignment, it becomes vulnerable to injury. A person wouldn't sit on a chair that has a wobbly leg because she wouldn't want the chair to break. The same rule applies to the human body. If the body is not aligned properly, it cannot appropriately absorb and distribute forces—and like the chair, it can break down.

Poor posture, as noted in the examples above, highlights muscles that may be shortened and muscles that are lengthened. In other words, poor posture can highlight an individual's muscle imbalances. Muscle imbalances affect the way a client moves and will affect the way a client responds to exercise or present a predisposition for injury. It is important to note that a static postural assessment may not be able to specifically identify whether a problem is structural in nature or whether it is derived from muscle imbalances. However, a static postural assessment provides excellent indicators of problem areas that must be further evaluated to clarify the postural imbalances that may be present. This provides a basis for developing an exercise strategy to target causative factors of faulty movement and neuromuscular inefficiency.

Common Postural Distortion Patterns

Postural distortion patterns are common postural malalignments and muscle imbalances that individuals develop based on a variety of factors (e.g., lifestyle, occupation, etc.). These patterns were studied and described by Vladmir Janda in the early 1970s. A prominent researcher, Janda (2002) identified three basic distortion patterns: the **pronation distortion syndrome**, the **lower crossed syndrome**, and the **upper crossed syndrome**. Although there may be many more compensatory patterns, Janda found these three to be the most inherent to typical movements performed by individuals. Janda suggested that there was a cascading effect of alterations or deviations in static posture that would more likely than not present in a particular pattern. He studied these patterns at length, found that these imbalances and movement alterations predictably presented themselves, and therefore should be identified in a static postural assessment:

- ◆ *Pronation distortion syndrome*: A postural distortion syndrome characterized by foot pronation (flat feet) and adducted and internally rotated knees (knock knees).

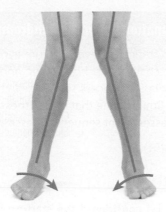

FIGURE 9.1 Pronation distortion syndrome.

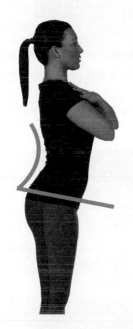

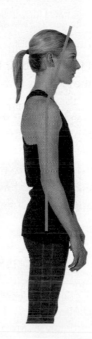

FIGURE 9.2 Lower crossed syndrome.

FIGURE 9.3 Upper crossed syndrome.

- ◆ *Lower crossed syndrome*: A postural distortion syndrome characterized by an anterior tilt to the pelvis (arched lower back).
- ◆ *Upper crossed syndrome*: A postural distortion syndrome characterized by a forward head and rounded shoulders.

The muscle imbalances associated with these distortion syndromes are shown in **Figures 9.1–9.3** and **Tables 9.1–9.3**.

Key Points to Remember When Observing Static Posture

Many elements are involved in conducting a detailed static postural assessment. The postural observations discussed here have been simplified but still provide the key information needed

TABLE 9.1 Pronation Distortion Syndrome

Short Muscles	Lengthened Muscles
Gastrocnemius	Anterior tibialis
Soleus	Posterior tibialis
Peroneals	Gluteus maximus
Adductors	Gluteus medius
Tension fasciae latae (TFL)	
Hip flexor complex	
Biceps femoris (short head)	

TABLE 9.2 Lower Crossed Syndrome

Short Muscles	Lengthened Muscles
Gastrocnemius	Anterior tibialis
Soleus	Posterior tibialis
Hip flexor complex	Gluteus maximus
Adductors	Gluteus medius
Latissimus dorsi	Transversus abdominis
Erector spinae	

TABLE 9.3 Upper Crossed Syndrome

Short Muscles	Lengthened Muscles
Upper trapezius	Deep cervical flexors
Levator scapulae	Serratus anterior
Sternocleidomastoid	Rhomboids
Scalenes	Mid-trapezius
Latissimus dorsi	Lower trapezius
Teres major	Teres minor
Subscapularis	Infraspinatus
Pectoralis major/minor	

to identify any of the three common postural distortion patterns. This will also make the assessment process more time efficient by only focusing on the areas specific to the common distortion patterns. As the fitness professional begins to understand the basic distortion patterns and the associated imbalances, he or she can begin to make some quick assumptions. For example, if the client's knees are internally rotated, the fitness professional can quickly determine that the client will most likely have flat feet as well.

The more the fitness professional performs these assessments, the better he or she will be at spotting postural distortion patterns, which will help to make the assessment process more time efficient. Fitness professionals should contact their clients prior to their first session to inform them that they will be performing postural assessments and that they should wear appropriate clothing (if they feel comfortable) to make it easier to identify postural imbalances.

Fitness professionals should not overanalyze, or make clients feel insecure by sharing too much information about the observations. No one wants to feel imperfect. Nor should clients

TRAINER TIPS ⊸⫞⊸⫞⊸

Note that clients may not feel comfortable being visually evaluated, so the more efficient the assessment can be, the better.

feel as if they are lab experiments, or that their structural "faults" are being exposed. The fitness professional should remember to keep the client's feelings in mind, and use this opportunity to show how an individualized program can be developed.

Performing a Static Postural Assessment

In general, when performing a static postural assessment, the fitness professional is checking for proper alignment of the kinetic chain checkpoints, **symmetry**, and specific postural distortion patterns. It is important that the client be viewed standing from multiple angles (anterior, posterior, lateral). The fitness professional should not "microanalyze" the client, but instead look for gross deviations in overall posture, meaning that any postural deviations noted during the assessment should be obvious. The fitness professional should look for natural deviations, and not force clients into positions they feel uncomfortable with when trying to identify any deviations. Clients should remove their shoes and socks for this assessment, as this will make it easier to assess the foot and ankle complex.

Postural assessments require observation of the kinetic chain. The use of kinetic chain checkpoints allows the fitness professional to systematically view the body in an organized fashion. The kinetic chain checkpoints are as follows:

- ◆ Foot and ankle
- ◆ Knee
- ◆ Lumbo-pelvic-hip complex (LPHC)
- ◆ Shoulders
- ◆ Head and cervical spine

As mentioned previously, a static postural assessment should assess an individual's posture from the front (anterior), side (laterally), and from behind (posterior). The following outlines what to look for from each view at each point of the kinetic chain:

Anterior view (**Figure 9.4**):

- ◆ *Foot/ankles*: Straight and parallel, not flattened or externally rotated (pronation distortion syndrome).
- ◆ *Knees*: In line with the foot (second and third toes), not adducted and internally rotated (pronation distortion pattern). One can also look to see if the knee falls on the inside of the big toe; if it does, then the knee is adducted and internally rotated.
- ◆ *LPHC*: Have the client stand against a wall with paper taped onto the wall behind the pelvis. Marks can then be placed on the paper at the level of either hip bone. It may become easier to see if the marks are aligned with each other and parallel to the ground then simply observing hip posture.
- ◆ *Shoulders*: Level, not elevated or rounded. A similar process to that used to assess the hips can be used to verify that the shoulders are level as well.
- ◆ *Head*: Neutral position, not tilted or rotated.

Lateral view (**Figure 9.5**):

- ◆ *Foot/ankle*: Neutral position, leg vertical at right angle to sole of foot.
- ◆ *Knees*: Neutral position, not flexed or hyperextended.
- ◆ *LPHC*: Pelvis neutral position, not anteriorly (lumbar extension) or posteriorly (lumbar flexion) rotated (lower crossed syndrome). The fitness professional can also teach the client how to perform an anterior and posterior tilt. One can use the analogy of the pelvis being a bucket of water and tipping the bucket forward to pour water out from the front and backward to pour water from the back. If the client is unable to easily rotate the pelvis forward, but can easily rotate it backwards, then he or she is probably already in an anterior tilt. If the client

TRAINER TIPS ◁▯─▯▷

If the fitness professional does not see the compensation, he or she should not force seeing it.

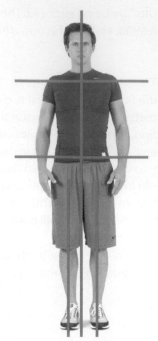
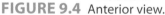

FIGURE 9.4 Anterior view.

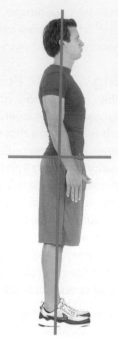

FIGURE 9.5 Lateral view.

Kyphotic curve

Outward curvature of the thoracic spine by which the spine is bent forward.

has a hard time rotating backwards, but can easily rotate forward, then the client is probably already in a posterior tilt.

◆ *Shoulders*: Normal **kyphotic curve**, not excessively rounded (upper crossed syndrome). The fitness professional can also have clients slowly raise their arms over their head to see if they can do so without arching their back. If they have to arch their back to do so, then they have limited range of motion at the shoulder and need to find more range through their lower back.

◆ *Head*: Neutral position, not migrating forward (upper crossed syndrome). The fitness professional should keep in mind that if the shoulders are rounded and the head is forward, then the ears and shoulders may line up. If the shoulders are rounded and the ears are aligned with the shoulders, then the head is more than likely forward as well.

Posterior view (**Figure 9.6**):

◆ *Foot/ankle*: Heels are straight and parallel, not overly pronated (pronation distortion syndrome). The fitness professional can also ask the client to try and flatten his or her arch (pronate), and then "build" the arch (supinate). If there is not much movement when flattening the feet but the client can easily "build" the arch, then the client probably has flattened feet.

◆ *Knees*: Neutral position, not adducted or internally rotated (pronation distortion syndrome). The fitness professional should see what happens at the knees (internal or external rotation) when the client adjusts his or her arches. If the knees do not move much when the client tries to flatten the feet, but they move a lot (externally rotate) when "building" the arch, then the knees are probably already internally rotated. This can also be done from the anterior view.

◆ *LPHC*: The fitness professional can have the client stand against a wall with paper taped onto the wall behind the pelvis. Marks can then be placed on the paper at the level of either hip bone. It may become easier to see if the marks are aligned with each other and parallel to the ground then simply observing hip posture.

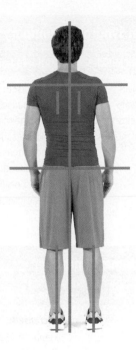

FIGURE 9.6 Posterior view.

◆ *Shoulders/scapulae*: Level, not elevated or protracted. Medial borders are essentially parallel and approximately 3–4 inches apart (upper crossed syndrome). Finger widths can be used to measure this distance.
◆ *Head*: Neutral position, neither tilted nor rotated.

Once this assessment has been performed, the fitness professional can begin to determine key areas that may need to be addressed through flexibility and strengthening techniques. **Tables 9.4–9.6** provide a summary of the three postural distortion patterns, along with the associated muscle imbalances for each distortion syndrome. In general, muscles that are identified as short (tight) should be stretched through the use of self-myofascial release (foam-rolling) and static stretching. Muscles that are identified as lengthened (weak) should be addressed through the use of strengthening techniques (core and balance exercises). Various movement-preparation strategies can be implemented during the warm-up portion of the workout to prepare the client for the higher-intensity workout that is to come.

CHECK IT OUT

How to Use Tables 9.4 Through 9.6

Based on the information presented in Tables 9.4 through 9.6, clients who display pronation distortion syndrome would foam-roll and statically stretch their calves (gastrocnemius and soleus), adductors, TFL, hip flexors, and bicep femoris, which are the tight/shortened muscles. They would then strengthen their anterior tibialis (e.g. resisted dorsiflexion), posterior tibialis (e.g. single-leg calf raise), gluteus maximus (e.g. floor bridges), and gluteus medius (e.g. lateral tube walking), which are the lengthened/weaker muscles.

TABLE 9.4 Pronation Distortion Syndrome Summary

Short Muscles	Lengthened Muscles	Altered Joint Mechanics	Possible Injuries
Gastrocnemius Soleus Peroneals Adductors Tension fasciae latae (TFL) Hip flexor complex Biceps femoris (short head)	Anterior tibialis Posterior tibialis Gluteus medius/maximus Hip external rotators	**Increased:** Knee adduction Knee internal rotation Foot pronation Foot external rotation **Decreased:** Ankle dorsiflexion Ankle inversion	Plantar fasciitis Posterior tibialis tendonitis (shin splints) Patellar tendonitis Low back pain

TABLE 9.5 Lower Crossed Syndrome Summary

Short Muscles	Lengthened Muscles	Altered Joint Mechanics	Possible Injuries
Gastrocnemius Soleus Hip flexor complex Adductors Latissimus dorsi Erector spinae	Anterior tibialis Posterior tibialis Gluteus maximus Gluteus medius Transversus abdominis Internal oblique	**Increased:** Lumbar extension **Decreased:** Hip extension	Hamstring complex strain Anterior knee pain Low back pain

TABLE 9.6 Upper Crossed Syndrome Summary

Short Muscles	Lengthened Muscles	Altered Joint Mechanics	Possible Injuries
Upper trapezius Levator scapulae Sternocleidomastoid Scalenes Latissimus dorsi Teres major Subscapularis Pectoralis major/minor	Deep cervical flexors Serratus anterior Rhomboids Mid-trapezius Lower trapezius Teres minor Infraspinatus	**Increased:** Cervical extension Scapular protraction/elevation **Decreased:** Shoulder extension Shoulder external rotation	Headaches Biceps tendonitis Rotator cuff impingement Thoracic outlet syndrome

TRAINER TIPS

Be sure to walk around the client as the exercise is being performed. Oftentimes form can look good from one view, but changing the view can help you spot technique flaws.

Movement Assessments

A person's posture is constantly changing to meet the demands placed on the kinetic chain. Thus, once the static postural assessment has been completed, the movement assessments should be performed. The findings from the movement assessments should further reinforce the observations made during the static postural assessment. Faulty body alignments not revealed during the static postural assessment may be noted during the dynamic postural observations. As such, the movement assessments are often the quickest way to gain an overall impression of a client's functional status. Because posture is dynamic, these observations show postural distortion and potential overactive and underactive muscles in a naturally dynamic setting.

Movement observations should relate to basic functions such as squatting, pushing, pulling, and balancing. In addition to providing crucial information about muscle and joint interplay, the observation process should search for any imbalances in anatomy, physiology, or biomechanics that may affect a client's results and possibly lead to injury (both in and out of the fitness environment). With the limited time that most fitness professionals have for observation, incorporating a systematic assessment sequence is essential.

Overhead Squat Assessment

Evidence supports the use of **transitional movement assessments** such as the **overhead squat assessment** (Zeller, McCrory, Kibler, & Uhl, 2003). These assessments appear to be reliable and valid measures of lower extremity movement patterns when standard protocols are applied. The overhead squat assessment is designed to assess dynamic flexibility, core strength, balance, and overall neuromuscular control. It has been shown to reflect lower extremity movement patterns during jump-landing tasks (Buckley, Thigpen, Joyce, Bohres, & Padua, 2007). **Knee valgus** during the overhead squat assessment is influenced by decreased hip abductor and hip external rotation strength, increased hip adductor activity, and restricted ankle dorsiflexion (Ireland et al., 2003; Bell & Padua, 2007; Vesci et al., 2007). Movement impairments observed during this transitional movement assessment may be the result of alterations in available joint motion, muscle activation, and overall neuromuscular control, which some hypothesize increases the risk of injury. For example, research has indicated that individuals who possess increased knee valgus are at greater risk for knee injury (Ford et al., 2015; Hewett, Myer, Heidt, et al., 2005). Being able to identify such compensations during the assessment allows the fitness professional to provide programming that can improve compensation and decrease the risk for knee injuries. See **Figures 9.7–9.10** for more on what to look for in an overhead squat assessment.

Position

1. The client should stand barefoot with hands overhead, arms lined up with the ear.
2. Eyes should be focused straight ahead on an object.
3. Feet should be pointed straight ahead, and the foot, ankle, knee, and LPHC should be in neutral position.

Transitional movement assessment

A type of assessment that evaluates dynamic posture.

Overhead squat assessment

A transitional movement assessment designed to assess dynamic flexibility, core strength, balance, and overall neuromuscular control.

Knee valgus

The process where the knees move forward and in, known as "knock knees."

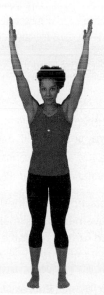

FIGURE 9.7 Overhead squat assessment start, frontal view.

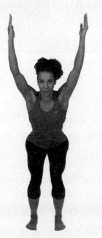

FIGURE 9.8 Overhead squat assessment finish, frontal view.

TRAINER TIPS

Adjusting the tempo, asking the client to move faster or slower, can highlight movement compensations if none are seen at the client's normal tempo.

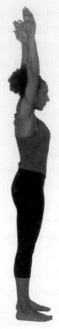

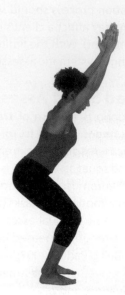

FIGURE 9.9 Overhead squat assessment start, lateral view.

FIGURE 9.10 Overhead squat assessment finish, lateral view.

Movement

1. Instruct the client to squat (at a natural pace) to roughly the height of a chair seat and return to the starting position.
2. Repeat the movement for five repetitions, observing from each position (anterior and lateral).

Views

1. View the feet, ankles, and knees from the front. The feet should remain straight, with the knees tracking in line with the foot (second and third toes).

CHECK IT OUT

When performing the overhead squat assessment, a common compensation that can occur is an individual's knees moving inward. This could be due to lack of range of motion at the ankle or weakness in the hips (or possibly both). A way to further investigate the primary area of focus that may be causing this compensation is to have the individual place his or her heels on a 2 × 4 board or weight plates, and then perform the assessment. This places the foot/ankle complex in a plantar-flexed position, providing more dorsiflexion range of motion. If the knees stay more in line with the feet, then the foot/ankle complex may be the source of the issue. If the knees still move inward, then the source may be weakness of the hips. A similar technique can be used when assessing the latissimus dorsi and its involvement when the low back arches. If the low back arches with the arms overhead, have the individual perform the squat with the hands on the hips. If the low back does not arch with the hands on the hips, then latissimus dorsi extensibility may be the issue, as the latissimus dorsi is in the stretched position with the arms overhead. If the low back still arches with the hands on the hips, then core weakness may be the primary issue.

2. View the LPHC, shoulder, and cervical complex from the side. The tibia should remain in line with the torso while the arms also stay in line with the torso.

Compensations: Anterior View
1. *Feet*: Do the feet flatten and/or turn out?
2. *Knees*: Do the knees move inward (adduct and internally rotate)?

Compensations: Lateral View
1. *LPHC*:
   a. Does the low back arch?
   b. Does the torso lean forward excessively?
2. *Shoulder*: Do the arms fall forward?

When performing the assessment, record all of the findings. Refer to **Table 9.7** and **Figures 9.11–9.15** to determine potential overactive and underactive muscles that will need

TABLE 9.7 Checkpoints for the Overhead Squat Assessment

View	Checkpoint	Compensation	Probable Overactive Muscles	Probable Underactive Muscles
Lateral	LPHC	Excessive forward lean	Soleus Gastrocnemius Hip flexor complex Abdominal complex	Anterior tibialis Gluteus maximus Erector spinae
		Low back arches (anterior pelvic tilt)	Hip flexor complex Erector spinae Latissimus dorsi	Gluteus maximus Hamstring complex Intrinsic core stabilizers (transverse abdominis, multifidus, transversospinalis, internal oblique pelvic floor)
		Low back rounds (posterior pelvic tilt)	Hamstring complex Rectus abdominis	Intrinsic core stabilizers (transverse abdominis, multifidus, transversospinalis, internal oblique pelvic floor) Gluteus maximus Erector spinae
Anterior	Feet	Turn out	Soleus Lateral gastrocnemius Biceps femoris (short head)	Medial gastrocnemius Medial hamstring complex Gracilis Sartorius Popliteus
	Knees	Move inward	Adductor complex Soleus/gastrocnemius Biceps femoris (short head) Tensor fasciae latae Vastus lateralis	Gluteus medius/maximus Vastus medialis oblique (VMO)

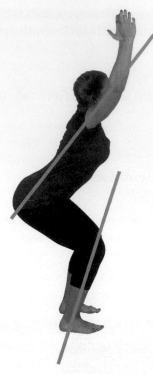

FIGURE 9.11 Excessive forward lean.

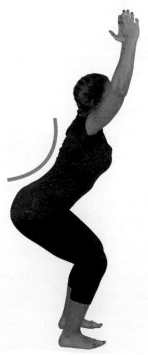

FIGURE 9.12 Low back arches.

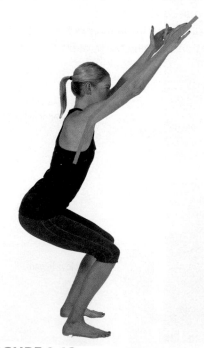

FIGURE 9.13 Arms fall forward.

to be addressed through corrective flexibility and strengthening techniques to improve the client's quality of movement, decreasing the risk for injury and improving performance.

Single-Leg Squat Assessment

The single-leg squat assessment also assesses dynamic flexibility, core strength, balance, and overall neuromuscular control. Evidence supports the use of the **single-leg squat assessment** as a transitional movement assessment (Zeller et al., 2003). This assessment appears to be a reliable and valid measure of lower extremity movement patterns when standard application protocols are applied. Knee valgus has been shown to be influenced by decreased hip abductor and hip external rotation strength, increased hip adductor activity, and restricted ankle dorsiflexion (Ireland et al., 2003; Bell & Padua, 2007; Zeller et al., 2003). These results suggest that the movement impairments observed during this movement assessment may be the result of alterations in available joint motion, muscle activation, and overall neuromuscular control. See **Figures 9.16** and **9.17** for the movements associated with this assessment.

Single-leg squat assessment

A transitional assessment performed on one leg to assess dynamic flexibility, core strength, balance, and overall neuromuscular control.

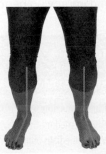

FIGURE 9.14 Feet turn out.

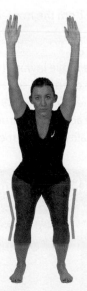

FIGURE 9.15 Knees move inward.

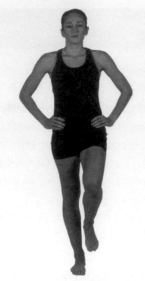

FIGURE 9.16 Beginning of single-leg squat assessment.

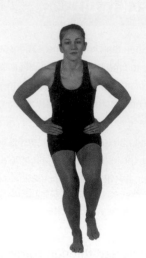

FIGURE 9.17 End of single-leg squat assessment.

Position

1. The client should stand barefoot with hands on the hips and eyes focused straight ahead on an object.
2. Feet should be pointed straight ahead, and the foot, ankle, knee, and LPHC should be in neutral position.

Movement

1. Have the client slowly squat to a comfortable level and return to the starting position at a comfortable pace.
2. Perform up to five repetitions before switching sides.

Views

View the knee from the front. The knee should track in line with the foot (second and third toes).

Compensation

Does the knee move inward (adduct and internally rotate)?

As with the overhead squat assessment, the fitness professional should record his or her observations. Refer to **Table 9.8** to determine potential overactive and underactive muscles that will need to be addressed through corrective flexibility and strengthening techniques to improve the client's quality of movement, decreasing the risk for injury and improving performance.

TABLE 9.8 Checkpoints for the Single-Leg Squat Assessment

Checkpoint	Compensation	Probable Overactive Muscles	Probable Underactive Muscles
Knee	Move inward	Adductor complex Biceps femoris (short head) Tensor fasciae latae Vastus lateralis	Gluteus maximus Gluteus medius Vastus medialis oblique (VMO)

CHECK IT OUT

For some individuals, the single-leg squat assessment may be too difficult to perform (e.g., elderly client). Other options include using outside support for assistance or simply performing a single-leg balance assessment to assess movement compensation and the ability to control the body in a relatively unstable environment.

Pushing Assessment

Like the overhead and single-leg squat assessments, the pushing assessment evaluates movement efficiency and potential muscle imbalances during pushing movements.

Position

Instruct the client to stand with abdomen drawn inward, feet in a split stance and toes pointing forward.

Movement

1. Viewing from the side, instruct the client to press the handles forward (at a 2/0/2 tempo) and return to the starting position.
2. Perform up to 20 repetitions in a controlled fashion. The lumbar and cervical spines should remain neutral while the shoulders stay level.

Compensations

1. *Low back*: Does the low back arch?
2. *Shoulders*: Do the shoulders elevate?
3. *Head*: Does the head migrate forward?

The fitness professional should record his or her observations. Refer to **Table 9.9** and **Figures 9.18–9.22** to determine potential overactive and underactive muscles that will need to be addressed through corrective flexibility and strengthening techniques to improve the client's quality of movement, decreasing the risk for injury and improving performance.

TABLE 9.9 Checkpoints for the Pushing Assessment

Checkpoint	Compensation	Probable Overactive Muscles	Probable Underactive Muscles
LPHC	Low back arches	Hip flexors Erector spinae	Intrinsic core stabilizers
Shoulder complex	Shoulder elevation	Upper trapezius Sternocleidomastoid Levator scapulae	Mid/lower trapezius
Head	Head migrates forward	Upper trapezius Sternocleidomastoid Levator scapulae	Deep cervical flexors

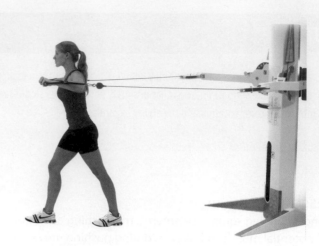

FIGURE 9.18 Beginning of pushing assessment.

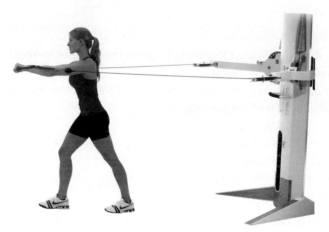

FIGURE 9.19 Ending of pushing assessment.

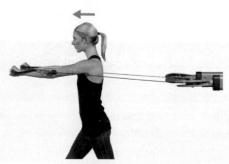

FIGURE 9.20 Pushing assessment forward head.

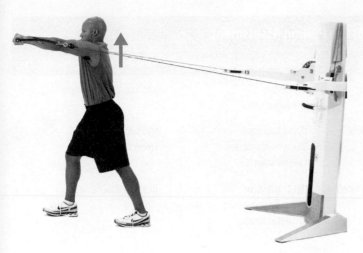

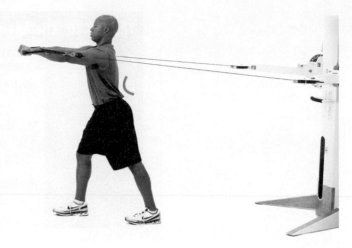

FIGURE 9.21 Pushing assessment elevated shoulders.

FIGURE 9.22 Pushing assessment low back arch.

CHECK IT OUT ✓

Although it is best to perform the pushing assessment in a standing position to obtain a better representation of the client's overall functional status, this assessment can also be performed on a machine. Push-ups may also be used to perform this assessment; however, many individuals do not have the capabilities to perform a traditional push-up, so modifications may need to be incorporated (e.g., push-up on knees, hands on a bench with feet on the floor).

Pulling Assessment

The purpose of this assessment is to observe movement efficiency and potential muscle imbalances during pulling movements.

Position

Instruct the client to stand with abdomen drawn inward, feet in a split stance and toes pointing forward. This assessment can be done using a cable apparatus or tubing as resistance.

Movement

1. Viewing from the side, instruct the client to pull the handles toward the body (at a 2/0/2 tempo) and return to the starting position. Like the pushing assessment, the lumbar and cervical spines should remain neutral while the shoulders stay level.
2. Perform up to 20 repetitions in a controlled fashion.

Compensations

1. *Low back*: Does the low back arch?
2. *Shoulders*: Do the shoulders elevate?
3. *Head*: Does the head migrate forward?

TABLE 9.10 Checkpoints for the Pulling Assessment

Checkpoint	Compensation	Probable Overactive Muscles	Probable Underactive Muscles
LPHC	Low back arches	Hip flexors Erector spinae	Intrinsic core stabilizers
Shoulder complex	Shoulder elevation	Upper trapezius Sternocleidomastoid Levator scapulae	Mid trapezius Lower trapezius
Head	Head protrudes forward	Upper trapezius Sternocleidomastoid Levator scapulae	Deep cervical flexors

The fitness professional should record his or her observations. Refer to **Table 9.10** and **Figures 9.23–9.27** to determine potential overactive and underactive muscles that will need to be addressed through corrective flexibility and strengthening techniques in order to improve the client's quality of movement, decrease the risk for injury, and improve performance.

CHECK IT OUT

Like the pushing assessment, the pulling assessment can also be performed on a machine. Keep in mind that the more stable the environment, the less likely you will see compensations in the lower extremities and core.

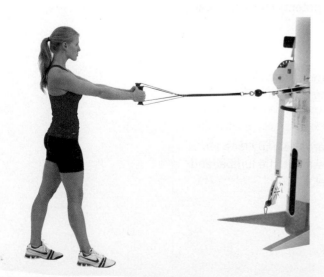

FIGURE 9.23 Beginning of pulling assessment.

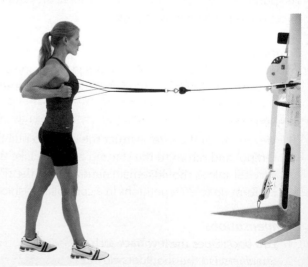

FIGURE 9.24 End of pulling assessment.

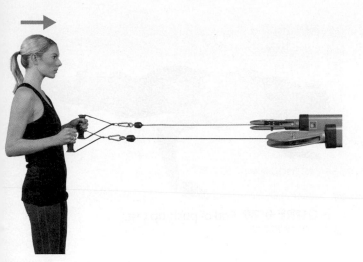

FIGURE 9.25 Pulling assessment forward head.

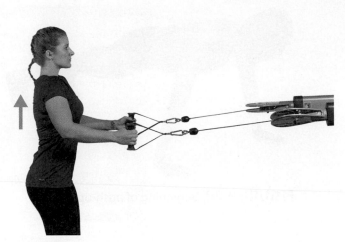

FIGURE 9.26 Pulling assessment elevated shoulders.

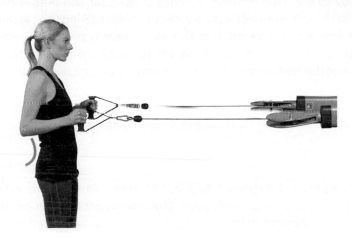

FIGURE 9.27 Pulling assessment low back arch.

Performance Assessments

Performance assessments are optional and can be used for clients looking to improve their athletic performance. These assessments measure upper extremity stability and muscular endurance, lower extremity agility, and overall strength. Basic performance assessments include the push-up test, Davies test, shark skill test, vertical jump test, 40-yard dash, pro shuttle, LEFT test, broad jump, bench press strength assessment, and squat strength assessment. This section will also review cardiorespiratory assessments, such as the YMCA 3-minute step test and the Rockport walk test.

Push-up Test

The push-up test is used to measure muscular endurance of the upper body; primarily the pushing muscles (**Figures 9.28** and **9.29**). Based on the positioning of the body (prone), this assessment can also be used to assess core stability endurance.

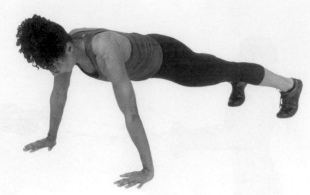

FIGURE 9.28 Beginning of push-up test.

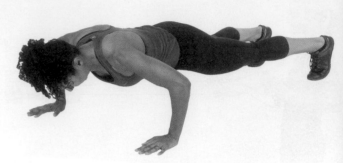

FIGURE 9.29 End of push-up test.

Procedure

1. In push-up position (ankles, knees, hips, shoulders, and head in a straight line), the client lowers the body so the chest is within 3 inches of the floor and pushes back up again, repeating for 60 seconds or to exhaustion without compensating (e.g., arching low back, extending cervical spine). A variation of this assessment is performing push-ups from a kneeling position or with one's hands on a bench with the feet on the floor. Whichever method is performed, be sure to use the same procedure during the reassessment process.
2. Record the number of actual repetitions.
3. The client should be able to perform more push-ups when reassessed.

Davies Test

The purpose of this assessment (**Figures 9.30** and **9.31**) is to measure upper extremity agility and stabilization (Hewett, Myer, Ford, et al., 2005). This assessment may not be suitable for clients or athletes who lack shoulder stability.

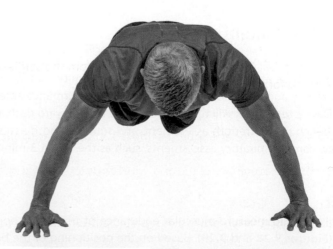

FIGURE 9.30 Beginning of Davies test.

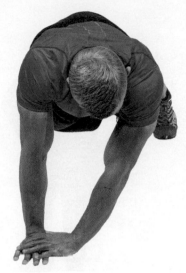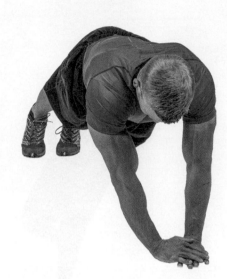

FIGURE 9.31 Davies test movement.

Position
1. Place two pieces of tape on the floor, 36 inches apart. If this distance is too difficult for the individual due to short arm length, the tape can be brought in closer; however, it is important to measure the distance used and record the distance in the notes, as this distance will need to be used again when the client is reassessed.
2. Have the client assume a push-up position, with one hand on each piece of tape.

Movement
1. Instruct the client to quickly move his or her right hand to touch the left hand.
2. The right hand should return back to the tape, and then repeat for the left hand.
3. Perform alternating touches on each side for 15 seconds.
4. Repeat for three trials.
5. Reassess in the future to measure improvement in the number of touches.
6. Record the number of lines touched by both hands.

Shark Skill Test
The purpose of this test is to assess lower extremity agility and neuromuscular control (**Figures 9.32–9.34**). It should be viewed as a progression from the single-leg squat and, as such, may not be suitable for all individuals.

Position
1. A nine-box grid is taped out on the floor. The grid is 3 × 3 boxes, with each box measuring 12 × 12 inches.
2. Position the client in the center box of the grid, with hands on hips and standing on one leg.

Movement
1. Instruct the client to hop to each box in a designated pattern, always returning to the center box.
2. Perform one practice run through the boxes with each foot.

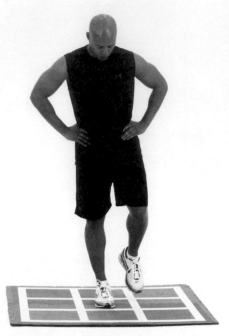

FIGURE 9.32 Beginning of Shark skill test.

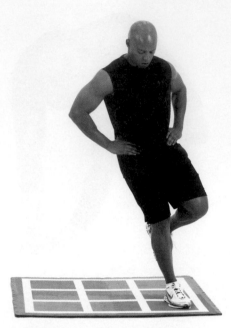

FIGURE 9.33 Shark skill test movement.

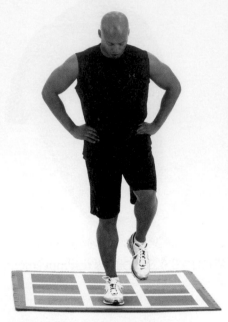

FIGURE 9.34 Shark skill test.

3. Perform the test twice with each foot (four times total), and keep track of the time for each repetition.
4. Record the times.
5. Add 0.10 seconds for each of the following faults:
   a. Non-hopping leg touches ground.
   b. Hands come off hips.
   c. Foot goes into the wrong square.
   d. Foot does not return to center square.
6. The client is later reassessed for improvements in time and fewer faults.

Upper Extremity Strength Assessment: Bench Press Test

The purpose of the bench press test is to estimate the one-rep maximum on overall upper body strength of the pressing musculature (**Figures 9.35** and **9.36**). This test can also be used to determine training intensities of the bench press. This is considered an advanced assessment (for strength-specific goals) and, as such, may not be suitable for many clients.

Position
Position the client on a bench, lying on his or her back. Feet should be pointed straight ahead. The low back should be in a neutral position.

Movement
1. Instruct the client to warm up with a light resistance that can be easily performed for 8–10 repetitions.
2. Take a 1-minute rest.
3. Add 10–20 pounds (5–10% of initial load), and perform 3–5 repetitions.
4. Take a 2-minute rest.

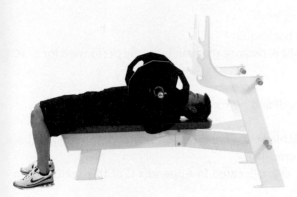

FIGURE 9.35 Beginning of bench press test.

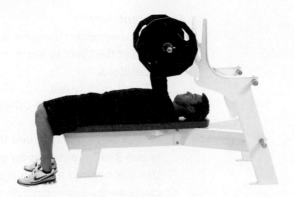

FIGURE 9.36 End of bench press test.

5. Repeat steps 3 and 4 until the client achieves failure between 2 and 10 repetitions (between 3 to 5 repetitions for greater accuracy).
6. Use the one-rep maximum estimation chart (located in Appendix C of this textbook) to calculate one-repetition max.

Lower Extremity Strength Assessment: Squat Test

The purpose of the squat test is to estimate the one-repetition squat maximum and overall lower body strength (**Figures 9.37** and **9.38**). This test can also be used to determine training intensities for the squat exercise. This is considered an advanced assessment (for strength-specific goals) and, as such, may not be suitable for many clients.

Position

Feet should be shoulder-width apart, pointed straight ahead, and with knees in line with the toes. The low back should be in a neutral position.

TRAINER TIPS

The bench press and squat tests are time-consuming assessments. The client may run out of time or become exhausted before reaching the end of the assessment. If this happens, the assessment can resume at a later date.

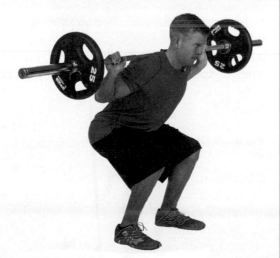

FIGURE 9.37 Beginning of squat test.   **FIGURE 9.38** End of squat test.

Movement

1. The movement is the same as a barbell back squat.
2. Instruct the client to warm up with a light resistance that can be easily performed for 8–10 repetitions.
3. Take a 1-minute rest.
4. Add 30–40 pounds (10–20% of initial load) and perform 3–5 repetitions.
5. Take a 2-minute rest.
6. Repeat steps 4 and 5 until the client achieves failure between 2 and 10 repetitions (between 3 to 5 repetitions for greater accuracy).
7. Use the one-rep maximum estimation chart (located in Appendix C of this textbook) to calculate the one-repetition max.

Vertical Jump Test

The purpose of the vertical jump test is to assess lower extremity power (**Figure 9.39**).

Position

The client stands side next to a wall and reaches up with the hand closest to the wall. Keeping the feet flat on the ground, the point of the fingertips is marked or recorded. This is called the *standing reach height*.

Movement

1. The client then stands away from the wall, and leaps vertically (without stepping) as high as possible, using both arms and legs to assist in projecting the body upwards, and touches the wall.
2. Mark the location where the client touched.
3. The difference in distance between the standing reach height and the jump height is the score. The best of three attempts is recorded.
4. When reassessing, the individual's jump height should be higher.

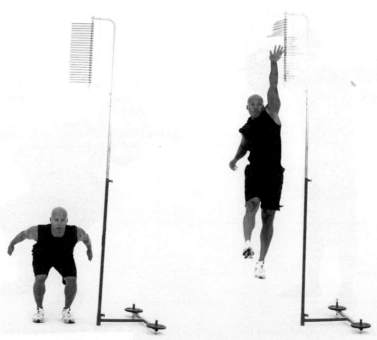

FIGURE 9.39 Vertical jump test.

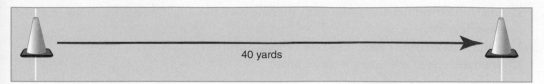

FIGURE 9.40 40-yard dash.

40-yard Dash

The purpose of the 40-yard dash is to assess acceleration and speed. This assessment is best performed on a track or field of at least 60 yards. The professional should also have a stopwatch and set up cones 40 yards apart (**Figure 9.40**).

Position

The client starts from a comfortable, stationary, three-point-stance position with the front foot behind the starting line. This starting position should be held for 3 seconds prior to starting.

Movement

1. When ready, the client sprints to the end cone.
2. Begin timing at the client's first movement and stop timing the moment the client's chest crosses the end cone.
3. Typically, two trials are allowed, with the best time recorded.
4. When reassessing, the individual's time should be less.

Pro Shuttle Test

The purpose of the pro shuttle test is to assess speed, explosion, body control, and the ability to change direction (agility) (**Figure 9.41**). The fitness professional will need a stopwatch and three cones. The assessment should be performed on a flat, nonslip surface.

Position

1. Three marker cones are placed along a line 5 yards apart.
2. The client stands at the middle cone.

Movement

1. On the signal "Go" the client turns and runs 5 yards to the right side and touches the line with the right hand.
2. Client then runs 10 yards to the left and touches the other line with the left hand.

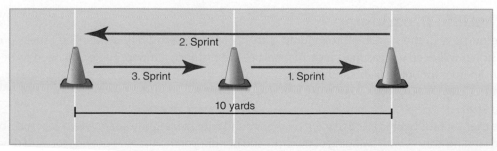

FIGURE 9.41 Pro shuttle test.

3. Finally, the client turns and finishes by running back through the start/finish line (the middle cone).
4. The best time seen in three trials is recorded.
5. When reassessed, the time should be lower.

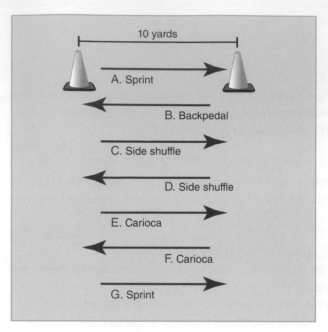

FIGURE 9.42 LEFT test.

LEFT Test

The purpose of the LEFT test is to assess agility, acceleration, deceleration, and neuromuscular control (**Figure 9.42**). The fitness professional will need a stopwatch and two marker cones. The assessment should be performed on a flat, nonslip surface.

Position

Two marker cones are placed 10 yards apart.

Movement

1. On the signal "Go," the client sprints from cone 1 to cone 2, backpedals back to cone 1, side shuffles to cone 2 then to cone 1, cariocas to cone 2 then to cone 1, and finishes with a sprint to cone 2.
2. The time is recorded.
3. When reassessed, the time should be lower.

Standing Broad Jump

The purpose of the standing broad jump is to assess lower extremity power. The fitness professional will need a measuring tape to measure the distance jumped. There will need to be a nonslip floor for both takeoff and landing.

Position

The client stands behind a line marked on the ground with feet slightly apart. A two-foot take-off and landing is used, with swinging of the arms and bending of the knees to provide forward drive.

Movement
1. The client attempts to jump as far as possible, landing on both feet without falling backwards.
2. Three attempts are allowed, and the longest jump is recorded, measuring from the starting point to where the heels land.
3. When reassessed, the distance should be greater.

Cardiorespiratory Assessment

Cardiorespiratory assessments help the fitness professional identify safe and effective starting exercise intensities, as well as appropriate modes of cardiorespiratory exercise for clients. Recall that the best measurement of cardiorespiratory fitness is $\dot{V}O_{2max}$. However, it is not always practical to measure $\dot{V}O_{2max}$ because of the equipment requirements, time involved, and willingness of clients to perform at maximal physical capacity. Therefore, submaximal tests are often the preferred method for determining cardiorespiratory functional capacity and fitness.

Submaximal testing allows for the prediction or estimation of $\dot{V}O_{2max}$. These tests are similar to $\dot{V}O_{2max}$ tests, but they differ in that they are terminated at a predetermined heart rate intensity or time frame. Multiple submaximal tests have been shown to be valid and reliable predictors of $\dot{V}O_{2max}$, and these tests are often categorized by type (run/walk tests, cycle ergometer tests, and step tests). Any of these tests can be used; however, the space or equipment constraints and specific population (e.g., elderly, youth) to be tested should be considered. Two common submaximal tests for assessing cardiorespiratory efficiency are the YMCA 3-minute step test and the Rockport walk test.

YMCA 3-Minute Step Test

The YMCA 3-minute step test is designed to estimate an individual's cardiorespiratory fitness on the basis of a submaximal bout of stair climbing, at a set pace for 3 minutes.

1. The client will perform 24 steps per minute on a 12-inch step for a total of 3 minutes (roughly 96 beats/steps per minute). It is important that the client performs the step test with the correct cadence. A metronome or simply stating out loud "up, up, down, down" can help keep the client stepping at the correct pace.
2. Within 5 seconds of completing the exercise, the client's resting heart rate is measured for a period of 60 seconds and recorded as the recovery pulse.
3. Locate the recovery pulse number in one of the categories shown in **Table 9.11**.
4. Determine the appropriate starting program based on the following categories:
   - **Poor:** Zone 1 (65–75% HR_{max})
   - **Fair:** Zone 1 (65–75% HR_{max})
   - **Average:** Zone 2 (76–85% HR_{max})
   - **Good:** Zone 2 (76–85% HR_{max})
   - **Very good:** Zone 3 (86–95% HR_{max})
5. Determine the client's maximal heart rate by using the age-predicted maximum heart rate regression formula: $208 - (0.70 \times Age)$.
6. **Zone 1:**
   - Maximal heart rate $\times$ 0.65
   - Maximal heart rate $\times$ 0.75
7. **Zone 2:**
   - Maximal heart rate $\times$ 0.76
   - Maximal heart rate $\times$ 0.85

TABLE 9.11 Recovery Pulse Table for YMCA 3-Minute Step Test						
Age	18–25	26–35	36–45	46–55	56–65	65+
Men						
Excellent	50–76	51–76	49–76	56–82	60–77	59–81
Good	79–84	79–85	80–88	87–93	86–94	87–92
Above average	88–93	88–94	92–88	95–101	97–100	94–102
Average	95–100	96–102	100–105	103–111	103–109	104–110
Below average	102–107	104–110	108–113	113–119	111–117	114–118
Poor	111–119	114–121	116–124	121–126	119–128	121–126
Very poor	124–157	126–161	130–163	131–159	131–154	130–151
Women						
Excellent	52–81	58–80	51–84	63–91	60–92	70–92
Good	85–93	85–92	89–96	95–101	97–103	96–101
Above average	96–102	95–101	100–104	104–110	106–111	104–111
Average	104–110	104–110	107–112	113–118	113–118	116–121
Below average	113–120	113–119	115–120	120–124	119–127	123–126
Poor	122–131	122–129	124–132	126–132	129–135	128–133
Very poor	135–169	134–171	137–169	137–171	141–174	135–155

8. **Zone 3:**
   - Maximal heart rate $\times$ 0.86
   - Maximal heart rate $\times$ 0.95

These zones will be used for the development of an integrated cardiorespiratory training program in addition to identifying a starting point for the client.

Rockport Walk Test

The Rockport walk test is also designed to estimate a cardiovascular starting point. The starting point is then modified based on ability level. This is a good alternative assessment for those unable to perform the 3-minute step test.

1. Record the client's weight.
2. Have the client walk 1 mile, as fast as he or she can control, on a treadmill. Record the time it takes the client to complete the walk. Immediately record the client's heart rate (beats per minute) at the 1-mile mark.
3. Use the following formula to determine the oxygen consumption (O_2) score:
   O_2 score = 132.853 – (0.0769 $\times$ Weight) – (0.3877 $\times$ Age) + (6.315 $\times$ Gender) – (3.2649 $\times$ Time) – (0.1565 $\times$ Heart rate)

Where:
- Weight is in pounds (lbs).
- Gender is Male = 1 and Female = 0.
- Time is expressed in minutes and 100ths of minutes.
- Heart rate is in beats/minute.
- Age is in years.

For example, the O_2 score for a 150-pound, 50-year-old female who completed the walk in 15 minutes and had a heart rate of 130 beats per minute would be calculated as follows:

$132.853 - (0.0769 \times 150) - (0.3877 \times 50) + (6.315 \times 0) - (3.2649 \times 15) - (0.1565 \times 130) = 32$

4. Locate the O_2 score in one of the categories shown in **Table 9.12**.

TABLE 9.12 O_2 Scoring Table for the Rockport Walk Test

Men

Age	Poor	Fair	Average	Good	Very Good
20–24	32–37	38–43	44–50	51–56	57–62
25–29	31–35	32–36	43–48	49–53	54–59
30–34	29–34	35–40	41–45	46–51	52–56
35–39	28–32	33–38	39–43	44–48	49–54
40–44	26–31	32–35	36–41	42–46	47–51
45–49	25–29	30–34	35–39	40–43	44–48
50–54	24–27	28–32	33–36	37–41	42–46
55–59	22–26	27–30	31–34	35–39	40–43
60–65	21–24	25–28	29–32	33–36	37–40

Women

Age	Poor	Fair	Average	Good	Very Good
20–24	27–31	32–36	37–41	42–46	47–51
25–29	26–30	31–35	36–40	41–44	45–49
30–34	25–29	30–33	34–37	38–42	43–46
35–39	24–27	28–31	32–35	36–40	41–44
40–44	22–25	26–29	30–33	34–37	38–41
45–49	21–23	24–27	28–31	32–35	36–38
50–54	19–22	23–25	26–29	30–32	33–36
55–59	18–20	21–23	24–27	28–30	31–33
60–65	16–18	19–21	22–24	25–27	28–30

5. Determine the appropriate starting program using the following categories:
   - **Poor:** Zone 1 (65–75% HR_{max})
   - **Fair:** Zone 1 (65–75% HR_{max})
   - **Average:** Zone 2 (76–85% HR_{max})
   - **Good:** Zone 2 (76–85% HR_{max})
   - **Very good:** Zone 3 (86–95% HR_{max})
6. Determine the client's maximal heart rate by using the age-predicted maximum heart rate formula: $208 - (0.70 \times Age)$. Then, take the maximal heart rate and multiply it by the following numbers to determine the heart rate training ranges for each zone:
7. **Zone 1:**
   - Maximal heart rate $\times$ 0.65
   - Maximal heart rate $\times$ 0.75
8. **Zone 2:**
   - Maximal heart rate $\times$ 0.76
   - Maximal heart rate $\times$ 0.85
9. **Zone 3:**
   - Maximal heart rate $\times$ 0.86
   - Maximal heart rate $\times$ 0.95

These zones will be used for the development of an integrated cardiorespiratory training program in addition to identifying a starting point for the client.

Translating Assessment Results into a Robust Goal Plan for the Client

Once all of the necessary assessments are performed, the fitness professional must compile that information and determine the best strategy to help improve the client's movement inefficiencies and muscle imbalances. When performing multiple assessments, many different compensations may be seen based on the demands of the assessment and the individual's physical capabilities. As mentioned earlier in this chapter, other compensations can be predicted based on the findings of the overhead and single-leg squat assessments. This section will review some of the potential compensations the fitness professional may see when performing the overhead and single-leg squat assessments.

Foot, Ankle, and Knee

Two common compensations seen at the foot, ankle, and knee when performing the overhead and single-leg squat assessments are the feet turning out and the knees caving inward. This compensation typically occurs due to lack of ankle range of motion, weakness of the hip musculature, or both (Bell & Padua, 2007; Vesci et al., 2007). Because of this, any assessment that involves the lower extremities may present such compensations. If this compensation is present during the overhead and/or single-leg squat assessments, it should be watched for in assessments such as the shark skill test, the Rockport walk test, and the YMCA 3-minute step test. As mentioned earlier in this chapter, compensations seen in the overhead and single-leg squat assessments can determine if other assessments should or should not be performed. For example, an athlete whose knee excessively adducts during the single-leg squat assessment should probably not do a shark skill test, because not only will the client's performance be hindered, it may increase the risk of injury due to the dynamic nature of the assessment. Another option may be to perform the shark skill test using two legs versus one if the assessment is key to the client's programming and demands of his or her sport. In this case, the fitness professional would note on the assessment form that it was modified in order to meet the client's needs.

Lumbo-Pelvic-Hip Complex

The primary compensations to watch for at the LPHC during the overhead squat assessment include the anterior tilting of the pelvis or excessive forward lean. This may be indicative of poor core control (i.e., weak transverse abdominis, gluteals). As such, any other assessment that places an emphasis on the core could elicit similar compensations as those seen during the overhead squat. For example, these compensations may also be seen in the push-up assessment, Davies test, standing pulling assessment, and standing pushing assessment. Gravity is a constant downward directed force that can have a great impact on the demands of the core, particularly in the prone position. If individuals have a difficult time controlling their core in a standing position (such as during the overhead squat), they are more than likely going to have a difficult time in a prone position. The force of gravity can be manipulated to lessen the demands on the core by decreasing the body's lever length in relation to gravity. This can be done by putting an individual in a more inclined position (e.g., hands on a bench with feet on the floor) or bringing the pivot point closer to the center of gravity (e.g., performing prone assessments with knees on the floor).

Shoulder Complex and Cervical Spine

Compensations seen in the shoulder complex and cervical spine regions during an overhead squat include the arms falling forward and the head migrating forward. With regards to the shoulders, this compensation is typically due to lack of strength in the scapular stabilizers and tightness in the anterior shoulder complex. Although this specific compensation may not be seen in other assessments, the lack of shoulder stability and range of motion that leads to the arms falling forward may be observed in other assessments that involve the upper extremities. For example, when performing the Davies test, the pushing assessment, the pulling assessment, or the push-up test, these imbalances may be displayed in the form of the shoulders elevating during the assessment: **scapular winging**, and the head migrating forward. When the arms fall forward and the head migrates forward during the overhead squat, these other compensations should be watched for as "supplementary" compensations that may be related to the compensations seen in the overhead squat.

Table 9.13 provides a summary of some of the common compensations seen in the overhead and single-leg squat assessments and how they translate to compensations seen in other assessments.

Prioritizing the Compensations

When performing movement assessments, it can be challenging for the fitness professional to determine which compensations are the most important to address. With so many compensations to look for, and the variety of assessments that can be performed, it can become a daunting task. As mentioned previously, the fitness professional should first focus on the most

TRAINER TIPS

Any assessment can be modified as long as the same protocols are followed each time.

Scapular winging

The scapula protrudes from the back in an abnormal position.

TABLE 9.13 Common Compensations Seen in Overhead and Single-Leg Squat Assessments

Observed Compensation	Probable Overactive Muscles	Probable Underactive Muscles	Other Assessments That May Show Similar Compensation
Low back arches	Hip flexor complex Erector spinae Latissimus dorsi	Gluteus maximus Hamstring complex Intrinsic core stabilizers (transverse abdominis, multifidus, transversospinalis, internal oblique pelvic floor)	Low back arches during Davies test, push-up test, standing pushing assessment, and/or standing pulling assessment
Arms fall forward	Latissimus dorsi Teres major Pectoralis major/minor	Mid/lower trapezius Rhomboids Rotator cuff	Shoulders elevate/head migrates forward/scapular winging during the Davies test, push-up test, standing pushing assessment, and/or standing pulling assessment
Turn out	Soleus Lateral gastrocnemius Biceps femoris (short head)	Medial gastrocnemius Medial hamstring complex Gracilis Sartorius Popliteus	Feet flatten during the shark skill test, Rockport walk test, 3-minute step test
Knees move inward	Adductor complex Soleus/gastrocnemius Biceps femoris (short head) Tensor fasciae latae Vastus lateralis	Gluteus medius/maximus Vastus medialis oblique (VMO)	Knees move inward during the shark skill test, Rockport walk test, 3-minute step test, and/or lower extremity strength test

CHECK IT OUT

In some instances individuals may have multiple compensations in the same region. For example, some people may exhibit an arching of the back at the beginning of the assessment, and then round the back towards the end of the assessment. Or, the knees may move inward initially, and then move outward as they move further into the squat. Common elements need to be addressed in both scenarios. For example, the gluteals would need to be addressed from a strengthening standpoint when the knees move in or out, and the calf complex and short head of the biceps femoris would need to be addressed from a flexibility standpoint. If the low back arches and rounds, strengthening of the core would be necessary in both scenarios. In such situations, first focus on the elements that would need to be addressed in both situations. This, in combination with proper technique coaching, can help to improve both issues.

obvious compensations and try not to microanalyze the client. If the compensations are evident in the overhead squat, more often than not they will be evident when performing other assessments where the client is in even more challenging positions (e.g. on one leg, prone position). Sometimes it is helpful for the fitness professional to assign a severity score to the various movement compensations. This can help with the prioritization process and also serve as a means of a baseline for future evaluations.

Something else to consider is that issues in the upper extremities can be due to imbalances in the lower extremities, and also due to compensations of the lower extremities as they manifest themselves as imbalances in the upper extremities. For example, a lack of range of motion at the ankle can result in the knee adducting and/or the torso leaning forward during an overhead squat. Addressing issues at the lower extremities (increasing ankle range of motion, increasing hip range of motion, strengthening the LPHC) could help to improve upper extremity function.

Knowing what the client is doing the majority of his or her day will also help to identify the client's priorities. For example, if a client sits behind a desk and wears heeled shoes the majority of her day, then the focus will more than likely be to address ankle range of motion (stretch the calves), hip range of motion (stretch the hip flexors), and shoulder range of motion (stretch the pectorals and latissimus dorsi), and also to strengthen the lumbo-pelvic-hip (spinal stabilizers and gluteals) region and scapular retractors.

In summary, Tables 9.4–9.7 show some of the commonalities among the compensations listed. For the most part, these issues are addressed by improving range of motion at the ankles, hips, and shoulders, while improving strength in the hips, core, and scapular retractors. In fact, if fitness professionals focused on simply stretching their clients' calves, hip flexors, latissimus dorsi, and pectorals and strengthening the gluteals, intrinsic core stabilizers, and scapular stabilizers, they would make huge gains in the functional status of the majority of their clients.

Reassessing Clients and Evaluating Progress

Although there are no set rules as to when fitness professionals should reassess their clients, a general guideline is that clients should be reassessed every 4 weeks. When it comes to performance assessments, progress is easy to measure based on the results of the first assessments. When reevaluating performance assessments, the score a client receives should be better than at the previous assessment. However, it can be more challenging to determine improvement when reassessing movement, particularly from a client's point of view. One of the most effective ways to show improvement is by recording and scoring the client's first assessment, recording and scoring the assessments thereafter in the same place, and comparing the different results. This is a great way for clients to see how much they have improved, versus it simply being verbalized by the fitness professional.

Using mirrors may also be a way for clients to visually see their improvement; however, if the client does not remember what he or she looked like during the first assessment, the client may find it difficult to correlate improvements during the reassessment. Fitness professionals can also take photos of their clients in order to show before and after improvements; however, permission must be obtained before photographing any client.

In addition, a client's "feel" can also provide key information on his or her progress. Many times, clients will express certain sensations they may feel when performing certain movements, such as, "I feel a little twinge in my knee when I squat down" or "My shoulders feel tight when I raise them overhead." It is important for the fitness professional to write these comments down, as the individual can refer back to them when performing a reassessment. Asking the client if she still feels the "twinge in the knee" or the "tightness in the shoulder" can determine how she is progressing. More often than not, clients will say that those sensations no longer exists, which could be a sign they are moving more efficiently, with less stress being placed on their structure and connective tissues.

Every workout can be considered an assessment. Fitness professionals should always be monitoring their clients' technique, and as technique improves exercises can be progressed, which translates into improvements in clients' movement quality. Conversely, if technique is poor, then exercise should be regressed to match the individual's physical capabilities, and then progressed accordingly from there. Although this may not be considered a "formal" reassessment, fitness professionals are constantly assessing. For example, if a client's knees move inward during an overhead squat assessment, that compensation should be watched for and addressed if performing squatting-type motions in the workout. This could be addressed by placing a resistance band around the client's knees and cueing him to press the outside of his knee against the band (which is trying to force the knees inward). This can provide tactile cueing on proper knee position during the squat, while also helping to strengthen the client's hip musculature (a common region of weakness with this compensation).

Assessment Modifications for Specific Populations

The assessments presented thus far and the steps necessary to execute them assume that the clients are healthy adults. However, fitness professionals work with a wide variety of clients with varying physical capabilities. Because of this, modifications may be required to meet each individual's unique capabilities.

Adjustments for the Youth Population

Strength deficits may be a factor for the youth population. When performing an assessment such as the push-up assessment, modifications should be implemented, such as performing it on the knees or with hands on a bench and feet on the floor. The pushing and pulling assessments may be better performed using tubing, because machines are often not designed to properly fit the dimensions of the young client. In addition, machines can be intimidating for this population. Due to the structural and neurological development occurring in this population, performing one-repetition maximum strength assessments should be avoided, because these can increase the risk of injury. The main element that should be integrated into the assessment process with this group is fun!

Adjustments for the Pregnant Population

Relaxin

Hormone produced during pregnancy that loosens and softens ligaments.

Assessment modifications for the pregnant client will depend on which trimester she is in. For example, few modifications may be required for a woman in her first trimester. However, as she advances into her second and third trimesters, modifications will need to be applied. Performing explosive-type movements is not recommended during the second and third trimesters due to increased levels of **relaxin**, a hormone that loosens and soften ligaments (American College of Obstetricians and Gynecologists, 2002). Because of this, many of the power and speed assessments will need to be eliminated if these assessments are consistent with the client's goals. As the fetus grows, there is more mass that now must be moved and stabilized, so modifications to the push-up assessment will also need to be applied (performing on knees, hands on bench). The single-leg squat assessment may need to be modified to a single-leg balance, as the growth of the fetus can alter a woman's center of gravity, making it more difficult for her to control balance in the more unstable environment. Adjustments to range of motion of the overhead squat may also need to be applied due to the new "anatomical barrier" that has been created.

Adjustments for the Senior Population

The senior population varies widely. Some senior clients may be very active and in excellent physical shape, in which case modifications to assessments may be few. In other cases, the individual may be very inactive, possess certain medical conditions, and/or be taking medications, in which case modifications will need to be applied. The focus of this section will be on the second scenario, as this is where the most modifications will be required. In fact, for some older adults it may not be necessary to perform certain performance assessments due to their capabilities and goals.

The range of motion for the overhead squat may need to be adjusted due to lack of strength and flexibility. Older clients may also need more coaching on how to squat during the assessment. Using cues such as "squat down as if you are sitting in a chair" or even placing a bench or chair behind them as a reference point may be helpful. The single-leg squat may also need to be regressed to a single-leg balance, as performing a squat on one leg may be too difficult to control. As with other special populations, push-up assessments may need to be performed either on the knees, or with the hands on a bench and feet on the floor due to strength and stabilization capabilities. If performing other pushing assessments, then the push-up test may not be needed. When performing the 3-minute step test, coordination capabilities should be considered, in which case the step may need to be lowered, or the client can simply perform the Rockport walk test. Older clients who are unfamiliar with the treadmill should grasp the side rails for stability until they feel more comfortable walking without them.

It is not uncommon for senior clients to be on medications when working with a fitness professional. Because of this, it is crucial that fitness professionals be familiar with some of the common medications seniors may be taking and their effects on heart rate and blood pressure, as this may dictate adjustments to assessments. **Table 9.14** provides a summary of common medications and their effects on blood pressure and heart rate.

TABLE 9.14 Effects of Medication on Heart Rate and Blood Pressure

Medication	Heart Rate	Blood Pressure
Beta-blockers	Decrease	Decrease
Calcium-channel blockers	Increase or No effect or Decrease	Decrease
Nitrates	Increase or No effect	No effect or Decrease
Diuretics	No effect	No effect or Decrease
Bronchodilators	No effect	No effect
Vasodilators	Increase or No effect or Decrease	Decrease
Antidepressants	Increase or No effect	No effect or Decrease

CHECK IT OUT

Because beta-blockers decrease blood pressure, an activity that requires an older client to be on the ground and eventually stand up, such as the push-up test (which can further decrease one's blood pressure, leading to dizziness) may need to be adjusted. For example, this activity could be performed with the hands on a bench or by simply performing the pushing assessment using cables, tubing, or a machine, depending on the client's capabilities.

Adjustments for the Obese Population

The primary focus with obese clients is to decrease weight. Obese individuals may not be physically capable of performing many of the assessments listed in this chapter. Moreover, with the additional mass the individuals may be carrying, being able to see compensations during many of the movement assessments may not be possible. In such cases, it may make more sense to focus less on movement compensations and to focus more on using the assessments as a workout to get the individual moving. For example, rather than performing an overhead squat to assess compensations, the fitness professional could have the client perform bodyweight squats for a given period of time (30–60 seconds). The number performed during this time period can be recorded and reassessed at a later date. The fitness professional can still observe the client's lower extremities for compensations while performing the assessment, but the focus is on getting the individual to move. This can also be done with the pushing and pulling assessments. With these two assessments, it may be better for the client to use cables or tubing rather than machines, because some larger people may not fit comfortably in traditional machines. The YMCA 3-minute step test may also be difficult for this population, so the Rockport walk test may be the preferred cardiorespiratory assessment. A single-leg squat assessment may also be too challenging and increase the risk of injury, so a single-leg balance may be a better choice to assess balance instead. Push-ups may require modifications of placing hands on a bench or even hands on a wall with the feet placed behind them.

Adjustments for Common Injuries

If a new client presents an injury, the fitness professional should refer that individual to the appropriate medical professional. However, some clients will report a past injury (e.g., low back pain) that they no longer experience or have gone to physical therapy to address (e.g., ACL tear). In such cases, modifications to assessments may need to be made to match the individual's capabilities. More important, focusing on certain regions of the body when performing particular assessments will be key, as these injuries may have been a result of, or lead to, certain compensations that can be seen during movement assessments. For example, if an individual has experienced foot, ankle, and knee injuries, then looking for the feet flattening and the knees caving inward during an overhead or single-leg squat would be something to watch for. Care should also be taken when performing performance assessments with this group, particularly during speed, agility, and quickness assessments that require rapid changes in direction. For clients who have experienced low back pain, it is important to watch for anterior or posterior rotation of the pelvis during the overhead squat, pushing, and pulling assessments, as this may indicate core weakness. The push-up position may be too difficult due to the demands on the core, in which case it may be more appropriate for clients to perform this assessment on their knees or with their hands on a bench. For those who have experienced shoulder injuries, it is important to watch for the arms falling forward during the overhead squat and/or the shoulders elevating and the head migrating forward during pushing and pulling assessments. Placing individuals in positions in which a large amount of stress is being placed on the shoulder complex (e.g., one-rep-max bench press, push-ups) may be eliminated or adjusted to decrease stress to the area.

Conclusion

Through proper assessment of a client's goals, needs, and abilities, the fitness professional can create an appropriate program for each client he or she works with. With a particular focus on postural and movement assessments, one can better assess how to address each client individually or in a group setting. Using this information, the fitness professional can move forward toward creating a specific program designed to meet each client's unique needs.

Case in Review

Although Jennifer may be expressing her excitement to begin working out, it is important to perform some essential human movement system assessments that will help you better understand the key areas you should be designing her training program around. You should conduct the following assessments:

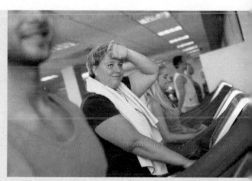
© StockLite/Shutterstock

- Overhead squat

- Single-leg squat

- Push

- Pull

During the assessments, you should be looking for compensations associated with the specified assessments listed in the charts provided. This will help you to fully understand and conceptualize what is going on within her human movement system. Ultimately, the assessment results will guide the program design, so that you address the compensations and prevent potential injuries.

These assessments are important for you, as a fitness professional, to get an overall idea of how well your client moves. They will help you to design a program that will address any movement impairments your client is exhibiting. Not only will you be better equipped to design a program that can prevent injuries, but it will enable you to address needs that Jennifer may not even know she has. Ultimately it will help you help your client reach her goals more effectively and efficiently.

References

American College of Obstetricians and Gynecologists. (2002). Exercise during pregnancy and the postpartum period. *Obstetrics and Gynecology, 99*, 171–173.

Bell, D. R., & Padua D. A. (2007). Influence of ankle dorsiflexion range of motion and lower leg muscle activation on knee valgus during a double-legged squat. *Journal of Athletic Training, 42*, S84.

Buckley, B. D., Thigpen, C. A., Joyce, C. J., Bohres, S. M., & Padua, D. A. (2007). Knee and hip kinematics during a double leg squat predict knee and hip kinematics at initial contact of a jump landing task. *Journal of Athletic Training, 42*, S81.

Bullock-Saxton, J. E. (1994). Local sensation changes and altered hip muscle function following severe ankle sprain. *Physical Therapy, 74*, 17–31.

Bullock-Saxton, J. E., Janda, V., & Bullock, M. I. (1993). Reflex activation of gluteal muscles in walking. An approach to restoration of muscle function for patients with low back pain. *Spine, 18,* 704–708.

Ford, K. R., Nguyen, A. D., Dischiavi, S. L., Hegedus, E. J., Zuk, E. F., & Taylor, J. B. (2015). An evidence-based review of hip-focused neuromuscular exercise interventions to address dynamic lower extremity valgus. *Open Access Journal of Sports Medicine, 6*, 291–303.

Fredericson, M., Cookingham, C. L., Chaudhari, A. M., Dowdell, B. C., Oestreicher, N., & Sahrmann, S. A. (2000). Hip abductor weakness in distance runners with iliotibial band syndrome. *Clinical Journal of Sport Medicine, 10*, 169–175.

Graven-Nielsen, T., & Mense, S. (2001). The peripheral apparatus of muscle pain: Evidence from animal and human studies. *Clinical Journal of Pain, 17*, 2–10.

Hewett, T. E., Myer, G. D., Heidt, R. S. Jr., Colosimo, A. J., McLean, S. G., van den Bogert, A. J., Paterno, M. V., & Succop, P. (2005). Biomechanical measures of neuromuscular control and valgus loading of the knee predict anterior cruciate ligament injury risk in female athletes: A prospective study. *American Journal of Sports Medicine, 33*(4), 492–501.

Hewett, T. E., Myer, G. D., Ford, K. R., Heidt, R. S. Jr., McLean, S. G., van den Bogert, A. J., Paterno, M. V., & Succop, P. (2005). Biomechanical measures of neuromuscular control and valgus loading of the knee predict anterior cruciate ligament injury risk in female athletes: A prospective study. *American Journal of Sports Medicine, 33*(4), 492–501.

Hodges, P. W., & Richardson, C. A. (1996). Inefficient muscular stabilization of the lumbar spine associated with low back pain. A motor control evaluation of transversus abdominis. *Spine, 21*, 2640–2650.

Hodges, P. W., & Richardson, C. A. (1997). Contraction of the abdominal muscles associated with movement of the lower limb. *Physical Therapy, 77*, 132–144.

Hodges, P., Richardson, C., & Jull, G. (1996). Evaluation of the relationship between laboratory and clinical tests of transversus abdominis function. *Physiotherapy Research International, 1*, 30–40.

Ireland, M. L., Willson, J. D., Ballantyne, B. T., & Davis, I. M. (2003). Hip strength in females with and without patellofemoral pain. *Journal of Orthopaedic and Sports Physical Therapy, 33*, 671–676.

Janda, V. (1983). *Muscle function and testing.* London, UK: Butterworth.

Janda, V. (2002). Muscles and motor control in cervicogenic disorders. In R. Grant (Ed.), *Physical therapy of the cervical and thoracic spine* (pp. 182–199). St. Louis, MO: Churchill Livingstone.

Kedgley, A., Mackenzie, G., Ferreira, L., Johnson, J. A., & Faber, K. J. (2007). In vitro kinematics of the shoulder following rotator cuff injury. *Clinical Biomechanics, 22*, 1068–1073.

Kim, Y., Lim, J. M., & Yoon, B. (2013). Changes in ankle range of motion and muscle strength in habitual wearers of high-heeled shoes. *Foot and Ankle International, 34*(3), 414–419.

Kucera, K. L., Marshall, S. W., Kirkendall, D. T., Marchak, P. M., & Garrett, W. E. Jr. (2004). Injury history as a risk factor for incident injury in youth soccer. *British Journal of Sports Medicine, 39*, 462–466.

Mense, S., & Simons, D. (2001). *Muscle pain. Understanding its nature, diagnosis, and treatment.* Philadelphia, PA: Williams & Wilkins.

Newmann, D. (2010). *Kinesiology of the musculoskeletal system: Foundations for physical rehabilitation* (2nd ed.). St. Louis, MO: Mosby.

Nyland, J., Smith, S., Beickman, K., Armsey, T., & Caborn, D. N. (2002). Frontal plane knee angle affects dynamic postural control strategy during unilateral stance. *Medicine and Science in Sports and Exercise, 34,* 1150–1157.

Powers, C. (2003). The influence of altered lower-extremity kinematics on patellofemoral joint dysfunction: A theoretical perspective. *Journal of Orthopaedic and Sports Physical Therapy, 33,* 639–646.

Powers, C. M., Ward, S. R., Fredericson, M., Guillet, M., & Shellock, F. G. (2003). Patellofemoral kinematics during weight-bearing and non-weight-bearing knee extension in persons with lateral subluxation of the patella: A preliminary study. *Journal of Orthopaedic Sports Physical Therapy, 33,* 677–685.

Sahrmann, S. A. (1992). Posture and muscle imbalance: Faulty lumbo-pelvic alignment and associated musculoskeletal pain syndromes. *Orthopaedic Division of the Canadian Physical Therapy, 12,* 13–20.

Sahrmann, S. A. (2002). *Diagnosis and treatment of movement impairment syndromes.* St. Louis, MO: Mosby.

Silva, A. M., de Sigueira, G. R., & da Silva, G. A. (2013). Implications of high-heeled shoes on body posture of adolescents. *Revista Paulista de Pediatria, 31*(2), 265–271.

Terada, M., Pietrosimone, B. G., & Gribble, P. A. (2014). Alterations in neuromuscular control at the knee in individuals with chronic ankle instability. *Journal of Athletic Training, 49*(5), 599–607.

Van der Windt, D. A., Thomas, E., Pope, D. P., de Winter, A. F., Macfarlane, G. J., Bouter, L. M., & Silman, A. J. (2000). Occupational risk factors for shoulder pain: A systematic review. *Occupational and Environmental Medicine, 57,* 433–442.

Vesci, B. J., Padua, D. A., Bell, D. R., Strickland, L. J., Guskiewicz, K. M., & Hirth, C. J. (2007). Influence of hip muscle strength, flexibility of hip and ankle musculature, and hip muscle activation on dynamic knee valgus motion during a double-legged squat. *Journal of Athletic Training, 42,* S83.

Yanagawa, T., Goodwin, C., Shelburne, K., Giphart, J. E., Torry, M. R., & Pandy, M. G. (2008). Contributions of the individual muscles of the shoulder to glenohumeral joint stability during abduction. *Journal of Biomechanical Engineering, 130,* 21–24.

Yasojima, T., Kizuka, T., Noguchi, H., Shiraki, H., Mukai, N., & Miyanaga, Y. (2008). Differences in EMG activity in scapular plane abduction under variable arm positions and loading conditions. *Medicine and Science in Sports and Exercise, 40,* 716–721.

Zeller, B., McCrory, J., Kibler, W., & Uhl, T. (2003). Differences in kinematics and electromyographic activity between men and women during the single-legged squat. *American Journal of Sports Medicine, 31,* 119–156.

10

INITIALIZING PROGRAM DESIGN

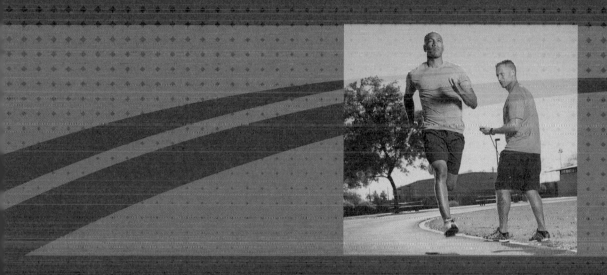

OBJECTIVES

After studying this chapter, you will be able to:

1. **Summarize** the components and outcomes of each level of the Optimum Performance Training™ (OPT™) model.

2. **Explain** the importance of systematic and progressive program design.

3. **Describe** how to use the OPT model template.

4. **Classify** movement assessment outcomes into specific programming.

5. **Apply** session flow and structure to the various needs of clients.

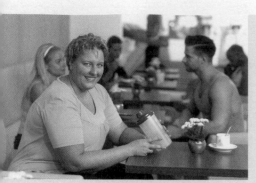

© StockLite/Shutterstock

Case Scenario

You have become familiar and comfortable with conducting and interpreting postural and basic movement assessments with your friends and family. You now have the ability, when conducting these assessments, to identify overactive and underactive muscles, and to recognize the possible causes based on conversations about their daily lives and the interviewing strategies you have learned.

Your client, Jennifer, has mentioned that she has never performed fitness assessments like those you have conducted on her, and she is not sure how you are going to use the results to design a program specific to her needs and fitness goals. With some skepticism on the value of the assessments you conducted last week, Jennifer wants to see how you integrated your observations into the program you designed for her.

After conducting a movement assessment, you noticed that from an anterior view Jennifer's knees move inward, and from a lateral view she leans forward.

- Based on this movement assessment, what would you discuss with Jennifer?

- How would you use this information to justify a particular program design?

- What additional information is needed to develop programming that is specific to Jennifer's needs, and why?

Progressive Program Design and the OPT Model

Using the results of an assessment, the fitness professional will have the information necessary to begin program design. Fitness professionals who have an understanding of each level of the OPT model are able to design systematic and progressive programs that address the needs and desires of their clients. First, however, the fitness professional must have an understanding of progressive program design.

The human body is constantly adapting and changing to the environment around it. Anything that creates a stress may eventually lead to an adaptation. These changes occur slowly over a period of time. The body is capable of adapting to almost anything, as long as the stress is applied gradually and includes physical activity through the general adaptation syndrome; which is the foundation for program design.

Exercise provides a stress that leads to adaptation. The program should follow a simple set of rules that prevents overtraining, but continuously allows the stresses to accumulate;

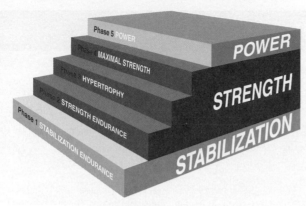

FIGURE 10.1 The OPT model.

resulting in the desired change. Therefore, the design of exercise programs follows a systematic approach. The OPT model is a system that provides a methodical approach for providing the proper progressions over time (**Figure 10.1**). The OPT model utilizes various exercise modalities (e.g., suspension training, dumbbells, body weight, etc.), but the results come from following the recommended acute variables throughout the program.

The OPT model is designed with the acute variables already programmed in, according to the needs of the different levels. The progression through each level and each phase is systematic and organized based on current evidence. The OPT model allows fitness professionals to coach their clients on lifestyle behaviors that can help them reach their goals sooner, rather than spending an excessive amount of time developing each part of a client's program.

The principle of **progressive resistance exercise (PRE)** for increasing strength and force production in muscles has not changed in many years (Taylor, Dodd, & Damiano, 2005). This principle begins with lower loads and higher repetitions and makes weekly progressions. These progressions occur over time, increasing the resistance by a small percentage each week and decreasing the repetitions as necessary. Maximal strength adaptations are achieved by ending with lifting the maximum weight possible for as few as 1–5 repetitions. In most cases, these progressions occur over 12–16 weeks, depending on the individual's goals. It is also important to note that progressive training has been shown to be one of the safest forms of resistance training in a variety of adult populations, as well as with young people (Taylor et al., 2005).

Progressive resistance exercise (PRE)
A method of increasing the ability of muscles to generate force. The progressions within the OPT model are divided up to support each component of integrated fitness training (flexibility, cardio, core, balance, reactive, SAQ, and resistance training) and each level (Stabilization, Strength, and Power).

Acute Variables

The acute variables are the most fundamental component in designing a training program. They determine the amount and kind of stress placed on the body, and ultimately what changes the body will experience. The body adapts to the demands placed on it, which is known as the principle of specificity (SAID Principle). For example, a client who lifts heavy weights with low repetitions will develop strength. Conversely, a client who focuses on light intensity and high repetitions will develop endurance. The OPT model provides the framework for the systematic progression of the acute variables. The following are the most commonly addressed acute variables: exercise selection, order of exercises performed, load (weight/resistance), volume (repetitions × sets), rest periods, and tempo (Hayes, Bickerstaff, & Baker, 2013).

Volume

Training volume is the total amount of work performed within a specified time. Training volume is typically the number of repetitions multiplied by the number of sets in a training session.

Training volume
The total amount of work performed within a specified time; typically the number of repetitions multiplied by the number of sets in a training session.

CHECK IT OUT

Load vs. Volume

As the load increases, the number of repetitions decreases. For example, a weight approximately 50% of one's maximum intensity could be lifted for several repetitions. If the weight is increased to 80% maximum intensity, then the repetitions would have to decrease. However, a client could increase the total volume by performing more sets. This would require significantly more rest between sets.

Load vs. Rest Period

Load and rest period are directly related. As load or intensity increases, the rest period must also increase. This is due to the amount of adenosine triphosphate (ATP) accessible to the muscles during activity. At 100% intensity, ATP typically depletes in a matter of seconds. Conversely, with intensities closer to 50% the body is capable of using oxygen to produce more ATP, so the rest period can decrease. At higher loads, rest periods could be up to 5 minutes, whereas at lower loads rest may not even be required.

It could also be considered over several training sessions. For example, if performing three sets of squats for 12 repetitions for three sessions during a week, the total training volume of squats for the week is 108 repetitions.

More training volume leads to better strength adaptations. In a recent study, participants who performed three sets increased strength over those who performed two sets, and those who performed two sets increased strength more than those who performed one set (Krieger, 2009). However, untrained individuals may achieve small increases in strength with performing one set.

Tempo

Repetition tempo refers to the speed with which each repetition is performed. This is an important variable for achieving specific training goals such as endurance, muscle growth, strength, and power. The movement occurs at different speeds in order to get the appropriate results from the training. The speed of the contraction used during exercise can affect the neural, hypertrophic, and metabolic response to resistance training, and is inversely related to training volume (Ballor, Becque, & Katch, 1987; Cronin, McNair, & Marshall, 2003; Hakkinen, Komi, & Alen, 1985; Mazzetti, Douglass, Yocum, & Harber, 2007; Sakamoto & Sinclair, 2006).

Slower training tempos are better for increasing endurance and initially developing motor control. Additionally, the eccentric portion of the contraction has been shown to have more force than the concentric phase of the contraction (Keogh, Wilson, & Weatherby, 1999). A slower tempo, especially during eccentric contractions, is recommended for stabilization training and with untrained individuals. The slower tempo also corresponds with the higher repetition ranges and decreased intensities of phase 1 of the OPT model.

Moderate training tempos have been shown to increase strength better than slow or fast tempos (Kanehisa & Miyashita, 1983). Therefore, a moderate training tempo is recommended for strength training.

Fast training tempos have been shown to produce better strength results when using maximal intensities, and the intent to lift the weight as fast as possible may be critical to maximizing performance gains (Jones, Hunter, Fleisig, Escamilla, & Lemak, 1999).

See **Table 10.1** for an overview of the assigned tempos for each phase of the OPT model.

TRAINER TIPS

A major benefit of using a slow tempo is the ability for the client to feel when his or her form is breaking down and to correct it. For example, if a client is using a faster tempo, it is very difficult to feel if the knees are caving in. By going slowly, a client can reinforce good movement patterns that will allow the use of faster tempo in later phases of the OPT model.

TABLE 10.1 Assigned Tempos for Each Phase of the OPT Model		
Tempo	**Adaptation**	**Phases**
Slow (4/2/1)	Endurance	1, 2
Moderate (2/0/2)	Strength	2, 3, 4
Fast (x/x/x)	Max strength, power	4, 5

CHECK IT OUT

The tempo is listed with three numbers (4/2/1, 2/0/2, etc.) The first number represents the seconds for the eccentric portion of the exercise. The middle number represents an isometric hold at the transition point of the exercise. The last number represents the number of seconds spent on the concentric portion of the exercise. The tempo x/x/x indicates that the exercise should be performed as fast as can be controlled.

Load and Intensity

Load is the amount of weight lifted, resistance used, or stability challenged, during training. Altering the load may affect an individual's hormonal, neural, and cardiovascular responses to exercise (Hayes et al., 2013). **Training intensity** is defined as an individual's level of effort compared to his or her maximal effort. This is usually represented as a percentage of the estimated one-repetition maximum (1RM). The load or training intensity used is dependent on several other acute variables, such as exercise selection, exercise order, volume, and rest period. It is important to consider the direct relationship load has to rest period, and the indirect relationship it typically has with volume, as shown in **Table 10.2**.

Rest Periods

A **rest period** is the time taken between sets or exercises to rest or recover. The amount of time taken for rest can significantly influence the adaptations and response to exercise. Rest periods are directly related to bioenergetic pathways and energy production, and are indirectly related to load and training intensity. Exercises performed at lower intensity can be performed for longer periods of time because the body is able to utilize oxygen, and therefore does not require much rest to recover. In contrast, when exercises are performed at much higher intensity for shorter periods of time, the body is not able to use oxygen and energy stores are quickly

Load
The amount of weight lifted or resistance used during training.

Training intensity
An individual's level of effort, compared with his or her maximal effort, usually expressed as a percentage.

Rest period
The time taken between sets or exercises to rest or recover.

TABLE 10.2 Load and Intensity	
As Load Increases	**As Load Decreases**
Volume decreases	Volume increases
Rest period increases	Rest period decreases

TABLE 10.3 Rest Period and Percent Recovery	
Amount of Rest	**Percent Recovery**
20–30 seconds	50%
40 seconds	75%
60 seconds	85–90%
3–5 minutes	100%

TABLE 10.4 Rest Period by Phase	
Phase of OPT Model	**Rest Period**
Muscular endurance and stabilization	0–90 seconds
Hypertrophy	0–60 seconds
Maximal strength	3–5 minutes
Power	3–5 minutes

depleted; thus the body requires longer rest periods. **Table 10.3** provides suggested recovery times following depletion of ATP (Harris et al., 1976).

The percentages shown in Table 10.3 are estimates. Recovery time can change based on conditioning. The more someone trains a particular energy system, the more efficient recovery becomes.

The recommendations presented in **Table 10.4** are based on the primary adaptation a client is seeking. This will be based on the goals of the training session and the phase of the OPT model.

The rest period is the most commonly misinterpreted acute variable during training sessions. Many exercise participants are relatively untrained and have an expectation of needing to take a break regularly throughout their sessions. However, only those individuals who are training close to their maximum effort need longer rest durations.

Exercise Selection

Exercise selection is the process of choosing exercises that allow for achievement of the desired change, or adaptation. Exercises should be specific to the client's desired training goals. The OPT model uses an integrated approach by applying exercises from all components of fitness (i.e., core, balance, reactive, resistance, and speed, agility, and quickness [SAQ] training). The primary adaptations follow the levels of the OPT model: Stabilization, Strength, and Power. The choice of exercise determines the muscle groups to be worked and the position in which they will be worked. For example, consider a squat compared to a seated knee extension. A squat is a multi-joint movement that uses large muscles in a complex fashion, requiring coordination with the goal of increasing strength. In contrast, a seated knee extension isolates one muscle, requires little coordination, and may result in increased hypertrophy of only the quadriceps. Both exercises are essentially for the lower body, but each achieves a different result.

Exercise selection

The process of choosing exercises that allow for achievement of the desired adaptation.

Order of Exercises

The order in which exercises are programmed can have an impact on the results of the training session. It has been found that the number of repetitions and sets (volume) was greater for those exercises performed at the beginning of a session compared to those performed at the end (Simao, Freitas de Salles, Figueiredo, Dias, & Willardson, 2012). Therefore, greater strength gains were seen in the first exercise of the training program. Similarly, it was discovered that during a circuit training session the exercises performed first had more repetitions than those performed last, regardless of the number of joints used or the size of the muscles involved (Piraua et al., 2013). Both of these studies suggest that the order of the exercise makes the difference, not the number of joints included, as has been previously taught. Exercises should be prioritized according to the individual's needs and training objectives.

Starting Program Design

Program design is the creation of a purposeful system or plan to achieve a goal. The OPT model is a proven, easy-to-use system of **periodization** that can be used to create a program for almost any client. When designing a program, the fitness professional must consider the following three questions:

1. Is it safe?
2. Is it based on findings from a comprehensive assessment?
3. Does it align with the client's goals?

Fitness professionals' most important job is to keep their clients safe when performing physical activity. Many injuries occur due to improper use of equipment, or use of equipment that has not been properly maintained. It is the fitness professional's responsibility to check the equipment before use. If employed in a health club, the fitness professional should also be proactive and check the equipment on a daily basis to ensure member safety.

Linear Periodization

Periodization refers to the planned changes in the acute variables of the training program. The planned changes are designed to result in physical changes that align with clients' goals. One of the most important aspects of periodization is to prevent injuries that can occur due to overtraining.

Linear periodization refers to classic or traditional strength and power training programming. It begins with high-volume, low-intensity training and progresses toward low-volume, high-intensity training. For example, many traditional strength athletes begin with lighter weight and higher repetitions. They slowly progress by decreasing repetitions as weight is added. With linear periodization, there will be slight percentage increases every week, with the majority of the training session being exactly the same. This type of programming usually lasts for many months and consists of 4–6 weeks of training in specific phases (see Figure 10.1). Each phase of training has unique goals to be achieved.

Following the OPT model from Phase 1 through Phase 5 is an example of linear periodization (**Figure 10.2**). Clients move to the next phase in the progression every 4–6 weeks based on their progress. The program begins at a level of low intensity and high volume, moves to moderate intensity and moderate volume, and ends at high intensity and low volume. The program is designed to first achieve the goal of stabilization, then to increase strength, ending with

Client Name:		Day 1	Day 2	Day 3	Day 4	Day 5	Day 6	Day 7
Start Date: Jan 31	Phase	Phase 2		Phase 2		Phase 2		
Progress Tracking Weight: 150 Body Fat: 33% Blood Pressure: N/A Resting HR: 70 Main Dysfunction: Knee Adduction		Super Sets 10 Reps 2 Sets 75%	Client Cardio and Corrective Flexibility Program Homework	Super Sets 10 Reps 2 Sets 75%	Client Cardio and Corrective Flexibility Program Homework	Super Sets 10 Reps 2 Sets 75%	Client Cardio and Corrective Flexibility Program Homework	Rest Day Light Cardio and Corrective Flexibility Program Homework
Cardio List cardio exercises		Stage 2 Zone 1: 130 BPM Zone 2: 150 BPM	Stage 1 130 BPM 30 Minutes	Stage 2 Zone 1: 130 BPM Zone 2: 150 BPM	Stage 1 130 BPM 30 Minutes	Stage 2 Zone 1: 130 BPM Zone 2: 150 BPM	Stage 1 130 BPM 30 Minutes	30 minute walk
Flexibility List flexibility exercises		SMR and Active Isolated Calves, Add., Lats	SMR and Static Calves, Adductors, TFL	SMR and Active Isolated Calves, Add., Lats	SMR and Static Calves, Adductors, TFL	SMR and Active Isolated Calves, Add., Lats	SMR and Static Calves, Adductors, TFL	SMR and Static Calves, Adductors, TFL
Re-assessment List assessments conducted							OHS, Body Fat, Circumference	

FIGURE 10.2 Weekly program based on linear periodization.

developing power. Linear periodization is a great way to begin working with untrained clients. The systematic progression with its accompanying goals and objectives ensures that clients are properly adapted before they move to the next phase. Most strength experts use this form of periodization (Herodek, Simonovic, & Rakovic, 2012).

In addition, linear periodization is helpful in teaching clients new skills. Balance, for example, is a learned skill that many people take for granted. A new client will learn balance training quicker if it is practiced consistently several times per week, as opposed to varying up the training on a daily basis. Learning a new skill takes mindful repetition. However, although linear periodization has its benefits, it has not been scientifically proven to be more beneficial than other types of periodization.

Undulating Periodization

Undulating periodization, sometimes referred to as *nonlinear periodization*, is a form of periodization that provides changes in the acute variables of workouts to achieve different goals on a daily or weekly basis. The undulation stays within the set phases of training, but it allows some variation within the progressions. Undulating periodization allows the client to train at varying intensities during a specific training cycle. This allows for multiple adaptations to be addressed in a single cycle. A typical undulating program would follow a 14-day cycle, with three or four different workouts. An example of undulating periodization is for the client to perform a stabilization workout on Monday, a strength workout on Wednesday, and a power workout on Friday.

Undulating periodization has been found to be very effective. In some studies it has been shown to be as, or more, effective as linear periodization at building muscle and strength (Marx et al., 2001; Rhea & Alderman, 2004). In addition, it has also been suggested that this form of periodization could prove to be more flexible for the client in certain circumstances (Herodek et al., 2012). If the client was scheduled to perform a power workout on Friday but had unusual muscle soreness from Wednesday's workout, the client could perform a stabilization workout instead. The opposite is also true. If a client shows up to a session extraordinarily motivated, a more intense work could be performed than was originally planned. In addition, research supports the use of undulating training to help reduce accumulated neural fatigue (Komi, 1986).

Applying Undulating Periodization to the OPT Model

Undulating periodization can be incorporated into the OPT model in several different ways. The fitness professional may choose to change up any of the acute variables, either daily or weekly.

> **Undulating periodization**
>
> A form of periodization that provides changes in the acute variables of workouts to achieve different goals on a daily or weekly basis.

TRAINER TIPS

Undulated periodization is a great way to program for athletes. It can be used to help athletes peak on a weekly basis rather than on a seasonal basis. It can also help the multisport athlete who needs recovery time but may not experience extended off-season periods.

CHECK IT OUT ✓

Undulating periodization is not only effective, but also fun! Traditional planning, which can occur months in advance, is often rigid and does not allow for the variation necessary to work with each client. When using the OPT model, it is suggested that the client should be able to successfully complete the phase in which he or she has been placed. It is important to plan intelligently while allowing the client to experience different training phases safely and effectively.

For the general fitness client, the type of training chosen for the day should be focused on goals as well as how the client is feeling. Many clients have high levels of stress in their lives that can have a significant impact on their day-to-day progressions. Fitness professionals should use every opportunity to help their clients feel successful and teach them how to apply the training to their everyday lives. The fitness professional should be prepared to modify the session accordingly for each client each day.

This can also be referred to as flexible nonlinear periodization. This type of periodization uses undulating periodization but allows for changes based on the client's readiness. It is suggested to test clients prior to the training session in order to determine readiness for a specific phase of training. Although a test is an accurate way to measure a baseline, it is always recommended to speak to clients about their readiness and use the first few minutes of the exercise session to help determine what phase they should be in. For example, if a client cannot perform 10 repetitions of a weight done on a previous session, then he or she may be experiencing fatigue (Fleck, 2011). In addition, clients should not be expected to perform an exercise that is beyond their training threshold. For example, a client in Phase 1 should not perform a Phase 5 power workout with maximum intensity if she has never trained at maximum intensity previously. Instead, if the Phase 1 client has demonstrated the coordination and ability to handle increased loads with the rapid accelerations and decelerations necessary for power training, then she could perform a Phase 5 workout at 80% intensity and be safe.

All exercise programs should be based on a movement assessment of the client and muscle imbalances should be addressed as a part of the training program. It is not advised to include an exercise that the client cannot perform proficiently in the undulated training program. Whereas research has found that participants who performed undulating periodization with a fitness professional had greater increases in strength, power, lean body mass, and aerobic capacity compared those who did not. The study also consisted of 1 month of functional and core exercises to correct movement imbalances (Storer, Dolezal, Berenc, Timmins, & Cooper, 2014).

The OPT model can be used in an undulating, nonlinear fashion in two different ways:

1. Using weekly cycles composed of various phases of the OPT model.
2. Using weekly cycles composed of one phase of the OPT model, but with intensities and volume varied throughout the week.

See **Figures 10.3** and **10.4** for two examples of using undulating periodization with the OPT model.

Utilizing Templates for OPT Programming

Programming templates serve several different purposes. They offer guidance and structure to the fitness professional and client, allow for accurate record keeping, and preserve historical and critical data. One of the major hurdles fitness professionals face is that they cannot be with the client every day. However, fitness professionals who provide their clients with a detailed template will eliminate much of the error associated with free time. When the clients know when, where, how, and why they need to be performing something, they are much more likely to be compliant. The programming template provides the homework.

The client should be assigned homework as part of the professional training program. In many cases the exercises done on one day may simply be repeated by the client on the next gym day. This is more applicable for phase 1 where there is not as much of an increase in load and volume, but it can be used in any phase depending on the client's schedule. Remember

Client Name:	Week 1							Week 2							Week 3							Week 4						
Start Date:	M	T	W	T	F	S	S	M	T	W	T	F	S	S	M	T	W	T	F	S	S	M	T	W	T	F	S	S
Phase 1: Stabilization Training	X							X														X						
Phase 2: Strength Training			X							X							X							X				
Phase 3: Hypertrophy																												
Phase 4: Maximal Strength Training				X															X									
Phase 5: Power Training												X														X		

	Week 1	Week 2	Week 3	Week 4
Cardio List cardio exercises	Workout Specific	Workout Specific	Workout Specific	Workout Specific
Flexibility List flexibility exercises	SMR-Calves, Adductors, Lats Static-Calves, Adductors, Lats 5–7 days/week Active/DROM Workout Specific	SMR-Calves, Adductors, Lats Static-Calves Adductors, Lats 5–7 days/week Active/DROM Workout Specific	SMR-Calves, Adductors, Lats Static-Calves, Adductors, Lats 5–7 days/week Active/DROM Workout Specific	SMR-Calves, Adductors, Lats Static-Calves, Adductors, Lats 5–7 days/week Active/DROM Workout Specific
Re-assessment List assessments conducted	Weight-185 (No change) Body Fat%-16% (no change) RHR-68 (Down 2 BPM)	N/A	N/A	Reassess next week.

Notes and Observations:
Working on developing overall strength and power. Flexibility and cardio workouts need to be workout specific. Next assessments need to look at performance assessment measures including vertical jump and 40. Also need to reassess OHS to verify whether a full Phase 1 needs to be readdressed.

FIGURE 10.3 Undulating periodization: Weekly Program 1

	Week 1							Week 2							Week 3							Week 4						
Client Name:																												
Start Date:	M	T	W	T	F	S	S	M	T	W	T	F	S	S	M	T	W	T	F	S	S	M	T	W	T	F	S	S
Phase 1: Stabilization Training	X		X		X																							
Phase 2: Strength Training								X		X		X																
Phase 3: Hypertrophy																												
Phase 4: Maximal Strength Training															X		X		X									
Phase 5: Power Training																						X		X		X		

	Week 1	Week 2	Week 3	Week 4
Cardio List cardio exercises	Perform Stage 1 cardio utilizing client modality choice 3 times. THR-68-72%=127-135 30 Minutes	Perform Stage 2 cardio with intervals in workouts. Repeat Stage 1 workout on off-days.	Perform Stage 2 cardio with intervals in workouts. Repeat Stage 1 workout on off-days.	Perform Stage 3 cardio with intervals in workouts. Repeat Stage 1 workout on off-days.
Flexibility List flexibility exercises	SMR-Calves, Adductors, Lats Static-Calves, Adductors, Lats 5-7 days/week	SMR-Calves, Adductors, Lats Active Iso-Calves, Adductors, Lats Static: 5-7 days/week	SMR-Calves, Adductors, Lats Active Iso-Calves, Adductors, Lats Static: 5-7 days/week	SMR-Calves, Adductors, Lats DROM-Workout Specific Static: 5-7 days/week
Re-assessment List assessments conducted	Weight-185 (No change) Body Fat%-16% (no change) RHR-68 (Down 2 BPM)	N/A	N/A	Reassess next week.

FIGURE 10.4 Undulating periodization: Weekly Program 2.

Notes and Observations:
Week 1 and 2: Low Intensity Day 1, Medium Intensity Day 2, High Intensity Day 3
Week 3: Upper Body Medium Intensity Day 1, Lower Body Medium Intensity Day 2, Upper Body High Intensity Day 3, Lower Body High Intensity Day 4
Week 4: Low Intensity Day 1, Medium Intensity Day 2, High Intensity Day 3

that the focus of phase 1 is on learning proper movement patterns; therefore, repetition is necessary. However, the movement must be repeated properly, so the client may need more practice with the fitness professional before being on his or her own. The body adapts to continuous stimuli, so homework should be used to provide it on days between official meetings with the client. The best way to provide clients with selected exercises is to offer them a simple template with all the information needed.

Client Homework

Homework should include exercises that engage the clients and help them progress toward their goals. In many forms of psychotherapy, it has been found that the clients who are given work to do outside of the session have the best outcomes (Shaw, 1999). Several different factors should be considered when convincing clients to complete homework:

- *Client attitudes toward homework.* Try to avoid the negative connotation that often comes with the word "homework." It is important to get clients to realize that repetition enables them to progress more quickly.
- *Client goals.* Many clients pursuing a weight loss goal suffer from a lack of motivation or even anxiety toward exercise. Some will be motivated to go the gym and perform an hour-long workout session without the trainer, whereas others may prefer to perform flexibility and light cardio, such as a walk in the neighborhood. Studies suggest that involving the client in the planning will result in better completion rates compared to those who are not involved (Freeman & Rosenfield, 2002). In addition, a proper explanation of each exercise and an emphasis on a collaborative strategy yields better adherence to homework (Glaser, Kazantzis, Deane, & Oades, 2000).
- *Task difficulty.* Studies suggest that homework that is too difficult, or that provokes anxiety, is less likely to be completed than homework that is doable (Broder, 2000). To encourage completion, training should begin with simple tasks and fitness professionals should periodically assess the client's readiness to take on more complex exercises. In addition to the difficulty of the task, consider the client's comprehension of what is being assigned. The vocabulary professionals use is often very different from what clients understand. Therefore, consider using pictures and less formal terminology, where available, to support the homework.

Figure 10.5 is an example of a simple homework template for a client. It provides detail but is not overwhelming, and thus should be easily completed by most clients.

Trainer Templates and Record Keeping

In order to keep track of each client's progress, it is important to keep records of each session. This record keeping will be an asset to the client now and in the future. For the fitness professional, this is the foundation of a good business. Informative records do not ensure success, but success without them is unlikely. Think of training templates as being similar to a report card. With a record, the professional and the client can follow goal progression and adjust the program as necessary to achieve the goal. For example, keeping accurate templates may show that a client is progressing well with core work but not with balance. This would indicate a need to focus more on balance work while maintaining core adaptations.

Client Homework Program

Name:			
Date:			
Goal:			
Phase:			

WARM-UP

Exercise	Sets	Duration	Coaching Tip
SMR			
Flexibility			

MOVEMENT PREP

Exercise	Sets by Rep	Tempo	Rest	Coaching Tip

WORKOUT

Exercise	Sets by Rep	Tempo	Rest	Intensity	Coaching Tip

COOL-DOWN

Exercise	Sets	Duration	Coaching Tip

Notes and Observations:

FIGURE 10.5 Homework template.

A training template should track five items: phase of training, exercises used, intensity of exercise, volume (reps × sets), and a measure of the outcome (e.g., "great session" or "needs improvement"). Each of these is described in detail below:

1. *Phase of training*. Having the phase number on the top of the template will allow for quick reference when planning the program. Each time a phase is revisited it should be more challenging than the last time it was performed. The fitness professional can revisit older templates from the same phase to guide future programming.
2. *Exercise selection*. It is essential that the trainer know exactly what exercises were performed in the previous session, and how they were performed. A mistake many new fitness

professionals make is not accurately recording the exercises used. This may prevent the client from making the necessary progressions.

3. *Intensity*. The intensity of the training may be the most variable over time, and the fitness professional must have a record of the intended intensity for a training session as well as the intensity of the previous session.

4. *Volume*. The importance of recording this information again lies in the need for progression. Throughout the training, the fitness professional must always be aware of the current volume, to be able to determine how the next sessions can progress. For example, if a client in Phase 3 is performing three sets of 12 repetitions, then the next progression may be to increase to four sets and drop to six or eight repetitions.

5. *Outcome*. Success is measured by the client being able to perform, and his or her confidence in performing the exercises. Research suggests that one of the primary indicators of weight loss failure or weight regain is feeling unsure about the success of a future weight loss program (Byrne, Cooper, & Fairburn, 2004). Therefore, it would stand to reason that a client needs to feel as though he or she has completed the majority of tasks satisfactorily. At the conclusion of the session, the fitness professional should spend a few minutes getting the client's opinions on the session to make the necessary adjustments.

Templates for Fitness Professionals

It is important for the fitness professional to know how and when to use each template. This tracking, or record keeping, should begin with the daily routine and extend all the way through the entire year of training. All programs should be written in advance, but specific details need not be added until the training actually occurs. The templates should be a general overview for both the professional and the client. Think of them as a quick reference guide to know when and where the client will be in a specific week or month during the year.

Yearly Programming

Tracking annual progress is an important job for the fitness professional. In order to ensure that goals are met and lifestyle changes are being adopted, a long-term plan and tracking system should be in place. A year-long program can be created within minutes using the OPT model. This will show clients where they can be if they stay motivated and stick with the program.

When designing the yearly plan, also known as a *macrocycle*, simply consider the phase of training that should be followed based on the client's goals. For example, a client seeking fat reduction will be in Phases 1, 2, and 5. In between each phase is a scheduled assessment, and expected outcomes related to goals. The template in **Figure 10.6** is an example of a yearly

CHECK IT OUT

Some programming terms are interchangeable within the industry:

Annual plan = Macrocycle
Monthly plan = Mesocycle
Weekly plan = Microcycle

Client Name:	JAN	FEB	MAR	APR	MAY	JUN	JUL	AUG	SEP	OCT	NOV	DEC
Month Started ⟹	Jan-2											
Phase 1: Stabilization Training	X											
Phase 2: Strength Training		X		X			X			X		
Phase 3: Hypertrophy					X			X			X	
Phase 4: Maximal Strength Training												
Phase 5: Power Training			X			X			X			X
Cardio List the stage that your client focused on.	Stage 1	Stage 2	Stage 3 and Stage 1	Stage 2	Stage 2	Stage 3 and Stage 1	Stage 1	Stage 2	Stage 3 and Stage 1	Stage 2	Stage 2	Stage 3 and Stage 1
Future Planning List the goals that the client will accomplish throughout the year. **Main Goal to Lose 50 Pounds!**	194 (–6)	188 (–6)	182 (–6)	176 (–6)	170 (–6)	164 (–6)	158 (–6)	152 (–6)	150!! Readdress Goals	??	??	??

FIGURE 10.6 Annual program.

program for a client with a goal of losing 50 pounds over the next year. With proper training, program adherence, and nutrition, it is healthy to lose up to 2 pounds per week. However, the template in Figure 10.6 uses 1.5 pounds lost per week as an average. After that, the goals will be reevaluated and a maintenance goal may be set for the remainder of the year. The purpose of writing down the desired outcome is to encourage clients to think positively and see that their goal can become a reality much quicker than they think.

The yearly program template should be shared with clients at the beginning of their training. It is important that the fitness professional demonstrate his or her level of commitment. Templates should be available in digital format so that they can be easily modified for each client. In addition, they should also be printed out, placing one paper copy in the client's file and sending the other home with the client.

Monthly Programming

Monthly tracking should include more than a simple check-in with progress updates. Each month the fitness professional should perform objective assessments. These include re-measuring the client's body composition, weight, blood pressure (if necessary), and heart rate, and performing the overhead squat assessment and any other necessary movement assessments. These reassessments should be used to monitor progress toward the client's goals and will provide information as to whether the current program needs to be adjusted.

When clients know that a monthly assessment is scheduled and coming up, they will likely better adhere to the fitness professional's recommendations. These reassessments can also help to increase client participation by putting more responsibility on the clients, making them active participants in working toward their goals. Reassessing clients shows professionalism and increases client retention. This will help further establish the fitness professional's credibility and professionalism.

Several weekly cycles can be put together to make up a monthly cycle, also known as a *mesocycle*. This monthly plan should include the progress update; including the reassessment data for that particular month. **Figure 10.7** shows a template for a monthly program featuring nonlinear periodization.

Weekly Programming

The weekly template is used to lay out a specific workout along with rest periods throughout the week. This is often referred to as a *microcycle*. Tracking weekly progress and checking in with clients is a great way to be sure they are staying motivated. Part of motivation is understanding that small decisions add up to big changes. These could include things as little as progressing to a an exercise by one rep, to as big as losing a couple of pounds. In addition, weekly tracking should include a check-in on how the client is feeling about the training. Clients make a significant financial investment for personal training. The fitness professional should use this time to let them know they have made the correct investment by fulfilling the customer service component. If there is something the client is unsatisfied with, the professional should catch it and make any necessary adjustments. A simple way to gather feedback is through an electronic survey. This is something that clients may complete on their own time, but it is necessary to provide them with a "due date" to ensure they complete it.

Weekly programs should be designed with the movement assessment in mind, and the body should be trained accordingly throughout the week. Volume is an acute variable that many consider on a daily basis. However, the fitness professional should be considering it on a weekly or biweekly basis. For example, if a client is training 3 days per week, and leg exercises are included all 3 days, the volume for legs after 2 weeks will be very high. This allows for more variation and broader application of program design, especially when using the undulating periodization. **Figure 10.8** offers an example weekly programming template featuring nonlinear periodization.

	Week 1							Week 2							Week 3							Week 4						
Client Name:																												
Start Date:	M	T	W	T	F	S	S	M	T	W	T	F	S	S	M	T	W	T	F	S	S	M	T	W	T	F	S	S
Phase 1: Stabilization Training	A		B		A			A		B		A			A		B		A			A		B		A		B
Phase 2: Strength Training																												
Phase 3: Hypertrophy																												
Phase 4: Maximal Strength Training																												
Phase 5: Power Training																												

	Week 1	Week 2	Week 3	Week 4
Cardio List cardio exercises	Workout Specific	Workout Specific	Workout Specific	Workout Specific
Flexibility List flexibility exercises	SMR-Calves, Adductors, Lats Static-Calves, Adductors, Lats 5-7 days/week	SMR-Calves, Adductors, Lats Static-Calves, Adductors, Lats 5-7 days/week	SMR-Calves, Adductors, Lats Static-Calves, Adductors, Lats 5-7 days/week	SMR-Calves, Adductors, Lats Static-Calves, Adductors, Lats 5-7 days/week
Re-assessment List assessments conducted	Weight-200 (Down 4 pounds) Body Fat%-22% (Down 2%) RHR-68 (Down 2 BPM)	N/A	N/A	Reassess next week.

Notes and Observations:
Overall Goal-Weight Loss/Body Fat Loss
Alternate Days with A and B:
A: 50% Intensity   **B:** 70% Intensity
    15-20 Reps   12-15 Reps

FIGURE 10.7 Monthly program.

Client Name:		Day 1	Day 2	Day 3	Day 4	Day 5	Day 6	Day 7
Start Date: Jan 31	Phase	Phase 2				Phase 2		
Progress Tracking Weight: 150 Body Fat: 33% Blood Pressure: N/A Resting HR: 70 Main Dysfunction: Knee Adduction		Super Sets 10 Reps 2 Sets 75%	Client Cardio and Corrective Flexibility Program Homework	Super Sets 10 Reps 2 Sets 75%	Client Cardio and Corrective Flexibility Program Homework	Super Sets 10 Reps 2 Sets 75%	Client Cardio and Corrective Flexibility Program Homework	Rest Day Light Cardio and Corrective Flexibility Program Homework
Cardio List cardio exercises		Stage 2 Zone 1: 130 BPM Zone 2: 150 BPM	Stage 1 130 BPM 30 Minutes	Stage 2 Zone 1: 130 BPM Zone 2: 150 BPM	Stage 1 130 BPM 30 Minutes	Stage 2 Zone 1: 130 BPM Zone 2: 150 BPM	Stage 1 130 BPM 30 Minutes	30-Minute Walk
Flexibility List flexibility exercises		SMR and Active Isolated Calves, Add., Lats	SMR and Static Calves, Adductors, TFL	SMR and Active Isolated Calves, Add., Lats	SMR and Static Calves, Adductors TFL	SMR and Active Isolated Calves, Add., Lats	SMR and Static Calves, Adductors, TFL	SMR and Static Calves, Adductors, TFL
Re-assessment List assessments conducted							OHS, Body Fat, Circumference	

FIGURE 10.8 Weekly program.

CHECK IT OUT

Surveys can be created for free using various online tools. The survey should be short and take the client no longer than 5 minutes to complete. The client should be reminded that it is an anonymous survey aimed at improving the trainer's personal fitness training services. The following is a sample survey that could be used.

How satisfied are you with the results of the training?

Very satisfied   Satisfied   Neutral   Dissatisfied   Very dissatisfied

How satisfied are you with the cardio program?

Very satisfied   Satisfied   Neutral   Dissatisfied   Very dissatisfied

How satisfied are you with resistance training program?

Very satisfied   Satisfied   Neutral   Dissatisfied   Very dissatisfied

How satisfied are you with the health club?

Very satisfied   Satisfied   Neutral   Dissatisfied   Very dissatisfied

How satisfied are you with the locker rooms?

Very satisfied   Satisfied   Neutral   Dissatisfied   Very dissatisfied

How likely are you to suggest personal training to a friend or family member?

Very likely   Likely   Neutral   Unlikely   Very unlikely

In one to two sentences please tell us what would make the experience better.

TRAINER TIPS

When planning for workouts, the fitness professional should keep in mind that sometimes a particular piece of equipment may not be available. The planned exercise does not always have to be identified by the specific piece of equipment used, but could rather include the joint action needed and a descriptor. For example, as opposed to writing a chest exercise as *standing cable chest press*, write the intended outcome, *unstable chest exercise*, and when the time comes the specific exercise can be noted. This allows some freedom to choose different options during the workout based on the availability of the equipment.

This template shows the phase, goal, intended intensity and repetitions, as well as the primary movement compensation being addressed. Much more could be filled in on this template, but as such it allows the professional to see the week ahead and communicate it effectively to the client. Notice the variation of intensity and volume throughout the week. The phase stays consistent for a new client, but the change in other variables follows the principles for nonlinear periodization.

Daily Programming: Designing the Workout

Daily programming is the most specific programming for the fitness professional. The fitness professional will use the weekly program as a guide and then select the exercises as needed to meet the client's goals. The daily program includes the following variables: client information (e.g. name, goal), integrated programming, muscles/joints used, intensity, volume, tempo, and rest period.

Note that placing the client's name and goal at the top of the daily program allows for quick reference as to who the client is and his or her particular goals. The top of the daily program also includes the number of days per week that the client trains.

The second item listed on the daily program is the integrated program. It includes the following components:

◆ Flexibility
◆ Core

- ◆ Balance
- ◆ Reactive
- ◆ SAQ
- ◆ Resistance

Two to 3 muscles or body areas should be chosen to focus on for flexibility. It is important to remember the amount of time spent with the client, and to plan accordingly with regards to how much time to spend on flexibility. Some clients may need more time in flexibility than others.

The resistance training section will require the most amount of time with regards to planning and implementation. Within resistance training, the fitness professional will select total body, upper body, and lower body exercises. Programming must consider exercise order (e.g., multi-joint before single-joint) and plane of motion (sagittal plane, frontal plane, or transverse plane).

The last section of the daily template is the cool-down. The most important aspect of this section is to perform some additional flexibility to reduce the chance of additional muscle imbalance, as well as to help increase total body circulation to speed up the recovery process.

If used appropriately, the daily template is designed to guide the fitness professional and client through the session. The professional should be prepared to adapt selected exercises from the workout based upon time constraints, equipment availability, and the client's capability on that given day. When all components of the daily template are assembled, it will look similar to the template shown in **Figure 10.9**.

Recording Completed Training Sessions

Recording the actual training session involves providing detail as to what was accomplished during the workout. Due to changing circumstances, adaptations may have been made to the workout, and a record should be kept of the changes that were made. In addition, the outcome of the session should be noted on the daily template. This will help with future planning of workouts.

The completed daily programming template should include details so that it looks similar to the template shown in **Figure 10.10**.

The information recorded on the daily programming template after the session will include the exercises performed, their volume and intensity, and needed rest. This allows for easy progressions at the next session. For example, the rest period can play a vital role in intensity. On day 3, when this template is repeated, the intensity of the chest exercise may be increased by eliminating the rest period.

The monthly programming template should also be used as a tool to reflect on program adherence and updating accordingly. The outcomes of the monthly tracking tool will be recorded in the reassessment. The yearly programming template will be reflections of the program's overall success with goal setting.

Templates for Clients

Client templates are less detailed and more goal oriented. Clients should be provided with monthly and yearly programs. These can serve as a reminder for what the upcoming weeks and months will entail. Some of the details may be modified on the templates. Clients may or may not want a daily programming template. However, clients should be provided a workout template for their homework between sessions. It is recommended that the client's homework be written with the necessary details, but at a level to be properly understood.

TRAINER TIPS

A rest period is recommended if the client has been performing vertical loading for the resistance section. If using vertical loading, the client would have had minimal rest thus far. The client may have performed one set of core, balance, and then reactive exercises back-to-back. Therefore, taking a quick break here would be indicated before performing the second set of core, balance, and reactive. This should be used to reduce rest periods and use the time of the session more efficiently.

TRAINER TIPS

If your program does not include a total body exercise, then move the leg exercise up to the first spot as opposed to starting with the chest exercise on the template. Ideally, you start a program with the largest muscle group or most complex exercise and progress to smaller muscle groups and less complex movements.

WARM-UP			
Exercise	**Sets**	**Duration**	**Coaching Tip**
SMR Calves, Adductors, TFL	1	30 Seconds or Until Muscle Releases	
Flexibility Calves, Adductors, TFL	1	30-Second Static Hold	

MOVEMENT PREP				
Exercise	**Sets by Rep**	**Tempo**	**Rest**	**Coaching Tip**
Prone Iso-abs	1 × 12	15 s Hold	15 s	
Supine floor bridge	1 × 20	4/2/1	15 s	
SL reach	1 × 8 ea. Leg	4/2/1	15 s	
Squat jump hold	1 × 8	3-5 s Hold	15 s	
Ladder 1 ins	1 × 2	Controlled	N/A	Focus on Form

RESISTANCE					
Exercise	**Sets by Rep**	**Tempo**	**Rest**	**Intensity**	**Coaching Tip**
Squat to row	1 × 17	4/2/1	0 s	30	
Push-up	1 × 17	4/2/1	0 s	BDW	
SL Wide Row	1 × 17	4/2/1	0 s	15	
SL DB scaption	1 × 17	4/2/1	0 s	8	
SL DB curl	1 × 17	4/2/1	0 s	12	
SL triceps ext.	1 × 17	4/2/1	0 s	12	
Lunge to balance	1 × 8 ea. Leg	4/2/1	30 s	BDW	

COOL-DOWN			
Exercise	**Sets**	**Duration**	**Coaching Tip**
Calves, Adductors, TFL	1	30 s	SMR
Calves, Adductors, TFL	1	30 s	Static Stretch

Notes and Observations:
Focus on Knees Adduction Correction

FIGURE 10.9 Daily program.

CHECK IT OUT

Flexibility, core, balance, reactive, and SAQ training can be combined and referred to as *movement prep*. These exercises are optional depending on the phase of the OPT model and can also be carried in their own individual workouts. When used in conjunction with a resistance training workout, they can serve as part of the movement prep warm-up to prepare the body for the work that is to come during the resistance portion of the workout.

WARM-UP			
Exercise	**Sets**	**Duration**	**Coaching Tip**
SMR Calves, Adductors, TFL	1	30 Seconds or Until Muscle Releases	
Flexibility Calves, Adductors, TFL	1	30-Second Static Hold	

MOVEMENT PREP				
Exercise	**Sets by Rep**	**Tempo**	**Rest**	**Coaching Tip**
Prone Iso-abs	1 × 12	15 s Hold	15 s	Had trouble with LB arch
Supine floor bridge	1 × 20	4/2/1	15 s	Looked good
SL reach	1 × 8 ea. Leg	4/2/1	15 s	Increase to 10 reps next
Squat jump hold	1 × 8	3-5 s Hold	15 s	Knees still add. on landing
Ladder 1 ins	1 × 2	Controlled	N/A	Focus on form

RESISTANCE					
Exercise	**Sets by Rep**	**Tempo**	**Rest**	**Intensity**	**Coaching Tip**
Squat to Row	1 × 17	4/2/1	0 s	30	Maintained weight
Push-up	1 × 17	4/2/1	0 s	BDW	Watch LB arch
SL Wide row	1 × 17	4/2/1	0 s	15	Actual 12 pounds
SL DB scaption	1 × 17	4/2/1	0 s	8	Actual 10 pounds
SL DB curl	1 × 17	4/2/1	0 s	12	Stayed
SL triceps ext.	1 × 17	4/2/1	0 s	12	Stayed
Lunge to balance	1 × 8 ea. Leg	4/2/1	30 s	BDW	Watch knee adduction

COOL-DOWN			
Exercise	**Sets**	**Duration**	**Coaching Tip**
Calves, Adductors, TFL	1	30 s	SMR
Calves, Adductors, TFL	1	30 s	Static Stretch

Notes and Observations:
Focus on Knees Adduction Correction.
Client felt tired today. Overall good workout. Nutrition sounds good. Need to continue to monitor nutrition logs. Still having trouble with the knees caving in. Client is getting better with movement patterns. Down 3 pounds on wide row. Probably due to energy levels. Monitor. Increase weight on DB scaption for next workouts. Increase reps of SL reach.

Due for OHS reassessment next week!!!

FIGURE 10.10 Daily program with actual training notes.

Yearly Programming Template for Clients

The yearly program provided to the client is similar to the template used by the fitness professional. The training phases are marked, and a spot for outcomes to be written every month is included (**Figure 10.11**). It is broken down into short, achievable goals associated with an action plan. However, if the first few target weights are not met, the yearly plan should be modified for the client. Do not let this turn into a reminder of unmet goals! The client can keep this document as a reminder of his or her long-term goals and the commitment the professional has made.

Client Name:	JAN	FEB	MAR	APR	MAY	JUN	JUL	AUG	SEP	OCT	NOV	DEC
Month Started ⇧	Mar-15											
Phase 1: Stabilization Training	X			X			X			X		
Phase 2: Strength Training		X			X			X			X	
Phase 3: Hypertrophy												
Phase 4: Maximal Strength Training												
Phase 5: Power Training			X			X			X			X
Cardio List the stage that your client focused on.	Stage 1	Stage 1	Stage 2	Stage 1	Stage 2	Stage 1 and Stage 3	Stage 1	Stage 2	Stage 3 and Stage 1	Stage 1	Stage 2	Stage 1 and Stage 1
Future Planning List the goals that the client will accomplish throughout the year. **LOSE 50 POUNDS!!**	Start 200								GOAL Date!! 150!!			
Progress Tracking Write down your client's measurable progress. PERSONAL TRACKER FOR YOU!! Record your weight here	Weight: 196	Weight: 194	Weight: 190	Weight: 185								

FIGURE 10.11 Yearly program for the client.

Monthly Programming Template for Clients

In an effort to make clients active participants, it is necessary for the fitness professional to provide a plan of action. The client should know what to expect over the next month. This includes the scheduled training days with the professional, cardio days (with intensity), active recovery days, and the scheduled reassessment. This will set the expectations for an entire course of training. It could be said that the monthly program for the client is the most important, yet most overlooked, aspect of success for the client. Many fitness professionals do not take the time to offer a monthly program, but they should strongly consider it.

Figure 10.12 is a monthly template that can be used by the client. The example template provides adequate detail about what will be occurring each day of the month in calendar form. In addition, there is a place for the client to fill in the cardio days with the actual time and intensity. This template can be hung somewhere in plain view for the client to see and review several times per day. The fitness professional can easily create a digital document that takes minimal time to edit and provide it to the client on the first session of each month.

The yearly and monthly program documents are vital for the clients. Everyone needs a plan and a method of tracking action steps needed to reach their goals. If a fitness professional is expecting a client to adhere to the program and be successful, the client must be provided with the necessary tools. The program begins with a hard document that explains the plan. Many organizations are moving toward providing all clients with digital copies of this information. This is adequate if it is updated and used properly.

SUN	MON	TUE	WED	THU	FRI	SAT
	1 Training Session A Light Day High Reps	**2** Flex Cardio 150 bpm 30 min	**3** Training Session B Moderate Day Lower Reps	**4** Flex Cardio 150 bpm 30 min	**5** Training Session A Light Day High Reps	**6** Flex Cardio 150 bpm 30 min
7 Active Recovery Foam Roll 45-minute walk	**8** Training Session B Moderate Day Lower Reps	**9** Flex Cardio 150 bpm 30 min	**10** Training Session A Light Day High Reps	**11** Flex Cardio 150 bpm 30 min	**12** Training Session B Moderate Day Lower Reps	**13** Flex Cardio 150 bpm 30 min
14 Active Recovery Foam Roll 45-minute walk	**15** Training Session A Light Day High Reps	**16** Flex Cardio 155 bpm 30 min	**17** Training Session B Moderate Day Lower Reps	**18** Flex Cardio 155 bpm 30 min	**19** Training Session A Light Day High Reps	**20** Flex Cardio 150 bpm 30 min
21 Active Recovery Foam Roll 45-minute walk	**22** Training Session B Moderate Day Lower Reps	**23** Flex Cardio 155 bpm 30 min	**24** Training Session A Light Day High Reps	**25** Flex Cardio 155 bpm 30 min	**26** Training Session B Moderate Day Lower Reps	**27** Flex Cardio 150 bpm 30 min
28 Active Recovery Foam Roll 45-minute walk	**29** Reassessment!	**30** **New Program**				

FIGURE 10.12 Monthly program for the client.

Assessment Outcomes and Program Design

Exercise programs should be designed based on the client's specific movement patterns. This is a key concept for program design, but unfortunately it is often either forgotten or overlooked. In fact, some fitness professionals may program exercises that make movement patterns worse! The movement assessment can serve two functions when it comes to programming: it shows the client's movement compensations and muscle imbalances, and it is an indication of how well the client can perform certain movements. If a client has a tough time performing the overhead squat, the professional should regress to an easier exercise until the movement compensations have been addressed.

Movement and Muscle Balance

The outcome of the program design is based on the client's ability to move efficiently. This will help the client to progress through the OPT model and reach the desired goals. Note that the *quality* of the movement should be considered over the *quantity*. All too often, quantity is the focus in an effort to maximize calorie burn or to focus on volume, and quality is neglected. In the initial phases of the OPT model, a focus on quantity over quality will slow the results and interfere with the development of a strong foundation.

Muscle imbalances can in large part be attributed to the client's lifestyle and daily activity pattern. There is no amount of foam-rolling, stretching, or strengthening that can correct poor daily habits. This is often seen when the client is not progressing after 1 month of proper training. If the overhead squat assessment is not getting better, either the program design needs to be considered or the daily patterns that occur outside of the gym need to be addressed by the fitness professional.

Fitness professionals should teach their clients how to move to when performing basic tasks throughout their day. The client learning how to move properly when not in the gym may be the most important factor when considering muscle imbalances. In fact, research suggests the majority of movement results can be attributed to how the client moves outside the presence of a fitness professional or physical therapist (Sahrmann, 2002). This will require the fitness professional to provide the client with movement-specific homework. For example, clients who are required to spend a great deal of time seated should be shown how to sit with better posture. It has been found that specific positioning of the computer screen, chair, and feet can have a profound impact on the mechanics of the body over time (Oha, Animagi, Paasuke, Coggon, & Merisalu, 2014).

CHECK IT OUT

Improper walking patterns can be caused by the shoes a person wears, leading to shortened calves over time, or by weakness in certain muscles around the hips and pelvis. Weak gluteals, for example, can lead to a decreased ability to push off during walking. In turn, the calves may become short and tight, causing the feet to turn out.

Assessment Considerations: Cardio

As with any form of exercise, the client's movement assessment needs to be considered when designing the cardiorespiratory programs. Many forms of cardio are effective at training the cardiorespiratory system, but may place undue stress on the musculoskeletal system. This stress can lead to common repetitive injuries, because the type of training may exacerbate the poor posture the client has throughout the day. For example, consider a sedentary office worker cycling. The position on the bike is often similar to sitting at a desk. Therefore, this individual may experience extra stress and discomfort near the low back, shoulders, and neck.

Fitness professionals should explain to the client why posture is an important consideration during cardio activities. Proper posture and form during cardio will help the body to use the correct muscles, leading to better movement, more calories burned, decreased chance of injury, and overall longevity and satisfaction with exercise. The following are some of the most common examples of poor cardio choices based on movement assessments along with recommendations for better options.

Cardio Considerations: Clients with Feet Turned Out

Clients whose feet turn out need to carefully consider all cardio that uses the lower extremities. Proper flexibility protocols must be adhered to before the activity. This would include self-myofascial release (SMR) and stretching for problematic muscles. Some types of cardio equipment are better than others for people with turned out feet. The following are considerations for clients with turned out feet:

◆ *Treadmill*: Treadmill use may need to be withheld for a short time for clients who cannot maintain their feet in a neutral position while walking.
◆ *Stair climber*: Stair climbers are a great form of exercise when used correctly (i.e., feet straight, knees in alignment, not slouching). However, with the feet turning out, the calves are usually overactive. On most stair climbers only the ball of the foot may be able to step on the platform. Every step will be relying heavily upon the calf muscles, which may make the movement compensation worse.

The following are suggested cardio activities for clients with turned out feet:

◆ *Treadmill*: Clients can use the treadmill *after* doing flexibility and if the speed is a level at which they can focus on keeping the five kinetic chain checkpoints aligned.
◆ *Elliptical trainer*: The elliptical trainer can be a great complement to clients with lower body compensations because it has a foot pad. When the client is on the elliptical, the foot can be positioned straight and the pad will help maintain it. In addition, the elliptical

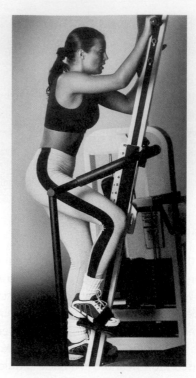

FIGURE 10.13 Versa climber.
© Stockbyte/Thinkstock

can be effective at engaging more of the glutes and posterior muscles, which may help improve the compensation.

◆ *Rowing machine*: Rowing machines can also be great for lower leg compensations. The foot is in a position that does not require as much control. However, the rowing machine may be very hip flexor centric, and if the tensor fascia latae (TFL) is causing the foot to turn out this may not be the best form of cardio.

◆ *Versa climber*: Versa climbers are another recommended form of cardio for the client with the feet turning out. The versa climber uses a foot pad that can assist in maintaining a neutral foot position (**Figure 10.13**)

Cardio Considerations: Clients with Anterior Pelvic Tilt

The fitness professional has more to consider when it comes to cardio for those clients who display an anterior pelvic tilt during the movement assessments. In order to avoid continuing to shorten the hip flexors and lengthen the hip extensors, seated positions should be replaced by upright positions whenever possible. This should be a main focus when programming for cardio with this compensation. The following should be kept in mind with regard to clients with anterior pelvic tilt:

◆ *Stationary bike/cycling*: The stationary bike or cycling is one of the more popular forms of cardio (**Figure 10.14**). Cycling is quadriceps and hip flexor dominant. Although there may be some gluteal and hamstring activity, the majority of the work is in the quadriceps. The ideal coordination for these activities is that as the individual is pressing down on the pedal the quadriceps should be working with the gluteals and calves (force-couple) to produce a powerful motion. However, in the client with anterior pelvic tilt, the quads are doing the majority of the work, and likely interfering with the ability of the gluteals to do their part. Therefore, time should be spent fixing the movement compensations to improve technique and power production if the client is going to participate in this activity.

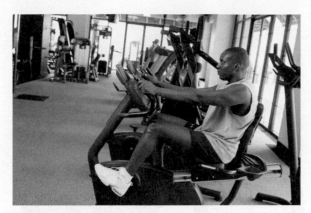

FIGURE 10.14 Recumbent bike.
© kenhurst/Shutterstock

- *Rowing machine*: Rowing machines are very quad and hip flexor dominant. Rowing should be withheld until the pelvic tilt is corrected or significantly reduced.
- *Stair climber or stepper*: Stair climbers or steppers could be great for gluteal activation and possibly reducing the pelvic tilt if the client can maintain the neutral pelvis during the activity. Unfortunately, most either cannot control or forget to control their pelvic position during the activity and perform the activity with the compensation present. This is still an effective method of burning calories, but it comes at the expense of form and function, likely making the movement compensation worse over time.
- *Treadmill*: Similar to the stair climber, if the client performs the recommended flexibility work and maintains the treadmill at a speed that is controllable, the treadmill is a recommended form of cardio. During proper gait, the hip should be able to extend and rely on the gluteal muscles to push the body forward. Clients should remain at a speed and incline that allows them to remain in control without holding on to the machine.

The following are suggested cardio activities for clients with anterior pelvic tilt:

- *Elliptical trainer*: The elliptical trainer is a great exercise as long as proper form is maintained.
- *Treadmill*: Treadmills can be suggested if performed *after* doing flexibility and if the speed is a level that the client can focus on keeping the five kinetic chain checkpoints aligned.

Cardio Considerations: Clients with Arms Falling Forward or Rounded Posture

Arms falling forward and rounded posture is another common compensation the fitness professional should be mindful of when programming cardio exercises. Many cardio exercises can be performed with good upper body posture as long as the individual is aware of it. The following are some exercises in which it is challenging to maintain good upper body posture:

- *Stationary bike/cycling*: In cycling, the aerodynamic position is to be rounded forward toward the handle bars (**Figure 10.15**). Although this may help reduce drag and increase speed, it is unfortunately a poor position for the upper body. Cycling with upright posture would be better for the client with upper body compensations.
- *Stair climber*: If performed correctly, the stair climber can be a great form of cardio for the person with upper body compensation. However, many people lean and slouch over the front of the machine. Doing this allows the upper body to take some of the weight off of the legs. Standing upright is better for the upper body and puts the weight back on the legs where it should be.

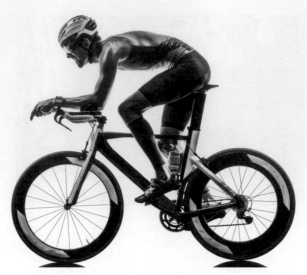

FIGURE 10.15 Cyclist in good aerodynamic form.
© ostill/Shutterstock

- *Treadmill*: Using a speed that is too high or an incline that is too steep will put clients in a situation in which they hold onto the machine to keep up with the belt. This holding on often pulls the upper body forward into the compensation.
- *Anything with a television*: Watching television is a popular way to pass time when performing steady-state cardio. However, the position of the TV may put the client into a bad position. If the TV is positioned too high, the individual may have to put the head into excessive extension, leading to the head protruding forward.

For those clients with arms falling forward or rounded posture, any form of cardio can work if proper posture is maintained. This is a mindful activity. If the client is not thinking about the upper body posture, then any form of cardio can make the compensation worse.

Assessment Considerations: Flexibility

Flexibility is the first opportunity the fitness professional has to improve quality of movement. If exercises are not performed correctly, it is likely that the movement compensations will never improve and may even get worse. The following should be considered with regard to flexibility:

- *Feet turn out*: The standing calf stretch (**Figure 10.16**) is intended to increase the length of the calf muscles, therefore reducing the compensation. When performing a standing calf stretch, the rear foot (leg being stretched) must be perfectly straight or slightly turned in. It is common for the client and trainer alike to let the toes turn out. This is moving through the compensation and possibly making it worse, not reducing it.
- *Anterior pelvic tilt*: The anterior pelvic tilt is typically caused by, or leads to, short and restricted hip flexors. Therefore, hip flexor stretches are usually the most beneficial stretch to include (**Figure 10.17**). It is common problem to perform this stretch with an anterior pelvic tilt. In order to reduce this, have the client perform a posterior tilt of the pelvis before moving too far into the stretch.

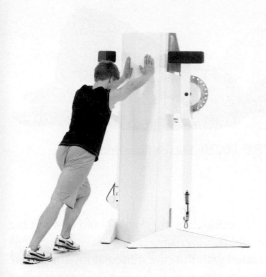

FIGURE 10.16 Standing calf stretch.

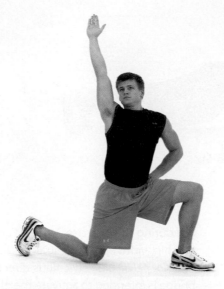

FIGURE 10.17 Kneeling hip flexor stretch.

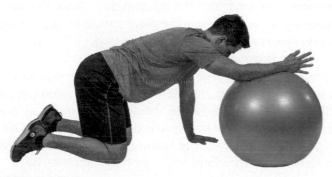

FIGURE 10.18 Ball lat stretch.

◆ *Arms falling forward*: Performing a latissimus dorsi (lats) stretch is a great way to combat this compensation (**Figure 10.18**). During the lat stretch, the hips must remain neutral. The lats attach to the arm and to the posterior aspect of the hips. Therefore, the position of the hips is important during the lat stretch. The fitness professional should have the client maintain a neutral position at the pelvis, or even go into a posterior tilt.

Assessment Considerations: Core

It is likely the client will have a weak or dysfunctional core and will want to use compensations to get through many of the core exercises. Therefore, it is important for the client maintain ideal alignment to avoid injury. Two valuable core exercises to consider are the supine bridge (**Figure 10.19**) and the prone iso-abs (**Figure 10.20**).

The following should be considered with regard to core exercises:

◆ *Feet turn out*: During the supine bridge, many clients will position their feet greater than hip width apart and rotated out. In order to activate the correct muscles the client should move the feet to hip width and keep them straight. It is common to see the toes turned

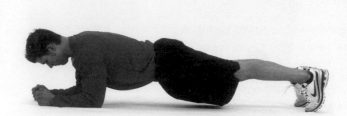

FIGURE 10.19 Prone iso-abs.

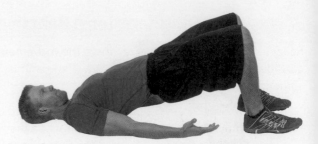

FIGURE 10.20 Supine floor bridge.

out during this exercise. To avoid activating the adductors the client should position the feet hip width apart and straight during the bridge.

- *Anterior pelvic tilt*: Pelvic tilt is directly associated with the core musculature. The supine bridge is intended to activate the gluteal muscles. However, those with an anterior pelvic tilt are likely to perform the exercise with an anterior pelvic tilt. This neglects the gluteals and increases tension in the low back. Clients should set their hips to neutral before performing this exercise and maintain this position throughout the movement. The prone iso-abs exercise is very similar, in that the client should be cued in the same manner as supine bridge to avoid compensations in the low back.

- *Arms falling forward*: Oftentimes, the lats are short, which will cause clients to arch their low back during the supine floor bridge. The fitness professional needs to consider hand position. A common hand and arm position during the prone iso-abs is to bring the hands together, internally rotating at the shoulders (also known as "praying hands"). This is an attempt to use the upper to body to compensate for the core. This position shortens the lats and pectorals, which may lead to the arms falling forward. The arms should run parallel to each other when performing the prone iso-abs exercise.

Assessment Considerations: Balance

Throughout the OPT model, balance training is an important component that helps to teach coordination and proprioception. Therefore, maintaining ideal form is essential. Consider the single-leg balance exercise:

- *Feet turn out*: With this compensation, the foot will turn out with the increased challenge of balance training in an attempt to increase the base of support. If this is allowed, then the compensation may become worse.

- *Anterior pelvic tilt*: Single-leg balance is an exercise that can be incredibly demanding on the muscles around the hips and spine. Therefore, it is not unusual to see a client demonstrate compensations around the hips during this exercise. During single-leg stance the gluteal muscles need to work with the abdominal muscles to keep the hips and the stance leg in proper position.

- *Arms falling forward*: Single-leg balance may not present as many challenges for the compensation of arms falling forward. If a client does well on single-leg balance, adding in some arm motion may help to decrease this compensation. For example, having a client perform single-leg balance with a scaption raise is a great way to reduce this compensation.

Assessment Considerations: Reactive Training

Reactive training is another area where the movement compensation needs to be taken into consideration due to the fact that the client will usually be performing faster motions and sometimes jumping:

- *Feet turn out*: When the client is jumping it is easier for the feet to turn out. In Phase 1, the recommended 3- to 5-second hold is when the client needs to focus on turning the feet back in. The focus should be on developing good foot-landing mechanics.
- *Anterior pelvic tilt*: The client with an anterior pelvic tilt will usually show one of two different movement impairments during reactive exercises. First, the client may not be able to fully extend the hips during a jump. This will result in the client flexing the hips all the way through the motion. The second impairment will be the client demonstrating an anterior tilt upon landing. Remember, this is why the 3- to 5-second hold is so valuable. Use this time to have the client reset the hips to neutral.
- *Arms falling forward*: The arms falling forward compensation during reactive exercises is similar to that seen with balance. Reactive training typically focuses on the lower body, so upper body compensation may not be as apparent. However, the upper body does play a role in lower body function during reactive exercises.

Assessment Considerations: Resistance

The demands of resistance training will change as the client progresses through the OPT model. Maintaining proper form will be more challenging during the beginning phases. Phase 1 will have a primary focus of form and decreasing movement compensations. By the time clients reach Phase 5 they should be able to maintain better form with less conscious thought. The following are considerations for resistance training:

- *Feet turn out*: This compensation will have the largest effect on exercises requiring a staggered stance. During the staggered stance, it is very common for the rear leg to turn out, exacerbating the compensation of the feet turning out. The rear leg should be straight, and if necessary the client can get the rear leg into a triple-extended position.
- *Anterior pelvic tilt*: Similar to the feet turning out, the staggered stance is a challenging position for the client with an anterior pelvic tilt. It presents a challenge because in order for the rear leg to be positioned properly the hip will need to extend. If the hip flexors are restricting this motion, then the front of the hips will likely be pulled down, exacerbating the compensation. In addition, the fitness professional will need to pay particular attention to the hips during lower body exercises. Squats and lunges, for example, are great exercises, but a client with this compensation may never fully extend the hips. This often results in a client performing many repetitions but none of them truly helping the client to reduce the compensation.
- *Arms falling forward*: The compensation of arms falling forward should be considered when choosing upper body exercises. Performing many repetitions of lat pull-downs, pull-ups, or heavy chest exercises may make the compensation worse. For example, a close-grip row is a great back exercise but it concentrates a lot of the tension onto the lats. By switching to a wide-grip row, the client can concentrate the tension onto the rear deltoid. If the client's arms fall forward, the fitness professional needs to pay close attention to form when performing overhead activities, such as a shoulder press. It is necessary for a person with this movement compensation to also monitor the hips during overhead press because of the attachment of the lats. If the client moves into an anterior pelvic tilt, overhead movements should be avoided until proper extensibility has been restored to the lats and pectorals.

Exercise Selection and Movement Dysfunction

The results of the movement assessments will help the fitness professional select exercises that will increase the quality of movement and to avoid those exercises that will not. If a client will be expected to repeat the exercises as homework, the exercises should be simple enough to execute safely. Always reflect back on the client goals and movement assessment when choosing exercises.

Common Exercises

A common question in fitness is "What is the best exercise for . . . ?" However, there is not a "best" exercise. Everyone moves slightly different and has different goals. A "best exercise" depends on several factors, one of the most important being the movement assessment. As with stretches, common strengthening exercises can be applied based on common movement compensations. The following is a list of 10 exercises that are effective in most individuals:

1. *Supine floor bridge*: Engages the gluteal muscles, which should be a very powerful muscle. Gluteal weakness is very common in the sedentary population.
2. *Prone Iso-abs*: Teaches the muscles that are designed to stabilize the spine to engage.
3. *Scaption*: Has been used for shoulder rehabilitation in physical therapy for many years. This has been proven to be an effective and safe shoulder exercise because it uses the entire shoulder girdle in the most functional plane of motion.
4. *Single-leg balance reach*: This is the recommended beginning exercise for most clients once the client is able to coordinate the muscular activity. In a forward reach, the center of gravity will shift forward, which means the muscles on the back of the body will have to increase their activity to offset the difference.
5. *Squat jump to stabilization*: Can be used with any movement compensation as long as the client can safely perform it. The goal of the squat jump in the initial phases is to teach deceleration.
6. *Back row*: Rowing motions will teach scapular retraction and depression as well as strengthen muscles that are often weak.
7. *Squat to row*: Uses two of the largest muscle groups in the body, the back and the gluteals, as well as all of the muscles around the core. In addition, this exercise can be used throughout the OPT model.
8. *Squat*: One of the foundational exercises in fitness. The squat requires work from many very large muscles and adequate range of motion in some very important joints.
9. *Lunge*: The lunge is another staple to training. Think of the lunge as a squat with a different footprint, requiring many of the same muscles and range of motion.
10. *Deadlift*: The deadlift is yet another foundational movement. The deadlift becomes very important for clients who do not have the range of motion to squat but still need to work their gluteal muscles. This is a great exercise to teach the body how to hinge at the hips with the spine stable and increase strength in the gluteals.

Exercises to Avoid

Just as movement assessments can guide the fitness professional to recommend certain exercises, the assessments can guide them to avoid certain exercises. If the professional knows what muscles may already be overactive, then exercises can be avoided that may exacerbate the muscle imbalances. Other exercises may be avoided due to the potential of muscle imbalances leading to incorrect exercise form. The following is a list of exercises to consider avoiding until specific movement compensations are corrected:

Feet Turning Out

- *Calf raises*: The feet typically turn out because the calves are shortened and overactive. More time should be spent on lengthening the calves. Calf raises should be avoided until the calf muscles are elongated.

Knees Caving In

- *Adductor machine*: The knees cave in because the adductors are already overactive, thus the adductor machine will likely make this worse.
- *Abductor machine*: The abductor machine may appear to be indicated with the knees caving in. However, the abductor machine usually places the hip close to a 90-degree angle. This will often place the gluteal muscles (the primary abductors) in a position that is too long to contract properly. Therefore, the abductor machine becomes a piriformis- and TFL-strengthening machine. The TFL is a contributor to the knees caving in and should not be strengthened. The piriformis is a hip rotator that is not designed for strength training, but instead to be a fast stabilizer and would be trained more efficiently on a proprioceptive device.
- *Leg extension*: Leg extension machines focus on the quadriceps muscle group. The largest and most powerful quadriceps is the vastus lateralis. It is also a muscle that is overactive during the compensation of knees falling inward. Therefore, to isolate the quads with that movement compensation could potentially make it worse.

Anterior Pelvic Tilt

- *Leg press*: The leg press is a quad-dominant machine and does not allow the gluteal muscles to work to their full potential. An exercise such as a squat, that uses the hips to full extension, would be recommended over a leg press until better movement is achieved.
- *Adductor machine*: Some of the adductors also serve as hip flexors (pectineus and adductor brevis). Isolating the adductors will potentially make the compensation worse.
- *Leg raises*: Oftentimes these are performed as abdominal exercises. However, the abs are not activated during this exercise, as they are in hip flexion. The hip flexors are overactive in an anterior pelvic tilt. Strengthening the hip flexors with this exercise may exacerbate the movement dysfunction.
- *Leg extension*: Leg extension is designed to isolate the quadriceps. One muscle of the quadriceps, the rectus femoris, is also a hip flexor. Therefore, isolating the quadriceps is not recommended in the presence of an anterior pelvic tilt.
- *Leg curl*: This exercise may be performed incorrectly due to the inflexibility of the quadriceps and hip flexors, the weakness of the hamstrings, and overactivity of the low back muscles; all indicated by anterior pelvic tilt. The most common compensation during the leg curl exercise is arching of the back. If this occurs, it is recommended to work on flexibility and core stabilization before returning to the leg curl.

Arms Falling Forward

- *Lat Pull-down*: Muscles that control the scapula in upward rotation should be worked on before performing lat strengthening work. If performing back exercises, choose a wide-grip row over a narrow-grip row. The wide grip will help to teach retraction of the shoulder blades and strengthen the rear deltoids, without also strengthening the lats.
- *Chest press machine*: The chest press is a great exercise to use with the arms falling forward if used with good form. An exercise such as a standing cable press will help to stabilize the core and use the shoulder girdle muscles correctly. The chest press machine, however, is often used with a significant amount of weight. This will increase the strength of the prime movers (pectorals) without teaching proper stabilization.

TRAINER TIPS

Transparency is paramount when working with your clients. They should always be provided with the "why" as they progress or regress throughout the phases.

◆ *Shoulder press*: The shoulder press is not harmful, but if the lats are inflexible then clients will likely arch their low back (relative flexibility) in order to successfully execute the shoulder press. Performing scaption raises or lateral raises is recommended until proper flexibility can be restored.

Communicating the Implementation and Progression of the OPT Model

Knowledge of the OPT model means little if the fitness professional is unable to communicate it to the client. It is vitally important to review the goals and intended outcomes of each phase with the client. Reviewing the goals and goal-setting process is recommended at the beginning of each phase, during reevaluation, and as part of movement assessments. Client success is largely dependent on the client's understanding of the outcomes.

A simple 5-minute conversation will have the client mentally prepared for the progressions to the next phase of training. This also shows the client that the fitness professional is invested and has planned for his or her continued success. When discussing homework, provide the client with the necessary templates and information to be successful. A great first month, with homework that includes flexibility, cardio, and active rest days, can easily become a great second month if the simple actions become habits.

Fitness professionals may sometimes encounter clients who do not understand the value of following proper progressions or solutions that are rooted in science. It is common for a client to obtain a gym membership and seek the assistance of a professional to quickly achieve a goal. The fitness professional will need to be prepared to address the questions and concerns that a client may have in regards to the scientific rationale behind integrated and progressive program design.

CHECK IT OUT

Consider the following example of transparent, informative communication with a client:

"Congratulations on doing such a great job in Phase 1, Mrs. Jones. As we move on to Phase 2, I would like to share a few things with you. The workouts are going to become a little harder. We will be performing back-to-back exercises with little to no rest in between. These will include exercises such as a squat followed by a single-leg deadlift."

"We are doing this because increasing the workload is going to help you lose more weight and further decrease body fat. This is a natural progression from Phase 1, so we have already worked on a lot of these exercises. In addition, we are going to go ahead and change up your cardiorespiratory program. Remember, we have been working on steady-state cardio to be sure your heart and lungs are able to work as efficiently as possible. Now, we are again going to bump up the intensity for a few minutes but then let you recover. This will be stage 2 in our stage training. Here is your copy of the cardio homework (including flexibility based on the movement assessments and active rest days) for the month. This increase in intensity is also going to help us burn more calories while we are still improving your overall health. These improvements, along with your nutrition, are going help you get about four to six more pounds off. This will have you around 155 pounds and closer to 25% body fat. Do you have questions before we get started?"

Exercise is a science, and one of the most important responsibilities of the fitness professional is to educate the client. The point of educating the client is to provide the information necessary for successful completion of the program. Even if these conversations are unsuccessful, they will still likely help the client to develop more trust and respect for the fitness professional.

Some of these conversations may be more challenging than others, and some may end with the client seeking out a fitness professional who will do what they want. But these conversations are important to ensure ethical and sound training standards. Fitness professionals do not want to get into situations where they let the client determine how the training will go. The OPT model is a proven system that was designed to take the guess work out of personal training. Fitness professionals should use effective communication and have confidence that the model will work. Encouraging patience and compliance are important to continuous successful outcomes.

The OPT Model and Client-Specific Goals

The OPT model is designed to be flexible and can be applied to achieve any goal. Whether the client is looking to improve overall performance or is just looking to lose weight, the OPT model will provide the guidance necessary to reach the goal while establishing a strong base for injury prevention.

Weight Loss Goal

Many factors play a role in successful weight loss. The one that fitness professionals can have the most impact with is the law of thermodynamics. If a person uses more calories than are consumed, weight loss will result. The best way to increase the number of calories burned is to move more. When combined with cardiorespiratory training, weight training provides an extremely potent means to burn calories by maintaining, or even increasing, lean muscle tissue. More activity and greater amounts of lean body mass result in more calories burned during exercise, and throughout the day. Resistance training also provides the added benefit of increased muscle strength.

A client only seeking to reduce body weight would not need to perform the hypertrophy training in Phase 3, or the maximum strength training in Phase 4. Therefore, the suggested phases would be Phases 1, 2, and 5. The client will be in Phase 1 for 4–6 weeks before entering Phase 2, and in Phase 2 for 4 weeks before entering Phase 5. Remember, undulating periodization may be performed within each phase. After the completion of Phase 5, the client would cycle back through with Phase 1. Between each phase (every 4–6 weeks) the client needs to be reassessed. This enables the fitness professional to ensure that muscle imbalances are being addressed, and to provide feedback to the client as to if he or she is headed in the right direction.

Along with the resistance training, the client will be performing cardiorespiratory training. Cardiorespiratory training helps to maximize calories burned and also helps to improve overall health. The client will perform stage training, beginning with Stage 1, Phase 1, and progressing through each stage along with the levels of the OPT model. The following describes the importance of each phase to weight loss:

◆ *Phase 1*: Increased caloric expenditure occurs as a result of achieving the endurance and stabilization goals. The addition of resistance training will provide a potent means to burn calories. The acute variable requirements in Phase 1 can provide a large metabolic demand during resistance training. This, combined with cardiorespiratory training, will

TRAINER TIPS

Some clients may want to build strength and hypertrophy in addition to losing weight. For these clients, going through Phases 3 and 4 is acceptable. The trainer may want to suggest that these clients focus on losing weight first, as they may already have the muscle mass they desire, they just lack muscle definition due to the extra weight.

optimize calorie burn. Keep in mind that Stage 1 cardio training will work to develop a sound aerobic base. Learning how to use oxygen efficiently will maximize calorie burn.

◆ *Phase 2*: This phase will increase calorie burn potential by increasing the metabolic demand and volume for increased caloric expenditure. Additionally, the increased intensity and volume may increase lean body mass. Cardio training will be increased to Stage 2. Stage 2 cardio training will introduce intervals by progressing the intensity into Zone 2 with recovery in Zone 1. This will add to the increased calorie burn and greater overall calorie deficits, leading to increased weight loss.

◆ *Phase 5*: The power phase focuses on high-force and high-velocity training. This will increase metabolic demand, requiring more energy and burning more calories. The required superset in Phase 5 consists of one strength exercise followed by one power exercise. The strength exercise being performed at a near maximal intensity, and the power exercise being performed at a near maximal speed, is where the increased metabolic demand comes from. Additionally, cardio training is progressed to Stage 3. This stage may be considered high-intensity interval training, with the client moving through Zones 1, 2, and 3 of the target heart rates, and undulating between Zone 2 and Zone 3. Zone 3 will be working up to 90% of maximum heart rate, increasing metabolic demand and requiring more calories to meet this demand.

Increase Lean Body Mass

Hypertrophy training

The chronic enlargement of muscles.

Increasing lean body mass, or **hypertrophy training**, can be defined as the chronic enlargement of muscles. To accomplish this goal, training programs need to progress with moderate volumes to force muscles to regenerate their cellular makeup and grow in size. In addition, nutrition is as important, if not more important, than with weight loss. In order for body tissue to grow, there must be a surplus of energy (in the form of calories). The calories must be of high quality and provided in a sufficient amount for the body to use them to grow muscle tissue.

Building muscle presents one of the greatest challenges in personal training and exercise. Under the right conditions the body can use excess calories to build lean body mass. The most important of these conditions is to have the extra energy (calories) for the body to actually add mass and build muscle. The next most important consideration is the load that is applied to the body and if the stimulus is appropriate for muscle growth.

It is recommended that Phases 1, 2, and 3 of the OPT model be utilized for lean tissue growth. Phases 1 and 2 provide the foundation to optimize muscle building upon entering phase 3. Phase 3, hypertrophy training, is designed to provide the volume and intensity that will lead to the cellular adaptation of muscle growth. This is approximately 75–85% one-rep maximum for 3 to 5 sets. Also, the rest period in this phase is *up to* 60 seconds. The key being that not more than 60 seconds can be taken in order to maximize the potential for muscle growth. This stimulus leads to hypertrophy.

Cardio should also be performed in hypertrophy training for overall health. In addition, the more efficient the cardiorespiratory system functions, the more effective the training sessions can be. However, the cardio may need to be performed less frequently, as the increased calorie burn may interfere with weight gain goals.

The nutritional recommendations for muscle growth begin with energy balance. To build muscle, more calories need to be consumed than are burned each day. The macronutrient breakdown and timing of nutrients becomes increasingly important for muscle growth. Muscle growth becomes even more complicated considering the extra calories to be spent in accordance with physical demands from the human movement system. If this is not accomplished, the excess calories will be converted and stored as fat. For more information on this topic, refer to a registered dietitian (RD).

CHECK IT OUT

Some clients will attempt to gain muscle while simultaneously losing fat. Due to the paradox of the necessary energy balances for each of these goals, this is very challenging, and is usually not the most effective way to go about training. Ideally, the two goals would be divided up into different mesocycles. One mesocycle would focus on gaining muscle, including the positive energy balance required to maximize muscle gain. The next mesocycle could then increase caloric expenditure and reduce calorie consumption in an effort to maintain as much muscle as possible while reducing body fat. Additionally, it is unlikely that trained athletes, who already have low percentages of body fat, can reduce body mass without losing some lean muscle.

Improve Sports Performance

The goal of improving general sports performance requires the client to increase overall proprioception, strength, and power output (or rate of force production). The training will need to be progressed from stabilization through the power phase of training. The client can be cycled through the entire OPT model depending on his or her particular needs and wants. However, for the typical client, Phases 1, 2, and 5 will be the most important. Because Phase 3 is dedicated to maximal hypertrophy, it will not be necessary for the goal of performance. In some cases, increased size may even inhibit maximal performance. For an athlete needing to make a goal weight, a boxer for example, hypertrophy training could be detrimental to his or her overall goals. Phase 4 can be used in moderation to help increase the initial strength levels required to optimize the adaptation necessary for phase 5.

In the OPT model, the client would begin in Phase 1 and remain there for 4–6 weeks before moving on to Phase 2. Phase 1 is vital for the performance client because it will prepare the connective tissues and muscles for the higher demands of training to follow. This is important because the majority of injuries do not occur to the muscle, but to the nonvascular connective tissues that support the muscle. Phase 1 provides time to ensure that these specific tissues increase their tensile strength to support the rest of the training. Phase 2 will promote greater overall strength endurance to prepare the client for the greater demands of Phase 5. As mentioned earlier, Phase 4 may also be used to increase strength without adding size, but is optional. After completing Phase 5 the client should cycle back through Phase 1.

Cardio can also be paired with Phase 5 training. However, high-intensity cardio sessions may be better suited for non-resistance training days. High-intensity cardio on the same days as Phase 5 resistance training could lead to overtraining.

Nutrition is also a major contributor to overall performance. The role of sports nutrition is to support the training program. Therefore, the nutrition for performance will change as the program changes. Poor nutrition can lead to fatigue, poor recovery, and injury, all of which will have a major impact on an individual's performance (Rosenbloom & Coleman, 2012). Many clients will have sports performance goals that coincide with general health goals. Although the general client's sport may not have the same demands as an athlete whose primary goal is sport-specific training, a similar approach can be taken to their nutrition planning. Many clients participate in year-round sports, but most participate in a sport that has traditional progression of a preseason, a competitive season, and an off-season. The nutrition and training should be adjusted for the sport season.

The **preseason** consists of different goals depending on the sport. Training goals usually consist of working in various phases of the OPT model to improve endurance, strength, power,

Preseason
The period immediately before the beginning of a new competitive season.

Competitive season

The period that consists of regulated games or competitions of a particular sport; the period of time featuring the most competitive activity.

Off-season

The period of the sports year when an activity or sport is not engaged in; the period of time when the most training can be performed.

and flexibility. Additionally, many clients may seek changes in body composition during this time. Macronutrient intake will be modified to support these goals.

The **competitive season** is often more demanding from an energy perspective due to the higher training load. Many clients performing in a sport may have higher training loads coupled with more frequent competitions that require different macronutrient needs. The in-season is typically a maintenance phase in the OPT model, ideally fluctuating between Phases 1 and 2.

The **off-season** is also known as *transition* or *postseason*. This period often presents nutritional challenges for clients who participate heavily in sports. The off-season comes with a decrease in training frequency, and for many clients this comes with the need to decrease overall food intake. Some clients will have hypertrophy goals and need the extra calories, but most will be recovering and just need to maintain their fitness levels; therefore, they will need to adjust their food intake to prevent excessive weight gain.

Muscle-Building Athletes

Athletes seeking to increase lean body mass, such as bodybuilders, should follow the balanced nutrition recommendations from the USDA. However, each macronutrient will be increased accordingly to create the positive energy balance needed for muscle growth. The bodybuilder should eat four to six times per day. Protein intake will need to be spread throughout the day. Ingestion of a carbohydrate and protein mixture should be consumed within 90 minutes of a workout to increase recovery and maximize gains. Protein recommendations for those seeking muscle growth range from 0.5 to 0.8 grams per kg (Rosenbloom & Coleman, 2012). The fitness professional should keep in mind that carbohydrates and fat are also required for muscular hypertrophy.

Endurance Athletes

Endurance athletes likely have the greatest energy demands, and thus the most detailed and extensive nutrition plans. The duration of endurance events increases all metabolic process; therefore endurance athletes require higher amounts of each macronutrient. An athlete participating in a sport lasting longer than 4 hours requires the greatest amount of carbohydrates, usually requiring 11 grams per kilogram of bodyweight per day to maintain energy demands. The current recommended daily allowance for protein for the average individual is 0.8 grams per kilogram per day; however, the endurance athlete requires 1.2–1.4 grams per kilogram per day (Rosenbloom & Coleman, 2012). Again, the demands of endurance sports increase the rate of protein synthesis, thereby requiring greater quantities of protein to maintain tissue repair and overall health.

No matter the goal, the fitness professional should tailor education to specific populations and their needs. However, all individuals should be advised on how to improve their foundational nutrition, nutrient timing and type, and be provided information on proper use and misuse of supplements.

Session Structure and Flow

Traditional training sessions need to have structure and flow. The investment made by the client requires that time and attention be paid to each aspect of the program. This includes everything from pre-session questions (e.g., "How was your cardio yesterday?"), to the details of each component of the integrated training session. Each session should include a warm-up with SMR and stretching, followed by core, balance, and reactive exercises. SAQ training should then be performed (if appropriate), followed by resistance training, a cool-down, and a homework assignment. Although this may sound like a lot, with a little practice and preparation each session will flow smoothly with more than enough time to complete everything.

Training vs. Coaching

To better utilize their time, fitness professionals should consider having coaching sessions in addition to training sessions. It is common to use these two terms interchangeably, but coaching and training involve different plans and different outcomes. Both training sessions and coaching sessions have their place when working with clients. Training is used for what would be considered the traditional aspect of personal training. The two main components of a training session are learning and practice. This includes learning new skills, new techniques, new programs, and practicing new skills. Training sessions will include the workouts, and the fitness professional will be the motivator for the client to reach his or her goals and push past self-induced barriers. It can be thought of in terms of the physical work that is performed throughout the session and in homework, as well as the recommendations for appropriate nutrition to follow outside the session. Coaching, on the other hand, focuses on the time spent in consultation, with the fitness professional and client working together to discuss potential obstacles to success and triggers to initiate forward momentum. Here the professional can work with the client to create effective lifestyle plans, and implement behavior modification techniques that will increase the likelihood of carrying out healthy actions outside of the gym.

Session Structure and Flow: 60-Minute Traditional Training Session

The first session may include more teaching than what is normally considered "training." For example, the majority of clients will need to be taught self-myofascial release and proper stretching technique. Once they have learned how to properly execute these tasks they should then be able to complete them on their own as homework. However, if the fitness professional does not observe the intended response (i.e., better movement capabilities), then the client's form and implementation may need to be revisited. Each session may vary slightly based on the client, but the sessions should follow a general format. The following is a suggested format for a 60-minute training session:

- The fitness professional should prepare by reviewing the planned session, the last two to three sessions, and the cardio homework. The fitness professional will set up the equipment for the session and ensure that the selected equipment is available or modifications are made as necessary.
- The *first 10 minutes* should be used for the warm-up (i.e., flexibility and cardio). Along with this should be a recap of what the client has done since the last session, following up on homework, nutrition, and any other pertinent factors, such as stress management. This may be performed before the flexibility work begins with a new client, or during the flexibility section with a more experienced client. In many cases, a new client will need to focus on those individual aspects without the distraction of trying to learn new exercises. In addition, if using core, balance, and reactive exercises in place of cardio, then no more than 5 minutes may be necessary here.
- The *next 10 minutes* may be spent on core, balance, and reactive exercises, as well as speed, agility, and quickness, if prescribed. A maximum of 10 minutes is needed, but less time is acceptable if the client completes all of the tasks.

◆ The *next 30 minutes* should be spent on the resistance training portion of the program. Keep in mind that the amount of time spent on resistance training will vary based on the client's goal. For example, 30 minutes of resistance training for a deconditioned client in Phase 1 seeking to lose weight could be plenty of time. However, a client in phase 4 may need to devote much more time to the resistance portion and less time to the details of core, balance, and reactive training.

◆ The *last 10 minutes* of the session will be devoted to the client cool-down, which consists of revisiting the SMR and static stretching techniques. Also during this time the fitness professional should remind the client of what the next few days will look like until he or she is back for the next scheduled session.

Session Structure and Flow: 25- to 30-Minute Traditional Training Session

Not everyone will want or have the luxury to participate in 60-minute sessions. Thirty-minute sessions can also be extremely effective, but they require some strategic planning, and require more effort on the part of the client. A training package with 30-minute sessions should begin with the intent of teaching the client the tools he or she will need to be successful. It is all too common for clients and fitness professionals alike to see the 30 minutes as an opportunity to merely train as hard as possible. This approach can lead to wasted time, client frustration, and possible injury. Each session should be planned with a particular learning objective:

◆ *Session 1*: The learning objective of the first session should be flexibility. The goal is for the client to feel comfortable performing the flexibility exercises on his or her own.
- The *first 10 minutes* may be used to thoroughly explain why and how the client will foam-roll and stretch the areas indicated by the movement assessment. This will be vitally important, because after the first session clients should perform the flexibility on their own before the training session.
- The *remaining 20 minutes* will be used to perform core, balance, and reactive training. If time allows, resistance training may be introduced as well.
- The cool-down can be performed by the client alone; however, this should be time to reinforce the flexibility.

◆ *Session 2*: The learning objective of the second session is core, balance, and reactive training. The goal is for the client to feel comfortable executing one or two exercises for each domain. It is important for the fitness professional to keep these exercises specific to the client, but to keep them basic, with minimal moving parts, so the client will be able to repeat them with good form.
- The *first 10 minutes* will focus on the details and rationale behind core, balance, and reactive training. Although clients do not need to know all the details of a prescribed exercise, they will need to know why it will benefit them and how to perform it correctly.
- The *remaining 20 minutes* may be used for resistance training. It is recommended to take one or two exercises (preferably total body exercises such as a squat to press or squat to row) and spend extra time teaching them to the client. The goal will be for the client to get more comfortable with each exercise. In the future, the client will get resistance exercises to perform as homework.
- The client will perform the cool-down on his or her own.

◆ *Session 3*: The third session is the session that sets the pace for the remainder of the training program. In this session, the client is expected to show up at least 15–20 minutes early to perform the flexibility, core, balance, and reactive exercises. These exercises will be a

CHECK IT OUT ✓

It is important for the fitness professional to maintain control over the direction of the sessions. If the client begins to come in late, skipping the essential parts of the warm-up, suggesting they are not needed or are a waste of time and they just want to train hard, then it is advised that the fitness professional not continue the training. If the client is not complying with the recommendations, he or she will not get the intended results. Anytime a client is unsuccessful, the professional is also unsuccessful. If the client is not willing to listen to the trainer and apply the recommendations, then it might be warranted to schedule a coaching session to discuss outcomes and the effort needed to accomplish those outcomes.

simple repeat of what the client learned in the first two sessions. If the client does not show up early and perform these exercises, then it should be mandatory in the training session.

- The *first 3–5 minutes* will be a recap of the warm-up. The professional will need to answer any questions the client has about form or technique. Also, the fitness professional should begin to get more inquisitive about what the client spends his or her time doing outside of the gym. If necessary, a coaching session can be scheduled to learn more about the client.
- The *next 25 minutes* will be used for resistance training. More exercises can be chosen, and more sets and reps can be completed, if desired.
- The cool-down will remain the same, with self guided flexibility.

Session Structure and Flow: Coaching Sessions (30 and 60 Minutes)

Coaching, sometimes more appropriately referred to as *lifestyle* or *fitness coaching*, evolved from fitness professionals needing to find a better way to connect with their clients. The International Coaching Federation (ICF) has defined **fitness coaching** as "partnering with clients in a thought-provoking and creative process that inspires them to maximize their personal and professional potential" (Cross, 2011). A coaching session is typically used to help motivate the client or to create change. Lifestyle or fitness coaching should not be confused with *life coaching*. Life coaching is more of a holistic approach to assisting clients to navigate themselves toward personal and professional fulfillment. This is beyond the scope of the fitness professional–client relationship. However, lifestyle or fitness coaches can apply various behavior change and communication strategies with their clients in order to obtain desired fitness results.

Coaching sessions should be used to review overall performance and progress. Sometimes clients advance their fitness knowledge to a level where they can apply program design principles, but still seek the accountability and motivation that a professional can provide.

A coaching session can be much like a conversation but the focus is on helping clients to discover the answers for themselves. Coaching is geared to help clients reach their full potential. This begins with the fitness professional working on effective communication and guiding conversations. Fitness and lifestyle coaching can be delivered in many different ways, including in person, over the phone, and via the Internet.

Fitness professionals must understand their scope of practice before beginning to engage in fitness coaching sessions. A coaching session is not intended to diagnose or treat any medical

Fitness coaching
The application of various behavior change and communications strategies with clients that leads to increased accountability and motivation, thus supporting their desire to achieve fitness goals.

conditions. Fitness professionals should have a network of healthcare professionals to refer clients to if needed and exercise caution if working with clients whose medical needs may exceed their training. Similarly, nutrition advice should not be provided beyond that which a fitness professional can give. Coaching sessions should be used to help guide the clients to their own solutions about change that needs to occur.

The first coaching session is very important because it sets the tone for the rest of the coaching sessions. Coaching sessions should be scheduled for the same amount of time that the traditional training sessions typically last. That being said, 30 minutes is usually sufficient, but it is never appropriate to have to rush the end of a coaching session. Coaching sessions should occur on a regular basis.

In the first session the fitness professional begins by trying to build a relationship with the client. This includes getting to know the client and his or her particular needs and goals. In this session it, is the coach's job to determine the client's readiness to exercise and decide what stage of change the client is in. This information will be used to assist in developing the client's program. The following should be part of an initial 60-minute coaching session:

- Engaging in detailed and collaborative discussion
- Focusing on the client's needs, desires, goals, and strategies
- Discovering areas of opportunity for making change and identifying the client's readiness for change
- Helping the client to create a vision, and then turning the vision into goals
- Creating a plan to meet these goals
- Setting weekly and monthly goals
- Helping the client feel supported and accomplished as he or she progresses through coaching and personal training

There is no set time that should be spent on each component of the session and the fitness professional should make note-taking a priority. These notes will be used for reflection and showing support by communicating effectively with the client.

Coaching sessions should be scheduled regularly. However, they should occur more frequently in the beginning, perhaps once a week. Then, the frequency can decrease over time and sessions can even occur over the phone or online. They do not always have to done in person. In fact, it has been suggested that the majority of fitness coaching sessions occur online and over the phone (Cantwell & Rothenberg, 2000).

Session Structure and Flow: Training and Coaching Combo Sessions (30 and 60 Minutes)

Training and coaching can be addressed in the same session, but there should be a clear delineation between the two. Coaching should not occur during training, and training should not occur during coaching. The two have different outcomes and different learning objectives. Too much overlap between the two blurs the lines of the objectives, and often leads to a lack of focus and an unclear vision.

A great opportunity to mix training and coaching is on the initial assessment and on all reassessment days. The initial assessment is a coaching session of sorts due to the collection of information and data regarding the client and the intended goals. On reassessments or re-evaluations, the coaching session will come after all other data has been collected. This coaching session will be imperative to review the previous month's goals and compare the actual outcomes with the intended outcomes. Often, this is where the difficult conversations emerge. These conversations will typically revolve around why or why not certain goals were obtained. Again, communication plays a large part in this. At the reevaluation the client should have a better grasp of what will be covered and how it will be covered.

Fitness professionals should complete an advanced course in behavior change prior to conducting coaching, or training and coaching combo sessions.

Session Structure and Flow: Training and Corrective Combo Sessions

The typical client will require a focus on correcting movement impairments at the beginning of their program. Therefore, the beginning weeks or even months may need to include pieces of corrective exercise in an effort to get the most out of each session. This is easily broken down by integrating some corrective strategies into the personal training session. However, corrective exercise is a detailed look at movement assessments, with the goal of narrowing down the exact cause of movement dysfunction through assessment modification, joint range of motion testing, and manual muscle testing. Fitness professionals interested in this approach should seek out an additional certification in corrective exercise.

Think of the specific warm-up in each session being a form of "corrective exercise." The main difference between an entirely "corrective" session versus a "normal" training session is the client's long-term goals and movement assessments. For example, if a client has just come to a fitness professional after being released for normal physical activity by her doctor because of an injury, then she would begin with an entirely corrective session. The movement would be evaluated, the causes of the dysfunction would be identified, and a program would be designed for that impairment. Fitness professionals work with "apparently healthy individuals", but movement still has to be taken into consideration. Therefore, flexibility, core, balance, and reactive exercises can be designed to be "corrective" in nature. The intent of these sessions is to reintegrate proper nervous system control and coordination of the musculoskeletal system.

The amount of time of each session can vary, but what is completed must remain consistent. If a client chooses to participate in shorter sessions, that does not mean he or she does not need corrective work. It means that the client will have more responsibility. If the client is not holding up his or her end of the training agreement, consider longer sessions or training more frequently. With proper assessments and integrated program design that follows the OPT model, each session will deliver exactly what the client needs.

It is highly recommended that fitness professionals complete an advanced program, course, or credential that specifically addresses corrective exercise prior to conducting training and corrective combo sessions.

Conclusion

Using the components and outcomes of each OPT level to create a progressive program design helps the fitness professional to create a plan that addresses the needs and wants of each individual client. This chapter has provided additional knowledge and concepts to help the fitness professional prepare for the implementation of program design, including useful templates and session structure and flow for different time frames. From here, each level of the OPT model (stabilization, strength, and power) will be covered in additional depth.

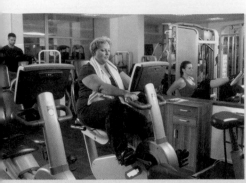

© StockLite/Shutterstock

Case in Review

When working with Jennifer, you discuss with her that the assessments conducted show some muscle imbalances that could possibly lead to injury if not addressed. You tell her because her knees move inward she is placing a great deal of stress upon the internal structures of the knee, which could lead to possible ligament injuries. Most of these types of injuries happen without contact, which means that if those muscle imbalances are not corrected, she may be susceptible to major knee injuries during normal functional movement. You talk with her as though you are here to help, siding with her on the notion that you have her best interests in mind, and that her goal should be to function without fear of injury on a daily basis. In addition to the knees, you discuss her forward lean. From the assessments, you suggest to her that she has weak core stabilizers and tight hip flexors, immediately following up that it could lead to low back pain.

It becomes increasingly evident that she is now listening to you and understands the importance of the assessments you performed. However, without proper programming, you will not address and/or correct the muscle imbalances that you have identified in Jennifer. To begin, you recommend the following programming strategies to address the assessment results:

- SMR and stretch the calves and hip adductors.

- Strengthen the external rotators of the hips through exercises such as lateral tube walking.

- Strengthen the core stabilizers though exercises such as prone-iso abs.

- SMR and stretch the lats and hip flexors.

References

Ballor, D. L., Becque, M. D., & Katch, V. L. (1987). Metabolic responses during hydraulic resistance exercise. *Medicine and Science in Sports and Exercise, 19*(4), 363–367.

Broder, M. S. (2000). Making optimal use of homework to enhance your therapeutic effectiveness. *Journal of Rationale-Emotive and Cognitive-Behavioral Therapy, 18*(1), 3–18.

Byrne, S. M., Cooper, Z., & Fairburn, C. G. (2004). Psychological predictors of weight regain in obesity. *Behaviour Research and Therapy, 42*, 1341–1356.

Cantwell, S., & Rothenberg, R. (2000). The benefits of lifestyle coaching. *IDEA Personal Trainer, 11*(7), 24–35.

Cronin, J. B., McNair, P. J., & Marshall, R. N. (2003). Force-velocity analysis of strength-training techniques and load: Implications for training strategy and research. *Journal of Strength and Conditioning Research, 17*(1), 148–155.

Cross, K. (2011). How to become a lifestyle coach. *IDEA Health and Fitness Library*. Available at: http://www.ideafit.com/fitness-library/how-to-become-lifestyle-coach (accessed January 10, 2016).

Fleck, S.J. (2011). Non-linear periodization for general fitness and athletes. *Journal of Human Kinetics Special Issue, 29A*, 41–45.

Freeman, A., & Rosenfield, B. (2002). Modifying therapeutic homework for patients with personality disorders. *Journal of Clinical Psychology, 58*(5), 513–524.

Glaser, N. M., Kazantzis, M., Deane, F. P., & Oades, L. G. (2000). Critical issues in using homework within cognitive-behavioral therapy for schizophrenia. *Journal of Rationale-Emotive and Cognitive-Behavioral Therapy, 18*(4), 247–261.

Hakkinen, K., Komi, P. V., & Alen, M. (1985). Effect of explosive type strength training on isometric force and relaxation-time electromyographic and muscle fiber characteristic of leg extensor muscles. *Acta Physiologica Scandinavica, 125*(4), 587–600.

Harris, R. C., Edwards, R. H., Hultman, E., Nordesjo, L. O., Nylind, B., & Sahlin, K. (1976). The time course of phosphorylcreatine resynthesis during recovery of the quadriceps muscle in man. *Pflugers Archive: European Journal of Physiology, 28*(367), 137–142.

Hayes, L. D., Bickerstaff, G. F., & Baker, J. S. (2013). Acute response exercise program variables and subsequent hormonal response. *Journal of Sports Medicine and Doping Studies, 3*(2), 1–10.

Herodek, K., Simonovic, C., & Rakovic, A. (2012). Periodization and strength training cycles. *Activities in Physical Education and Sport, 2*, 254–257.

Jones, K., Hunter, G., Fleisig, G., Esamilla, R., & Lemak, L. (1999). The effects of compensatory acceleration on upper-body strength and power in collegiate football players. *Journal of Strength and Conditioning Research, 13*(2), 131–143.

Kanehisa, H., & Miyashita, M. (1983). Specificity of velocity in strength training. *European Journal of Applied Physiology and Occupational Physiology, 52*(1), 104–106.

Keogh, J. W., Wilson, G. J., & Weatherby, R. P. (1999). A cross-sectional comparison of different resistance training techniques in the bench press. *Journal of Strength and Conditioning Research, 13*(3), 247–250.

Komi, P. V. (1986). Training of muscle strength and power: Interaction of neuromotoric, hypertrophic, and mechanical factors. *International Journal of Sports Medicine, 7*(1), 10–15.

Krieger, J. W. (2009). Single versus multiple sets of resistance exercise: A meta-regression. *Journal of Strength and Conditioning Research, 23*(6), 1890–1901.

Marx, J. O., Ratamess, N. A., Nindl, B. C., Gotshhalk, L. A., Volek, J. S., Dohi, K., . . . Kraemer, W. J. (2001). Low volume circuit versus high-volume periodized resistance training in women. *Medicine & Science in Sports and Exercise, 33*(4), 635–643

Mazzetti, S., Douglass, M., Yocum, A., & Harber, M. (2007). Effect of explosive versus slow contractions and exercise intensity on energy expenditure. *Medicine and Science in Sports and Exercise, 39*(8), 1291–1301.

Oha, K., Animagi, L., Paasuke, M., Coggon, D., & Merisalu, E. (2014). Individual and work-related risk factors for musculoskeletal pain: A cross-sectional study among Estonian computer users. *BMC Musculoskeletal Disorders, 15*, 181.

Piraua, A. L., Beltrao, N. B., Alves Araujo de Lima Jr., D. R., Reis de Queiroz, G., Gomes de Souza, J., Melo, B. M., & Cappato de Araujo, R. (2013). Effect of exercise order on the resistance training performance during a circuit training session. *Brazilian Journal of Kineanthropometry and Human Performance, 16*(3), 325–333.

Rhea, M. R., & Alderman, B. L. (2004). A meta-analysis of periodized versus nonperiodized strength and power training programs. *Research Quarterly for Exercise and Sports, 75*(4), 413–422.

Rosenbloom, C. A., & Coleman, E. J. (2012). *Sports Nutrition: A Practice Manual for Professionals* (5th ed.). Washington, DC: Academy of Nutrition and Dietetics.

Sakamoto, A., & Sinclair, P. J. (2006). Effect of movement velocity on the relationship between training load and the number of repetitions of bench press. *Journal of Strength and Conditioning Research, 20*(3), 523–527.

Sahrmann, S. A. (2002). *Diagnosis and Treatment of Movement Impairment Syndromes*. Philadelphia, PA: Mosby, Elsevier.

Shaw, B. F. (1999). Therapist competence ratings in relation to clinical outcome in cognitive therapy of depression. *Journal of Consulting and Clinical Psychology*, *67*(6), 837–846.

Simao, R., Freitas de Salles, B., Figueiredo, T., Dias, I., & Willardson, J. M. (2012). Exercise order in resistance training. *Sports Medicine Research*, *42*(3), 251–265.

Storer, T. W., Dolezal, B. A., Berenc, M., Timmins, J. E., & Cooper, C. B. (2014). Effect of supervised, periodized training versus self-directed training on lean body mass and other fitness variables in health club members. *Journal of Strength and Conditioning Research*, *28*(7), 1995–2006.

Taylor, N. F., Dodd, K. J., & Damiano, D. L. (2005). Progressive resistance exercise in physical therapy: A summary of systematic reviews. *Journal of the American Physical Therapy Association*, *25*, 1208–1223.

CHAPTER 11

THE OPTIMUM PERFORMANCE TRAINING™ (OPT™) MODEL: APPLYING STABILIZATION

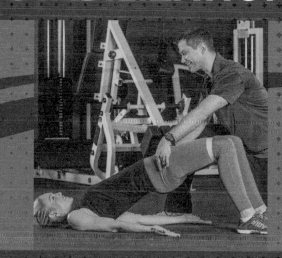

OBJECTIVES

After studying this chapter, you will be able to:

1. **Describe** the goals and outcomes of the Stabilization Level of the Optimum Performance Training (OPT) model.

2. **Explain** how stabilization goals are achieved.

3. **Utilize** stabilization acute variables on various client types.

4. **Implement** appropriate cardio protocols for the Stabilization Level.

5. **Implement** appropriate movement prep protocols for the Stabilization Level.

6. **Implement** appropriate resistance training protocols for the Stabilization Level.

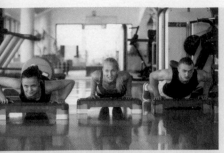

© fotoinfot/Shutterstock

Case Scenario

You have begun to build your pipeline, having acquired and assessed three new clients who are looking for help to accomplish three very different fitness goals. You have basic program design knowledge, and can put together a fitness program based on the objective assessments you conducted during the consultation stage with each client. You now have to address each client's goals, in addition to correcting muscle imbalances identified in the assessments and minimizing potential injury.

Your first client, Roderick, has been an avid gym-goer and is ready to take his training to the next level. Roderick goes to the gym daily, predominately lifting weights, in hopes of entering a bodybuilding competition that is 9 months away.

Your second client, Mary, has avoided the gym because she feels intimidated by the others working out and feels self-conscious when working out next to someone who she feels is in better shape than her. Recently, Mary's primary doctor has recommended that she should seek out a personal trainer to help her lose 20 pounds.

Your third client, Ashley, has overcome many weight issues, but has been a victim of yo-yo dieting and workout programs she feels have not provided the results she has been looking for. Over time, Ashely's persistence to improve her health has sparked a passion for long-distance running and biking. She is highly committed and is willing to put in the time required to reach her goals. Feeling a need to challenge herself further, Ashley has registered to run a marathon in 4 months.

- How would you describe the adaptations of OPT Phase 1: Stabilization Endurance in a manner that aligns with each of your clients' fitness goals?

- How would you use the acute variables within the Stabilization Level for each of your clients?

- What movement prep and resistance training exercises would you use for each client?

Introduction to the Stabilization Level of the OPT Model

The Stabilization Level is the first of the three levels of the OPT (Optimum Performance Training) model (**Figure 11.1**). The three levels represent the primary adaptations, and then the levels are split into smaller phases to achieve more specific goals. Altogether, the OPT model has

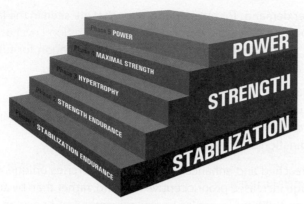

FIGURE 11.1 The OPT Model: Stabilization.

three levels that build upon one another with five phases spread throughout them. The Stabilization Level has one primary adaptation of stabilization endurance. This means that the Stabilization Level only has one phase, Phase 1: Stabilization Endurance. It is important not to confuse the levels of the OPT model with the phases. Even though it might seem straightforward now, the Strength Level will contain multiple phases. It is helpful to think of the title of the level (e.g., Stabilization), and then the phase in which clients are being trained (e.g., Phase 1: Stabilization Endurance).

The Stabilization Level of the OPT model is the foundational level for all subsequent training phases. Phase 1: Stabilization Endurance is found within the Stabilization Level of the OPT model. It has the goal of increasing and maintaining optimal levels of stabilization for prolonged periods of time while concurrently developing the highest levels of coordinated movement, good form/technique, and structural integrity. These outcomes are strategically honed through this phase's controlled tempos and high repetitions.

Oftentimes stabilization training is thought of as core training, focusing only on the lumbo pelvic-hip complex (LPHC). Although the LPHC is involved in every aspect of this level of training, stabilization is not limited to that region. Additional joints, particularly highly mobile ones like the ankles, hips, and shoulder girdle, need stability and coordination for balance.

Stabilization training is the base upon which the Strength and Power Levels are built. Performing chest exercises with cables, or executing a push-up on a stability ball, are both examples of unstable exercises that can be seen in the gym. It is more difficult to lift heavier weight in these conditions.

Goals and Adaptations in the Stabilization Level

Clients and fitness professionals alike need to know that even though the Stabilization Level is the starting point of the OPT model, it does not mean that it is the easiest level. The neurological, metabolic, and physiological demands can be quite high, which makes it difficult for many individuals to endure when training protocols are properly applied.

The direct goals of stabilization training include increased stability, **muscular endurance**, control in all planes of motion, and coordination of movement. However, the indirect goal is

---

TRAINER TIPS

Stability is determined by the client, not by a particular exercise. Sometimes a movement may not appear to be a stability exercise, but the focus is to create controlled instability. This could be seen in the example of a client performing a seated machine row without allowing the chest to touch the front support pad, as this could be the most unstable surface a client could control.

TRAINER TIPS

Before progressing to more creative exercises, make sure that the client has mastered the basic movements. For example, learning to perform a squat correctly before loading the movement will help prevent injury and allow you to use more complex exercises with the client in the future.

Muscular endurance

(1) A muscle's ability to contract for an extended period. (2) The ability to produce and maintain force production over prolonged periods of time.

Proprioception
The ability to recognize bodily movement and position.

to progress to greater demands for other adaptations that are seen in the latter phases of OPT. Therefore, it is important to consider Phase 1 of the Stabilization Level as having critical and immediate benefits, but also offering the promise of a foundation for future outcomes. The goals of Phase 1 are as follows:

◆ Increase stability.
◆ Increase muscular endurance.
◆ Increase control in all planes of motion.
◆ Increase coordination of movement.

These goals are reached and enhanced by selecting exercises unique to Phase 1 and progressing them through increased proprioceptive demand, rather than by adding external load. **Proprioception** is the ability to recognize bodily movement and position. Recall that placing an individual in an unstable, yet controllable, environment will challenge the individual's proprioception. An example of this would be to progress a push-up on the floor to a push-up with hands or feet on a stability ball.

The client's form should be closely monitored to ensure that proprioceptive progressions are executed safely, but still present a challenge. In order to progress to the Strength and Power Levels of the OPT model, it is important to develop neuromuscular efficiency through Phase 1 training first. If clients have poor form when performing an exercise with light to moderate weights, it is likely that poor form will continue through increases in resistance, leading to greater risks of injury.

Scientific Principles of Stabilization Training

Neuromuscular efficiency is the ability for all the muscles to efficiently work together in all three planes of motion. This is the ultimate goal of all movement. The Stabilization Level of the OPT model is designed to enhance stability and coordination, along with the endurance to maintain these outcomes for a prolonged period of time. In order to create these adaptations, the Stabilization Level will require different variations of the acute variables. Note that these variables must be applied correctly to achieve the desired responses. The variables work together to develop muscular stabilization and neuromuscular coordination over extended periods of time. The correct use and application of acute variables in this level serves as the supporting scientific principle in the Stabilization Level.

CHECK IT OUT

At the beginning of exercise, an individual will not be taking in enough oxygen to meet the immediate demands for ATP production for the aerobic energy system. This lack of oxygen is called the *oxygen deficit*. In the same way, when exercise ceases the individual's oxygen intake will not immediately return to baseline. Heavy breathing will occur until oxygen levels return to normal. This is called *excess post exercise oxygen consumption* (EPOC). During this window, metabolism will remain elevated and extra calorie burn will take place. This concept is important for understanding and applying intervals, specifically high-intensity interval training.

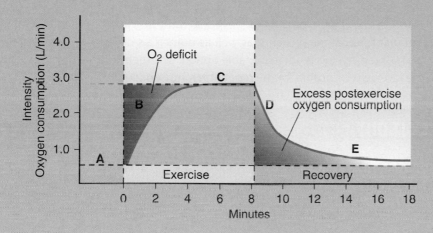

TRAINER TIPS

High repetitions and low rest time make Phase 1 ideal for clients trying to lose weight.

The tempo of the repetitions performed is important, because muscular endurance is best developed with slow repetitions. Stabilization endurance resistance training will often apply a 4/2/1 tempo. The numbers in the tempo are associated with specific muscle actions and are always labeled E/I/C (eccentric/isometric/concentric).

EPOC The repetition range for stabilization training is necessary to build proper connective tissue strength and muscular endurance. The elevated number of repetitions is also important when developing motor patterns for new movements or exercises.

Additionally, in support of endurance improvement, the repetition range in the Stabilization Endurance Phase is 12–20 reps. Combined with a 4/2/1 tempo, this repetition range can be taxing metabolically due to the continuous demands placed on the body.

This is one reason why the amount of sets for muscular endurance is limited to 1–3. **Time under tension (TUT)**, which is the amount of time from the beginning of one resistance training set to the end without breaking, is very high because of the slow tempo and high repetition range. This requires a lower set range.

Time under tension (TUT)

The amount of time from the beginning of one resistance training set to the end without breaking.

CHECK IT OUT

Note that how the tempo is labeled does not necessarily correlate to the way an exercise is initiated. E/I/C stays constant so all researchers and practitioners have a standard for labeling tempo. Squats start with the eccentric phase of the exercise—the descent into the squat—which is a 4-second count. A deadlift starts with the concentric phase of movement—the lift—which is a 1-second count. Also, some researchers will notate tempo as E/I/C/I to indicate that there are two different places within a lift where an isometric hold will be placed.

Timed hold

An acute variable where the requirement is to hold a specific pose or posture for a specified period of time.

TRAINER TIPS

Intensity levels in the stabilization Endurance Phase are determined by the amount of instability or proprioception that is added or removed.

The Stabilization Level has an acute variable that is important to the specific adaptations required in this particular phase. This variable is a **timed hold**. Some exercises in the Stabilization Level are not designed to be repetitious, but rather simply held for a certain amount of time for sets.

Timed holds are highly indicated in the Stabilization Level of training, because they require the neuromuscular system to stabilize a particular postural position. Timing of the hold is important to quantify in order to compare it to standards and past performance, or to set goals for specific poses to be held.

Another variable in this level of the OPT model is training intensity, and it is important to address it in all training phases as well. Stabilization training will work at intensities between 50–70% of the one-repetition maximum (1RM).

To find 50–70% of a client's 1RM, the professional must first find the client's 1RM. However, keep in mind that for beginning clients, as well as numerous others that have little desire to ever lift at 100% intensity, this is not reasonable option. One method to estimate this number is to look at the inverse relationship for the repetition range and intensity (**Table 11.1**).

CHECK IT OUT

Timed holds may include:
- Pallof press hold.
- Prone iso-abs.
- Single-leg balance.
- Squat jump to stabilization (repetition and timed holds combined).

CHECK IT OUT

Timed holds can be held for 20–30 seconds for clients just starting a stabilization training program. However, as clients progress, the core training recommendations for timed holds can be manipulated:

Tempo 4/2/1 $=$ 7 seconds

Repetition range $=$ 12–20

$7 \times 12 =$ **84 s**

up to

$7 \times 20 =$ **140 s**

It is important for the fitness professional to watch to ensure that the client is stabilizing in optimal alignment; otherwise, he or she may be prepping to be stable in a poor position.

TABLE 11.1 Training Intensity	
Repetitions	**Intensity**
12 is equivalent to	75%
20 is equivalent to	50%

Because of the correlation between repetitions and intensity, the client can simply focus on 12–20 repetitions and generally fall within 50–75% intensity of the 1RM. It is important to determine whether the client has reached momentary muscular fatigue, or voluntary fatigue at the conclusion of each set. If 20 repetitions are completed, but the client could do another 5, then the client is not within the intensity range for the completion of the set.

Rest intervals in the Stabilization Level of the OPT model are relatively short. However, individuals just starting an exercise routine may respond better to longer rest periods until they adjust to the demands of their program. Longer rest periods also help to ensure proper exercise technique. By reducing the amount of fatigue experienced, the client may be able to perform each exercise with greater precision. More advanced clients in this level will benefit from shorter rest intervals. Rest periods for the Stabilization Endurance Phase are 0–90 seconds. This does not mean to do a set of push-ups and rest zero seconds before doing another set of push-ups. Zero seconds indicates a circuit where there is no rest between an exercise for a body part or movement, and another for a different body part or movement. A deconditioned client may need up to 90 seconds between sets, with some clients needing even more rest than 90 seconds. However, one way to progress the exercise programming without increasing external resistance would be to decrease the rest period between sets. This can be progressed until there are zero seconds between exercises in a total body circuit, and the 90-second break can be applied at the end of the sequence.

Training volume is the total amount of work performed within a specified time (Fleck & Kraemer, 1997; Kraemer et al., 2000; Tan, 1999). The OPT model presents training variable guidelines in order to prevent overtraining, as all training is cumulative. Training volume varies among individuals based on the client's (Campos et al., 2002; Kraemer et al., 2002; Marx et al., 2001; Spiering & Kraemer, 2008):

- Training phase.
- Goals.
- Age.
- Work capacity or training status.
- Recoverability.
- Nutritional status.
- Injury history.
- Life stress.

A conditioned client may be able to perform a specific exercise at 60% of maximum with a total volume of 36–60 repetitions (three sets of 12–20 reps). Each phase in the OPT model will have training goals that dictate repetitions, sets, intensity, rest, and tempo, and these combined dictate the volume (Campos et al., 2002; Kraemer et al., 2000; Spiering & Kraemer, 2008; Tan, 1999).

CHECK IT OUT

In the Stabilization Level, sets are generally horizontally loaded for deconditioned clients or clients working on form, technique, and/or corrective movements. **Horizontal loading** is when sets are followed immediately by rest intervals until the set range is complete for an exercise or body part. **Vertical loading** is a type of circuit applied to more conditioned clients, allowing alternating body parts to be trained from set to set starting from the upper extremity and moving to the lower extremity with little to no rest in between.

Horizontal loading

Performing all sets of an exercise or body part before moving on to the next exercise or body part.

Vertical loading

Circuit applied to more conditioned clients allowing alternating body parts to be trained from set to set, starting from the upper extremity and moving to the lower extremity with little to no rest in between.

Training frequency
The number of training sessions performed during a given period, usually 1 week.

Training duration
(1) Length of workout from beginning to end. (2) Amount of time spent in a particular phase of training.

 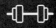
Training frequency is another variable in the Stabilization Level. It refers to the number of training sessions performed during a given period, usually 1 week. New clients may begin training their entire body two times per week, and conditioned clients up to four times per week.

Training duration is an acute variable with two different meanings. The first meaning is the length of the workout from beginning to end. Personal training sessions are usually 1 hour in duration, though session duration may vary.

The second meaning of duration is the amount of time spent in a particular phase of training. Typically, a phase of training will last 4 weeks, as this is the general time frame for the body to adapt to a given stimulus. Afterward, the training stimulus will have to be raised to achieve further adaptations (Bompa, 1993; Enoka, 1988; Sale, 1988). It is recommended that a client remain in Phase 1 for 4–6 weeks.

Exercise selection is where most of the acute variables are applied, including repetitions, tempos, timed holds, sets, and intensities. Exercise selection in the Stabilization Level is specific to the client's needs. This means that what are chosen as chest exercises in the Stabilization Level are, and should be, different from the chest exercises chosen for the Strength Level. Stabilization exercises seldom require the use of a machine, because of the focus on intermuscular coordination. These exercises are selected to challenge the individual's proprioception.

Tracking Progress in the Stabilization Level

Tracking a client's workouts allows the fitness professional and the client to see evidence that the programming is delivering quantifiable results. A challenge that fitness professionals face, when demonstrating to their clients that they are progressing, is explaining that the most important improvements in this level are seen in movement quality and the ability to stabilize joint motion. To see these results, and speak to them, the fitness professional should view each workout and exercise as a series of movement assessments.

Other advancements are seen in the client's ability to better stabilize and perform motions in proprioceptively enriched environments. For example, if a new client advances from performing a standing single-arm cable chest press to a standing single-arm, single-leg chest press, then, assuming stability is maintained, progress is demonstrated. Providing this type of feedback to the client is helpful in the early stages of training so that improvement is recognized and, in turn, is motivating.

Progress tracking in the Stabilization Level can also be seen in terms of increasing intensity, volume, and so on. However, clients will not always realize the inverse relationships between certain acute variables, and thereby might become demotivated. The fitness professional should maintain transparency on the rationale and ultimate outcome of each session, in order to keep the client engaged and ensure that overall progress is being tracked.

In terms of progression, it is important to note that no level, phase, exercise, or outcome should ever come at the expense of safe movement patterns. For this reason, the fitness professional may not want to always drive the client using acute variables as demonstration of improvement or for motivation.

Cardiorespiratory Training Protocols in the Stabilization Level

Cardiorespiratory training is subject to the same Specific adaptation to imposed demands (SAID) principle as other forms of training. Bodies will adapt to the modality, intensity, and environment in which they train. Changing these variables will continue to illicit stress, to which the body will continually work to adapt. Varying cardiorespiratory training can also minimize the potential for overtraining. Therefore, the three different stages of cardiorespiratory training will mirror the three levels of the OPT model in terms of progression.

As with resistance training, warm-ups are important for cardiorespiratory workouts. A 5- to 10-minute general warm-up is suggested in this phase, to be performed at a low to moderate intensity (20–60% heart rate reserve [HRR], 35–69% maximum heart rate [HR_{max}], or 10–13 on the Rated Perceived Exertion [RPE] scale).

In Phase 1, cardiorespiratory training will be Stage I, and should involve base training in Zone 1. This will develop the cardiorespiratory base adaptations that are required to begin more intense methods of training. The goal is to get clients to a point where they can success-fully complete 30 minutes of cardio exercise without stopping, at 65–75% of their HR_{max}. This may be completed by initially programming for 10-minute cardio workouts, then working up to the full 30 minutes and beyond. Clients should be able to maintain their heart rate within this zone (not going over or below) for the full 30 minutes. Some clients will be able to accomplish this feat in the first few of weeks of training. These clients may require longer periods for their exercise programming. Some clients will need more time (e.g., 6–8 weeks) to achieve this goal. The guideline should be that clients cannot move to the next level of the OPT model until this goal has been met.

Depending on the client's goals, needs, and wants, these recommendations can be modified by either extending or reducing the time allotted to the warm-up period. Modifications can be made to activities based on any known or suspected medical, health, or physical limitations a client may have or present. New clients who are sedentary or have medical and health lim-itations, or those with limited previous exercise experience, may initially require up to half or more of their dedicated workout time to be directed to warm-up activities. Clients who have numerous postural issues and low fitness will need additional time during the warm-up to work on aligning their body and activating muscles.

The goal in Stage I is to improve aerobic cardiorespiratory fitness levels in apparently healthy, yet sedentary, clients by maintaining a target heart rate of 65–75% of HR_{max}, or approximately 12–13 on the RPE scale. If the talk test is employed to monitor training intensity, the client should have increased respiratory rate, but still be able to carry on a conversation.

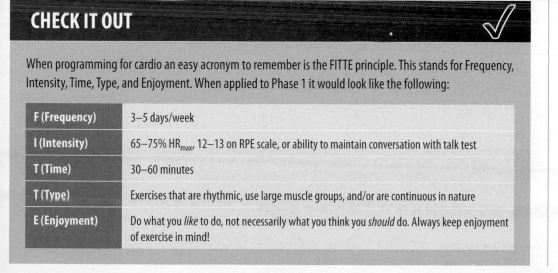

CHECK IT OUT

When programming for cardio an easy acronym to remember is the FITTE principle. This stands for Frequency, Intensity, Time, Type, and Enjoyment. When applied to Phase 1 it would look like the following:

F (Frequency)	3–5 days/week
I (Intensity)	65–75% HR_{max}, 12–13 on RPE scale, or ability to maintain conversation with talk test
T (Time)	30–60 minutes
T (Type)	Exercises that are rhythmic, use large muscle groups, and/or are continuous in nature
E (Enjoyment)	Do what you *like* to do, not necessarily what you think you *should* do. Always keep enjoyment of exercise in mind!

Movement preparation

The systematic implementation of flexibility, core, balance, reactive, and SAQ (as applicable) training principles prior to completing the remaining majority portion of the workout (e.g., resistance training).

Fascia

A web of connective tissue that wraps and surrounds muscle fibers, bones, nerves, and blood vessels. The myofascial system covers individual muscles as well as connecting groups of larger muscles together.

Davis's law

Soft tissue will align along the lines of stress that are placed upon it.

Because most clients present muscle imbalances, it is advised that clients perform corrective flexibility programs *prior* to completing their cardio sessions during the Stabilization Level. Performing cardio, even a light warm-up, without proper flexibility can further enhance muscular dysfunction. Thus, it is advisable that cardio training should only be performed after standard Stabilization Level flexibility protocols have been conducted.

Movement Preparation in the Stabilization Level

Individuals in the Stabilization Level of training should incorporate all forms of movement preparation. **Movement preparation**, often called *movement prep*, is an important addition to the fitness professional's systematic implementation of the workout protocol. It implements applications of flexibility, core, balance, reactive, and speed, agility, and quickness (SAQ) training principles. Note, however, that SAQ is optional with Stabilization clients. The goal is to prime the body for the remaining higher intensity portion of the workout. The systematic and specific implementation of the NASM movement prep protocol provides a safe and effective way to minimize injury risks. It consists of activating underactive muscles, increasing range of motion (ROM), neuromuscular efficiency, structural stability, inter- and intramuscular stabilization, intervertebral stabilization, and hip and scapular stability, as well as coordinating functions between highly mobile body segments such as ankles, hips, or the LPHC.

SMR and Flexibility Protocols in the Stabilization Level

When programming for flexibility, it is important to follow the integrated flexibility continuum. In Phase 1: Stabilization Endurance, this is called *corrective flexibility* and requires a combination of self-myofascial release (SMR) and static stretching (**Table 11.2**).

SMR is a flexibility technique that focuses on the neural, muscular, and fascial systems in the body. By applying gentle force to adhesions, or "knots," the elastic muscle fibers are altered from a bunched-up position into a straighter alignment to the direction of the muscle, or **fascia** (**Davis's law**). The relaxation response in SMR, commonly referred to as *foam-rolling*, is achieved through autogenic inhibition. The Golgi tendon organs (GTOs), when stimulated with pressure or tension for longer than 30 seconds, will show an inhibitory or relaxation response. This is critical in maximizing time spent in SMR. Clients should apply the pressure to the adhesion for a minimum of 30 seconds in order to achieve the desired response, rather than rolling back and forth.

TABLE 11.2 Phase 1: Stabilization Endurance Flexibility Acute Variables							
Reps	Sets	Tempo	Intensity	% Interval	Rest Frequency	Duration	Exercise Selection
1	1–3	30-second hold	N/A	N/A	3–7 times/week	4–6 weeks	SMR and static stretching

Individuals typically conceptualize flexibility training as just static stretching. This requires the individual to stretch a muscle and hold it for a prolonged period of time to initiate the autogenic inhibition response, allowing the muscle to relax. Research has shown that this prolonged period is approximately 30 seconds (Chaitow, 1997; Etnyre & Abraham, 1986).

Static stretching is a corrective modality designed to mitigate the effects of poor posture, shortened muscles, and decreased ROM. The focus of flexibility in the Stabilization Level is primarily corrective, so static stretching is indicated for this level/phase of training, and implemented based on the assessment results. In addition to holding the identified muscles in a stretched position, contracting the antagonistic muscles while holding a static stretch can reciprocally inhibit the muscles being stretched. This allows them to relax and further enhances the stretch. For example, when performing a kneeling hip flexor stretch, fitness professionals can instruct their clients to contract their hip extensor (gluteus maximus) to reciprocally inhibit the hip flexors (psoas, rectus femoris), allowing for additional lengthening. Another example would be contracting the scapular retractors (middle trapezius and rhomboids) to reciprocally inhibit the pectoralis major. **Figures 11.2–11.4** highlight some common static stretching techniques.

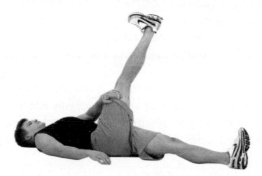

FIGURE 11.2 Static supine biceps femoris stretch.

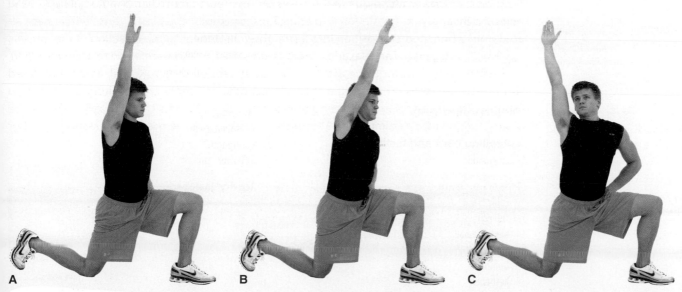

A   B   C

FIGURE 11.3 Static kneeling hip flexor stretch.

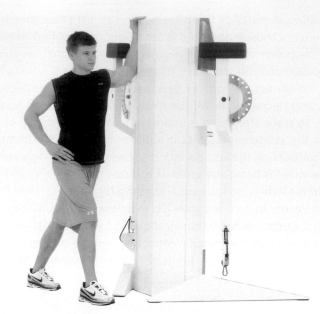

FIGURE 11.4 Static pectoral stretch.

Core Protocols in the Stabilization Level

NASM defines the core as the LPHC and the thoracic and cervical spine. The parameters and acute variables for core stabilization training are respectively noted in **Tables 11.3 and 11.4**. Prone iso-abs is an excellent exercise for discussion of core stabilization. Prone iso-abs (plank) often is performed with timed holds of 30 seconds or more. However, shorter time periods

TABLE 11.3 Core Training Parameters	
Variables	**Exercise Selection**
Plane of motion • Sagittal • Frontal • Transverse	**Progressive** • Easy to hard • Simple to complex • Known to unknown • Stable to unstable
Range of motion (ROM) • Full • Partial • End range	**Systematic** • Stabilization • Strength • Power
Type of resistance • Cable • Tubing • Medicine ball • Power ball • Dumbbell • Kettlebell	**Activity/goal-specific**

TABLE 11.3   Core Training Parameters (*cont.*)

Variables	Exercise Selection
Body position • Supine • Prone • Side-lying • Kneeling • Half-kneeling • Standing • Staggered stance • Single leg • Standing progression on unstable surface	**Integrated**
Speed of motion • Stabilization • Strength • Power	**Proprioceptively challenging** • Stability ball • Balance plate • Wobble board • Half foam roll • Balance pad
Duration	**Based in current science**
Frequency	**2–4 times/week**
Amount of feedback • Fitness professional's cues • Kinesthetic awareness	

TABLE 11.4   Core Stabilization Acute Variables

Reps	Sets	Tempo	Intensity	% Interval	Rest Frequency	Duration	Exercise Selection
12–20	1–4	4/2/1	N/A	0–90 seconds	2–4 times/week	4–6 weeks	1–4 core stabilization

can be held for repetitions, such as a 5-second timed hold repeated for 10–15 repetitions. The plank position is used to give the core strength and endurance in a neutral position, and while performing other exercises, such as push-ups or standing push-type exercises, where sagittal plane anterior stabilization is needed. Timed holds for the plank teach the core to stay strong for the duration of these other exercises. The following are other exercises that produce an external force, against which the core must create an internal resistance to hold the spine and LPHC in place:

◆ Supine floor bridge (**Figure 11.5**)
◆ Supine floor bridge with marching (**Figure 11.6**)
◆ Side Iso-abs (**Figure 11.7**)

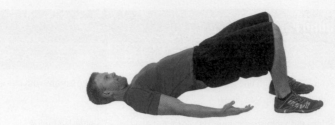

FIGURE 11.5 Supine floor bridge.

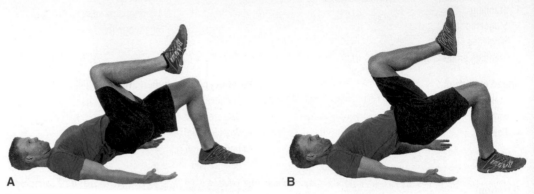

A   B

FIGURE 11.6 Supine floor bridge with marching.

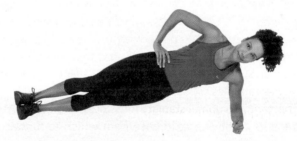

FIGURE 11.7 Side Iso-abs.

When identifying the need for core stabilization based on compensations found in the movement assessments, it is important to observe the direction of unwanted movement. The fitness professional should observe if the client is moving forward or backward, side to side, or rotating. This allows the fitness professional to know in which plane of motion the compensation takes place. Once the plane and direction of compensation are identified, a corrective preparation exercise can be added to the workout to better prepare the body for overload in resistance training. It is important that fitness professionals be able to recognize unwanted movements before being able to identify muscles. The following are some examples of compensations and associated planes:

- ◆ Anterior pelvic tilt: Sagittal plane compensation
- ◆ Hip shift: Frontal/transverse plane compensation
- ◆ Hip rotation: Transverse plane compensation

It is important to note that compensations in undesired planes of motion may be caused by instability or lack of ROM in the desired plane (see **Table 11.5**).

TABLE 11.5 Plane Stability

Sagittal Plane Stability	Frontal Plane Stability	Transverse Plane Stability
Prone Iso-abs (aka plank)	Prone iso-abs with one leg elevated and abducted Side iso-abs (aka side plank)	Prone iso-abs with one leg elevated
Bridge	Bridge with mini-band around knees (above or below, not on, the knees)	Single-leg bridge
Stability ball roll outs	Suitcase holds/carries	Pallof press Antirotational hold Single-arm fly
Quadruped	Quadruped opposite leg reach with abduction	Quadruped opposite leg reach
Marching	Side-lying hip abductions Side-lying single-leg marching	Sandbag pull-through

Balance Protocols in the Stabilization Level

Balance is a person's ability of keep his or her **center of gravity (CoG)** over the base of support. The smaller and more unstable the base of support, the more challenging the exercise becomes. It is important to point out the performance goal measures and performance production measures. The goal in balance training is indeed to keep the CoG over the base of support. The parameters for balance stabilization training are listed in **Table 11.6**. The production of those goals, or how well the exercises are performed, is of great importance for fitness professionals. If the balance exercises are not performed well, then the professional should regress the exercise to the most unstable balance exercises that can be safely, efficiently, and effectively produced. The acute variables for balance stabilization are listed in **Table 11.7**.

Core stability is important, but spinal stability must be reinforced soundly by the hip, knee, foot, and ankle for the core to have a solid base from which to function. Core and balance

Center of gravity (CoG)

The area within an object at which the weight is equally balanced in all directions. In a person, this is generally around the navel, but can change depending on the posture/movement of the body.

TABLE 11.6 Balance Training Parameters

Exercise Selection	Variables
Safe	**Plane of motion** • Sagittal • Frontal • Transverse
Progress • Easy to hard • Simple to complex • Stable to unstable • Static to dynamic • Slow to fast • Two arms/legs to single-arm/leg • Eyes open to eyes closed • Known to unknown (cognitive task)	**Body position** • Two legs/stable • Single leg/stable • Two legs/unstable • Single leg/unstable

(continued)

TABLE 11.6 Balance Training Parameters (*cont.*)

Exercise Selection	Variables
Proprioceptively challenging • Floor • Balance beam • Half foam roll • Foam pad* • Balance disc* • Wobble board* • BOSU ball	

*These modalities come in many shapes and sizes that will dictate proper progression.

TABLE 11.7 Balance Stabilization Acute Variables

Reps	Sets	Tempo	Intensity	% Interval	Rest Frequency	Duration	Exercise Selection
12–20 or 6–10 each side for single leg	1–3	4/2/1, if applicable 0- to 60-second timed holds if tempo is not applicable	N/A	0–90 seconds	2–4 times/week	4–6 weeks	1–4 balance stabilization

stability are closely related and should be integrated together into a progressive system, in order to develop the motor skills to support the structural integrity and neuromuscular efficiency of the human movement system.

Balance exercises can be applied in a progressive format to allow for static, transitional, and dynamic control. In balance stabilization training, the fitness professional will look to challenge the client's static balance with very little to no movement of the stance leg (**Table 11.8**).

In order to ensure neuromuscular efficiency, and simultaneously help clients understand their proprioceptive limitations, controlled instability is implemented as the balance portion for the Stabilization Level. This is also how exercises are progressed in the Stabilization Level. Individuals' needs and abilities differ, so the fitness professional should follow a systematic and progressive approach when incorporating balance training into the program. Balance stabilization training exercises are designed to improve reflexive joint stabilization contractions to increase joint stability. This is done by maintaining a neutral position of the stance leg with little to no movement. Example balance stabilization exercises include:

- ◆ Single-leg balance (**Figure 11.8**)
- ◆ Single-leg lift and chop (**Figure 11.9**)
- ◆ Single-leg hip internal and external rotation (**Figure 11.10**)

TABLE 11.8 Balance Posture

| The balance posture should follow several basic principles:
• Feet pointed straight ahead
• Knees stay aligned with 2nd and 3rd toes
• LPHC stays level on top of the leg
• Body parts may move to increase challenges to balance stability, but the knee must stay in line with the center of the foot while the foot is pointing straight ahead. | See Figure 11.8 for an example of good balance posture during a single leg balance. |

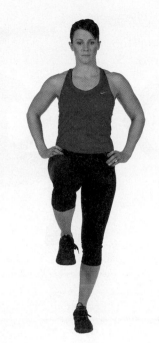

FIGURE 11. 8 Single-leg balance.

CAUTION

A number of training modalities are available on the market today that challenge one's balance, and they can all be very useful tools. However, to ensure the safety and effectiveness of balance training, individuals must start in an environment they can safely control and go through a systematic progression (e.g., floor → balance beam → half foam roll → balance disk). Not following the proper progression can cause movement compensations and improper execution of the exercise, decreasing the effectiveness of the exercise and increasing the risk for injury.

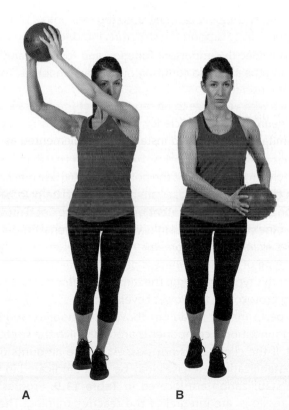

A   B

FIGURE 11.9 Single-leg lift and chop.

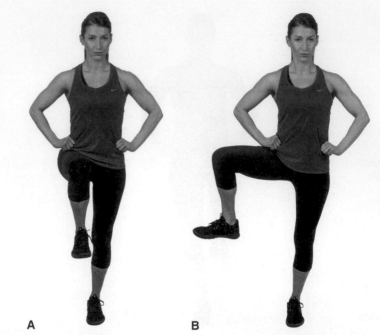

A   **B**

FIGURE 11.10 Single-leg hip external rotation.

Reactive Protocols in the Stabilization Level

Reactive stabilization provides the important function and focus of landing mechanics, with the purpose of enhancing the ability to control ground reaction forces. The following are possible reactive stabilization exercises:

- Single-leg box hop-up with stabilization (**Figure 11.11**)
- Box jump-up with stabilization (**Figure 11.12**)
- Box jump-down with stabilization (**Figure 11.13**)

The 3- to 5-second hold on the landing is the point at which these mechanics can and should be addressed with the client. These exercises are not meant to be plyometric workouts, especially in the Stabilization Level. Rather the intention is to develop good movement patterns and landing motions so that the client can avoid injury. The professional fitness industry sometimes uses the words *reactive training* and *plyometric training* interchangeably; however, reactive training is a particular type of training, whereas plyometrics is a specific set of exercises and protocols that fall under this type of training. The term *plyometric* has been reserved specifically for the reactive training protocols in the Power Level.

NASM's integrated performance paradigm shows core stability and neuromuscular stability (balance) as the foundational components around which the stretch–shortening cycle should be developed. If the client does not possess ample amounts of core and balance stabilization, reactive-stabilization exercises may be contraindicated in the program. Acute variables for reactive stabilization are located in **Table 11.9**. Progressions, and perhaps more importantly regressions, are integral to the reactive training. The NASM OPT model provides a systematic approach to reactive training, starting with stabilization and landing mechanics. **Table 11.10** provides regressed to progressed versions of reactive-stabilization exercises.

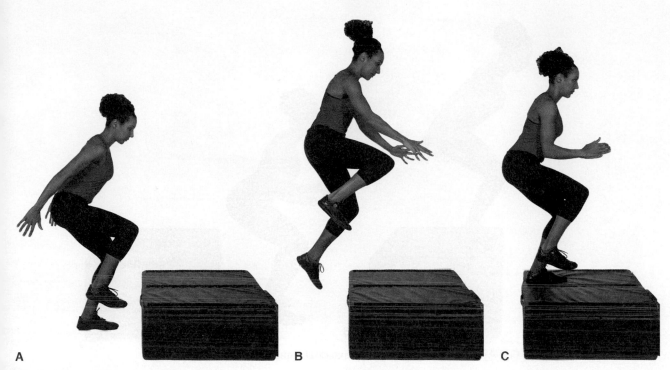

A   B   C

FIGURE 11.11 Single-leg box hop-up with stabilization.

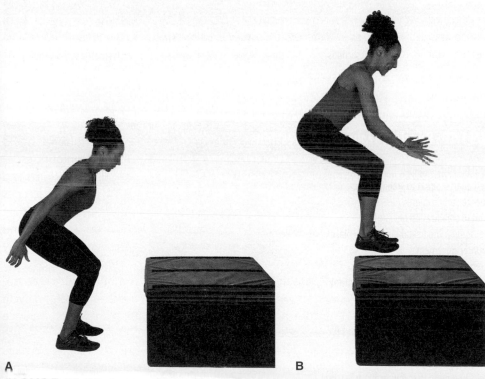

A   B

FIGURE 11.12 Box jump up with stabilzation.

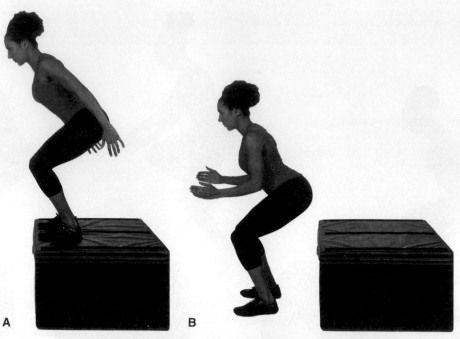

FIGURE 11.13 Box jump down with stabilization.

TABLE 11.9	Reactive Stabilization Acute Variables						
Repetitions	**Sets**	**Tempo**	**Intensity**	**% Interval**	**Rest Frequency**	**Duration**	**Exercise Selection**
5–8	1–3	3- to 5-second hold on landing	N/A	0–90 seconds	2–4 times/week	4–6 weeks	0–2 plyometric stabilization

TABLE 11.10 Reactive Training Progressions
Squat hold for stabilization
Single-leg quarter squat to stabilization
Drop squat to stabilization
Drop squat to stabilization one leg
Low-level squat jump to stabilization, in place:
• No countermovement
• Countermovement
Low-level squat jump to stabilization, sagittal:
• No countermovement
• Countermovement
Low-level squat jump to stabilization, frontal:
• No countermovement
• Countermovement
Low-level squat jump to stabilization, transverse:
• No counter movement
• Counter movement

TABLE 11.10   Reactive Training Progressions (*Cont.*)

Small box (3–6 inches) step down to stabilization:
- Sagittal
- Frontal
- Transverse

Small box step down stabilization, single leg:
- Sagittal
- Frontal
- Transverse

CHECK IT OUT

Ground contact should take place with the reactive portion of the foot upon landing. This is just in front of the medial longitudinal arch, and behind the ball of the foot. Landings should be "soft." Think about the "egg toss" game. The goal is not necessarily how far an individual can throw the egg, but rather how gently the egg is caught uncracked. Much like the human body, the egg does not crack from being thrown (the jump), but from a poor landing. Once the initial range has been found to toss the egg, the individual can progress the distance in between the thrower and catcher. The simple rules laid out in egg toss can also be applied to exercise:

- Start at a safe distance.
- Focus more on landing than jumping.
- Progress slowly to keep focus on how well the client decelerates force.

TRAINER TIPS

Your client can revisit earlier OPT phases, but it is unwise to progress forward until the client is ready. It may be beneficial to use Phase 1 exercises in later phases. If a client is feeling rundown on a particular day, you do not want to have the client engage in high-intensity exercise. Regressing back to a squat jump with stabilization on the ground instead of performing box jumps may be necessary for the client in this case.

Once clients have developed the ability to absorb forces, they can progress to the Strength Level of reactive training where they can start to add the stretch–shortening cycle with a focus on concentric force production.

SAQ Protocols in the Stabilization Level

Speed, agility, and quickness training is often referred to by the acronym SAQ. SAQ is optional in the Stabilization Level, but it can be implemented. The goal is to initiate a base level of agility and quickness for the client to be able to move at functionally applicable speeds in a dynamic environment. In order to reduce the chance of injury, exercises with limited horizontal inertia and unpredictability should be chosen, such as cone shuffles and agility ladder drills. Balance components may be added to agility ladder drills, such as in-in-out to balance. The quickness component would be when the client holds the balance until the fitness professional gives the audible to "stop" to balance and the "go" to continue. See **Table 11.11** for acute variables used in SAQ stabilization programming.

SAQ training should not be limited to athletes, as it is a fun way to include conditioning exercises into any integrated fitness program. Clients and athletes alike must first have sufficient core and balance stabilization prior to engaging in SAQ drills, which is why it is considered optional. Once core and balance stabilization can support the dynamics of SAQ (and reactive

TABLE 11.11 SAQ Stabilization Acute Variables

Reps	Sets	Tempo	% Intensity	Interval	Rest Frequency	Duration	Exercise Selection
2–3	0–2	Controlled for effective movement patterns	N/A	0–90 seconds	2–4 times/week	4–6 weeks	4–6 drills with limited horizontal inertia and unpredictability

training), SAQ training can be added. Clients who can control core and balance stabilization exercises for recommended repetitions, sets, and tempos should be able to effectively control SAQ stabilization exercises. Example SAQ exercises for stabilization include:

- Ladder drills-one-ins
- Ladder drills-two-ins
- Accelerators
- Form running drills

The common thread of each of these exercises is the ability to provide a particular output per unit of time, which is why they are often coupled together in training. Multilimb coordination, controlled precision, aim, steadiness, stabilization, and balance of movement, without the need to produce high-end speed, is the goal of this level of SAQ training (**Tables 11.12** and **11.13**).

TABLE 11.12 SAQ Training

Speed, in an athletic context, is defined as the "rate of performance" of an activity. It is the ability to achieve high velocity of movement.

Agility is the ability to accelerate, decelerate, stabilize, and change direction quickly while maintaining proper posture.

Quickness is the ability to *react* and change body position with maximum rate of force production, in all planes of motion, from all body positions, during functional activities.

Important components of SAQ stabilization:
- Coordinating arm/leg movement
- Aiming foot contacts to specific locations
- Maintaining neutral LPHC stability while multiple limbs are moving
- Minimizing horizontal inertia and unpredictability

TABLE 11.13 SAQ Stabilization Parameters

SAQ Stabilization Exercise Selection	Variables
Safe **Done with supportive shoes** **Performed on a proper training surface** • Grass field • Basketball court • Tartan track surface • Rubber track surface • Performed with proper supervision	**Plane of motion** • Sagittal • Frontal • Transverse **ROM** • Full • Partial

Progressive
- Easy to hard
- Simple to complex
- Known to unknown
- Stable to unstable
- Body weight to loaded
- Activity specific

Type of resistance
- Medicine ball
- Balance band

Type of implements
- Tape
- Cones
- Boxes

Muscle action
- Eccentric
- Isometric
- Concentric
- Speed of motion
- Duration
- Frequency
- Amplitude of movement

Resistance Training Protocols in the Stabilization Level

After all elements of movement prep have been applied, and potentially cardiorespiratory training as well, the client's human movement system should be well primed to perform the rest of the workout. In the general population, the remainder of the workout will focus on resistance training.

Resistance training in the Stabilization Level of the OPT model will continue to provide both stabilization and endurance. Stabilization is the human movement system's ability to provide optimal dynamic joint support to maintain correct posture during all movements. It requires high amounts of endurance for optimal recruitment of prime movers to increase force production and force reduction. Consistent training with controlled, unstable exercises, like the stability ball and/or single-leg exercises, for example, increase the body's ability to stabilize and balance itself (Behm, Anderson, & Curnew, 2002; Cosio-Lima et al, 2003; Heitkamp et al, 2001). Conversely, if training is not performed with controlled unstable exercises, clients will not gain the same level of stability (Bellew, Yates, & Gater, 2003; Cressey et al, 2007; Heitkamp et al., 2001). Research shows that improper stabilization can negatively affect a muscle's force production (Edgerton et al, 1996). Muscular endurance is the ability to produce and maintain force production for prolonged periods of time. Improving endurance is vital to the maintenance of proper and prolonged stability of the core and joints, as well as being the foundation on which hypertrophy, strength, and power are built.

Application of the acute variables in Stabilization Level resistance training will need to be applied specifically and progressively. Due to the inverse relationships between some of the acute variables, such as intensity, repetitions, tempo, and total volume, it is sometimes helpful to manipulate and progress one acute variable at a time in order to see the improvements and achievements. For example, repetitions might stay in relatively the same range while intensity is consistently increased. Similarly, repetition ranges and intensity can remain the same, while reducing the amount of recovery time. **Table 11.14** identifies the acute variables associated with resistance training in the Stabilization Level. Resistance training exercises for the Stabilization Level are shown in **Figures 11.14–11.16**.

TABLE 11.14 Resistance Training Acute Variables

	Reps	Sets	Tempo	% Intensity	Interval	Rest Frequency	Duration	Exercise Selection
Resistance	12–20	1–3	4/2/1	50–70%	0–90 seconds	2–4 times/week	4–6 weeks	1–2 stabilization progression
Flexibility	1	1–3	30-second hold	N/A	N/A	3–7 times/week	4–6 weeks	SMR and static
Core	12–20	1–4	4/2/1	N/A	0–90 seconds	2–4 times/week	4–6 weeks	1–4 core-stabilization
Balance	12–20 or 6–10 each side for single leg	1–3	4/2/1 if applicable 0- to 60 60-second timed holds if tempo is not applicable	N/A	0–90 seconds	2–4 times/week	4–6 weeks	1–4 balance-stabilization
Reactive	5–8	1–3	3- to 5-second hold on landing	N/A	0–90 seconds	2–4 times/week	4–6 weeks	0–2 plyometric-stabilization
SAQ	2–3	1–2	Controlled for effective movement patterns	N/A	0–90 seconds	2–4 times/week	4–6 weeks	4–6 drills with limited horizontal inertia and unpredictability

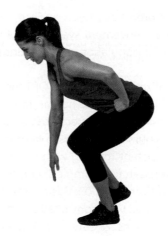

FIGURE 11.14 Single-leg squat touchdown.

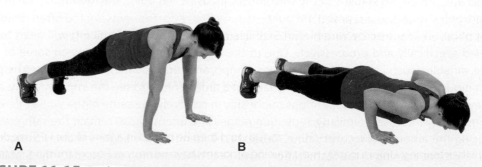

A   B

FIGURE 11.15 Push-up.

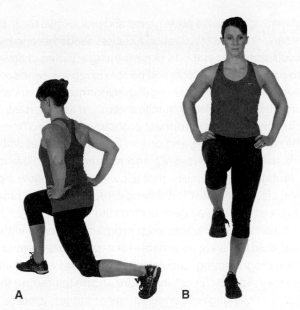

FIGURE 11.16 Transverse plane lunge to balance.

Common Mistakes Made in the Stabilization Level

Applying concepts related to program design and execution can always be disrupted by common mistakes that are made when working with clients. As a fitness professional, it is important to be aware of the pitfalls others have fallen into and actively make efforts to avoid them. The following are common mistakes that can be made in the Stabilization Level by fitness professionals:

◆ Underutilized assessments
◆ Lack of protocol, programming, or formulated means of progression
◆ Desire to progress too soon
◆ Focusing on stabilization or endurance, but not on both

Underutilized Assessments

As a professional in any career, it is important to have a wide range of data to pull from, so the optimal choices for a particular person and situation are provided. This is best done through a well-designed assessment. Too often, assessments are not utilized, or, more likely, not applied or followed up on. Assessments only work if they are used. Also, the only way to truly gauge a client's progress is to reassess and measure progress. These components are too often removed from training programs, limiting the value of what the fitness professional offers.

Lack of Protocol, Programming, or Formulated Means of Progression

Once assessments are implemented the client should then be placed in a level of the OPT model to begin their training. Unfortunately, most training programs have no protocol, programming, systems, or formulated means of progression or regression. They are often workouts that need refinement, preparation, and development to reach a professional and progressive means of delivering service. Often these exercise programs bypass stabilization exercises altogether and put clients at risk when performing their workouts, engaging in sports, or performing activities of daily living. Therefore, it is important to be able to properly assess clients and be able to regress exercises to provide service to a broad spectrum of clients. Though niche training (e.g., performance enhancement) can and should be sought out within the athletic population, stabilization is just as important, if not more so.

Sometimes the lack of protocol or appropriate programming stems from whether the fitness professional knows the reason, rationale, and proper form for exercises within each component (flexibility, cardio, core, balance, reactive, SAQ, and resistance). Stabilization Endurance training provides specific foundational exercises that allow clients to follow a path of progression. Proper form in this level creates the best stability possible as the client progresses through the OPT model. The professional must be diligent in checking form.

Well-designed warm-ups and movement prep programs are used with the most elite athletes in the world, so it should not seem reasonable for a traditional client or recreational athlete to bypass this part of the programming. Clients like to "feel" the workout and muscles working. Movement prep allows specific muscles to work more and be felt during the exercise program. If the gluteus maximus is not engaging during squats or lunges, it needs movement prep to help it prior to actually squatting.

Adding in the movement prep will provide insight to what the upcoming workout may look like. Good scapular stabilization in the movement prep may indicate an upper body focus. The movement prep will also help the professional in cuing the workout.

Desire to Progress Too Soon

Whether requested by the client or the fitness professional, training in the Stabilization Level is often accompanied with a desire to move faster than the adaptations occur and progressions allow. It is important to take the time to develop the necessary adaptations within each phase of training, not just Phase 1. If the progressions occur too rapidly, the client is at risk for injury, burnout, or drop out. It is the responsibility of the fitness professional to ensure that the client is ready for the next progression or phase prior to advancing forward.

The inability to stabilize joints while controlling bodily deceleration has led to a targeted focus on eccentric training in a controlled environment. A notable benefit of the slow eccentric movement is that it is the phase of the muscle action spectrum where most strength is developed. The slow and controlled rehearsal of deceleration allows the fitness professional to focus on building strength while minimizing the chance of injury.

The muscles of stabilization have specific responsibility to efficiently provide static and dynamic support to joints. When this phase of training is overlooked before moving into strength- or power-based programming, the stabilizers may be poorly equipped to support the stabilization needs of the body during the excess strength demands, external loads, and rate of force production.

Focusing Only on Stabilization or Endurance, But Not Both

Stability training and endurance training are not the same, but they complement each other well. Cutting down rest time, increasing repetitions, and adding sets may increase endurance, but not stability. Standing on one leg, using tools to challenge the body's ability to stabilize (e.g., stability ball), and doing unilateral presses or pulls while practicing antirotational exercise are all great, but they do not necessarily increase repetition, set, or work capacity endurance. Fitness professionals should practice both stabilization and endurance, and use the range

TRAINER TIPS

Perhaps a game of "You Pick One, I Pick One," where clients pick an exercise they want to do and the fitness professional supersets it with a stability exercise, can build excitement in Phase 1. If the client picks a bench press, the fitness professional could superset it with a push-up on a stability ball. Give clients a little of what they want and a bit of what they need.

CAUTION ⚠

An important note to make regarding the slow eccentric phase: it is the phase where most soreness is developed as well, so keeping the set range low in the initial workouts with clients is important to be able to gauge their reaction to the training.

CHECK IT OUT

The following are examples of common client objections to performing stability exercises and responses to negate them.

"I want to build muscle."

Stabilization Level training is important because symmetry is highly regarded in bodybuilding, recreational or professional. Activating the correct muscles, protecting the joints, and building a base before building the body is critical. With appropriate nutritional support, hypertrophy is still attainable in this level.

"I play(ed) competitive team sports."

It does not matter which sport is played, the importance of stabilization training for all competitive sports cannot be overstated. Precision and control of the body specific to the environment, reaction to the moving components of competition, and reaction to competitive cues all hinge on the neuromuscular system's ability to produce, reduce, and stabilize itself in multiple planes, at various speeds, in a safe and coordinated manner. As the NASM integrated performance paradigm states, force production and reduction depend on how well the body can stabilize and balance itself.

"I want to lose weight."

This is the easiest of all potential client resistances to answer. The slow tempos suggested in the Stabilization Level of the OPT model keep the client under tension for long periods of time. This, plus the high repetition range, and the common implementation of short rest periods between sets, or circuits, will increase the metabolic furnace. The client will increase heart rate, respiratory rate, sweat, and feel the burn (**acidosis**) in the muscles.

"This is easy."

All sets should end in momentary muscular, or volitional, fatigue. This means that no additional reps can be completed in the set before the loss of form or giving up.

"I'm bored."

This is possible for any level of training. The problem with bored clients is that they soon become someone else's clients, or stop training altogether. This is where periodization comes into play. The body and the brain may plateau, so be sure to find out what the client likes, and add it to their programming.

Acidosis

The accumulation of excessive hydrogen ions in the body, causing increased acidity of the blood and muscle

CHECK IT OUT

The OPT model provides the fitness professional with the freedom to work within it and through it. It is a repeatable system of progression with proven outcomes. It is important to maintain the preset variables such as tempo, sets, repetitions, etc. With all the different types of training tools and styles that exist, many fitness professionals ask, "What does NASM think of this exercise?" An exercise is not inherently good or bad, rather it should be asked if the exercise is appropriate for the client based on the client's assessments, goals, and phase of the OPT model.

TABLE 11.15 The Progression Continuum

Modality	Lower Body	Upper Body
Floor	Two-leg stable	Two arm
⇩	⇩	⇩
Sport beam	Staggered-stance stable	Alternating arms
⇩	⇩	⇩
Half foam roll	Single-leg stable	Single arm
⇩	⇩	⇩
Foam pad*	Two-leg unstable	Single arm with trunk rotation
⇩	⇩	
Balance disc*	Staggered-stance unstable	
⇩	⇩	
Wobble board*	Single-leg unstable	

*These modalities come in many shapes and sizes that will dictate proper progression.

CHECK IT OUT

Benefits of Phase 1 training for weight loss clients:

- Muscular endurance
- Increased time under low tension
- Lower rest intervals
- Core activation
- Increased caloric expenditure

of acute variables to adjust the programs and exercise selection specifically for their clients. **Table 11.15** shows how to effectively progress core, balance, and resistance training exercises.

Integrating the Stabilization Level with Other Phases

The levels of the OPT model are not "all or nothing," so incorporating more than one phase may be a point of preference that is well indicated. Stabilization Level training is excellent for neuromuscular efficiency, so it may be beneficial for clients to perform core stabilization prior to strength or power work. Performing small, specific exercises from the Stabilization Level, while in preparation for more intense training phases, may be necessary to facilitate the neural support to the local and global stabilization systems.

The eventual addition of undulating periodization into the client's program is a common way to continually touch base with their Phase 1 training once per week, while cycling through other phases of training on subsequent days. This variety can help keep clients stay engaged in the workouts while still supplying results-driven programming.

Corrective Strategies for Stabilization Clients

Each level of the OPT model is associated with a category of flexibility training, along with different techniques within each category. The category of flexibility training that correlates to Phase 1 training is called *corrective flexibility*. Using different techniques ((e.g., SMR, static stretching), the fitness professional can help correct muscle imbalances identified during static postural and dynamic movement assessments. Once the assessments have been performed and short and/or overactive muscles have been identified, the stretches can be implemented.

With each short and/or overactive muscle there are lengthened and/or underactive muscles that lack the strength to keep the associated joint(s) in proper alignment. For instance, if the knees fall inward during a squat, there are muscles that are pulling the knees together (muscles to be inhibited/stretched), and there are antagonist muscles lacking the strength to hold the knees in alignment (muscles to be activated). It is within the Stabilization Level that these issues will be addressed. Certainly, there is a professional obligation to help clients optimize movement, but progressing someone to the Strength or Power Level while their knees adduct in a squat is potentially dangerous.

Conclusion

The Stabilization Level of the OPT model provides the foundation for all subsequent training modalities. It is from this foundation that the successful fitness professional can safely build to address each client's individual needs and goals. Building from this level, continued reading will explore the goals and outcomes for the Strength Level of the OPT model.

Case in Review

As you begin to work with your three clients, it is important to describe the Stabilization Level and to explain how Phase 1 will be used to help them reach their fitness goals. Regardless of each client's abilities or previous experience with exercise, you explain the role that stabilization plays as you progress to higher levels of the OPT model. The following are examples of how you would approach each client identified within the case scenario:

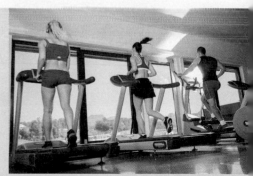

© fotoinfot/Shutterstock

- **Roderick, the bodybuilding client:** "In order to produce more force for the competition, the core needs to be stable and strong. Phase 1 will develop the core stabilization you need to produce more force in your powerlifts."

- **Mary, the weight loss client**: "Phase 1 may not seem like an intense workout. However, with the assigned acute variables, there is little rest and a great deal of time under tension for the muscles. Not only does this increase the intensity of the work, but it will also increase the caloric load of the workouts."

- **Ashley, the marathon client**: "In order to maintain a long-term event, you need to develop endurance, especially through the core of your body. The core will be the stable place from which the levers of your body will push from to propel you forward. Stability should be a high priority so that you do not lose energy through the use of your limbs when running. This will also require endurance that is developed during Phase 1."

When using the acute variables within the Stabilization Level, refer and follow the recommendations provided for Phase 1. You will want to progress your clients on an individual basis by periodically assessing each client, as well as determining the client's ability level. When addressing movement prep and resistance training within the Stabilization Level, you implement the following exercises based on each of your client's fitness goals:

- **Roderick, the bodybuilding client**: Focus on stabilization pushing and pulling exercises such as the single-leg cable chest press and single-leg cable row. Also, focus on stabilization hip hinge exercises, single-leg Romanian dead lift, and single-leg squat touchdown.

- **Mary, the weight loss client**: Perform circuits, with no rest between each exercise, of single-leg squat to row, single-leg balance reach, ladder drills (two feet each box, one foot each box), and squat jump with hold.

- **Ashley, the marathon client**: Single-leg balance with running arms, multiplanar single-leg balance reach, multiplanar hop with stabilization, multiplanar hop up with stabilization, ladder drills (two-feet each box, one foot each box), squat jump with hold, single-leg balance with opposite arm opposite leg reach.

References

Anderson, G., Gaetz, M., Holzmann, M., & Twist, P. (2011). Comparison of EMG activity during stable and unstable push-up protocols. *European Journal of Sport Science, 13*(1), 1–7. doi: 10.1080/17461391.2011.577240

Behm, D. G., Anderson, K., & Curnew, R. S. (2002). Muscle force and activation under stable and unstable conditions. *Journal of Strength Conditioning Research, 16*, 416–422.

Bellew, J. W., Yates, J. W., & Gater, D. R. (2003). The initial effects of low-volume strength training on balance in untrained older men and women. *Journal of Strength Conditioning Research, 17*, 121–128.

Bompa, T. O. (1993). *Periodization of strength: The new wave in strength training.* Toronto, ON: Verita Publishing.

Campos, G. E., Luecke, T. J., Wendeln, H. K., Toma, K., Hagerman, F. C., Murray, T. F., . . . Staron, R. S. (2002). Muscular adaptations in response to three different resistance-training regimens: Specificity of repetition maximum training zones. *European Journal of Applied Physiology, 88*, 50–60.

Chaitow, L. (1997). *Muscle energy techniques.* New York, NY: Churchill Livingstone.

Cosio-Lima, L. M., Reynolds, K. L., Winter, C., Paolone, V., & Jones, M. T. (2003). Effects of physioball and conventional floor exercises on early phase adaptations in back and abdominal core stability and balance in women. *Journal of Strength and Conditioning Research, 17*, 721–725.

Cressey, E. M., West, C. A., Tiberio, D. P., Kraemer, W. J., & Maresh, C. M. (2007). The effects of ten weeks of lower-body unstable surface training on markers of athletic performance. *Journal of Strength and Conditioning Research, 21*, 561–567.

Edgerton, V. R., Wolf, S. L., Levendowski, D. J., & Roy, R. R. (1996). Theoretical basis for patterning EMG amplitudes to asses muscle dysfunction. *Medicine and Science in Sport and Exercise, 28*(6), 744–751.

Enoka, R. M. (1988). Muscle strength and its development: New perspectives. *Sports Medicine, 6*, 146–168.

Etnyre, B. R., & Abraham, L. D. (1986). Gains in range of ankle dorsiflexion using three popular stretching techniques. *American Journal of Physical Medicine, 65*, 189–196

Fleck, S. J., & Kraemer, W. J. (1997). *Designing resistance training programs* (2nd ed.). Champaign, IL: Human Kinetics.

Heitkamp, H. C., Horstmann, T., Mayer, F., Weller, J., & Dickhuth, H. H. (2001). Gain in strength and muscular balance after balance training. *International Journal of Sports Medicine, 22*, 285–290.

Kraemer, W. J., Adams, K., Cafarelli, E., Dudley, G. A., Dooly, C., . . . Triplett-McBride, T. (2002). American College of Sports Medicine position stand. Progression models in resistance training for healthy adults. *Medicine and Science in Sport and Exercise, 34*, 364–380.

Kraemer, W. J., Ratamess, N., Fry, A. C., Triplett-McBride, T., Koziris, L. P., . . . Fleck, S. J. (2000). Influence of resistance training volume and periodization on physiological and performance adaptations in collegiate women tennis players. *American Journal of Sports Medicine, 28*, 626–633.

Marx, J. O., Ratamess, N. A., Nidl, B. C., Gotshalk, L. A., Volek, J. S., . . . Kraemer, W. J. (2001). Low-volume circuit versus high-volume periodized resistance training in women. *Medicine and Science in Sport and Exercise, 33*, 635–643.

Park, S. Y., & Yoo, W. G. (2011). Differential activation of parts of the serratus anterior muscle during push-up variations on stable and unstable bases of support. *Journal of Electromyography and Kinesiology, 21*, 861–867.

Sale, D. G. (1988). Neural adaptation to resistance training. *Medicine and Science in Sport and Exercise, 20*(Suppl), S135–S145.

Spiering, B. A., & Kraemer, W. J. (2008). Resistance exercise prescription. In: Chandler, T. J., & Brown, L. E. (Eds.), *Conditioning for strength and human performance* (pp. 273–291). Baltimore, MD: Wolters Kluwer, Lippincott Williams & Wilkins.

Tan, B. (1999). Manipulating resistance training program variables to optimize maximum strength in men: A review. *Journal of Strength and Conditioning Research, 13*, 289–304.

CHAPTER 12

THE OPTIMUM PERFORMANCE TRAINING™ (OPT™) MODEL: APPLYING STRENGTH

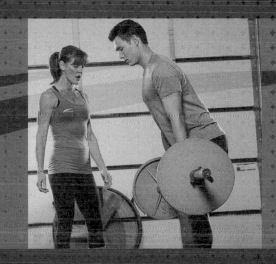

OBJECTIVES

After studying this chapter, you will be able to:

1. **Describe** the goals and outcomes of the Strength Level of the Optimum Performance Training (OPT) model.

2. **Explain** how strength goals are achieved.

3. **Utilize** strength acute variables on various client types.

4. **Implement** appropriate cardio protocols for the Strength Level.

5. **Implement** appropriate movement prep protocols for the Strength Level.

6. **Implement** appropriate resistance training protocols for the Strength Level.

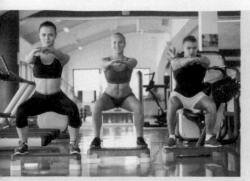
© fotoinfot/Shutterstock

Case Scenario

Think back to the three new clients you have acquired, assessed, and introduced to the Stabilization Level of the OPT model. Now that you have helped your clients prepare a stable base, preparing their bodies for the demands of higher training intensities, you feel that each of your clients can now move onto the Strength Level of the OPT model.

Your client's profiles and fitness goals are as follows:

- **Roderick** has been an avid gym-goer and is ready to take his training to the next level. Roderick goes to the gym daily, predominately lifting weights in hopes of entering an annual bodybuilding competition that is 9 months away.

- **Mary** has avoided the gym because she feels intimidated by the others working out and becomes self-conscious when exercising next to someone who she feels is in better shape. Recently, Mary's primary care physician has recommended that Mary seek a personal trainer to help her lose 20 pounds.

- **Ashley** has overcome many weight issues, but has been a victim of yo-yo dieting and workout programs she feels have not provided the results she is looking for. Over time, Ashely's desire to improve her health has sparked a passion for long-distance running and biking. She is highly committed and is willing to put in the time required to reach her goals. Feeling a need to challenge herself further, Ashley has registered to run a marathon in 4 months.

Consider the following questions:

- What are some possible client objections that you may experience as you progress to higher phases within the OPT model?

- How would you explain the purpose of each of phases of the Strength Level as they relate to each of your clients' fitness goals?

- How would you use the acute variables within the Strength Level for each of your clients?

- What movement prep and resistance training exercises would you use for each client?

- How is the Stabilization Level still used even though the clients are now in the Strength Level?

Introduction to the Strength Level of the OPT Model

With the foundational knowledge of the goals and outcomes of the Stabilization Level, the fitness professional can move forward to learning the protocols and applications of the Strength Level of the optimum performance training (OPT) model (**Figure 12.1**). The Strength Level is different from the Stabilization and Power Levels in that it is composed of three different phases: Phase 2: Strength Endurance, Phase 3: Hypertrophy, and Phase 4: Maximal Strength. The Strength Level of training is designed to maintain stability, while increasing the amount of stress placed on the body for improved muscle size and strength. This period of training is a progression from stabilization training, and promotes additional muscular fitness adaptations that support optimal function. This chapter will explore how various strength goals are achieved as well as appropriate protocols, movement prep exercises, and resistance training exercises for the Strength Level.

The capacity of the human body to stabilize itself against external forces, complete complex movements, and respond to a variety of stresses is remarkable. Force generation is governed by the central nervous system to enable the human body to complete a variety of tasks, including incredible feats of strength such as a power-lifter completing a 1,200-pound back squat, as well as the precise control of motion demonstrated by a ballerina during an arabesque. The manner in which the body creates, governs, and coordinates forces to function so effectively, as well as how it adapts to the stresses it faces, are important areas of study for the fitness professional.

Goals and Adaptations in the Strength Level

The Strength Level of the OPT model focuses on strength development to promote optimal performance of the body. In this level of training, the focus is to:

◆ Increase the ability of the core musculature to stabilize the lumbo-pelvic-hip complex (LPHC) and spine under heavier loads and through more complex ranges of motion (strength endurance).
◆ Improve **metabolic conditioning**.

Metabolic conditioning
Exercise that improves effective and efficient energy storage and delivery for physical activity.

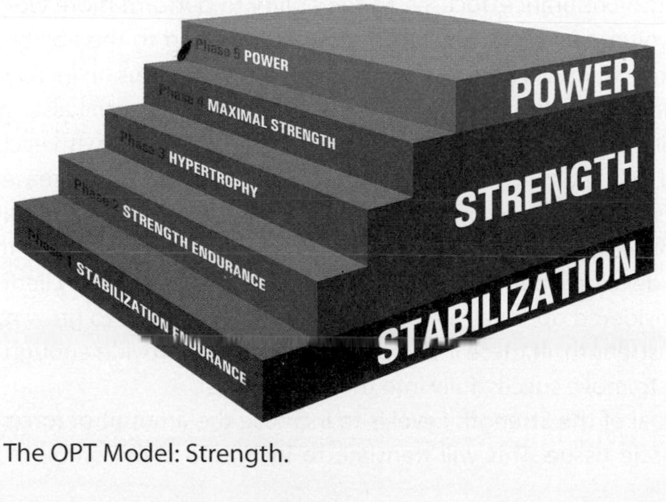

FIGURE 12.1 The OPT Model: Strength.

- ◆ Increase the load-bearing capabilities of muscles, tendons, ligaments, and joints (strength endurance and hypertrophy).
- ◆ Increase the volume of training to stimulate muscle tissue growth (hypertrophy).
- ◆ Increase motor unit recruitment, frequency of motor unit activation, and motor unit synchronization (maximal strength).

Muscular weakness has been linked to frailty and functional impairments that occur with aging, whereas muscular strength has been shown to help maintain mobility and movement efficiency across the lifespan (Pendergast, Fisher, & Calkins, 1993; Peterson, Rhea, Sen, & Gordon, 2010; Rantanen et al., 1999). The loss of muscle mass that accompanies physical inactivity is seen as a predictor of weakness, disability, and diminished autonomy among older adults, and diminished strength has been identified as a principle limiting factor in functionality later in life (Dehail et al., 2007; Hughes, Myers, & Schenkman, 1996; Peterson, Sen, & Gordon, 2011). Therefore, strength development and maintenance is vital to healthy aging and continued function throughout the lifespan. Resistance exercise has been shown to increase lean body mass, and improvements in strength also serve as the foundation for power improvements (Harris, Stone, O'Bryant, Proulx, & Johnson, 2000; Peterson, Alvar, & Rhea, 2006; Peterson et al., 2011).

Given the connection between strength and functionality, and the correlation between strength and power, the Strength Level in the OPT model is vital to the proper and orderly development of muscular fitness. Each phase is designed to stimulate a specific group of adaptations in the neuromuscular system, with the end result being improved ability to exert force in a controlled, coordinated fashion. Without sufficient development of total body strength, postural alignment may become flawed, activities of daily living and many occupational demands will be difficult to complete, and power potential will be limited. Additionally, muscles and connective tissue such as tendons and ligaments may not be adequately prepared for the progression in training that occurs in the Power Level, increasing the risk of injury both in training and during the performance of power-related tasks. The underlying goals of the Strength Level, how the body generates force and adapts with improved abilities when confronted with proper stresses, and effective strategies for implementing the phases of the Strength Level in an organized training plan will be discussed.

The Strength level has three phases, each with a slightly different focus, but building on the previous phase to culminate in maximal strength development. Improving the ability to produce force over extended periods of time, increasing muscle mass, and enhancing maximal force capacity has valuable health and fitness benefits. Fitness professionals should keep these goals in mind and understand how each phase helps their clients to achieve these goals.

Phase 2, Strength Endurance, focuses on the ability to perform more work, and to tolerate greater exercise volume and intensity. These adaptations lead to the ability to train at higher loads and at greater volume in Phase 3: Hypertrophy, with the focus on increasing muscle mass. As muscle mass increases during Phase 3, force production potential also increases, as more muscle mass results in more myofilaments pulling across each other with each muscle contraction. This will lead into Phase 4: Maximal Strength. Phase 4 stimulates increased neuromuscular performance. This, accompanied by the growth of muscular tissue from Phase 3, will provide the adaptations necessary for maximal strength gain. Thus, all the phases in the Strength Level build toward the development of maximal strength. Depending of the client's goals, Phases 3 and 4 may be considered optional, as some may not have a desire to grow muscle or develop maximal levels of strength. In these instances, Phase 2 would provide enough strength adaptation for the client to move successfully into the Power Level.

The primary goal of the Strength Level is to increase the amount of force capable of being produced by muscle tissue. This will translate to increased stabilization of joints, improved

CAUTION

Skipping the Strength Level may result in increased risk of injury during the performance of power-related tasks.

CHECK IT OUT

Goals during Phase 2: Strength Endurance, include:

- Increased work capacity and **exercise tolerance**.
- Improvement in the core musculature's ability to stabilize the pelvis and spine under heavier loads, through complete ranges of motion.
- Increased load-bearing capabilities of the muscles, tendons, ligaments, and joints.

As these goals are met, the client is better prepared to move to Phase 3: Hypertrophy, where the primary goals include:

- Increased muscle mass.
- Increased connective tissue strength and mass.
- Increased metabolism through increased muscle mass.

Phase 4: Maximal Strength, continues the adaptations from Phases 2 and 3 and features the following goals:

- Increased **motor unit activation**.
- Increased motor unit synchronization.
- Increased **muscle coordination**.
- Enhanced force production in preparation for the Power Level.

Exercise tolerance

Increased ability to perform more exercise in less time, without undue fatigue or excessive soreness.

Motor unit activation

Increased recruitment of motor units and/or recruitment of motor units rapidly and repeatedly.

Muscle coordination

Complex neurological control of motor units, ensuring effective contraction and relaxation of muscle tissue across agonist and antagonist muscle groups.

posture, and enhanced movement control. The end goal is to enhance the function of the human body through strategic management of training stress.

The majority of the adaptations that occur in the initial weeks of training are attributed primarily to neurological changes in the activation and coordination of motor units (Folland & Williams, 2007; Ruther et al, 1995). After periods of training, it appears that the level of motor unit activation increases, thus increasing the amount of force produced (Folland & Williams, 2007). One study found diminished co-activation of agonist and antagonist muscles after only 1 week of resistance training, suggesting improved coordination of the activation of specific muscle tissue during a desired movement (Carolan & Cafarelli, 1992). This may be a protective mechanism implemented by the brain to prevent excessive amounts of tension from being generated before the muscle and tendon are prepared to handle such forces.

Over time, changes begin to occur in the structure of the muscle tissue, enabling greater amounts of tension to be created. Hypertrophy, or an increase in muscle size, is a common outcome following resistance training programs in most populations, due to the addition of new myofilaments within the muscle fiber (Folland & Williams, 2007). A strong correlation exists between muscle cross-sectional area and muscular strength (Maughan, Watson, & Weir, 1983). The addition of these filaments results in greater numbers of contractile elements in the muscle, dramatically increasing force potential.

In addition to the alteration in the structure of muscle tissue, other soft tissue will be able to experience higher amounts of tension without being damaged. As a result of strength training, tendons increase in thickness and rigidity, and bones increase in density (Almstedt et al, 2011; Ashe et al., 2013; Folland & Williams, 2007; Hinton, Nigh, & Thyfault, 2015; Humphries et al, 2009). As bones increase in density they become better able to safely handle the lifting of heavier weight, decreasing the risk of fractures, and as tendons become thicker they are better able to handle high loads and greater amounts of stress.

TRAINER TIPS

As long as a client can perform an exercise safely, the client can be progressed to Phase 2 quickly. Phase 2 is a superset with Phase 1 exercises, so the client is still getting the adaptations of strength endurance and stabilization.

CHECK IT OUT

Wolf's law states that bone will build upon the lines of stress that are applied to it. This is the reason why strength training is so important to older adults. As they lose bone mineral density it becomes important for them to continually load the bones with weight in order to decrease the amount of bone mineral loss. Davis's law is the same for soft tissue and shows the evidence for the adaptations of tendons and muscle with strength training. These tissues will build upon their lines of stress as well.

Strength endurance

The ability of the body to repeatedly produce high levels of force for prolonged periods.

These adaptations ultimately result in improved muscular function in several ways. **Strength endurance** is enhanced as muscles become more efficient, meaning that less muscle tissue is needed to move a certain amount of resistance, or to support the body. Research has shown that muscular endurance is highly trainable, with improvements ranging from 5–50% after 6–24 weeks of exercise (Arazi, Rahmati, & Zaheri, 2013; Figueiredo et al., 2011; Rhea, Alvar, Burkett, & Ball, 2003). Improved strength endurance results in less fatigue during activities of daily living, increased capacity for exercise, and improved posture throughout the day.

Hypertrophy may be a desired outcome for some clients regardless of the change in muscle function. Research has shown increases in muscle cross-sectional area ranging from 1–14% among the general population (Peterson et al., 2011; Ruther et al., 1995). Women generally experience far less hypertrophy than men due to having lower blood androgen levels (Brown & Wilmore, 1974). However, women are capable of increasing muscle mass with positive implications for health and function, with long-lasting effects as aging naturally results in some deterioration in muscle tissue. Therefore, hypertrophy should remain as a potential goal of the Strength Level for women of all ages. Maximal strength improves with each of the adaptations described. Research has demonstrated improvements in strength ranging from 5–55% following strength training programs of up to 24 weeks (Peterson, Rhea, & Alvar, 2004; Rhea & Alderman, 2004; Rhea, Alvar, et al., 2003). With improved maximal strength, submaximal tasks become less stressful and work capacity is improved.

TRAINER TIPS

Strength training will not produce large amounts of muscle growth in women. Understanding that the androgen levels of women will not produce large muscular growth adaptations is important when clients are nervous about putting on muscle mass.

Scientific Principles of Strength Training

The application of stress to promote improved function is guided by several key scientific principles, which provide important direction to the fitness professional when planning and implementing an effective training program. These scientific principles should be considered when creating the program, as well as when influencing alterations in the training plan over time. Fitness professionals must be familiar with each principle and know how each relates to a successful training program.

Overload Principle and Strength Training

When beginning a resistance training program following a period of inactivity, a client does not need a great deal of added stress to trigger improvements in structure and function. A client who has been training consistently for many years will require a greater amount of stress to overload the muscles, due to the body's familiarity with training stress. In one study, low-volume, low-intensity resistance training, performed by untrained populations, resulted in more strength improvements than in lifters who had been training consistently for at least

6 months (Rhea, Alvar, et al., 2003). The study also suggests that different degrees of overload can stimulate different amounts of strength improvements. Additionally, individual differences in response can influence the degree of improvement seen with a specific training stress (Fluck, 2006; Mann, Lamberts, & Lambert, 2014). It is therefore vital that the fitness professional prescribe the right amount of stress to stimulate the desired gain in fitness, requiring individual monitoring and alterations with training.

Progression

With consistent exercise, the amount of stress needed to overload the systems of the body must increase, or progress, in order to continue to see improvements in fitness. Research has shown a need to increase volume and intensity of resistance training in order to continue to stimulate strength improvements (Peterson et al., 2004; Rhea, Alvar, et al., 2003). The muscular system becomes accustomed to resistance training stress, and improved structure and function ceases, or at least slows. As this occurs, training stress must be increased to promote continued gains in strength and hypertrophy.

The principle of progression also suggests a gradual, continuous increase in stress rather than drastic, rapid changes. The increase in stress should allow the body to initiate and execute changes in structure and function. Applying the correct amount of stress to initiate changes without excessively overloading the muscular system is vital to safety and effectiveness. Thus, progression should occur gradually over a long period of time for the best improvements.

Muscular Force Production

Strength represents the ability to generate force (Siff, 2001). This force is a result of tension created in muscles when activated by the nervous system. The activated muscle tissue creates tension by pulling toward the midline of the muscle belly. As muscles shorten, the tension created is transferred to the skeletal system through the tendons, which attach muscles to bones. This tension, transferred through the tendons to the bone, produces movement around the joints of the skeletal system.

Muscle contractions are signaled via an electrical impulse from a motor nerve, which controls a group of muscle fibers. Inside each muscle fiber are filaments (actin and myosin) that engage when prompted and pull across each other, resulting in the shortening of the muscle fiber. The pulling of many filaments throughout the muscle develops tension in the tissue and exerts force on the bones to which they attach.

The amount of force produced at a given time is determined by a number of factors, including the size and number of motor units recruited, activation of those motor units, and the level of **neural drive**. Recruiting a greater number of motor units, and/or recruiting larger motor units, results in a greater number of filaments generating tension within the muscle. As more motor units are activated, more filaments become engaged and contract within the muscle or muscle groups, creating higher levels of tension (**Figure 12.2**). Sending a higher frequency of signals in rapid succession, or increasing neural drive, compounds the contraction force and can increase muscle tension (Folland & Williams, 2007). Thus, the brain can regulate force production depending on the task and level of tension needed (Zatsiorsky, 1995). Additionally, the neuromuscular system must be able to stabilize the body, or specific segments of the body, while force is being created by muscle contractions. Failure to stabilize during force production results in increased risk of injury and poor execution of tasks.

Neural drive
The frequency of activation signals sent to muscle fibers via motor neurons.

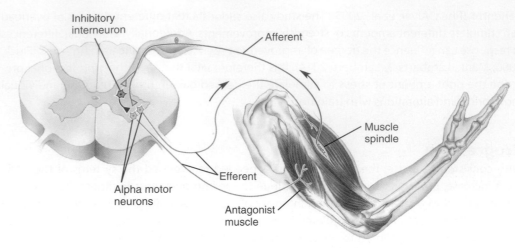

FIGURE 12.2 Motor unit activation.

Tracking Progress in the Strength Level

Specific goals in each phase of the Strength Level will determine the appropriate tests to monitor progress. Many of the goals involve complex physiological processes, which cannot be tested without access to an advanced lab or testing center. Instead, fitness professionals can monitor the expression of these adaptations through a variety of field tests. Tracking progress, along with interpreting improvements in relation to expected changes, are important roles of the fitness professional. Each phase has specific methods for tracking progress through the levels of the OPT model. However, sometimes the client has other goals, such as losing weight. In these instances, it is important to track the adaptations that the phase aims to accomplish as well as the client's individualized goal.

During Phase 2, documenting the maximum number of repetitions a client can perform at a submaximal weight is a good way to measure strength endurance and track progress. Examining core stability during complex load-bearing exercises, such as the squat, can provide valuable information in the evaluation and tracking of progress in this regard. Clients should be able to safely stabilize lighter loads during complex exercises prior to progressing to heavy loads.

Circumference measurements and body composition assessments are valuable during Phase 3: Hypertrophy (**Figure 12.3**). The goal in this phase is to increase muscle mass. Circumference measurements can be tracked over time to monitor progress, and should be evaluated in conjunction with body composition assessments, as reductions in body fat will cause circumference to decrease. Theoretically, body fat may decrease while muscle mass is increasing, with a result of no change in circumference measurement. Either way, the end result is positive and should be explained to the client as such. Also note that changes in body composition, specifically the increase of muscle mass, may take a long time to achieve, so it is best to keep clients' expectations reasonable to prevent discouragement.

Various measures of strength should be conducted during Phase 4: Maximal Strength. The one-repetition maximum (1RM) test has been used frequently in the literature (Rhea, Alvar, et al., 2003). Research has shown that in untrained populations improvements in strength over 12 weeks range between 5–55% depending on training volume, intensity, and frequency (Rhea, Alvar, et al., 2003; Seitz et al, 2014).

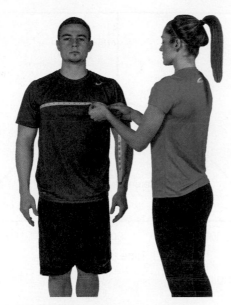

FIGURE 12.3 Circumference measurement.

CHECK IT OUT

Increased muscle mass is almost nonexistent in untrained exercisers during the first few months of training (Schoenfeld, 2010). After the first few months, where the majority of improvement in muscular fitness results from neurological changes, hypertrophic responses to training begin to appear. However, it appears that increases in muscle mass do not occur as rapidly as other muscular adaptations, with changes of 0.5–10% being reported after about 12 weeks of training in various populations (Arazi et al., 2013; Goto et al., 2004; Peterson et al., 2010; Ruther et al., 1995). Fitness professionals should be prepared to discuss the rate of increase in muscle mass with their clients.

Another method of tracking improvements in strength is to monitor and record the weight used during certain exercises for a certain number of repetitions. For instance, in week 1 of Phase 4 a client may perform eight repetitions on the chest press machine at 45 pounds. In week 3, the same exercise for eight repetitions was also performed and the client was able to lift 60 pounds, representing a 15-pound increase (33%). In week 12, the chest press was again performed for eight repetitions and the client was able to lift a maximal weight of 75 pounds (a 66% increase from week 1). Monitoring the weight performed in the same exercise, for the same number of repetitions, allows for the identification and evaluation of improvements.

For all testing, untrained clients will most likely see greater improvements during the Strength Level than will highly-trained clients. As the body becomes better conditioned, improvements in fitness are more difficult to achieve. Thus, the rate of improvement slows over time, representing **diminishing returns** (Figure 12.4). Due to this, more work is needed to achieve any improvement in fitness, with the total potential improvement declining as the individual becomes more accustomed to training. Fitness professionals must be prepared to educate clients regarding the anticipated rate of improvement and total amount of improvement over time, in order to motivate clients and make alterations to training as needed.

Diminishing returns

As the systems of the body become more developed, the rate of improvement in fitness slows.

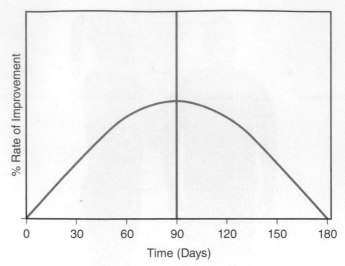

FIGURE 12.4 Diminishing returns.

Cardiorespiratory Training Protocols in the Strength Level

Optimum fitness and performance result from well-rounded training, focusing on all aspects of fitness. During the Strength Level, it is important that cardiorespiratory exercise continues to be included in the training program to ensure progress in all fitness areas. Multicomponent fitness training must be done in the proper manner to avoid conflicting stimuli and overtraining. The fitness professional must balance training stresses, to ensure proper progression without undermining the goals of the Strength Level.

All clients should perform an appropriate amount of cardiorespiratory exercise, even those seeking maximal strength development, such as strength athletes and weightlifters. The majority of clients can perform cardiorespiratory exercise at higher intensities and volumes, and greater frequencies, while still achieving considerable strength improvements. For those in the general population, the mixture of both cardiorespiratory exercise and resistance training throughout the Strength Level is appropriate. This is where Stage II cardiorespiratory training will become important (**Figure 12.5**). The focus is to increase the workload of cardio training in a way that will help clients alter their heart rate in and out of Zones 1 and 2. Stage II is the introduction to interval training, in which intensities are varied throughout the workout. As with resistance training, it needs to be understood that a client will not be ready to move directly into high levels of high-intensity interval training (HIIT). They must utilize the general adaptation syndrome (GAS) in order to achieve the adaptations necessary for higher levels of intensity in their interval training. The prudent fitness professional will understand this, and progress the client through the stages of cardiorespiratory training in order to avoid injury and early burnout. A typical Stage II workout is structured as follows:

1. Warm-up in Zone 1 for 5–10 minutes (65–75%)
2. Move into a 1-minute interval in Zone 2. The client should reach Zone 2 within that minute (76–85%).

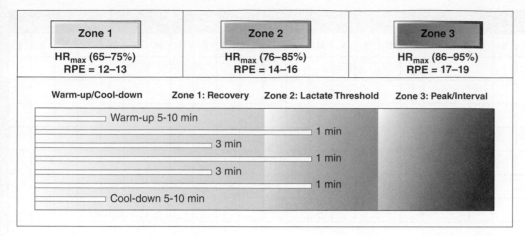

FIGURE 12.5 Stage II cardiorespiratory training.

3. After the 1-minute interval the client should return to Zone 1 for 3 minutes.
4. Repeat this as long as the client has recovered back to Zone 1 within the 3-minute period.
5. Repeat this pattern for a 30-minute workout. Finish with a 5- to 10-minute cool-down.

The timing of the intervals can be changed and adjusted to vary the workout. The goal is to maintain a 1:3 work-to-rest ratio. For instance the client can be asked to work in Zone 2 for 30 seconds and the recovery period reduced from 3 minutes to 90 seconds. The fitness professional should ensure that the client is achieving the Zone 2 goal in the 30-second work period and recovering to Zone 1 within the 90-second recovery period. The fitness professional can also utilize the first session of Stage II training to gain a more accurate view of the fitness level of the client and make adjustments accordingly.

TRAINER TIPS

You might consider splitting the cardio up into segments: 15 minutes before the workout and 15 minutes after. This provides a warm-up and cool-down for the client, and it is perfect for the low intensity needed to preserve muscle gains in this phase.

CHECK IT OUT ✓

1. If the client was not able to reach the predicted Zone 2 range in 1 minute, then use the heart rate he or she was able to reach as the client's "85%."
2. Take 9% off this number to get the lower end of the client's readjusted zone.
3. For example, if 150 beats per minute (bpm) was the predicted 85% of HR_{max}, but the client was only able to work up to 145 bpm during the 1-minute push, 145 bpm should now be considered that client's 85% HR_{max}.
4. Take 9% off 145 (9% of 145 is 13 beats: 145 − 13 = 132). So, 132 bpm is 76% of the client's HR_{max}.
5. If the client gets into the readjusted Zone 2, and reaching this zone was fine, work slowly to increase the client's time in this zone.
6. If the client's heart rate goes above the predicted zone and he or she still can recover back to Zone 1 at the end, add a couple of beats per minute to the zone and then work on increasing the time.

In Stage II, it is important to alternate days of the week with Stage I training. This means alternating sessions every workout, as shown in **Figure 12.6**.

When cardio and resistance training are performed in the same session, fatigue may be an issue to consider when planning the order in which the different exercises should be

Week	Week 1							Week 2							Week 3							Week 4						
Day	M	T	W	T	F	s	s	M	T	W	T	F	s	s	M	T	W	T	F	S	S	M	T	W	T	F	s	s
Phase 1																												
Phase 2																												
Phase 3																												
Phase 4																												
Phase 5																												
Cardio	S1		S2		S1			S2		S1		S2			S1		S2		S1			S2		S1		S2		
Flexibility	X		X		X			X		X		X			X		X		X			X		X		X		

S1 = Stage I   S2 = Stage II

FIGURE 12.6 Monthly plan – Stage II cardio training.

Concurrent training

Training designed to maintain or improve multiple fitness components in the same training phase.

performed. The components of greatest priority should be performed first, in order to avoid fatigue and maximize the quality of the most important parts of the workout. For clients needing greater improvements in strength, strength training should be done first, followed by cardiorespiratory exercise. Those seeking greater improvements in cardiorespiratory fitness should perform endurance training early in the session, followed by resistance exercises for strength development. Simply altering exercise order and managing acute variables can enable **concurrent training** to occur within the same session.

CHECK IT OUT

In recent years, research has identified potential drawbacks of concurrent cardiorespiratory exercise and strength training. Concurrent training, defined as simultaneously incorporating both resistance and endurance exercise within a training regimen, should be carefully considered when designing the training program during the Strength Level of the OPT model, as variations in training volume, intensity, and exercise order can influence adaptations, it is important to minimize the negative impact of concurrent exercise (Fyfe, Bishop, & Stepto, 2014).

Resistance and endurance training represent divergent exercise modes, with opposing adaptations in muscular properties (Fyfe et al., 2014). Research has shown that concurrent training compromises the development of strength and muscle mass (Fyfe et al., 2014; Leveritt et al, 1999). However, it appears that acute training variables can be altered in order to minimize the impact of concurrent training on strength development and muscle mass. Cardiorespiratory exercise of high intensity, frequency, and volume appears to cause the greatest limitation to the development of strength and hypertrophy. Therefore, cardiorespiratory exercise during the Strength Level *for those clients seeking maximal strength gains* should involve the following:

1. Lower-intensity cardiorespiratory exercise (<75% of maximum oxygen uptake).
2. Frequencies of 3 days per week or fewer.
3. Volume of less than 45 minutes per day.

CAUTION

Fatigue from one form of training can influence the performance of other modalities later in the training session. When prescribing both cardiorespiratory exercise and resistance training in the same session, whichever component is of greatest priority should be completed first.

Movement Preparation in the Strength Level

Although the primary focus of the Strength Level is to increase force production, continued attention to other movement preparation components (i.e., flexibility, core, balance, reactive, and SAQ) can have a positive impact on strength development while also contributing to improvements in overall fitness. The movement preparation portion of the training session can be used to address each of these fitness components while also preparing the body for resistance training.

Fitness professionals should avoid a few of the common mistakes that are often made during the movement prep portion of the workout. Rushing through the movement prep in order to get to the resistance training may result in the incorrect performance of strength exercises, which may reinforce movement dysfunction. Training strength in the presence of unchecked movement impairments may then lead to altered force-couple relationships and synergistic dominance, further exacerbating the movement dysfunction. Another common mistake is failure to individualize the movement prep portion to the specific needs of each client. Implementing the same techniques for all clients may be an adequate general warm-up, but will not address the specific movement dysfunctions or limitations of each client. As with all portions of the training session, tailoring exercises to the needs of each individual client is vital to optimal fitness development. The movement prep plays a key role in this process and must be implemented accordingly.

SMR and Flexibility Protocols for the Strength Level

Self-myofascial release (SMR) techniques and flexibility exercises remain important during the Strength Level of the OPT model. SMR has become a tool that most fitness professionals now embrace and utilize in some manner (Stitz & Pelot, 2015). Some concern has been expressed regarding SMR prior to athletic or strength performance, but the most recent review suggests that it does not impede athletic performance acutely or in the short term (Janot et al., 2013; Peacock et al., 2014; Beardsley & Skarabot, 2015). In fact, SMR may increase muscular performance, aid in effective preparation for exercise and activity, improve movement efficiency, as well as increase efficiency of, and prolong, the stretch–shortening cycle (Beardsley & Skarabot, 2015; Bradbury-Squires et al., 2015). Increases in agility, strength, and speed resulting from the use of SMR and dynamic warm-up exercises have also been seen (Peacock et al., 2014). Therefore, SMR techniques are useful during both the warm-up/movement prep and cool-down portions of a workout during the Strength Level of the OPT model.

The optimal dose of SMR for improvements in range of motion (ROM) and muscular performance is a minimum of 30 seconds per set, with 1–2 sets per overactive muscle(s) (**Table 12.1**). SMR techniques should be chosen to target a variety of muscle groups (Peacock et al., 2014).

Active-isolated stretching allows for agonists and synergists to move a limb through a full ROM while the antagonists are being stretched. Active-isolated stretching is utilized for the Strength Level and its associated phases. Before workouts, 1–2 sets of active-isolated stretches should be performed at 5–10 repetitions with a 1- to 2-second hold for each.

TABLE 12.1. Flexibility Strength Acute Variables

	Reps	Sets	Tempo	% Intensity	Rest	Frequency	Duration	Exercise Selection
SMR	1	1–2	Minimum of 30-second holds	N/A	N/A	3–7 days/week	4 weeks	SMR
Active-isolated	5–10	1–2	2- to 5-second holds	N/A	N/A	3–7 days/week	4 weeks	Active-isolated

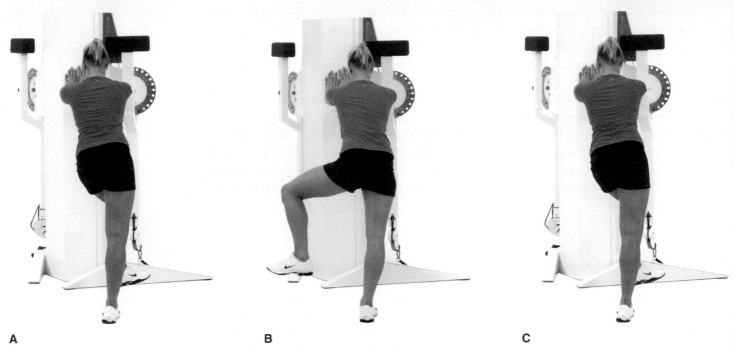

Active gastocnemius stretch with pronation and supination.

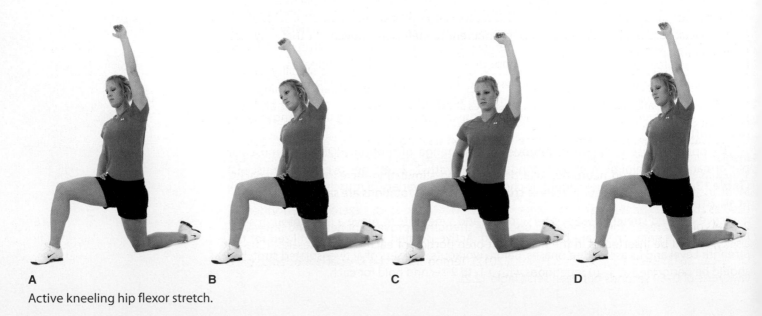

Active kneeling hip flexor stretch.

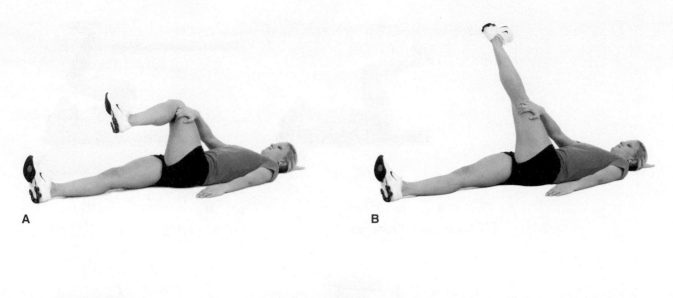

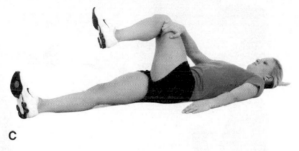

Active supine biceps femoris stretch.

Core Protocols for the Strength Level

The objective of core training is to uniformly strengthen the deep and superficial muscles that stabilize, align, and move the trunk of the body, especially the abdominals and muscles of the back. A weak core is a fundamental problem inherent to inefficient movement that may lead to predictable patterns of injury (Hewett, Paterno, & Myer, 2002; Hodges & Richardson, 1996; Leetun et al., 2004; Nadler, Malanga, et al., 2002; O'Sullivan et al., 1997). Core stability has important health implications but is also needed to ensure safety during resistance training.

In Phases 2, 3, and 4 of the OPT model, exercises should involve dynamic eccentric and concentric movements of the spine throughout a full ROM (including rotation) while performing the activation techniques learned in core stabilization training (Phase 1). Phases 2 through 4 involve increased training loads and faster tempos as compared to core training during Phase 1, resulting in enhanced neuromuscular demands and stimulating increased force capacity. Medicine ball hip to hip rotation, reverse crunches, and cable rotations are samples that can be used as core strengthening exercises (**Figures 12.7–12.9**). One to four exercises, performed for 2–3 sets of 8–12 repetitions, depending upon core strength improvement needs and time availability, should be inserted to in the movement prep portion of each training session (Chang, Lin, & Lai, 2015; Reed, Ford, Myer, & Hewett, 2012). Tempo should be kept at a moderate pace with rests of 0–60 seconds between sets (Table 12.2).

TRAINER TIPS ⫞

If clients are struggling with the stabilization exercise of the superset in Phase 2, prime them with a couple of targeted core exercises to warm-up with, and if they are still struggling, offer a regression for the exercise. For example, if they cannot stabilize with a ball push-up, perhaps have them do bench push-ups or regular push-ups first, and then once that is mastered, move them back into a ball push-up to reevaluate their ability to stabilize their core.

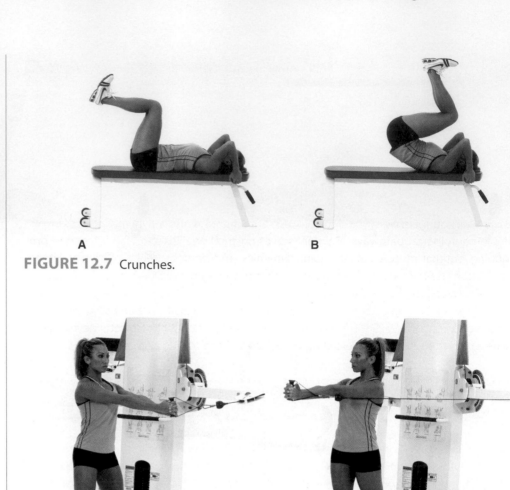

A   B

FIGURE 12.7 Crunches.

A   B

FIGURE 12.8 Cable rotations.

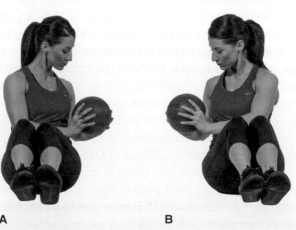

A   B

FIGURE 12.9 Medicine ball hip to hip rotation.

TABLE 12.2 Core Strength Acute Variables							
Reps	Sets	Tempo	Intensity	Rest	Frequency	Duration	Exercise Selection
8–12	2–3	2/0/2	N/A	0–60 seconds	2–4 days/week	4 weeks	1–3 core strength

Balance Protocols in the Strength Level

Balance is often thought of as only a static process, but balance is also a dynamic process involving multiple neurological pathways. Maintenance of postural equilibrium is an integrated process requiring optimal muscle balance, joint dynamics, and neuromuscular efficiency. Fitness professionals can use balance training protocols to promote improved performance in each of these areas. Research has shown that balance training improves sports performance and reduces sport-related injuries, and restores proprioception and neuromuscular function compromised by injuries (Bernier & Perrin, 1998; Elis & Rosenbaum, 2001; Hertel et al., 2006; Hewett, Meyer & Ford, 2005; McKeon & Hertel, 2008; Mansfield et al., 2015; Lesinski et al., 2015; Zech et al., 2009).

CHECK IT OUT

During activities of daily living, individuals may encounter the need to demonstrate balance, and athletes experience many balance demands during sport activities (Mansfield et al., 2015). Perturbations, such as external forces from an opposing athlete or tripping during walking over uneven surfaces, challenge the neuromuscular system as it attempts to stabilize the body through muscle activation and body positioning. Balance recovery reactions, such as swaying around the ankles or hips, taking a step, and shifting body weight, are executed to prevent falls and maintain stability (Mansfield et al., 2015). Strength plays an important role in these reactions as greater force production contributes to improved stabilization.

Balance training remains an important component of the Strength Level, contributing to the safety and effectiveness of resistance training for strength adaptations. Balance stabilization exercises, as performed in the Stabilization Level, are progressed to exercises that involve dynamic eccentric and concentric movements of the balance leg through a full ROM. These movements will require dynamic control in the mid-ROM, with isometric stabilization at the end ROM. Balance exercises in the Strength Level are designed to improve neuromuscular efficiency of the entire human movement system. The following is a sampling of balance strength exercises (**Figures 12.10–12.14**):

- Single-leg squat
- Single-leg squat touchdown
- Single-leg Romanian deadlift
- Single-leg Lift and Chop
- Multiplanar lunge to balance

Phases 2, 3, and 4 of the Strength Level should incorporate one to three balance strength exercises, in the movement prep portion of the training session, up to four times per week (Table 12.3). About 2–3 sets of each exercise (depending on the client's goals and amount of

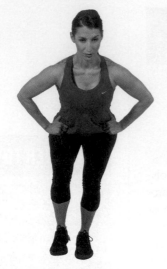

FIGURE 12.10 Single-leg squat.

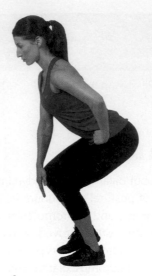

A

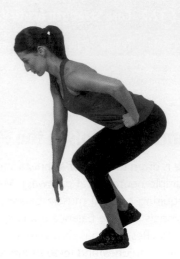

B

FIGURE 12.11 Single-leg squat touchdown.

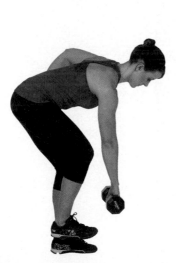

FIGURE 12.12 Single-leg romanian deadlift.

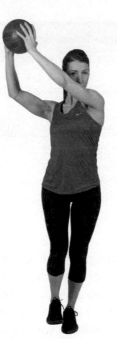

A

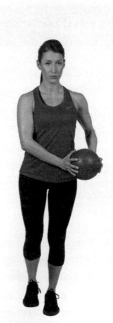

B

FIGURE 12.13 Single-leg lift and chop.

TABLE 12.3 Balance Strength Acute Variables

Reps	Sets	Tempo	Intensity	Rest	Frequency	Duration	Exercise Selection
8–12	2–3	2/0/2	N/A	0–60 seconds	2–4 days/week	4 weeks	1–3 balance strength

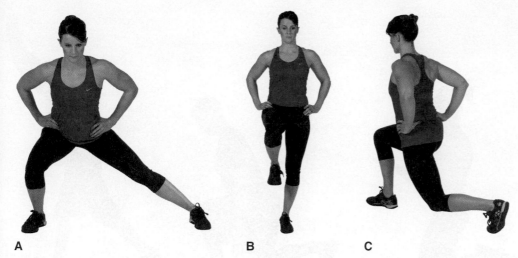

A   B   C

FIGURE 12.14 Multiplanar lunge to balance.

improvement needed) performed for 8–12 repetitions per set are optimal (Lesinski et al., 2015). The tempo should progress to 2/0/2 in order to increase the neuromuscular demand of each exercise. When training balance, fatigue should be kept to a minimum, thus 30–90 seconds of rest between sets should be provided to allow for sufficient recovery.

Reactive Training Protocols for the Strength Level

The inclusion of reactive training in the Strength Level should involve a progression from the Stabilization Level to the use of more dynamic eccentric and concentric movement through a full ROM. Speed and neural demand should also be progressed in this level by performing multiple repetitions in succession (without pausing between repetitions). Sample reactive strength exercises include (**Figures 12.15–12.17**):

- ◆ Tuck jump
- ◆ Butt kick
- ◆ Jumping lunges

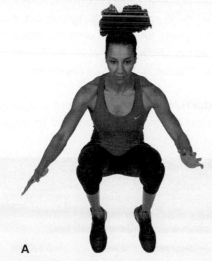
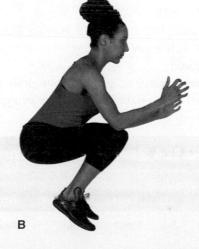

A   B

FIGURE 12.15 Tuck jump.

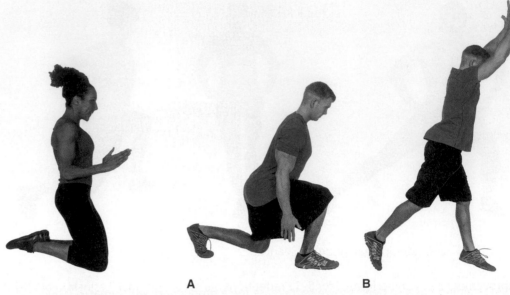

FIGURE 12.16 Butt kick.   **FIGURE 12.17** Jumping lunges.

Reactive training should be included in the movement preparation portion of training sessions 2–4 days per week (**Table 12.4**). One to three exercises should be performed for 2–3 sets of 8–10 repetitions per set. To reduce fatigue while still engaging the nervous system, 0–60 seconds of rest between sets should be allowed (Ramirez-Campillo et al., 2014). The tempo for these exercises should be repetitive, while still maintaining proper joint alignment and exercise technique. Selection of reactive exercises should relate to the resistance exercises to be performed during the training session to ensure neuromuscular activation in similar muscle groups.

SAQ Protocols for the Strength Level

Speed, agility, and quickness (SAQ) are important to both sports performance and activities of daily living. SAQ training is commonly included in sports conditioning programs to enhance athletic performance, and has been shown to have value in fall prevention programs among the elderly, and in rehabilitation programs for those suffering from knee osteoarthritis (Bloomfield et al., 2007; Holmberg, 2015; Polman, Bloomfield & Edwards, 2009; Talwar et al., 2015; Rogers et al., 2012). It is now clear that SAQ training is a valuable stimulus to promote improved physical function.

Agility exercises, such as cone drills or agility ladders, placed in movement preparation periods may enable clients who struggle with resistance exercise techniques to improve

TABLE 12.4 Reactive Strength Acute Variables

Reps	Sets	Tempo	Intensity	Rest	Frequency	Duration	Exercise Selection
8–10	2–3	Repeating	N/A	0–60 seconds	2–4 days/week	4 weeks	1–3 reactive strength

CHECK IT OUT

Not only does SAQ training improve speed and agility, it may also promote improved cognitive functioning (Lennemann et al., 2013) through stimulating the nervous system with both visual and auditory stimuli requiring cognitive responses. Agility exercises have been shown to positively affect the brain with improved spatial navigation (Lennemann et al., 2013), which may explain the improved balance, proprioception, and functional fitness observed in subjects completing an SAQ training program (Fitzgerald, Childs, Ridge, & Irrgang, 2002; Rogers et al., 2012).

performance through enhanced spatial awareness and proprioception. Other clients who suffer from functional impairments that may limit exercise technique or ROM may benefit from agility exercises that promote functional movement, making agility exercises a valuable addition to a training session.

SAQ training has also been shown to increase force production, which makes it a valuable supplement to strength training (Polman et al., 2009). Regardless of the mechanisms involved, it does appear that SAQ training may help the nervous system to respond or react more efficiently to demands placed on it, as well as enhance muscular recruitment and coordination (Brown, Ferrigno, & Santana, 2000).

SAQ exercises completed during movement prep may enable the neuromuscular system to perform optimally during the resistance training portion of strength sessions. By challenging the nervous system to coordinate muscle activation, as is required during SAQ drills, the body is ready to correctly execute resistance training mechanics. A variety of SAQ drills can be included in movement prep, including:

- Agility ladder drills.
- Cone drills.
- Hurdle drills.
- Reaction drills.

SAQ protocols should progress from stabilization exercises to include a greater amount of neurological challenge and dynamic movements (**Table 12.5**). Speeds should increase from the Stabilization Level to present a higher demand on neuromuscular coordination and fast-twitch muscle activation. This will optimally prepare the body for the strength development exercises performed in the strength training sessions.

Depending on the amount of time allotted for each session, six to eight SAQ drills may be included in the movement prep portion of each Strength Level workout. When used in

TABLE 12.5 SAQ Strength Acute Variables

Reps	Sets	Tempo	Intensity	Rest	Frequency	Duration	Exercise Selection
3–5 run throughs	3–4	Fast	N/A	0–60 seconds	2–4 days/week	4 weeks	6–8 drills allowing greater horizontal inertia but limited unpredictability

CHECK IT OUT

It is important for fitness professionals to differentiate between athletes and other clients when implementing SAQ drills. Athletes are often more coordinated, more highly trained, and more accustomed to SAQ protocols. General-population clients may not need to perform SAQ drills at fast speeds to gain the benefits, and each client will demonstrate a different capacity for such training. The goal of SAQ training is to provide an appropriate neuromuscular challenge for each client. Fitness professionals should encourage clients to perform each drill at a speed and level of exertion that is challenging but safely doable. Then, over time, each client should be motivated to increase their speed, while also adding cues or directions during a SAQ exercise, to continue to stimulate the nervous system to improve.

movement prep, SAQ drills should not generate a great deal of fatigue, thus 0–60 seconds rest between repetitions or drills is advisable. If SAQ drills are used to increase the metabolic demand of a workout, such as during Phase 2: Strength Endurance and Phase 3: Hypertrophy, shorter rest periods can be allowed with greater numbers of repetitions and drills included to increase training volume. Longer rest periods, allowing for greater recovery and the maintenance of high speeds and intensities, may be more appropriate during Phase 4: Maximal Strength, to avoid fatigue while stimulating the neuromuscular system for resistance training.

Resistance Training Protocols in the Strength Level

Resistance training has been identified as the optimal method of exercise for the development of muscular fitness in many different populations (Arnold, & Bautmans, 2014; Cheema et al., 2014; Cruickshank, Reyes, & Ziman, 2015; Kjolhede, Vissing, & Dalgas, 2012; Lonbro, 2014; Roig et al., 2009; Shaw, Shaw, & Brown, 2015; Skoffer, Dalgas, & Mechlenberg, 2015; Stewart, Saunders, & Grieg, 2014; Wen-hua et al., 2015). Various resistance training modalities, such as bodyweight, free weights, machines, and other implements provide opportunities to introduce stress to the neuromuscular system and promote adaptations in strength endurance, hypertrophy, and maximal strength. Strength level exercises are performed in a stable environment, therefore fitness professionals will need to alter acute training variables without increasing the proprioceptive demands of the exercises to promote specific adaptations (**Figures 12.18–12.20**).

Training in Phase 2: Strength Endurance, is a hybrid form of training that promotes increased stabilization endurance, hypertrophy, and strength. This entails the use of superset techniques in which a stable exercise (e.g., bench press) is immediately followed with a stabilization exercise with similar biomechanical motion (e.g., stability ball push-up).

Training in Phase 3: Hypertrophy, is specific for the adaptation of maximal muscle growth, focusing on high levels of volume with minimal rest periods to force cellular changes that result in an overall increase in muscle size. Acute variables in this phase can be progressed if a client, with the goal of increasing lean body mass and general performance, has successfully

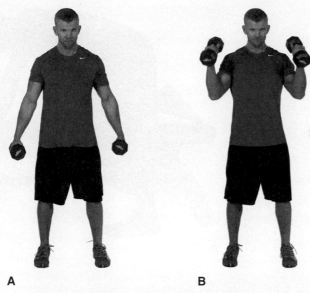

A   **B**

FIGURE 12.18 Standing dumbbell biceps hammer curl.

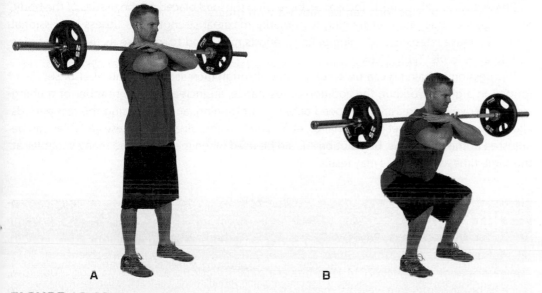

A   **B**

FIGURE 12.19 Front squat.

TABLE 12.6 **Resistance Strength Acute Variables**								
	Reps	**Sets**	**Tempo**	**Intensity**	**Rest**	**Frequency**	**Duration**	**Exercise Selection**
Phase 2: Strength Endurance	8–12	2–4	Strength: 2/0/2 Stabilization: 4/2/1	70–80%	0–60 seconds	2–4 times/week	4 weeks	1 Strength superset with 1 Stabilization
Phase 3: Hypertrophy	6–12	3–5	2/0/2	75–85%	0–60 seconds	3–6 times/week	4 weeks	2–4 Strength Level exercises/ body part
Phase 4: Maximal Strength	1–5	4–6	x/x/x	85–100%	3–5 min	2–4 times/week	4 weeks	1–3 Strength Level exercises

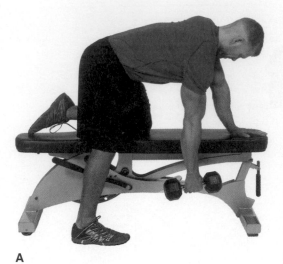

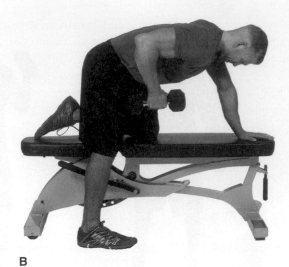

A   **B**

FIGURE 12.20 Dumbbell supported row.

completed Phases 1 and 2. Because the goal of this phase is primarily hypertrophy, the fitness professional will want to increase volume and intensity of the program.

Phase 4: Maximal Strength, focuses on increasing the load placed on the tissues of the body. As the goal of this phase of training is primarily maximal strength, the fitness professional should increase intensity and volume. Rest periods may need to increase as the client trains with heavier loads (Table 12.6).

Progression in training can be accomplished through increases in the number of sets performed in a given workout, the addition of resistance, an increase in the number of training session per week, increasing the speed or tempo of training, and decreasing the rest periods allowed between each set (Rhea, Phillips, et al., 2003). A combination of these variables can be adjusted at the same time, but caution should be used when increasing too many variables at the same time as overstress may result.

CHECK IT OUT

A common challenge faced by many fitness professionals is convincing women of the value of resistance training. Many have misconceptions about resistance training, including the fear that it will make them look masculine, will make them bulky, or even that it might be harmful to reproductive function. The values of resistance training among women have been well documented (Brady & Straight, 2014; Consitt, Copeland, & Tremblay, 2002; Gidycz & Dardis, 2014; Kelley & Kelley, 2009; Kraemer et al., 1991; Singh Paramanandam & Roberts, 2014; Zhao, Zhao, & Xu, 2015) and include:

- Increased strength.
- Improved quality of life.
- Increase or maintenance of bone mineral density.
- Decreased risk of falls during activities of daily living.
- Decreased risk of injury during sport activities.
- Improved blood cholesterol.
- Increased metabolic rate.

Fitness professionals can help their clients commit to resistance training by explaining why this form of training is so important. Resistance training is sometimes perceived as a training method used only by bodybuilders or athletes, and some clients may have incorrect notions about how it will affect their body. Clients should be reassured that the fitness professional will monitor their lifting technique, teach them proper training methods, and ensure that their training regimen is appropriate. With this information, the professional–client relationship will be strengthened, leading to increased confidence and commitment to training.

Common Mistakes Made in the Strength Level

Common mistakes that fitness professionals make in the Strength Level include:

- Failure to adjust training variables based on individual training status.
- Utilizing the same group of exercises for all clients regardless of their individual needs.
- Failure to alter training in a coordinated fashion over time.
- Prescribing training to muscular failure for lengthy periods of time.
- Creating excessive muscle soreness by overprescribing intense training.

Failure to Adjust Training Variables Based on Individual Status

The first common mistake made by fitness professionals when implementing the Strength Level is failing to connect the status and/or needs of the client with programming choices such as modality, volume, intensity, and frequency. For example, training status will greatly influence the appropriate training volume and intensity in the Strength Level. Applying too much volume is a common mistake professionals make when implementing a training plan for clients who have been inactive for long periods of time or are just beginning an organized exercise routine. The selection of sets, repetitions, intensity, tempo, and rest periods should all be influenced by the client's training status (Rhea, Phillips, et al., 2003). Lower ranges for each variable should be selected for clients just beginning a training program or just entering the Strength Level. As training status improves, gradual progression to the higher volumes and intensities at faster paces is appropriate and needed for continued improvement.

Using the Same Exercises for All Clients

While the ultimate goal of the Strength Level is to improve the client's ability to generate force, the methods implemented to reach that goal can greatly enhance the degree to which strength is improved. It can also enhance the degree to which increased force capacity improves performance for activities of daily living, occupational demands, or in sports. Fitness professionals should select the exercises and modalities that will allow for the greatest improvement in muscular fitness for each individual. A common mistake in the Strength Level is the reliance on a repeated set of exercises for all clients. Rather than altering exercises based on individual needs, some fitness professionals take all of their clients through the same exercises. This greatly decreases the overall value of strength training for each client.

Lack of Progressive Changes in Programming

Weekly, and even daily, alterations in workouts are important to develop fitness in various movement patterns and to manage training stress. Professionals should avoid the mistake of simply creating a 1-week plan that is repeated throughout the level. Variety, with a purpose, is key to fostering long-term adaptations and increasing adherence to the training plan. Variation in exercise selection will enable the body to adapt to a range of challenges, rather than just a single movement. Even slight alterations in volume, intensity, and rest periods can provide a significantly different training stress, which will in turn prompt continued adaptation by the body (Rhea, Ball, Phillips, & Burkett, 2002). Mapping out the entire Strength Level, with variations each week, will help the fitness professional identify the timing and degree to which training will be varied over time.

Prescribing Training to Muscle Failure

Muscular failure

A training approach that involves the completion of as many reps as possible until the individual is unable to complete a repetition due to fatigue.

Another potential mistake among fitness professionals when implementing the Strength Level is the prescription of training to **muscular failure**. In this training approach, the client performs repetitions to the point of voluntary failure, where he or she is not able to fully complete a repetition due to fatigue. This training approach appears to have begun due to the expectation that maximum stress placed on the neuromuscular system would result in maximal adaptations. In recent years, evidence has accumulated to discount this expectation (Medrano, 2010). It is important to note that improvements in strength and hypertrophy can be achieved without causing significant damage to muscle tissue (Close, Kayani, Vasilaki, & McArdle, 2005; Drinkwater et al., 2007; Goto et al., 2004; Speiring et al., 2008) and that improvements appear to match, or even exceed, those accomplished through training to failure. Additionally, training to muscular failure may have a negative impact on speed of execution, both during training and in the performance of sports-related tasks (Izquierdo, Gonazlez-Badillo et al., 2006; Izquierdo, Ibanez, et al., 2006). In essence, complete muscle fatigue and damage to muscle tissue is not necessary to trigger adaptations in strength endurance, hypertrophy, or maximal strength. Added risks that accompany training to muscular failure include increased blood pressure due to the Valsalva maneuver, improper exercise technique due to fatigue, and reduced effectiveness of joint proprioception (Rozzi, Lephart, & Fu, 1999). The added discomfort, potential soreness, and psychological demand of this approach can be a significant deterrent to long-term exercise adherence in the general population, and potentially lead to overtraining in athletes. Therefore, the risks far outweigh the benefits of this training approach.

TRAINER TIPS

When meeting with new clients, explain to them that, at minimum, 30 days of consistency will be required for them to start seeing noticeable change in their outward appearance. Thirty days of consistency equates to working out at least 4 days a week for 30 days.

Creating Excessive Muscle Soreness Through Aggressive Intensities

Rather than relying on high levels of fatigue and creating excessive soreness, fitness professionals should trust the OPT model and ensure gradual progression in training stress over time. This approach will result in improved muscular endurance, hypertrophy, and maximal strength while improving adherence to the exercise regimen. Fitness professionals should educate their clients regarding the proper amount of stress needed to promote adaptations, and dispel the "no pain, no gain" or "push to the limit" training philosophies that have existed for many years.

General Recommendations for Avoiding Mistakes in the Strength Level

Selecting the proper weight for each exercise is a challenge that requires some trial-and-error and a good familiarity of each client. At the beginning of a training program, and with the introduction of each new exercise, the fitness professional should start with a conservative amount of weight and gradually increase the weight until the proper intensity has been achieved. The fitness professional should keep detailed notes for each exercise with the amount of weight lifted for a given number of repetitions. Over time, these weights should gradually increase as muscular fitness improves. Relying on notes from past workouts can help the fitness professional identify the appropriate amount of weight needed to stimulate adaptations.

Especially with exercises that are challenging for a client, proper exercise technique must be taught, monitored, and maintained at all times. Improper lifting technique is the source of many lifting injuries, and clients should never be allowed to continue an exercise when improper technique is being used. These opportunities can be used to stop the client and review proper technique. It is better to reduce the weight and stop the workout, to ensure proper lifting technique, rather than rush through the workout with poor technique in an attempt to complete all of the planned work.

Pain is generally a sign of movement dysfunction or injury, and may require a consult with an orthopedic physician to ensure that exercise is not exacerbating an injury. At minimum, fitness professionals should alter exercise selection and ensure appropriate training loads to avoid pain. If these alterations do not result in pain-free exercise, the fitness professional should avoid stressing a particular joint or muscle until the client is checked and treated for the cause of the pain. When pain-free exercise is possible, fitness professionals should then ensure the exercises are performed with proper technique, with appropriate loads, through a full ROM.

Integrating the Strength Level with Other Phases

The OPT model represents an effective template for implementing a long-term training plan. But it should not be viewed as a rigid plan that cannot be adapted to a variety of needs or training goals. There may be instances where a concurrent training approach is needed, where multiple phases are combined into one. Firefighters, for instance, need adequate levels of endurance, strength, and power to perform their duties effectively (Rhea, Alvar, & Gray, 2004). Once a firefighter has achieved the necessary muscular fitness, maintaining fitness in all components becomes the goal. Undulated training can be implemented to maintain fitness, or even promote small improvements in each area of fitness (**Figure 12.21**; Peterson, Dodd, Alvar, Rhea, & Favre, 2008).

Research suggests that **maintenance** of muscular fitness requires less training volume for muscular endurance, hypertrophy, strength, and power (Viciana, Mayorga-Vega, & Cocca, 2013; Phillips, 2009; Ronnestad, Nymark, & Raastad, 2011; Santos & Janeira, 2011). Volume is reduced by either performing less work during each session or by decreasing the training frequency. Intensity, however, should be kept relatively high. For example, during periods of training aimed at developing maximal strength, 4–6 sets per exercise may be prescribed. However, to maintain current strength levels, 1–2 sets is sufficient as long as intensity is kept relatively high.

The number of sessions in a given week targeting specific components would be determined by individual needs. If maintenance of all muscular fitness components were desired,

---

TRAINER TIPS ⫞▯⫟

Proper form is paramount. Do not hesitate to interrupt the workout or tweak a variable in order to correct form. A great way to teach proper form is through *tell*, *show*, *do*. First *tell* the client what the exercise is and what correct form looks like. Then *show* the client what the exercise should look like. Finally, have the client *do* the exercise.

Maintenance
Sustaining developed levels of muscular fitness without improvement.

Client Name:	Week 1							Week 2							Week 3							Week 4						
Start Date:	M	T	W	T	F	S	S	M	T	W	T	F	S	S	M	T	W	T	F	S	S	M	T	W	T	F	S	S
Phase 1: Stabilization Training	X							X							X							X						
Phase 2: Strength Training			X							X							X							X				
Phase 3: Hypertrophy																												
Phase 4: Maximal Strength Training					X														X									
Phase 5: Power Training												X														X		

Cardio List cardio exercises	Workout Specific	Workout Specific	Workout Specific	Workout Specific
Flexibility List flexibility exercises	SMR-Calves, Adductors, Lats Static-Calves, Adductors, Lats 5–7 days/week Active/DROM Workout Specific	SMR-Calves, Adductors, Lats Static-Calves, Adductors, Lats 5–7 days/week Active/DROM Workout Specific	SMR-Calves, Adductors, Lats Static-Calves, Adductors, Lats 5–7 days/week Active/DROM Workout Specific	SMR-Calves, Adductors, Lats Static-Calves, Adductors, Lats 5–7 days/week Active/DROM Workout Specific
Re-Assessment List assessments conducted	Weight-185 (no change) Body Fat%-16% (no change) RHR-68 (Down 2 BPM)	N/A	N/A	Reassess next week.

Notes and Observations:
Working on developing overall strength and power. Flexibility and cardio workouts need to be workout specific. Next assessments need to look at performance assessment measures including vertical jump and 40. Also need to reassess OHS to verify whether a full Phase 1 needs to be readdressed.

FIGURE 12.21 Undulated training program template.

one session would target each component, progressing through the phases of the OPT model: Stabilization Endurance, Strength Endurance, Hypertrophy, Maximal Strength, and Power.

Different phases of the OPT model can even be implemented into the same session. If a client needs more focus on stabilization training, then Stabilization Level protocols can be implemented into the movement prep or cool-down portions of the workout. Similarly, some athletes may need to work on power, but may not have time to perform Power Level exercises on their own. A Power Level warm-up could be applied to a resistance strength workout. This would help with power adaptations, while still maintaining the strength focus of the program.

Corrective Strategies for Strength Clients

Continuous monitoring of posture, dynamic flexibility, core strength, balance, and overall neuromuscular control is advisable for all clients. Posture and movement assessments enable the fitness professional to create progress reports and monitor movement efficiency as a client progresses through the OPT model. During the Strength Level, changes in muscular fitness should promote, not impair, movement efficiency.

Strength training, when performed through full ROM, does not result in decreased soft tissue extensibility, and conversely may even promote improvements in flexibility (Leite et al., 2015; Simao et al., 2011). Some researchers have found a decrease in strength when stretching is performed immediately prior to testing, but there is a lack of evidence suggesting that stretching decreases improvements in strength over the course of a training program (Behm, Button, & Butt, 2001; Craemer, 2004; Kokkonen, Nelson, & Cornwell, 1998; Yamaguchi et al., 2006; Simao et al., 2011). No research has shown a detrimental effect from performing corrective techniques in conjunction with a strength training phase. Therefore, fitness professionals should include corrective techniques as needed throughout the Strength Level. For instance, if a strength imbalance is noted between different muscle groups, or different body segments, training can target the weaker muscle groups. Unilateral exercises can help identify strength differences, and exercise technique during complex exercises such as the squat can help identify weak links in the kinetic chain. If an imbalance exists, for example between the right and left quadriceps, added exercises for the weaker side can be included in a workout to promote strength balance. If a client struggles to maintain proper trunk posture during the squat, most likely a strength deficit in the core muscles exists. Exercises to promote core strength can then be added to the training plan to improve upon this weakness and enable proper squat execution.

Movement preparation, warm-up, and cool-down are good opportunities to incorporate corrective strategies. Not only will movement deficiencies be addressed, but the body will be better prepared for strength training following corrective exercise performed in the warm-up. Another effective strategy for including corrective exercise in the Strength Level is to perform supersets, combining a strength exercise and a corrective technique based on individual needs. This approach will allow for the development of strength, while promoting the proper application of increased force in correct movement patterns.

Conclusion

The OPT model stresses the safety needs of the client, as well as the scientific knowledge required for making informed decisions with regard to the needs and desires of each client. The Strength Level requires more than just a basic understanding of its goals and outcomes; it also requires implementation of appropriate protocols and exercises. With the understanding of both the Stabilization and Strength Levels, a fitness professional can move forward to the final level of the OPT model: Power.

TRAINER TIPS

At minimum, you should be performing movement assessments every 30 days and adjusting the corrective exercise strategies based on what you see. Incorporate corrective exercise into the warm-up and movement prep and as a superset with a strength exercise during the actual workout.

Case in Review

As you progress your clients, it is important to explain the purpose of the level they are training in to ensure that they understand the path that you have laid out for them. Also, ensure to remind your clients of where their training needed to start and how it must progress in order to achieve the goals they have set. Looking back at your three clients, they might object to their training program because they want to begin lifting heavier weights, worry that they might show muscle, and/or feel that greater muscle might hinder their performance. Even though your clients haven't expressed this, you want to

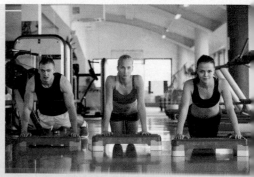
© fotoinfot/Shutterstock

continuously "paint" the path from where they started in their training and how Level 2, Strength, will help get them there.

To further explain the purpose of the phases within the Strength Level to your clients, you continue to relate the phases to your clients' fitness goals. To minimize objections, you describe your clients' need for the Strength Level using the following strategies:

- **Roderick, the bodybuilding client**: "Strength Endurance will continue to build upon the base that you developed in Phase 1. This phase will ensure that you are growing stronger while maintaining the ability to perform physical activity for a long period of time. While this is not the main goal of your competitions, it will help in your overall training ability and injury prevention."

- **Mary, the weight loss client**: "I understand your concern of building muscles, however, the hormonal balance of women will not allow for huge muscular growth. We would have to work very hard for that. I would rather focus on Phase 2 for you to continue the development of strength and endurance. Don't be intimidated by heavier loads. This will only help you to be able to better handle your activities of daily living. We will not put you in a situation where muscle growth will become an issue."

- **Ashley, the marathon client**: "Phase 2 is going to be vital for you. However, we will want you to grow strong as well. Not only will you be able to develop more power, and therefore more speed, with more strength, but you will also be better able to withstand injuries given your running regimen. This will be important for better performance and injury prevention."

When using the acute variables for the Strength Level, you might plan the following for each of your clients based on their fitness goals:

- **Roderick, the bodybuilding client**: Spend time in all three phases of the Strength Level in order to maximize strength gains.

- **Mary, the weight loss client**: Spend time in Phase 2 in order to develop her daily functional capacity.

- **Ashley, the marathon client**: Spend time in Phase 2 and Maximal Strength in order to fully develop her capabilities as an endurance athlete.

When addressing the movement prep and resistance training exercises associated with the Strength Level, you implement the following exercises based on each of your client's fitness goals:

- **Roderick, the bodybuilder**: Deadlift, bench press, squat, incline press, overhead press, Romanian deadlift, bent over row, triceps press down.

- **Mary, the weight loss focused client:** Squat, dumbbell row, dumbbell chest press, dumbbell deadlift, biceps curl, triceps extension, overhead press.

- **Ashley, the marathon runner:** Squat, Romanian deadlift, straight-arm pull down, seated row, overhead press.

It is important when working with any of the three clients that you incorporate Stabilization into Phase 2. Stabilization can be incorporated into movement prep or a modified Phase 1 workout can be completed on off days as active recovery.

References

Almstedt, H., Canepa, J. A., Ramirez, D. A., & Shoepe, T. C. (2011). Changes in bone mineral density in response to 24 weeks of resistance training in college-age men and women. *Journal of Strength and Conditioning Research, 25*, 1098–1103.

Arazi, H., Rahmati, S., & Zaheri, S. (2013). The effect of two sequence patterns in resistance training on strength, muscular endurance, and circumference in novice male athletes. *Croatian Sports Medicine Journal, 28*, 7–14.

Arnold, P., & Bautmans, I. (2014). The influence of strength training on muscle activation in elderly persons: A systematic review and meta-analysis. *Experimental Gerontology, 58*, 58–68.

Ashe, M. C., Gorman, E., Khan, K. M., Brasher, P., Cooper, D. M. L., McKay, H. A., & Liu-Ambrose, T. (2013). Does frequency of resistance training affect tibial cortical bone density in older women? A randomized controlled trial. *Osteoporosis International, 24*, 623–632.

Beardsley, C., & Skarabot, J. (2015). Effects of self-myofascial release: A systematic review. *Journal of Bodywork and Movement Therapies, 19*(4), 747–758.

Behm, D. G., Button, D. C., & Butt, J. C. (2001). Factors affecting force loss with prolonged stretching. *Canadian Journal of Applied Physiology, 26*, 261–272.

Bernier, J. N., & Perrin, D. H. (1998). Effect of coordination training on proprioception of the functionally unstable ankle. *Journal of Orthopaedic and Sports Physical Therapy, 27*, 264–275.

Bloomfield, J., Polman, R., O'Donoghue, P., & McNaughton, L. (2007). Effective speed and agility conditioning methodology for random intermittent dynamic type sports. *Journal of Strength and Conditioning Research, 21*, 1093–1100.

Bradbury-Squires, D. J., Noftall, J. C., Sullivan, K. M., Behm, D. G., Power, K. E., & Button, D. C. (2015). Roller-massage application to the quadriceps and knee-joint range of motion and neuromuscular efficiency during a lunge. *Journal of Athletic Training, 50*, 133–140.

Brady, A. O., & Straight, C. R. (2014). Review: Muscle capacity and physical function in older women: What are the impacts of resistance training? *Journal of Sport and Health Science, 3*, 179–188.

Brown, C. H., & Wilmore, J. H. (1974). The effects of maximal resistance training on the strength and body composition of women athletes. *Medicine and Science in Sports, 6*, 174–171.

Brown, L. E., Ferrigno, V. A., & Santana, J. C. (2000). *Training for speed, agility and quickness.* Champaign, IL: Human Kinetics.

Carolan, B., & Cafarelli, E. (1992). Adaptations in coactivation after isometric resistance training. *Journal of Applied Physiology, 73*, 911–917.

Chang, W. D., Lin, H. Y., & Lai, P. T. (2015). Core strength training for patients with chronic low back pain. *Journal of Physical Therapy Science, 27*, 619–622.

Cheema, B. S., Kilbreath, S. L., Fahey, P. P., Delaney, G. P., & Atlantis, E. (2014). Safety and efficacy of progressive resistance training in breast cancer: A systematic review and meta-analysis. *Breast Cancer Research and Treatment, 148*, 249–268.

Close, G., Kayani, A., Vasilaki, A., & McArdle, A. (2005). Skeletal muscle damage with exercise and aging. *Sports Medicine, 35*, 413–427.

Consitt, L. A., Copeland, J. L., & Tremblay, M. S. (2002). Endogenous anabolic hormone responses to endurance versus resistance exercise and training in women. *Sports Medicine, 32*, 1–22.

Craemer, J. T. (2004). Acute effects of static stretching on peak torque in women. *Journal of Strength and Conditioning Research, 18*, 236–241.

Cruickshank, T. M., Reyes, A. R., & Ziman, M. R. (2015). A systematic review and meta-analysis of strength training in individuals with multiple sclerosis or Parkinson disease. *Medicine* (Baltimore), *94*, e411.

Dehail, P., Bestaven, E., Muller, F., Mallet, A., Robert, B., Bourdel-Marchasson, I., & Petit, J. (2007). Kinematic and electromyographic analysis of rising from a chair during a "sit-to-walk" task in elderly subjects: Role of strength. *Clinical Biomechanics, 22*, 1096–1103.

Drinkwater, E. J., Lawton, T. W., McKenna, M. J., Lindsell, R. P., Hunt, P. H., & Pyne, D. B. (2007). Increased number of forced repetitions does not enhance strength development with resistance training. *Journal of Strength and Conditioning Research, 21*, 841–847.

Elis, E., & Rosenbaum, D. (2001). A multistation proprioceptive exercise program in patients with ankle instability. *Medicine and Science in Sports and Exercise, 33*, 1991–1998.

Figueiredo, T., Rhea, M. R., Bunker, D., Ingrid, D., Freitas, B., Fleck, S., & Simao, R. (2011). The influence of exercise order on local muscular endurance during resistance training in women. *Human Movement, 12*, 237–242.

Fitzgerald, G., Childs, J., Ridge, T., & Irrgang, J. (2002). Agility and perturbation training for a physically active individual with knee osteoarthritis. *Physical Therapy, 82*, 372–382.

Fluck, M. (2006). Functional, structural and molecular plasticity of mammalian skeletal muscle in response to exercise stimuli. *Journal of Experimental Biology, 209*, 2239–2248.

Folland, J. P., & Williams, A. G. (2007). The adaptations to strength training. *Sports Medicine, 37*, 145–168.

Fyfe, J. J., Bishop, D. J., & Stepto, N. K. (2014). Interference between concurrent resistance and endurance exercise: molecular bases and the role of individual training variables. *Sports Medicine, 44*, 743–762.

Gidycz, C. A., & Dardis, C. M. (2014). Feminist self-defense and resistance training for college students: A critical review and recommendations for the future. *Trauma, Violence, and Abuse, 15*, 322–333.

Goto, K., Nagasawa, M., Yanagisawa, O., Kizuka, T., Ishii, N., & Takamatsu, K. (2004). Muscular adaptations to combinations of high- and low-intensity resistance exercises. *Journal of Strength and Conditioning Research, 18*, 730–738.

Harris, G., Stone, M. H., O'Bryant, H., Proulx, C. M., & Johnson, R. (2000). Short-term performance effects of high speed, high force or combined weight training. *Journal of Strength and Conditioning Research, 14*, 14–20.

Hertel, J., Braham, R. A., Hale, S., & Olmsted-Kramer, L. C. (2006). Simplifying the star excursion balance test: Analyses of subjects with and without chronic ankle instability. *Journal of Orthopaedic and Sports Physical Therapy, 36*, 131–137.

Hewett, T. E., Myer, G. D., & Ford, K. R. (2005). Reducing knee and anterior cruciate ligament injures among female athletes: A systematic review of neuromuscular training interventions. *Journal of Knee Surgery, 18*, 82–88.

Hewett, T. E., Paterno, M. V., & Myer, G. D. (2002). Strategies for enhancing proprioception and neuromuscular control of the knee. *Clinical Orthopaedics and Related Research, 402*, 76–94.

Hinton, P. S., Nigh, P., & Thyfault, J. (2015). Effectiveness of resistance training or jumping exercise to increase bone mineral density in men with low bone mass: A 12-month randomized, controlled trial. *Bone, 79*, 203–212.

Hodges, P. W., & Richardson, C. A. (1996). Inefficient muscular stabilization of the lumbar spine associated with low back pain. A motor control evaluation of transversus abdominis. *Spine, 21*, 2640–2650.

Holmberg, P. M. (2015). Agility training for experienced athletes: A dynamical systems approach. *Strength and Conditioning Journal, 37*, 93–98.

Hughes, M. A., Myers, B. S., & Schenkman, M. L. (1996). The role of strength in rising from a chair in the functionally impaired elderly. *Journal of Biomechanics, 29*, 1509–1513.

Humphries, B., Fenning, A., Dugan, E., Guinane, J., & MacRae, K. (2009). Whole-body vibration effects on bone mineral density in women with or without resistance training. *Aviation, Space, and Environmental Medicine, 80*, 1025–1031.

Izquierdo, M., Gonzalez-Badillo, J. J., Hakkinen, K., Ibanez, J., Kraemer, W. J., Altadill, A., . . . Gorostiaga, E. M. (2006). Effect of loading on unintentional lifting velocity declines during single sets of repetitions to failure during upper and lower extremity muscle actions. *International Journal of Sports Medicine, 27*, 718–724.

Izquierdo, M., Ibanez, J., Gonzalez-Badillo, J. J., Hakkinen, K., Ratamess, N. A., . . . Gorostiaga, E. M. (2006). Differential effects of strength training leading to failure versus not to failure on hormonal responses, strength, and muscle power gains. *Journal of Applied Physiology, 100*, 1647–1656.

Janot, J. M., Malin, B., Cook, R., Hagenbucher, J., Draeger, A., Jordan, M., & Van Guilder, G. (2013). Effects of self myofascial release and static stretching on anaerobic power output. *Journal of Fitness Research, 2*, 41–54.

Kelley, G. A., & Kelley, K. S. (2009). Review: Impact of progressive resistance training on lipids and lipoproteins in adults: A meta-analysis of randomized controlled trials. *Preventive Medicine, 48*, 9–19.

Kjolhede, T., Vissing, K., & Dalgas, U. (2012). Multiple sclerosis and progressive resistance training: A systematic review. *Multiple Sclerosis, 18*, 1215–1228.

Kokkonen, J., Nelson, A. G., & Cornwell, A. (1998). Acute muscle stretching inhibits maximal strength performance. *Research Quarterly for Exercise and Sport, 69*, 411–415.

Kraemer, W. J., Godon, S. E., Fleck, S. J., Marchitelli, L. J., Mello, R., Dziados, J. E., . . . Fry, A. C. (1991). Endogenous anabolic hormonal and growth factor responses to heavy resistance training exercises in males and females. *International Journal of Sports Medicine, 12*, 228–235.

Leetun, D. T., Ireland, M. L., Wilson, J. D., Ballantyne, B. T., & Davis, I. M. (2004). Core stability measures as risk factors for lower extremity injury in athletes. *Medicine and Science in Sport and Exercise, 36*, 926–934.

Leite, T., Teixeira, A., Saavedra, F., Leite, R., Rhea, M. R., & Simao, R. (2015). Influence of strength and flexibility training, combined or isolated, on strength and flexibility gains. *Journal of Strength and Conditioning Research, 29*, 1083–1088.

Lennemann, L. M., Sidrow, K. M., Johnson, E. M., Harrison, C. R., Vojta, C. N., & Walker, T. B. (2013). The influence of agility training on physiological and cognitive performance. *Journal of Strength and Conditioning Research, 27*, 3300–3309.

Lesinski, M., Hortobagyi, T., Muehlbauer, T., Gollhofer, A., & Granacher, U. (2015). Dose-response relationships of balance training in healthy young adults: A systematic review and meta-analysis. *Sports Medicine, 45*, 557–576.

Leveritt, M., Abernathy, P. J., Barry, B. K., & Logan, P. A. (1999). Concurrent strength and endurance training: A review. *Sports Medicine, 28*, 413–427.

Lonbro, S. (2014). The effect of progressive resistance training on lean body mass in post-treatment cancer patients: A systematic review. *Radiotherapy and Oncology, 110*, 71–80.

Mann, T. N., Lamberts, R. P., & Lambert, M. I. (2014). High responders and low responders: Factors associated with individual variation in response to standardized training. *Sports Medicine, 44*, 1113–1124.

Mansfield, A., Wong, J. S., Bryce, J., Knorr, S., & Patterson, K. K. (2015). Does perturbation-based balance training prevent falls? Systematic review and meta-analysis of preliminary randomized controlled trials. *Physical Therapy, 95*, 700–709.

Maughan, R. J., Watson, J. S., & Weir, J. (1983). Strength and cross-sectional area of human skeletal muscle. *Journal of Physiology, 338,* 37–49.

McKeon, P. O., & Hertel, J. (2008). Systematic review of postural control and lateral ankle instability, Part 2: Is balance training clinically effective? *Journal of Athletic Training, 43,* 305–315.

Medrano, I. C. (2010). Muscular failure training in conditioning neuromuscular programs. *Journal of Human Sport and Exercise, 5,* 196–213.

Nadler, S. F., Malanga, C. A., Bartoli, L. A., Feinberg, J. H., Prybicien, M., & Deprince, M. (2002). Hip muscle imbalance and low back pain in athletes: Influence of core strengthening. *Medicine and Science in Sports and Exercise, 34,* 9–16.

Nadler, S. F., Moley, P., Malanga, G. A., Rubbani, M., Prybicien, M., & Feinberg, J. H. (2002). Functional deficits in athletes with a history of low back pain: A pilot study. *Archives of Physical Medicine and Rehabilitation, 83,* 1753–1758.

O'Sullivan, P. B., Phyty, G. D., Twomey, L. T., & Allison, G. T. (1997). Evaluation of specific stabilizing exercise in the treatment of chronic low back pain with radiologic diagnosis of spondylolysis or spondylolisthesis. *Spine, 22,* 2959–2967.

Peacock, C. A., Krein, D. D., Silver, T. A., Sanders, G. J., & von Carlowitz, K. P. A. (2014). An acute bout of self-myofascial release in the form of foam rolling improves performance testing. *International Journal of Exercise Science, 7,* 202–211.

Pendergast, D. R., Fisher, N. M., & Calkins, E. (1993). Cardiorespiratory, neuromuscular, and metabolic alterations with age leading to frailty. *Journal of Gerontology, 48,* 61–67.

Peterson, M. D., Alvar, B. A., & Rhea, M. R. (2006). The contribution of maximal force production to explosive movement among young collegiate athletes. *Journal of Strength and Conditioning Research, 20,* 867–873.

Peterson, M. D., Dodd, D. J., Alvar, B. A., Rhea, M. R., & Favre, M. (2008). Undulation training for development of hierarchical fitness and improved firefighter job performance. *Journal of Strength and Conditioning Research, 22,* 1683–1695.

Peterson, M. D., Rhea, M. R., & Alvar, B. A. (2004). Maximizing strength development in athletes: A meta-analysis to determine the dose-response relationship. *Journal of Strength and Conditioning Research, 18,* 377–383.

Peterson, M. D., Rhea, M. R., Sen, A., & Gordon, P. M. (2010). Resistance exercise for muscular strength in older adults: A meta-analysis. *Ageing Research Reviews, 9,* 226–237.

Peterson, M. D., Sen, A., & Gordon, P. M. (2011). Influence of resistance exercise on lean body mass in aging adults: A meta-analysis. *Medicine and Science in Sports and Exercise, 43,* 249–258.

Phillips, S. M. (2009). Physiologic and molecular bases of muscle hypertrophy and atrophy: Impact of resistance exercise on human skeletal muscle. *Applied Physiology, Nutrition, and Metabolism, 34,* 403–410.

Polman, R., Bloomfield, J., & Edwards, A. (2009). Effects of SAQ training and small-sided games on neuromuscular functioning in untrained subjects. *International Journal of Sports Physiology Performance, 4,* 494–505.

Ramirez-Campillo, R., Andrad, C., Alvarez, C., Henriquez-Olguin, C., Martinez, C., Baez-SanMartin, E., . . . Izquierdo, M. (2014). The effects of interest rest on adaptation to 7 weeks of explosive training in young soccer players. *Journal of Sports Science and Medicine, 13,* 287–296.

Rantanen, T., Guralnik, J., Sakari-Rantala, R., Leveille, S., Simonsick, E. M., Ling, S., & Fried, L. P. (1999). Disability, physical activity, and muscle strength in older women: The women's health and aging study. *Archives of Physical Medicine and Rehabilitation, 80,* 130–135.

Reed, C. A., Ford, K. R., Myer, G. D., & Hewett, T. E. (2012). The effects of isolated and integrated core stability training on athletic performance measures, a systematic review. *Sports Medicine, 42,* 697–706.

Rhea, M. R., & Alderman, B. L. (2004). A meta-analysis of periodized versus nonperiodized strength and power training. *Research Quarterly for Exercise and Sport, 75,* 413–422.

Rhea, M. R., Alvar, B., Burkett, L. N., & Ball, S. D. (2003). A meta-analysis to determine the dose response for strength development. *Medicine and Science in Sports and Exercise, 35,* 456–464.

Rhea, M. R., Alvar, B. A., & Gray, R. (2004). Physical fitness and job performance of firefighters. *Journal of Strength and Conditioning Research, 18*, 348–352.

Rhea, M. R., Ball, S. D., Phillips, W. T., & Burkett, L. N. (2002). A comparison of linear and daily undulating periodized programs with equated volume and intensity for strength. *Journal of Strength and Conditioning Research, 16*, 250–255.

Rhea, M. R., Phillips, W. T., Burkett, L. N., Stone, W. J., Ball, S. D., Alvar, B. A., Thomas, A. B. (2003). A comparison of linear and daily undulating periodized programs with equated volume and intensity for local muscular endurance. *Journal of Strength and Conditioning Research, 17*, 82–87.

Rogers, M. W., Tamulevicius, N., Semple, S. J., & Krkeljas, Z. (2012). Efficacy of home-based kinesthesia, balance, and agility exercise training among persons with symptomatic knee osteoarthritis. *Journal of Sports Science and Medicine, 11*, 751–758.

Roig, M., O'Brien, K., Kirk, G., Murray, R., McKinnon, P., Shadgan, B., & Reid, W. D. (2009). The effects of eccentric versus concentric resistance training on muscle strength and mass in healthy adults: A systematic review with meta-analysis. *British Journal of Sports Medicine, 43*, 556–568.

Ronnestad, B. R., Nymark, B. S., & Raastad, T. (2011). Effects of in-season strength maintenance training frequency in professional soccer players. *Journal of Strength and Conditioning Research, 25*, 2653–2660.

Rozzi, S. L., Lephart, S. M., & Fu, F. H. (1999). Effects of muscular fatigue on knee joint laxity and neuromuscular characteristics of male and female athletes. *Journal of Athletic Training, 34*, 106–114.

Ruther, C. L., Golden, C. L., Harris, R., & Dudley, G. A. (1995). Hypertrophy, resistance training, and the nature of skeletal muscle activation. *Journal of Strength and Conditioning Research, 9*, 155–159.

Santos, E., & Janeira, M. (2011). The effects of plyometric training followed by detraining and reduced training periods on explosive strength in adolescent male basketball players. *Journal of Strength and Conditioning Research, 25*, 441–452.

Schoenfeld, B. J. (2010). The mechanisms of muscle hypertrophy and their application to resistance training. *Journal of Strength and Conditioning Research, 24*, 2857–2872.

Seitz, L., Reyes, A., Tran, T., Villareal, E., & Haff, G. (2014). Increases in lower body strength transfer positively to sprint performance: A systematic review with meta-analysis. *Sports Medicine, 44*, 1693–1703.

Shaw, B. S., Shaw, I., & Brown, G. A. (2015). Resistance exercise is medicine: Strength training in health promotion and rehabilitation. *International Journal of Therapy and Rehabilitation, 22*, 385–389.

Siff, M. (2001). Biomechanical foundations of strength and power training. In Zatsiorsky, V. (Ed.), *Biomechanics in sport* (pp. 103–139). London: Blackwell Scientific Ltd.

Simao, R., Lemos, A., Salles, B., Leite, T., Oliveira, F., Rhea, M., & Reis, V. (2011). The influence of strength, flexibility, and simultaneous training on flexibility and strength gains. *Journal of Strength and Conditioning Research, 25*, 1333–1338.

Singh Paramanandam, V., & Roberts, D. (2014). Weight training is not harmful for women with breast cancer-related lymphoedema: A systematic review. *Journal of Physiotherapy, 60*, 136–144.

Skoffer, B., Dalgas, U., & Mechlenburg, I. (2015). Progressive resistance training before and after total hip and knee arthroplasty: a systematic review. *Clinical Rehabilitation, 29*, 14–30.

Spiering, B. A., Kraemer, W. J., Anderson, J. M., Armstrong, L. E., Nindl, B. L., Volek, J. S., & Maresh, C. M. (2008). Resistance exercise biology. *Sports Medicine, 31*, 863–873.

Stewart, V. H., Saunders, D. H., & Greig, C. A. (2014). Responsiveness of muscle size and strength to physical training in very elderly people: A systematic review. *Scandinavian Journal of Medicine and Science in Sports, 24*, 1–10.

Stitz, J., & Pelot, T. (2015). Self myofascial release as a tool to improve athletic readiness? *Olympic Coach, 26*, 1–3.

Talwar, J., Zia, N. U., Maurya, M., & Singh, H. (2015). Effect of agility training under single-task condition versus training under dual-task condition with different task priorities to improve balance in the elderly. *Topics in Geriatric Rehabilitation, 31*, 98–104.

Viciana, J., Mayorga-Vega, D., & Cocca, A. (2013). Effects of a maintenance resistance training program on muscular strength in schoolchildren. *Kinesiology, 45*, 82–92.

Wen-hua, L., Chen, J., Xin, C., Lin, L., Hai-yan, Y., Yu-qui, Z., & Rui, C. (2015). Impact of resistance training in subjects with COPD: A systematic review and meta-analysis. *Respiratory Care, 60*, 1130–1145.

Yamaguchi, T., Ishi, K., Yamanaka, M., & Yasuda, K. (2006). Acute effect of static stretching on power output during concentric dynamic constant external resistance leg extension. *Journal of Strength and Conditioning Research, 20*, 804–810.

Zatsiorsky, V. M. (1995). *Science and practice of strength training*. Champaign, IL: Human Kinetics.

Zech, A., Hubscher, M., Vogt, L., Banzer, W., Hansel, F., & Pfeifer, K. (2009). Neuromuscular training for rehabilitation of sports injuries: A systematic review. *Medicine and Science in Sports and Exercise, 41*, 1831–1841.

Zhao, R., Zhao, M., & Xu, Z. (2015). The effects of differing resistance training modes on the preservation of bone mineral density in postmenopausal women: A meta-analysis. *Osteoporosis International, 26*, 1605–1618.

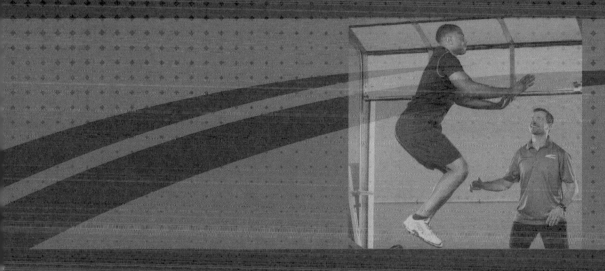

CHAPTER 13

THE OPTIMUM PERFORMANCE TRAINING™ (OPT™) MODEL: APPLYING POWER

OBJECTIVES

After studying this chapter, you will be able to:

1. **Describe** the goals and outcomes of the Power Level of the Optimum Performance Training (OPT) Model.

2. **Explain** how power training goals are achieved.

3. **Utilize** Phase 5 acute variables on various client types.

4. **Implement** appropriate cardio protocols for the Power Level.

5. **Implement** appropriate movement prep protocols for the Power Level.

6. **Implement** appropriate resistance training protocols for the Power Level.

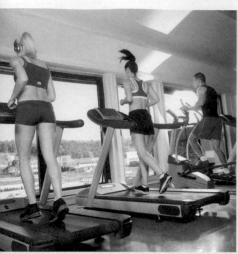

© fotoinfot/Shutterstock

Case Scenario

You have been able to build a good relationship with each of your three clients, progressing them through the first two levels of the OPT model: Stabilization and Strength. By training three clients with completely different fitness goals, you have gained insight as to why and how the first two levels of the OPT model can be used to reach an array of fitness accomplishments.

Let's return to your three clients and their fitness goals:

- **Roderick, the bodybuilder**, has been an avid gym-goer and is ready to take his training to the next level. Roderick goes to the gym daily, predominately lifting weights in hopes of entering an annual bodybuilding competition that is 9 months away.

- **Mary, the weight loss focused client**, has avoided the gym because she feels intimidated by others who are working out and feels self-conscious when exercising next to someone who she feels is in better shape than her. Recently, Mary's primary care physician has recommended that she should seek a personal trainer to help her lose 20 pounds.

- **Ashley, the marathon runner**, has overcome many weight issues but has been the victim of yo-yo dieting and workout programs she feels have not provided her the results she has been looking for. Over time, Ashley's desire to improve her health has sparked a passion for long-distance running and biking. She is highly committed and is willing to put in the time required to reach her goals. Feeling the need to challenge herself further, Ashley has registered to run a marathon in 4 months.

Consider the following questions:

- Aside from your client who is competing in a bodybuilding competition, how can you explain the rationale of applying the Power Level to your other two clients as it relates to their fitness goals?

- How would your clients use the Phase 5 acute variables?

- What movement prep and resistance training exercises would you use for each client?

- How are the other OPT levels used during Power?

Introduction to the Power Level of the OPT Model

The Power Level is the summit of the OPT model, and it is built upon the gains obtained in the previous two levels (**Figure 13.1**). This level relies heavily on the adaptations gained from the Stabilization and Strength Levels and applies them at functionally applicable (realistic) speeds and forces as seen in everyday life and sports. Unlike the Strength Level, the Power Level only has one phase, Phase 5: Power. Although power may be commonly believed to only apply to athletes, the fitness professional should understand the primary outcome of this level is to prepare the neuromuscular system to function safely and effectively at speeds that will be applied in a natural environment, rather than a controlled gym setting. This is accomplished by increasing the rate of force production (i.e., muscle contraction) within the kinetic chain. With a successful increase in the rate of force production, clients will be able to better perform their activities of daily living and significantly decrease their risk for injury.

Goals and Adaptations in the Power Level

The Power Level may be viewed as the most exciting level for the client to reach. This level is the culmination of a systematic progression and development of adaptations, which prepare the client to not only successfully complete Power Level training, but to also gain the most benefit from the associated exercise protocols. Sometimes trainers and clients want to rush into power training. This may lead to burnout and injury due to the client's lack of strength and stability. Therefore, the trainer should use appropriate caution and communication to ensure that the client is fully prepared for the demands of the Power Level.

The Power Level consists of one phase, Phase 5: Power, with the goal to increase the overall rate of force production. In order to achieve this goal, the fitness professional should strive to enhance the client's neuromuscular efficiency and prime mover strength. When these goals are

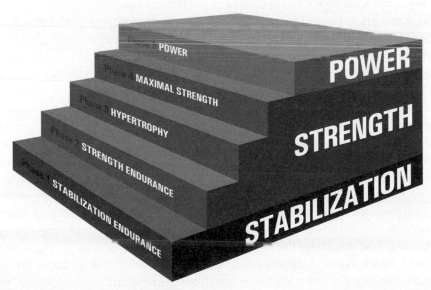

FIGURE 13.1 The OPT Model: Power.

combined and achieved, the client will be better prepared to move at functionally applicable speeds in his or her daily environment. The goals of Phase 5 are as follows:

- ◆ Enhance neuromuscular efficiency.
- ◆ Enhance prime mover strength.
- ◆ Increase the rate of force production.

Power is a correlation between speed and force and can be defined as force multiplied by velocity. Therefore, an increase in either force or velocity will produce an increase in power. This is accomplished by either increasing the load (i.e., force), as in progressive strength training, or increasing the speed at which the load is moved (i.e., velocity). The combined effect is a better rate of force production in daily activities and sporting events.

Whereas the Strength Level develops the force that is required by the power equation, the Power Level will require the individual to train at both heavy loads (85–100%) and light loads (30–45%) at high speeds. By working in this manner, the neuromuscular system will respond by increasing the number of motor units activated, the synchronization of those motor units, and the speed at which they are excited (Crewther, Cronin, & Keogh, 2005; Ebben & Blackard, 1997; Newton et al., 2002; Schmidtbleicher, 1992; Wilson, Murphy, & Giorgi, 1996). In order to work both velocity and force in this level, **supersets** are utilized. A high-force exercise is used immediately followed by a high-speed exercise to address both aspects of the development of power through an increased rate of force production. This type of superset application is used specifically in the resistance training portion of the Power Level.

The adaptations to Power Level training result in positive changes affecting muscles, tendons, bones, joints, nerves, and **proprioceptors**. Apart from strength training, dedicated power training produces specific adaptions that can reduce the incidence of injuries, improve rehabilitation treatment outcomes, enhance functional activities of daily living, and maximize sports performance.

Power training can significantly improve maximal and explosive muscular strength across a wide variety of clientele. While studies have shown mixed results, it has been found that muscle fibers can take on characteristics of faster type II fibers through power training (Kyrolainen et al., 2005; Markovic & Mikulic, 2010). Additionally, numerous studies have shown that power training can increase muscle–tendon stiffness and thereby improve power (Gambetta, 2007; Markovic & Mikulic, 2010; Sahrom et al., 2013; Turner & Jeffreys, 2010).

Just as in strength training, power training also has the potential to increase muscle size, or hypertrophy (Komi, 2003; Markovic & Mikulic, 2010). The development of hypertrophy through power training may also delay the progression of **sarcopenia**, or muscle loss, in older adults (Boyle, 2010; Hazell, Kenno, & Jakobi, 2007; Miszko et al., 2003; Orr et al., 2006). This is just one of the many benefits that older adults can gain from the adaptations provided by Power Level training. Recent research has confirmed that in the elderly muscle power is more predictive

Superset
One exercise immediately followed by another exercise with no rest.

Proprioceptors
Sensors in muscles and tendons that provide information about joint angle, muscle length, and muscle tension (i.e., muscle spindles, GTOs).

Sarcopenia
The loss of muscle tissue as a natural result of the aging process.

CHECK IT OUT

Stiff tendons are an important adaptation to the development of power. Imagine that a basketball represents a tendon. Consider dribbling an underinflated (compliant) basketball. It never seems to come back up to your hand, so you have to put more and more force into dribbling. In contrast, an overinflated (stiff) ball reacts quickly to the ground and pops up higher than you can handle! The compliant ball deforms and loses energy when it hits the ground, whereas the stiff ball immediately reacts to the ground force by bouncing up.

of success with performing activities of daily living than strength (Hazell et al., 2007). Exercise programming for this population should include high-velocity strength training to allow for transfer of resistance training strength gains into more functional, usable strength and power (Orr et al., 2006). This could result in quicker reactions, improved balance, increased levels of accident and fall prevention, and better recovery time from injury; all leading to higher levels of independence (Newton et al., 2002).

The Power Level will also play a role in adaptations for the development of both recreational and competitive athletes. Through improvements in strength, stability, and **anaerobic power** sports performance can be improved (Chu, 1998). A large number of studies have shown the positive performance benefits of Power Level training, including improvements in jumping, sprinting, agility, and endurance running (Markovic, 2007; Markovic & Mikulic, 2010; Paavolainen et al., 1999).

Although it may seem counterintuitive, power training has been shown to be an effective method to reduce the incidence of sports injuries, especially noncontact **anterior cruciate ligament (ACL)** injuries (Chu & Myer, 2013; Mandelbaum et al. 2005; Markovic & Mikulic, 2010; Figure 13.2). Most sports injuries in young athletes tend to take place during a deceleration

Anaerobic power

Maximum power (work per unit time) that is the result of all-out, high-intensity, physical output without the use of oxygen. It is a reflection of the short-term effects of the intramuscular high-energy phosphates—adenosine triphosphates (ATP) and phosphocreatine (PCr).

Anterior cruciate ligament (ACL)

One of the four ligaments in the knee that connects the femur to the tibia.

TRAINER TIPS

Work on jumping with seniors. Have them jump onto a stretching mat, which is a padded surface for impact, and only about an inch or two high. The focus is on jumping and landing with proper technique, not the height or speed.

FIGURE 13.2 ACL tear.

task (Chu & Myer, 2013). Eccentric strength is a focus in power training. The importance of eccentric strength in rehabilitation is now becoming widely accepted, as research has shown that the proper development of eccentric strength is a key ingredient in getting injured athletes back to their sport (Chu & Myer, 2013). These same injury prevention adaptations for athletes may be applied to other clients, including seniors, to ensure that they avoid injuries and receive better recovery during rehabilitation as well.

Scientific Principles for Power Training

In order to achieve the desired adaptations of the Power Level, the fitness professional should fully understand the scientific concepts that have led to the adaptations for every other level and phase of the OPT model. The use of the SAID principle, the General Adaptation Syndrome (GAS), the principle of overload, and the integrated performance paradigm laid the foundations in the previous levels, and they will still be used within the Power Level to produce adaptations. However, there are some scientific foundations that are specific to the adaptations sought within the Power Level of the OPT model that must be understood in order to apply the appropriate acute variables.

Force-Velocity Curve

The force-velocity curve simply describes the inverse relationship between the force a muscle can produce and the speed of a muscle contraction (**Figure 13.3**). The amount of force that can be generated by a concentric muscular contraction goes down as the velocity goes up, and vice versa (Haff & Nimphius, 2012). The implication here is that peak power output is not possible at maximal force. Peak power is best achieved at around 60–70% of maximal force and at about 30–40% of maximal velocity (Hazell et al., 2007).

This is why the OPT model relies on supersets during resistance training in the Power Level. The supersets are designed to be made up of one maximal strength exercise followed immediately by a power exercise using the same muscles. The client will be training for maximal force production followed immediately by maximal speed. This will focus on both adaptations in order to achieve maximal power.

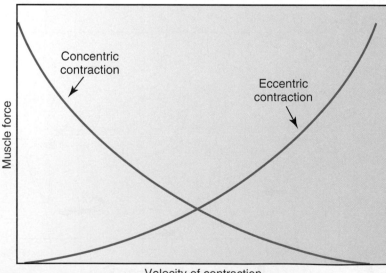

FIGURE 13.3 Force-velocity curve.

Size Principle

Force and power production can be maximized by increasing both the *number* of motor units recruited as well as the *frequency* of motor unit firing (Kraemer & Looney, 2012; McCardle, Katch, & Katch, 2000). The human body is efficient when it comes to exerting force. When muscles are used to produce force or power, all the motor units do not fire at once. Movements that require low force or power activate few motor units, whereas those requiring higher force or power recruit more motor units. Smaller and slower type I motor neurons are recruited first and motor units that are faster (type II), with larger axons, are subsequently recruited as more force and power are needed. This is referred to as **Henneman's size principle** (Figure 13.4; McCardle et al., 2000). This principle is important to keep in mind for optimizing the adaptations in the Power Level. If a client only lifts light weights, does primarily low-power exercises or aerobic activities, he or she will not activate the larger, faster, and more powerful type II fibers, and therefore the muscles needed for strength and power will essentially remain untrained (Kraemer & Looney, 2012). The optimal strength training variables required to recruit these type II fibers are greater than or equal to 85% of the one-repetition maximal (1RM), six or fewer repetitions, sets, and 2- to 5-minute rest periods (Turner & Jeffreys, 2010).

> **Henneman's size principle**
> Motor units which are under load are recruited from smallest to largest.

Role of the Proprioceptors in Power Production

The pre-stretch from the loading phase in a reactive exercise, such as a jump squat, leads to the stimulation of muscle spindles, which are being stretched and therefore react reflexively to protect the muscle by initiating a contraction (Kraemer & Looney, 2012). Power training has been shown to lead to increased stretch–reflex excitability, improving the muscle spindles' response to a rapid stretch, allowing for a rapid contraction and greater power development (Turner & Jeffreys, 2010).

Tracking Progress in the Power Level

Much of the progress in the Power Level will come from the way a client "feels." Clients may feel more coordinated, powerful, or agile when performing their activities of daily living; they may feel like they have more of a spring in their step or can move more quickly when required;

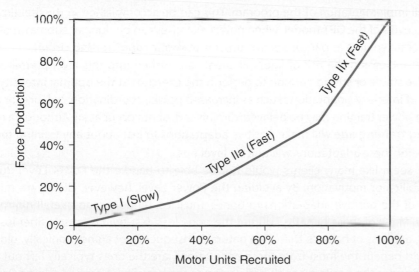

FIGURE 13.4 Henneman's size principle.

Intensity can be increased by adding light weights, using elastic resistance, raising the box height on a drop jump, going from a double-leg to a single-leg exercise, or jumping for a greater distance or height (Chu & Myer, 2013).

Drop jump

This plyometric drill consists of stepping off a box typically 18–24 inches high and immediately jumping up after landing. This is the most stressful and technically demanding plyometric drill. It is also known as a depth jump.

Metabolic conditioning circuit

A high-intensity exercise circuit designed to increase the storage and delivery of energy for any activity. It primarily conditions the phosphagen and glycolytic pathways.

Training age

Refers to the number of years a client has been training. A 12-year-old client who started training at 9 years old would have a training age of 3, whereas a 23-year-old who started training at age 22 would have a younger training age of 1.

and perhaps they will even be able to perform physical feats that they either have not been able to accomplish in a while or that they were never able to accomplish.

Although these are great ways to view progression in the Power Level, it is important for the trainer to be able to show specific and quantifiable results for the client. As with the previous levels this can be achieved simply through record keeping. Showing the clients how the acute variables have progressed is one way to show progress. The best way to show progress is through the use of performance assessments. Showing improvements in one's vertical jump or 40-yard dash will demonstrate increases in power. It is important when selecting these benchmarks to keep the client's abilities in mind. If the client does not have excellent landing mechanics, then a vertical jump test may not be the best assessment. Rather a 40-yard dash, or simply showing improvements in the acute variables, may be enough.

Whether clients opt for sophisticated tests or simply prefer to report how they feel, it is imperative to track this progress reliably over the course of the Power Level. Because this phase is more demanding and not as familiar to most clients, tracking progress will help them understand how the benefits of the Power Level specifically apply to them and why it is important not to skip this phase.

Problems Related to Avoiding or Rushing the Power Level

Rushing into the Power Level before the client is ready is setting him or her up for feelings of frustration as well as possible injury. Plyometric movements require smoothly coordinating all the limbs to maximize the intensity level. They also require eccentric control and strength, or the ability of a muscle to lengthen while under tension to properly land (Chu, 1998). Landing safely will minimize any negative impact to bones or soft tissues and is enhanced by good balance, body control, and spatial awareness, as well as eccentric muscle strength. Before starting the Power Level it is imperative that clients demonstrate competence in all these areas (Gambetta, 2007).

Core stability and lower-body strength are also important prerequisites for safe and effective power training. A **drop jump** from just 24 inches can produce a force up to five times a client's body weight (Chu & Myer, 2013). Having sufficient functional leg strength and core control will allow the body to properly dissipate these impact forces with minimal trauma to soft tissue or joints (Chu & Myer, 2013). Eccentric strength training and landing techniques should be taught before full implementation of the program. This can be accomplished in the Stabilization and Strength Levels of the OPT model, when power exercises can be done at submaximal intensity and moderate volume as part of a warm-up or **metabolic conditioning circuit**.

Besides increasing the risk of injury, if clients are rushed into this level prematurely, they may not be stable or strong enough to perform the exercises at the optimal intensity. Without this level of intensity, adaptations such as increased power, coordination, balance, or any other benefit of power training may be delayed, diminished, or not occur at all. Although a new client at a young **training age** will make positive adaptations to just about any training modality at any intensity, these adaptations will quickly level out.

It may seem like many clients would not be able to handle the Power Level due to age, athletic ability, or motivation. By avoiding the Power Level, however, clients are missing out on many of the positive adaptations to bones, muscles, tendons, and overall neuromuscular efficiency. Many of these benefits counter the bone loss, fast-twitch muscle fiber loss, slowed reactions, and loss of balance that are a natural consequence of aging. Ironically, older adults, who would benefit the most from these adaptations, are the ones typically left out of power training. Besides the positive health and performance benefits of properly doing Power Level training, clients will enjoy the change in their program and learn new skills and exercises.

Criteria for Participation in the Power Level

The minimum criteria for safely participating in the Power Level are core and joint stability, a good strength base, optimal range of motion (ROM) around key joints such as the hips and ankles, and good neuromuscular control (Chu & Myer, 2013).

The squat pattern is the most important indicator that a client is ready for explosive lower-body power exercises. An overhead squat or single-leg squat is a good option for screening. Points to look for that would require correction before transitioning to the Power Level include excessive forward trunk lean, knees falling inward (valgus), feet turning out, excessive forward lean, or the inability to get the thighs at least parallel to the ground.

Benefits of the Power Level

Fitness professionals can help their clients set goals that suit their specific situation and lifestyle needs. Based on the knowledge of the adaptations of the Power Level, there are numerous positive benefits that most clients can identify with. Communicating these adaptations are a great starting point for illuminating goals that clients may not have been aware of. Clients should start with just one or two goals in the beginning, and track the goals to ensure that progress is being made.

Increase Muscular Power and Strength

Numerous studies have demonstrated that power training can significantly improve both maximal and "explosive" muscular strength. These results have been noted across a wide spectrum of the population, from athletes to non-athletes, as well as males and females of all fitness levels. Power training results in slow-twitch muscle fibers taking on the characteristics of faster type II fibers (Kyrolainen et al., 2005; Markovic & Mikulic, 2010). Just as in strength training, power training has the potential to increase muscle size, or hypertrophy, but with the added benefit of preferentially affecting the fast-twitch type II fibers (Komi, 2003; Markovic & Mikulic, 2010). Additionally, numerous studies have shown that power training can increase muscle–tendon stiffness and thereby improve power (Gambetta, 2007; Markovic & Mikulic, 2010; Sahrom et al., 2013; Turner & Jeffreys, 2010).

The average client simply wants to feel better, lose some body fat, and enjoy recreational activities into their later years. The specific benefits of muscular strength and power that resonate with a client should be stressed by the fitness professional, which will help the client come up with his or her own attainable goals. For instance, becoming stronger and more powerful is a very time-efficient way of increasing the resting metabolic rate and contributing to long-term fat loss. Strength and power also result in more coordinated, powerful, and faster movements that may improve the performance of recreational activities or sports, as well as help prevent injury. Finally, being stronger and more powerful can offer a sense of well-being and confidence throughout the lifecycle, as well as in potentially dangerous or frightening life situations.

Improve Bone Health

Besides increasing muscular power and reactive abilities, a secondary benefit of power training is the positive effect it has on building bone mass. The direct impact through dynamic loading on long bones has been shown to be especially effective at increasing **bone mineral density** at the femoral neck, a common location for hip fractures (Markovic & Mikulic, 2010). This is particularly helpful for the elderly population in preventing a broken hip as the result of a fall, or from falling after breaking the hip.

Studies on school-based programs for children have shown a gain in bone mineral density as a result of reactive training. These school-based "jump" training programs have also been shown to improve overall bone structure as well as strength. The best benefits were for pre-pubescent and early pubescent children, as well as young and premenopausal women (Markovic & Mikulic, 2010).

Reduce the Effects of Aging

The normal aging process typically results in a yearly loss of muscle mass and strength. It has been reported that from 65 to 85 years of age strength and power decline every year, with power declining more quickly. From 20 to 70 years of age maximal anaerobic power has been shown to drop each decade (Boyle, 2010; Izquierdo et al., 1999).

Being physically active is not enough to stop this trend, as low-intensity activities do not seem to provide enough of a stimulus to maintain type II muscle fibers (Newton et al., 2002). However, recent studies have shown that power training for seniors has the potential to help slow or reverse this loss in power (Hazell et al., 2007; Izquierdo et al. 1999; Miszko et al., 2003; Newton et al. 2002; Orr et al., 2006). This could result in quicker reactions, accident avoidance, fall prevention, increased independence, improved balance, and better recovery times from injury (Newton et al., 2002).

Recent research has confirmed that in the elderly muscle power is more predictive of success with performing activities of daily living than strength (Hazell et al., 2007). It may be that exercise programming for this population should include high-velocity strength training to allow for transfer of the strength gains from resistance training into more functional, usable strength and power (Orr et al., 2006).

Bone mineral density (BMD)

Mineral matter per square centimeter of bone. It is an indirect indicator of osteoporosis and fracture risk.

TRAINER TIPS

Recommend to older adult clients that they take the stairs up and the elevator down. They will gain strength and cardiorespiratory performance by taking the stairs up and avoid the risk of injury due to deceleration by taking the elevator on the way down.

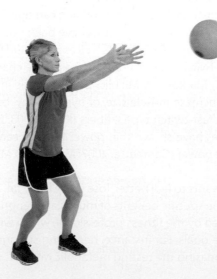

CHECK IT OUT

Even physically active people will experience *sarcopenia* with ageing, unless high-intensity activity is also part of the movement mix.

A study looking at the impact of power training on balance in older adults determined that lower muscular power was predictive of balance problems and fall risks, as rapid responses are needed to maintain postural stability (Orr et al., 2006). The study found that 10 weeks of power training with a low load and high velocity resulted in the greatest improvement in balance. Improved balance seemed to be associated with increased contraction velocity. Response times were reduced, postural muscles were optimally recruited, and sensory integration improved.

In another study on the effect of power training on physical function of older adults, the authors found that power training was more effective than strength training at improving scores on a validated test of functional ability (Miszko et al., 2003). They found that the velocity of movement and intensity of exercise improved function more than the total work performed, as the power training group actually performed less total work than the strength training group. They attributed the results to the greater neural activation that power exercises elicit in comparison to strength exercises, especially in regard to improvements in timed task performance. Evidence suggests that power training may help reduce the incidence of common sports injuries as well as reverse or slow age-related sarcopenia (Boyle, 2010; Hazell et al., 2007; Miszko et al. 2003; Orr et al., 2006).

Improve Sports Performance

Power training can play an important role in the success of many sports that require explosive vertical or linear movement. It is critical to understand, however, that power training is only part of what an athlete needs to be successful and reduce injury risk. A good base of stability, strength, and anaerobic conditioning are necessary before performance-level power training begins. Conversely, power training will ultimately lead to improvements in strength, stability, and anaerobic power (Chu, 1998). A large number of studies have shown the positive performance benefits of power training (Chu & Myer, 2013; Gambetta, 2007; Markovic & Mikulic, 2010):

- *Jumping*: Short-term power training has been shown to improve vertical jump height for a large cross section of the population, including children, young adults, males and females, athletes and non-athletes, and those with all levels of training experience (Markovic, 2007; Markovic & Mikulic, 2010).
- *Sprinting*: Sprinting performance can also improve with power training. A review of studies noted improvements in sprinting; while one study, sprint performance in 10- to 55-meter distances improved significantly (Markovic, 2007; Markovic & Mikulic, 2010). Strength and power training, therefore, are key training methods for improving the ability to transition from acceleration to maximal velocity on the field (Markovic, 2007).
- *Agility*: Because the majority of agility drills require a quick switch from eccentric to concentric muscle action, performance on these drills can improve as a direct result of power training (Markovic & Mikulic, 2010).
- *Endurance running*: Surprisingly, well-trained endurance athletes have been shown to improve with the addition of anaerobic power training. In a 1999 study, it was demonstrated that explosive power training, along with endurance training, improved running performance in 5Ks (Paavolainen et al., 1999).
- *Prevent injury and improve treatment outcomes*: Although it may seem counterintuitive, power training has been shown to be an effective method to reduce the incidence of

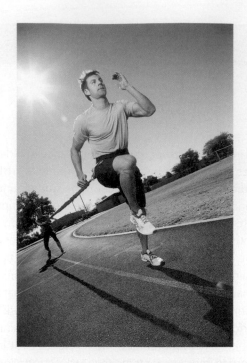

Eccentric strength

One of the three phases in the movement of a muscle. Refers to the action of a muscle while lengthening under load.

sports injuries, especially noncontact anterior cruciate ligament (ACL) injuries (Chu & Myer, 2013; Mandelbaum et al., 2005; Markovic & Mikulic, 2010; **Figure 13.2a**). Most sports injuries in young athletes tend to take place during a deceleration task (Chu & Myer, 2013). **Eccentric strength** is a focus in power training. The importance of eccentric strength in rehabilitation is now becoming widely accepted, as research has shown that the proper development of eccentric strength is a key ingredient in getting injured athletes back to their sport (Chu & Myer, 2013).

Based on each client's assessment results and goals, the fitness professional should explain the benefits of Power Level training which best fit the client's needs. It is best to use plain English without any jargon or technical words. Point out one or two "hot button" benefits, so that the client is not overloaded with information. Begin to stress these benefits before entering the Power Level and as reminders throughout the Power Level workout.

Cardiorespiratory Training for the Power Level

Parasympathetic nervous system

Stimulates rest and digestion physiological processes.

Because the Power Phase relies on the anaerobic energy systems for success, it makes sense to emphasize training the anaerobic system, rather than doing traditional long, slow, distance aerobic training. An aerobic base is important to establish before training begins at this phase, but doing too much aerobic training can in fact preferentially activate the **parasympathetic nervous system** and lead to less-than-optimal power output potential (Gambetta, 2007).

Ironically, anaerobic interval training can develop aerobic capacity as well as, if not better than, aerobic training. Interval training will also have the added benefit of burning more calories per unit of time, as well as raising the metabolic rate for a much longer post-exercise period than aerobic training (Boyle, 2010). Also, interval training can be done in much less time and yields faster results than aerobic training.

CHECK IT OUT

Example "hot button" issues include:

- Fat loss.
- Building muscle to "look good."
- Improving one's ability to hike, backpack, trek, or hunt.
- Improving race time in a 5K, 10K, half marathon, or marathon.
- Improving coordination ("too clumsy;" "not good at sports;" etc.)
- Becoming a better "weekend warrior": tennis tournaments, softball, soccer, etc.
- Reducing injuries (while playing sports, at work, etc.)
- Achieving elite status in sports (high school, college, or as a professional).
- Improving balance and reducing fall or accident risk.
- Being able to play with grandchildren (or children).
- Reducing the risks of osteopenia or osteoporosis.
- Reversing age-related muscle loss.
- Improving reaction ability to avoid accidents.
- Being able to continue working in a physically demanding career (firefighter, police officer, furniture mover, etc).

Therefore, Stage III cardiorespiratory training should be implemented during Power Level training (**Figure 13.5**). The client will warm-up in Zone 1 for up to 10 minutes. The workload should then increase every 60 seconds until the client reaches Zone 3 (86–95% HR_{max}). This will require a slow climb through Zone 2 for at least 2 minutes. The client will then spend 1 minute in Zone 3 before reducing the workload to allow the client to spend 1 minute in Zone 2. This process of performing intervals between Zones 2 and 3 can be repeated for up to 30 minutes. The time spent in each interval can be adjusted, but it should remain close to a 1:1 ratio. If the client cannot return to a Zone 2 heart rate in the time allotted, either the Zone 1 or Zone 2 interval periods need to be lengthened or the client could be entering into exhaustion and the intervals can be cut short through a cool-down.

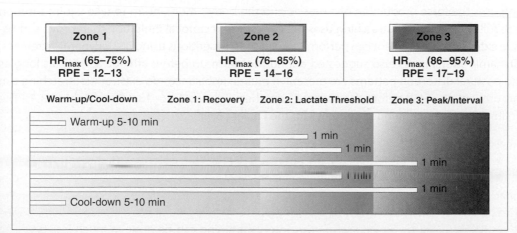

FIGURE 13.5 Stage III cardiorespiratory training.

CHECK IT OUT

The following are common interval variations:

- 15-second work interval: 3:1 ratio (45 seconds rest for beginner) *or* 2:1 ratio (30 seconds rest for advanced).
- 30-second work interval: 3:1 ratio (90 seconds rest) *or* 2:1 ratio (60 seconds rest) .
- 60-second work interval: 2:1 ratio (120 seconds rest) *or* 1:1 ratio (60 seconds rest).

As intervals progress within a session, the rest intervals should increase slightly due to the increased fatigue (Boyle, 2010). For instance, an interval training program with a 1:1 rest-to-work ratio could start with 30 seconds of work and 30 seconds of rest. By the second and third intervals, the rest period could go up to 45 seconds, and by the fourth and fifth intervals the rest could be as long as 60 seconds.

Movement Preparation in the Power Level

The most important reason for utilizing movement preparation in the Power Level is to prime the nervous system for the more rigorous work to come. Movement prep in the Power Level is equally as important as in the other levels and should never be minimized.

SMR and Flexibility Protocols for the Power Level

Optimal joint mobility and flexibility are crucial for the safe and effective performance of the strength and power exercises in the Power Phase. The protocols for flexibility are distinct depending on whether they are used as a warm-up or cool-down or whether they are done on off days to maintain tissue health. The SMR protocols are the same as those seen in the Stabilization and Strength Levels. The flexibility protocols should be done three times per week minimum, and as much as seven times per week depending on the client's needs and time constraints. Anywhere from 3–10 exercises for dynamic flexibility should be done for 10–15 reps. One to two sets is ideal.

Dynamic stretching is utilized during the Power Level of the OPT model. This type of stretching uses the force production of a muscle and the body's momentum to take a joint through the full ROM. Dynamic stretching uses the concept of reciprocal inhibition to improve soft tissue extensibility. The client can perform one set of 10 repetitions using 3–10 dynamic stretches. Dynamic stretching is also suggested during the warm-up before athletic activity, as long as no postural distortion patterns are present. If muscle imbalances do exist, static stretching can accompany the SMR before the dynamic stretches (**Figures 13.6–13.10** and **Table 13.1**). The following are recommended stretches for the Power Level:

- ◆ Prisoner squat.
- ◆ Multiplanar lunges.
- ◆ Single-leg squat touchdown.
- ◆ Tube walking.
- ◆ Medicine ball lift and chop.

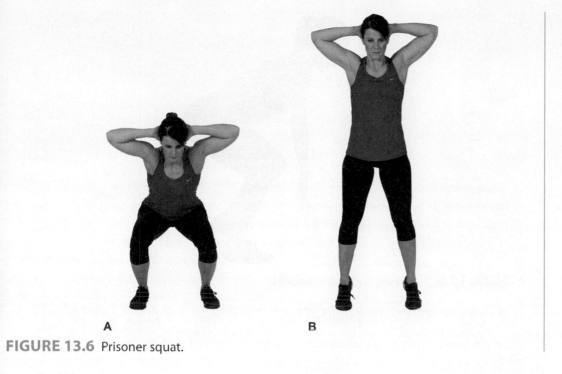

A   B

FIGURE 13.6 Prisoner squat.

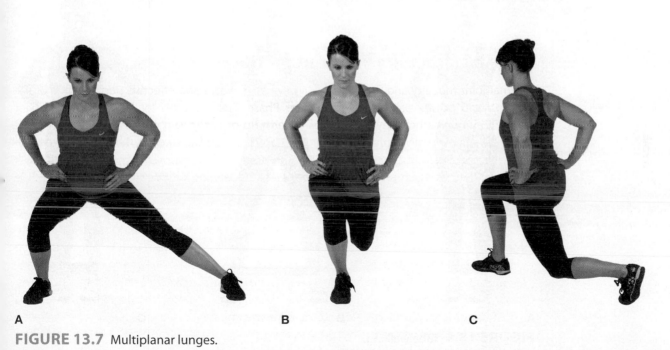

A   B   C

FIGURE 13.7 Multiplanar lunges.

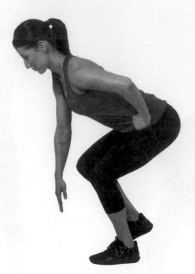

FIGURE 13.8 Single-leg squat touchdown.

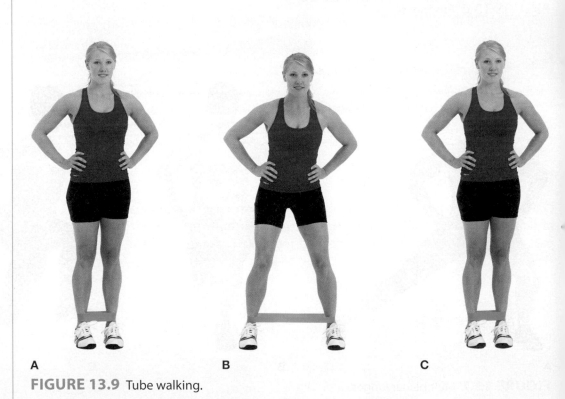

A

B

C

FIGURE 13.9 Tube walking.

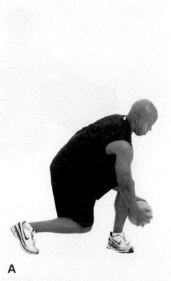
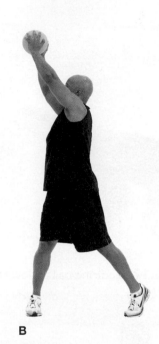

A   **B**

FIGURE 13.10 Medicine ball lift and chop.

TABLE 13.1 Flexibility Power Acute Variables

	Reps	Sets	Tempo	Intensity	Rest	Frequency	Duration	Exercise Selection
SMR	1	0–2	30–60 seconds	N/A	N/A	3–7 days/week	4 weeks	3 muscles
Dynamic stretches	10–15	0–2	Controlled	N/A	N/A	3–7 days/week	4 weeks	3–10 exercises

Core Protocols for the Power Level

Core exercises in the Power Phase involve trunk movements and are performed as quickly and as safely as possible with light resistance. These include exercises such as the rotation chest pass, medicine ball pullover throw, and soccer throw (**Figures 13.11–13.13**). 2–3 sets of up to

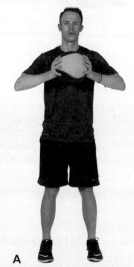
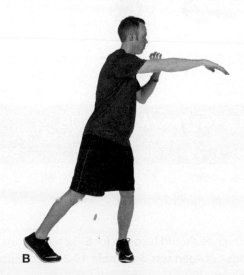

A   **B**

FIGURE 13.11 Rotation chest pass.

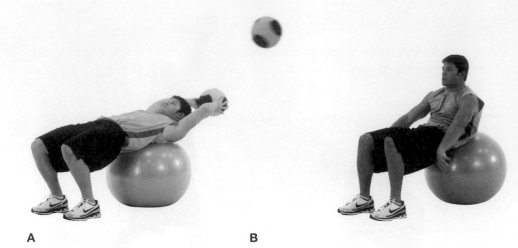

A   **B**

FIGURE 13.12 Medicine ball pullover throw.

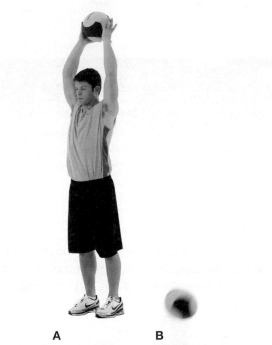
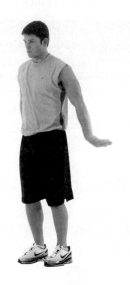

A   **B**

FIGURE 13.13 Soccer throw.

TABLE 13.2	Core Power Acute Variables						
Reps	Sets	Tempo	Intensity	Rest	Frequency	Duration	Exercise Selection
8–12	2–3	x/x/x	N/A	0–60 seconds	2–4 days/week	4 weeks	0–2 core power

two core exercises should be done for 8–12 repetitions. The rest period should be a range from 0–60 seconds between sets. See **Table 13.2** for core power acute variables.

Balance Protocols for the Power Level

Balance exercises in the Power Phase involve dynamic movements performed in a controlled manner. Multiplanar single-leg box hop up with stabilization and multiplanar single-leg proprioceptive plyometrics with stabilization (**Figures 13.14** and **13.15**) are examples of balance exercises for the Power Level. 2–3 sets of 1–2 balance-power exercises should be done for 8–12 repetitions. The rest period should be 0–60 seconds between sets. See **Table 13.3** for balance power acute variables.

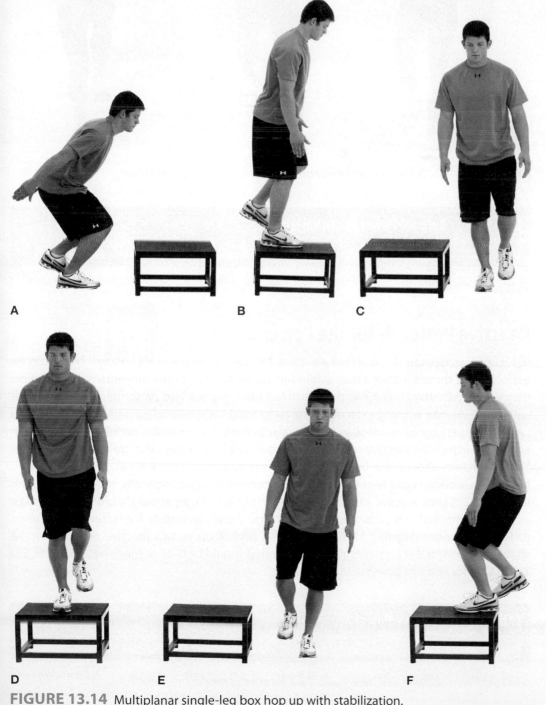

FIGURE 13.14 Multiplanar single-leg box hop up with stabilization.

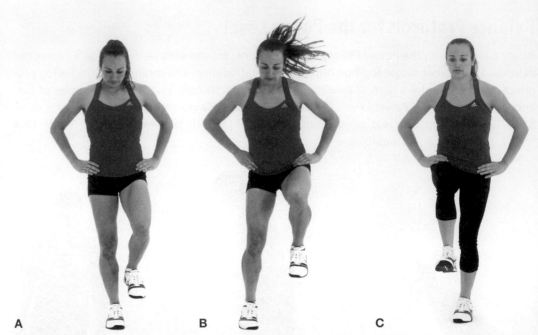

A　　　　　　　　　B　　　　　　　　　C

FIGURE 13.15 Single-leg proprioceptive plyometrics with stabilization.

TABLE 13.3	Balance Power Acute Variables						
Reps	**Sets**	**Tempo**	**Intensity**	**Rest**	**Frequency**	**Duration**	**Exercise Selection**
8–12	2–3	Controlled	N/A	0–60 seconds	2–4 days/week	4 weeks	0–2 balance power

Reactive Protocols for the Power Level

Reactive exercises are the required exercises for training in the Power Phase. These can be performed at three separate times within this phase. As part of the movement prep portion, they will prepare the body for further reactive work. They will also be combined in a superset with the resistance training exercises to develop maximal speed adaptations. These exercises can also be performed on off-days in their own true reactive workout, during which the focus should be on only the reactive exercises and should not involve any other training components. These workouts should also be followed by a rest day, because the neuromuscular demand from these workouts can lead to fatigue and potential injury. Specifically, the acute variables for movement prep reactive exercises begin with tempo. The exercises should be done as fast as can be controlled to reduce ground contact time. These can include ice skaters, squat jumps, or jumping lunges (Figures 13.16–13.18). 2–3 sets of up to two reactive power exercises should be done for 8–12 repetitions. The rest period should be 0–60 seconds between sets. See **Table 13.4** for reactive power acute variables.

TABLE 13.4	Reactive Power Acute Variables						
Reps	**Sets**	**Tempo**	**Intensity**	**Rest**	**Frequency**	**Duration**	**Exercise Selection**
8–12	2–3	x/x/x	N/A	0–60 seconds	2–4 days/week	4 weeks	0–2 reactive power

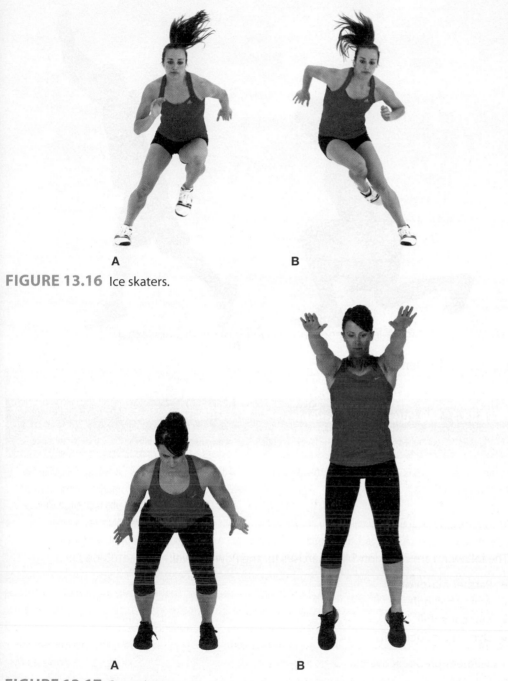

FIGURE 13.16 Ice skaters.

A   B

FIGURE 13.17 Squat jumps.

A   B

SAQ Protocols for the Power Level

Speed, agility, and quickness (SAQ) exercises done for movement prep involve drills emphasizing quick changes of direction in either a set pattern, as in using the agility ladder or cones, or in a reactive environment where clients would have to change direction in response to an auditory or visual stimuli. These should be done as fast as can be controlled. 3–5 sets of 6–10 agility drills should be done for 3–5 repetitions. The rest period should be 0–90 seconds between sets. See **Table 13.5** for SAQ power acute variables.

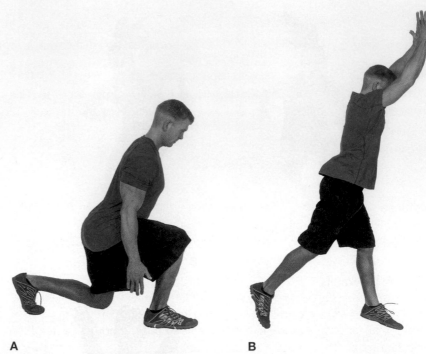

A   **B**

FIGURE 13.18 Jumping lunges.

TABLE 13.5 SAQ Power Acute Variables							
Reps	Sets	Tempo	Intensity	Rest	Frequency	Duration	Exercise Selection
3–5 run throughs	3–5	x/x/x	N/A	0–90 seconds	2–4 days/ week	4 weeks	6–10 drills allowing maximal horizontal inertia and unpredictability

The following are common SAQ exercises for the Power Level:

◆ Partner mirror drill
◆ Agility ball drill
◆ Star cone drill
◆ Dynamic ladder drills

Resistance Training Protocols in the Power Level

The resistance training protocol for the Power Phase utilizes a specified superset where a strength exercise is performed at near maximal resistance (85–100% of the one-repetition max-imum) followed by a power exercise that is biomechanically similar and performed explosively at 30–45% of the 1RM. For example, barbell squats would be followed by jump squats.

This training protocol is not only time efficient, but it is more effective than performing the strength and power exercises separately within one workout, or than simply doing a reactive

CHECK IT OUT

A study on upper body power found that using lower resistance for the strength exercise (65% of the one-repetition maximum, rather than 85%) still led to significant gains in power production. This has positive implications for clients who cannot lift near-maximal loads, because they will still benefit from doing the Power Phase supersets. A solid base of strength, however, is important to realize optimal gains in power at either heavy or moderate loads (Baker, 2003).

TRAINER TIPS

The average client is not hoping for a career in professional sports, and probably doesn't care about maximizing vertical jump performance. Your clients are usually very busy, however, so it is helpful to explain how doing Power Phase supersets is a more time-efficient way to get the results that are most important to them.

program without a strength training component (Baker, 2003; Chu & Myer, 2013; Ebben, 2002). Solid research confirms that combining strength with reactive training using supersets, as prescribed in the Power Level, leads to better results than either strength or power training done separately (Turner & Jeffreys, 2010). In a study of college football players on the effectiveness of using strength and power supersets, it was found that the athletes doing the supersets significantly improved performance on the vertical jump compared to those doing the power exercises separately following the resistance training exercises (Ebben, 2002).

Lifting heavy loads prior to a power exercise seems to put the body in a heightened state of neuromuscular excitability. The heavy resistance training increases the speed and efficiency of nerve impulses to the muscles, allowing for faster movement. This enhanced excitability has been shown to last 5–30 minutes (Horwath & Kravitz, 2008). Doing the strength exercise first allows the client to take advantage of this heightened state, which leads to better training outcomes for the power exercise that follows.

For strength exercises done as a part of the superset complex the range is 1–5 repetitions. This allows for the maximum amount of motor unit recruitment and force production with the least fatigue. The power exercise in the superset should be done for 8–10 repetitions. Power exercises are performed for more repetitions because the resistance is exceptionally lower.

CHECK IT OUT

Possible mechanisms that allow for superior results of the strength and power supersets, also known as *postactivation potentiation*, are (Baker, 2003; Chu & Myer, 2013; Santos & Janeira, 2008; Horwath & Kravitz, 2008):

- Increased neuromuscular stimulation that leads to slow-twitch type I fibers behaving more like fast-twitch fibers.
- More direct electrical stimulation (potentiation) to the muscle.
- Reflex potentiation (enhanced H-reflex), which increases the efficiency and rate of nerve impulses to the muscles.
- Increased synchronization of motor unit firing.
- Reduced inhibition from the GTOs.
- Enhanced reciprocal inhibition of the antagonist muscles.
- Increased phosphorylation (for ATP production) of myosin, during a maximal voluntary contraction (MVC), leading to faster rates of muscular contraction and tension.

CAUTION

It may not appear that older clients are moving fast enough, but it is important to match the expectations of speed and power with a client's age, level of experience, and specific chronic or acute injuries or conditions that may be present. As long as they are moving relatively faster than normal, they will derive benefits to some degree.

Open-chain exercises

Exercises where the foot or hand is free to move and usually not in contact with the ground. These exercises, such as a leg extension on a machine, are not as functional as closed-chain exercises such as squats.

If the resistance were too high, clients would not be able to move at their fastest, which would compromise the development of optimal speed and power.

The strength and power complex should be performed for 3–5 sets. For clients new to the Power Phase, start at the low end, 2–3 sets, and gradually increase to 4–5 sets. The goal of 4–5 sets places much more demand on the neuromuscular system and may best be implemented the second time a client goes through the Power Phase.

The strength and power exercises in the superset should be performed as fast as can be controlled. As the loads will be near maximal in the strength portion, those movements may not be very fast. The power exercises should be performed as fast as possible, with maximal effort, to realize the greatest gains in power development.

In strength training, the intensity is a direct result of the amount of weight lifted. In power training, the intensity is more a result of the type of exercise performed. The spectrum from easy to demanding power exercises will dictate the intensity.

The strength portion of the workouts should be performed at 85–100% of the 1RM. As described by Henneman's size principle, this ensures maximal motor unit recruitment, which will include the faster and larger type II muscle fibers necessary for optimal strength and power production. Peak power production has been determined to be greatest from 30–45% of the 1RM, or up to 10% of body weight (De Vos et al., 2005; Hazell, Kenno, & Jakobi, 2007; Izquierdo et al. 1999; Gambetta, 2007).

The rest interval between the strength and power exercise in the superset should be 1–2 minutes. The rest between circuits should be 3–5 minutes. Because power training is anaerobic it is important that sufficient recovery time is given. That way, energy stores are replenished enough for maximal strength and power production, and chance of injury or improper mechanics is minimized.

Power phase workouts should be performed 2–4 times per week. When doing full-body workouts, twice per week is ideal. If a body split is used, then four times per week would be best. Ideally, 48–72 hours of rest is needed for a full recovery before the next bout of exercise for the same muscle groups (Chu & Myer, 2013).

For the OPT model, each workout session, including warm-up and cool-down, should not exceed 60 minutes. Each phase will typically last 4 weeks. The average client should also work on landing and takeoff techniques as well as eccentric strength during all OPT phases leading up to the Power Level. This prepares clients for a 4-week cycle of the Power Phase, which reduces the risk of injury and helps produce optimal results. Some clients believe that more is better, and may want to work out longer than 60 minutes in one session, or more days per week than what the fitness professional has determined is optimal. They may even want to stay in the Power Phase for more than 4 weeks. It is important to stress, however, that in the Power Phase, the high neuromuscular demand requires even more rest and recovery to achieve results than in other phases. The focus should be on intensity and quality of movement rather than quantity.

Exercise choice will depend on the client's age, experience, specific goals (sport or activity), body weight, or injury limitations. For example, single-leg reactive exercises are more stressful than double-leg take-offs and landing (Gambetta, 2007).

Multi-joint strength exercises (e.g., squats) using barbells, dumbbells, or other free-weight implements are usually a better choice than an **open-chain**, single-joint exercise, or exercises on a machine. Single-joint exercises and exercise machines are fine for supplementary strength training and have their place in a program. In the power–strength superset, however, it is best to involve more joints of the body, in a closed-chain environment, for better functional crossover to sports, recreation, or activities of daily living (Chu & Myer, 2013). Using free weights requires the client to stabilize his or her joints under load, whereas machines stabilize the joints for the client. Creating maximal joint stability under load is an important prerequisite to the safe and effective execution of a high-power reactive exercise. See **Table 13.6** for resistance power acute variables.

Reps	Sets	Tempo	Intensity	Rest	Frequency	Duration	Exercise Selection
1–5 (Strength) 8–10 (Power)	3–5	x/x/x (Strength) x/x/x (Power)	85–100% (Strength) Up to 10% body weight or 30–45% 1RM (Power)	1–2 minutes between supersets 3–5 minutes between circuits	2–4 times/ week	4 weeks	1 strength superset with 1 power exercise

TABLE 13.6   Resistance Power Acute Variables

CHECK IT OUT

Clients often offer weight loss as one of their goals. If they improve their diet, they can lose weight. If they exercise in conjunction with an improved diet, however, they can prime their body to burn calories at a higher rate by increasing their resting metabolic rate. This makes the weight loss from dieting more effective and longer lasting. In much the same way, strength training done before power training in a superset primes the nervous system and allows for power adaptations to be more effective and longer lasting due to the increased neuromuscular stimulation and improved muscle stiffness resulting from the strength training set.

Common Mistakes Made in the Power Level

Because power training is the most advanced level of training in the OPT model, it requires special attention to detail by the fitness professional to maximize adaptations and performance outcomes as well as to reduce injury risk. The most basic mistake a fitness professional can make is not assessing or preparing a client properly for the Power Level. Even if a client does appear to be prepared for this level, it is critical to keep in mind any chronic or acute injuries that might require an exercise to be regressed, unloaded, or avoided altogether. The following are common mistakes that trainers should avoid in the Power Level:

- Too much volume
- Not using proper regressions
- Inappropriate exercise selection
- Not cueing intensity

Too Much Volume

The stimulus for adaptation in power training is intensity. Volume should be kept relatively low and intensity high. Higher volumes could create undo fatigue resulting in poor form, using incorrect motor patterns that may become permanent, and increasing the risk of injury. In general it is best not to exceed 150 repetitions in a session and allow at least 48 hours of rest between sessions (Gambetta, 2007).

Not Using Proper Regressions

Once a client's limitations are known, or if a client is new to the Power Level, it is important to properly regress a power exercise to ensure optimal safety and effective adaptations. The danger of too much too soon can set a client back or possibly lead to injury (Gambetta, 2007).

CHECK IT OUT

There is a continuum of intensity for power exercises. Choosing a less intense version of a similar exercise will accomplish comparable goals and prepare clients for more rigorous training when they are ready. For example, skipping could be a regression for alternate leg bounding, and double-leg hops can be substituted for single-leg bounds. It is useful to understand the basic continuum of power exercises based on intensity level to better know how to regress an exercise. A generalized scale of lower-body power exercise intensity from low to high would start with jumps in place and progress to standing jumps, multiple hops and jumps, box drills, and finally culminate with the highest intensity reactive exercise, drop (depth) jumps (Chu & Myer, 2013).

Reducing any of the training variables, such as frequency, intensity, or volume, can lessen the impact of a power exercise or protocol without overly compromising outcomes. Intensity can be decreased, for example, by "unweighting a client" (i.e., having the client hold on to the suspension straps or elastic bands while performing a jump squat, or doing a power push-up on a bench instead of the floor).

Inappropriate Exercise Selection

Fitness professionals should choose power exercises that are appropriate for their clients based on their clients' goals, physical limitations, sport, and body type. If their goals are improving balance and being able to accomplish simple activities of daily living, then box jumps are probably not the right choice. Light skipping or jumps in place might be better. If a client has rotator cuff impingement, then doing high-speed medicine ball overhead throws may put too much stress on the tendon. Instead, light medicine ball chest passes, resistance-band speed pulls, or skiers could be better choices. Avoiding upper-body reactives altogether may even be the best choice. In designing programs for a specialized athlete it is necessary to perform a needs analysis for the sport and the athlete. The fitness professional should understand the biomechanics involved in the sport and the forces necessary for success. For example, sprinters would need exercises that target the hip extensor complex, including the hamstrings, so spending more time on bounding or long jump drills would be more appropriate than medicine ball slams (Chu & Myer, 2013). An offensive lineman requires start speed from a crouching position, so working on vertical jumps is not as useful as doing standing long jumps, which develop horizontal power (Chu, 1998).

When considering body type it is most important to consider body weight. If a client is overweight or obese, then drop jumps, tuck jumps, single-leg hops, skipping, or even jumping jacks are inappropriate and dangerous. Clients may feel self-conscious, and this could result in a negative association with exercise and possibly to dropping out of the program. More importantly, the excessive ground reaction forces on impact can have progressive or immediate injury implications.

Not Cueing Intensity

Cueing is an art in training. Painting the right verbal picture can inspire clients to put their body in the right position at the right time to execute a movement with the optimal amount of force. Power training adaptations occur when a drill is performed with maximal speed or intensity.

CHECK IT OUT

For clients with joint issues or recovering from injuries, using more forgiving surfaces such as grass, sprung gym floors, or non-slip gym mats can be helpful to reduce impact forces and still make some progress. Keep in mind, however, that too soft a floor can reduce the elastic response and create a more concentric action, which would lessen the positive adaptations of power training (Gambetta, 2007). Studies have shown, however, that using non-rigid surfaces, such as sand training or aquatic training, results in similar increases in jumping and sprinting performance as traditional ground-based reactives, with the added benefit of less muscle soreness (Markovic & Mikulic, 2010).

Dynamic contractions recruit more motor units than even maximal strength efforts, and fast contractions recruit the most motor units (McGill, 2004). Research has proven that simply *trying* to move a load as fast as possible is beneficial, even if it doesn't happen! So, the intent and effort in attaining maximal velocity creates a focus and body awareness that improves the result (McGill, 2004). Many clients, however, will just go through the motions. It is up to the fitness professional to cue this intensity properly. Some cues that may resonate include "jump as high as possible" or "you are running from a tiger!" Clients could be asked to imagine that they must clear an obstacle, like a log or stream, for a long jump. Have fun with it and make it relevant to their interests. Remember, however, that maintaining proper form cannot be compromised in an attempt to achieve maximal power.

Integrating the Power Level with Other Phases

Power training can be intimidating to many clients. The human body has evolved to quickly and explosively run, bound, and jump to avoid danger or get around in an unforgiving environment. Simply observing young children at play confirms how humans are wired to run, hop, skip, jump, tumble, and roll. In the Stabilization and Strength Levels of the OPT model, it is essential to weave in power training drills and exercises to provide a well-rounded stimulus to improve overall functional human movement. These levels should serve as a training ground for reactive fundamentals such as takeoff and landing techniques and eccentric strength, or for just prepping the body for more intense dynamic movements to come with accessible and familiar drills such as jumping jacks, skipping rope, or in-place standing jumps.

In the Stabilization Level, reactive drills should only be used if a client has demonstrated adequate core stability and balance. The power exercises at this level should be at a lower intensity and focus on form, technique, and stable, balanced landings. Vertical jumps, horizontal jumps, or box jumps should end with the client holding a stable landing.

Another option is to combine reactive power drills and agility drills into a metabolic circuit for anaerobic conditioning before weight training begins. Various protocols can be used such as the Tabata protocol with a 2:1 work-to-rest ratio (20 seconds/10 seconds) for eight sets.

Reactive power exercises can also be incorporated as a "finisher" after resistance training for more advanced clients and athletes. This is a great way to use these more neurologically demanding exercises to expand a client's work capacity in a fatigued state, in order to match the demands of the client's sport or hobby.

Finally, when a client has progressed to the Power Level, it is important to return to Phase 1 or 2 on a scheduled and intermittent basis so the adaptations of Stabilization and Strength Endurance are not lost. Additionally, if a client arrives to a session feeling below average, rather than pushing through a Power Phase workout, the trainer should regress the session to a previous phase in the OPT model to avoid overtraining and/or injury.

Corrective Strategies for Power Clients

The formal assessment for new clients should serve as a guide for the implementation of exercises to correct deficiencies in stability or mobility, as well as any substantial asymmetries between limbs. It is also imperative to use each workout as a **formative assessment** to gauge progress and look for any compensations or new issues that arise, as well as to monitor progress in areas that need improvement.

Because of the demanding and technical nature of the Power Phase, it is especially important to address these concerns on an ongoing basis. Small improvements in hip mobility, for example, can reduce the amount of load on the low back or knees. The extra mobility in the hips will also allow for a bigger ROM for loading a reactive movement, resulting in the ability to produce more power.

SMR can be a good supplement to prepare the muscles and tendons for optimal proprioceptive responsiveness, as well as to move through a full ROM with less potential for compensations. It is also wise to foam-roll after Power Level training to begin the recovery process and help muscles, tendons, and joints function better for the next session. Good areas to roll for Power Level preparation are the bottom of the feet (plantar fascia), calves, hamstrings, IT band, piriformis, and the latissimus dorsi.

Static stretching should be used to achieve optimal flexibility as well as to correct left/right imbalances. Optimal ankle, knee, and hip flexion are important to load the body for a maximal jump. Full extension on takeoff at the ankle, knee, and hip, as well as the thoracic spine and shoulders, are also keys to maximize power potential. Stretching extensors, such as the hamstrings, will help with optimal loading while stretching flexors, such as the quadriceps and hip flexors, will help achieve maximal extension on takeoff. Static stretching, however, should be done on a separate day or at the end of a power training session, as it can have a detrimental effect on performance (Faigenbaum et al., 2005; McNeal & Sands, 2003).

Neuromuscular-based core training, which includes activating and stabilizing muscles of the trunk, abdominal wall and LPHC is critical for safe and effective power development. Combining whole-body dynamic balance and core stability exercises will help with dynamic core stability in response to the high forces generated by the limbs (Chu & Myer, 2013).

Conclusion

A deep understanding of the three levels of the OPT model is important for a successful fitness plan. By progressively and systematically working with clients, using the OPT model through the Stabilization, Strength, and Power Levels, the fitness professional can greatly assist clients in achieving their fitness goals. Once an understanding of the three levels of the OPT model has been achieved, the fitness professional can begin to learn how to implement these levels dynamically in the everyday setting.

Formative assessment

An informal, quick assessment of movement proficiency during a workout to gauge progress and screen for any new areas of concern.

TRAINER TIPS

To demonstrate the effectiveness of SMR with your clients, do an initial test with no movement prep activities (perhaps a body-weight squat) and record it (video or photo). Then, SMR the applicable areas and record the exercise being executed again. You may be able to show an improvement in the client's performance with just one round of SMR, which should reinforce the importance of SMR for the various activities.

Case in Review

As you progress your clients to the Power Level of the OPT model, you may find that some will question the need for, or the purpose of, the Power Level and/or the alignment of the Power Level with their fitness goals. Similar to the approach used to help convey the importance of the Strength Level, continue to describe and explain the need for the Power Level and how it is vital to making progress. For example, of the three clients you have currently been training, you may not get objections from Roderick, the bodybuilder, but you may feel resistance from your other two, Mary and Ashley. Continuing to explain the rationale for the Power Level, you could use the following strategy:

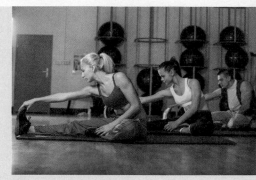
© fotoinfot/Shutterstock

- **Mary, the weight loss focused client**: "The Power Level will help you to better perform your daily tasks at functionally applicable speeds. This will prepare you for the dynamic world you live in and enable you to decelerate as well as produce forces needed to protect yourself from injury."

- **Ashley, the marathon runner**: "More power will provide you with more speed in your running. Phase 5 will ultimately help increase your speed and running economy, even if you are an endurance athlete."

While working with your clients, ensure that they utilize the acute variables in the manner that is recommended and referenced in this chapter. When addressing the movement prep and resistance training exercises associated with the Power Level, you implement the following exercises based on Mary and Ashley's fitness goals:

- **Mary, the weight loss focused client**: Side oblique medicine ball toss, ice skaters, multiplanar squat jumps, jump ups, jump downs.

- **Ashley, the marathon runner**: Jumping lunges, multiplanar hops, hop ups, hop downs, power step ups, soccer throws, overhead medicine ball throws,

Keep in mind that Strength Level exercises will be utilized in conjunction with Power Level exercises in the supersets of the resistance training scheme. Stabilization exercises can be utilized in movement prep or as active recovery on off days.

References

Baker, D. (2003). Acute effect of alternating heavy and light resistances on power output during upper-body complex power training. *Journal of Strength and Conditioning Research, 17*(3), 493–497.

Boyle, M. (2010). *Advances in functional training: Training techniques for coaches, personal trainers, and athletes.* Santa Cruz, CA: On Target Publications.

Cook, G. (2003). *Athletic body in balance: Optimal movement skills and conditioning for performance.* Champaign, IL: Human Kinetics.

Chu, D. A. (1998). *Jumping into plyometrics* (2nd ed.). Champaign, IL: Human Kinetics.

Chu, D. A., & Myer, G. D. (2013). *Plyometrics*. Champaign, IL: Human Kinetics.

Crewther B., Cronin, J., & Keogh, J. (2005). Possible stimuli for strength and power adaptation: Acute mechanical responses. *Sports Medicine, 35,* 967–989.

De Vos, N. J., Singh, N. A., Ross, D. A., Stavrinos, T. M. Orr, R., & Singh, M. A. F. (2005). Optimal load for increasing muscle power during explosive resistance training in older adults. *Journal of Gerontology: Medical Sciences, 60*(5), 638–647.

Ebben, W. P. (2002). Complex training: A brief review. *Journal of Sports Science and Medicine, 1*(2), 42–46.

Ebben, W. P., & Blackard, D. O. (1997). Complex training with combined explosive weight and plyometric exercises. *Olympic Coach, 7,* 11–12.

Faigenbaum, A. D., Bellucci, M., Bernieri, A., Bakker, B., & Hoorens, K. (2005). Acute effects of different warm-up protocols on fitness performance in children. *Journal of Strength and Conditioning Research, 19*(2), 376–381.

Gambetta, V. (2007). *Athletic development: The art and science of functional sports conditioning.* Champaign, IL: Human Kinetics.

Haff, G. G., & Nimphius, S. (2012). Training principles for power. *Strength and Conditioning Journal, 34*(6), 2–12.

Hazell, T., Kenno, K., & Jakobi, J. (2007). Functional benefit of power training for older adults. *Journal of Aging and Physical Activity, 15,* 349–359.

Horwath, R., & Kravitz, L. (2008). Postactivation potentiation: A brief review. *IDEA Fitness Journal, 5*(5), 21–23.

Izquierdo, M., Ibanez, J., Gorostiaga, E., Garrues, M., Zuniga, A., Anton, A., & Larrion, J. L. (1999). Maximum strength and power characteristics in isometric and dynamic actions of the upper and lower extremities in middle-aged and older men. *Acta Physiologica Scandinavia, 167,* 57–68.

Komi, P. V. (Ed.). (2003). *Strength and power in sport* (2nd ed.). Oxford, UK: Wiley-Blackwell.

Kraemer, W. J., & Looney, D. P. (2012). Underlying mechanisms and physiology of muscular power. *Strength and Conditioning Journal, 34*(6), 13–19.

Kyrolainen, H., Avela, J., McBride, J. M., Koskinen, S., Andersen, J. L., Sipila, S., & Takala, T. E. (2005). Effects of power training on muscle structure and neuromuscular performance. *Scandinavian Journal of Medicine and Science in Sports, 15,* 58–64.

Mandelbaum, B. R., Silvers, H. J., Watanabe, D. S., Knarr, J. F., Thomas, S. D., Griffin, L. Y., & Kirkendall, D. T. (2005). Effectiveness of a neuromuscular and proprioceptive training program in preventing anterior crochet ligament injuries in female athletes: 2-year follow-up. *American Journal of Sports Medicine, 33*(7), 1003–1010.

Markovic, G. (2007). Does plyometric training improve vertical jump height? A meta-analytical review. *British Journal of Sports Medicine, 41,* 349–355.

Markovic, G., & Mikulic, P. (2010). Neuro-musculoskeletal and performance adaptations to lower-extremity plyometric training. *Sports Medicine, 40*(10), 859–895.

McCardle, W. D., Katch, F. I., & Katch, V. L. (2000). *Essentials of exercise physiology* (2nd ed.). Baltimore, MD: Lippincott Williams & Wilkins.

McGill, S. (2004). *Ultimate back fitness and performance.* Waterloo, Canada: Wabuno Publishers.

McNeal, J. R., & Sands, W. A. (2003). Acute static stretching reduces lower extremity power in trained children. *Pediatric Exercise Science, 15,* 139–145.

Miszko, T. A., Cress, M. E., Slade, J. M., Covey, C. J., Agrawal, S. K., & Doerr, C. E. (2003). Effect of strength and power training on physical function in community-dwelling older adults. *Journal of Gerontology: Medical Sciences, 58*(2), 171–175.

Newton, R. U., Hakkinen, K., Hakkinen, A., McCormick, M., Volek, J., & Kraemer, W. J. (2002). Mixed-methods resistance training increases power and strength of young and older men. *Medicine and Science in Sports & Exercise, 34*(8), 1367–1375.

Orr, R., De Vos, N. J., Singh, N. A., Ross, D. A., Stavrinos, T. M., & Fiatarone-Singh, M. A. (2006). Power training improves balance in healthy older adults. *Journal of Gerontology: Medical Sciences, 61*(1), 78–85.

Paavolainen, L., Hakkinen, K., Hamalainen, I., Nummela, A., & Rusko, H. (1999). Explosive-strength training improves 5-km running time by improving running economy and muscle power. *Journal of Applied Physiology, 86*, 1527–1533.

Sahrom, S. B., Cronin, J. B., & Harris, N. K. (2013). Understanding stretch shortening cycle ability in youth. *Strength and Conditioning Journal, 35*(3), 77-88.

Santos, E. J. A. M., & Janeira, M. A. A. S. (2008). Effects of complex training on explosive strength in adolescent male basketball players. *Journal of Strength and Conditioning Research, 22*(3), 903–909.

Schmidtbleicher, D. (1992). *Training for power events*. In: Chem, P. V. (Ed.), *Strength and power in sports* (pp. 381–396). Boston, MA: Blackwell Scientific.

Turner, A. N., & Jeffreys, I. (2010). The stretch shortening cycle: Proposed mechanisms and methods for enhancement. *Strength and Conditioning Journal, 32*(4), 87–99.

Wilson, G. D., Murphy, A. J., & Girogi, A. (1996). Weight and plyometric training: Effects on eccentric and concentric force production. *Canadian Journal of Applied Physiology, 21*, 301–315.

CHAPTER 14

THE OPTIMUM PERFORMANCE TRAINING™ (OPT™) MODEL: EVERY DAY

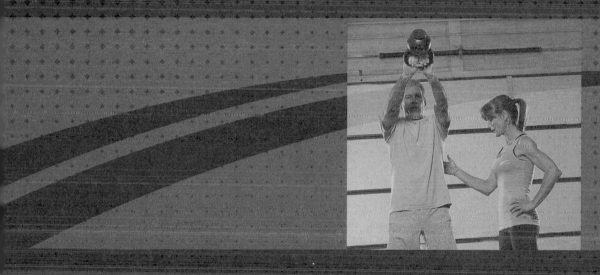

OBJECTIVES

After studying this chapter, you will be able to:

1. **Implement** various modalities into the different phases of the Optimum Performance Training (OPT) model.

2. **Create** group personal training programs that align with the OPT model.

3. **Describe** common special considerations that will be need to be made with various populations.

4. **Implement** appropriate program design protocols for various populations.

5. **Implement** OPT model programming as part of a larger, more holistic health and fitness program.

6. **Identify** common fitness technologies used by fitness professionals.

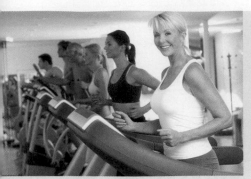

© Monkey Business Images/Shutterstock

Case Scenario

Over the past few months, you have been taking on more clients and building your pipeline. Using the OPT model to design integrated exercise programs has given you the confidence to develop workouts that help your clients achieve their specific goals. Because of your client diversity, you find the use of movement assessments and explanations of the OPT model to be effective strategies for selling professional services during orientation sessions with potential clients.

Through your experience of training a marathon runner, a bodybuilding contestant, and a client focused on weight loss, you have demonstrated your ability to design personalized fitness solutions. As you continue to acquire and work with new clients, you quickly realize there will be times that you might not have access to the optimal environment and/or equipment required for your clients' programs.

This past week you assessed five new clients focused on weight loss, who are all friends with each other. Although each member of the group shares the goal of wanting to lose weight, the path that lies ahead for each client will be different based on the results of each individual's assessment. To make things more difficult, they have expressed the importance of working out together, and can only do so during times the gym you normally work at is unavailable.

To explore your options, you will need to address the following:

- Explain the use of different modalities based on the resources that are available to you and the space requirements for five clients.

- Explain how both you and your clients can benefit from a group personal training program.

- Discuss how to use group personal training when the clients' abilities differ.

- Using each individual's subjective assessment (i.e., age, medical history, lifestyle questionnaire, PAR-Q), give examples of how that information will govern how you approach your programming considerations.

Introduction to Using the OPT Model Every Day

The OPT model is not a rigid set of steps that fitness professionals must adhere to in order for their clients to achieve the desired adaptations. Rather, the OPT model is a guide that should be molded and adjusted based on consideration of several factors. Schedules, equipment availability, injuries, and illness can all interfere with a program that was designed with the perfect application of the OPT model. When roadblocks arise, the fitness professional must be willing to adapt the model to meet the client's needs at that moment in time. Similarly, when various modalities are available, the fitness professional should use them to meet the needs of each individual client. Applying the OPT model every day will require the fitness professional to be creative and flexible in the application of the acute variables within the program to achieve results.

Introduction to Modalities and the OPT Model

The human body responds to appropriate levels of stress with improved performance. According to the *General Adaptation Syndrome*, the systems of the body will respond to stress with improved fitness and performance. Throughout history, various training modalities have been developed to introduce unique stresses to the body in an effort to promote improved function. Creativity, ingenuity, and innovation have resulted in the development of a variety of training tools that present different physical challenges to the neuromuscular system. Inventors and equipment manufacturers continue to evolve these **modalities** in ways that enhance the safety, effectiveness, and challenge of traditional exercises. It is important that fitness professionals become familiar with the various modalities used to promote fitness and function, know how to best incorporate them into a training regimen, and understand when their use is most valuable.

Arguments over which modality is best are common in the fitness industry. In reality, there is no "best" form of training for all populations and clients. Instead, fitness professionals should be concerned with selecting the appropriate modality based on the individual client's goals and phase of training. Understanding the history of each modality, along with knowledge of the benefits, risks, and correct techniques, will enable the fitness professional to make educated decisions about proper use and integration of different modalities throughout the OPT model.

Training modalities fall into the following categories:

◆ Bodyweight training
◆ Suspension training
◆ Free weights and implements
◆ Resistance machines
◆ Ropes
◆ Vibration exercise
◆ Rolling acute resistance

Oftentimes, trainers will become comfortable with the same type of workouts and rely too heavily on a limited number of modalities. Some circumstances may dictate heavy reliance on one form of training, and certain modalities may fit better during specific phases of the OPT model. A lack of access to certain equipment may also limit the choices available. However, fitness professionals should be familiar with each modality, comfortable teaching and refining proper technique, and skilled at integrating each tool into a well-rounded training program. The more accustomed a fitness professional becomes with each modality, the better they can be integrated into a workout as needed.

Modality
A form or mode of exercise that presents a specific stress to the body.

CAUTION

Fitness professionals should become familiar with the many different modalities; however, use of modalities without proper knowledge and experience is not recommended.

CHECK IT OUT

When constructing a training plan, fitness professionals should start by determining which modalities will be used. These decisions are based on the availability of exercise equipment and the client's goals, needs, and performance capabilities.

CHECK IT OUT

Different resistance training modalities are like tools in a toolbox. Each tool has a specific purpose and a specific type of job to accomplish. Just as an individual would not use a hammer for every task, relying solely on one modality is not advisable. Fitness professionals must be familiar with the various tools that they can use to help their clients achieve their training goals.

Bodyweight exercise

Form of resistance training where the source of resistance is the weight of the body.

Calisthenics

A form of bodyweight training that uses rhythmic full-body movements.

Bodyweight Training

Perhaps the least expensive, most accessible, and most versatile modality is **bodyweight exercise (Figure 14.1)**. In this form of resistance training, the source of resistance is the body. Rather than lifting external weights such as a barbell, strategic positions and movement patterns are used to activate and stress various muscle groups, with the source of resistance being gravity. **Calisthenics** and other bodyweight exercises such as push-ups and pull-ups have been used in fitness training for thousands of years. Gymnastics is a very dynamic form of bodyweight resistance training, requiring the gymnast to perform various movements that require extensive muscle activation, synchronization, and coordination. Various static holds used in yoga also represent a form of bodyweight resistance training, and numerous reactive exercises such as jumps, skips, and bounds represent good methods for improving strength and power without the need for equipment. Each of these forms of bodyweight resistance training can be incorporated into a training regimen at various stages of the OPT model to enhance the training experience.

The primary challenges with bodyweight exercise are progressing as muscular fitness improves, and being able to perform repetitions at full body weight in the early stages of training. In addition, body weight may provide too much load for those with a low ratio of strength to body weight. However, many bodyweight movements can be used to present progressive challenges to the neuromuscular system, including mountain climbers, lunge with rotation, and walking lunge with rotation. Additionally, burpees represent a challenging exercise for both the muscular system and metabolic processes (Ratamess et al., 2015).

TRAINER TIPS

You may not have certain resources and equipment at your disposal when training multiple clients at the same time. Having your clients use their body weight and gravity is often a go-to strategy. Keep in mind the use of this modality when putting together your clients' programs.

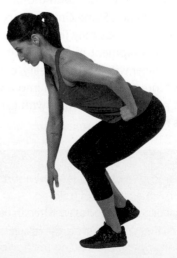

FIGURE 14.1 Bodyweight exercise.

CHECK IT OUT

The push-up is a common bodyweight exercise for the upper body. Over time, an exerciser should be able to increase the total number of push-ups in each set. Another way to progress the stress during this exercise is to elevate the feet by placing them in suspension straps. The elevation of the feet adds to the load by increasing the amount of body weight being lifted. The addition of instability by removing the feet from the ground also increases the demand on both the upper body and trunk musculature throughout the push-up. Increasing the portion of body weight providing resistance and introducing instability are great ways to progress to higher levels of challenge during bodyweight exercises.

Research has shown improvements in strength solely through the use of bodyweight training among the elderly, suggesting that reliance solely on this modality may be of value among less trained populations (Watanabe et al., 2015). For exercisers who are accustomed to heavier loads applied through other modalities, however, bodyweight training alone is unlikely to present sufficient overload to result in improvements in absolute strength. That said, it may be sufficient to improve muscular endurance, and it has been shown to improve functional movement (Daneshjoo, Mokhtar, Rahnama, & Yusof, 2012).

Although the loads placed on the body during bodyweight exercises are often lower than those applied with other modalities, it is still very important that fitness professionals instruct and ensure proper exercise technique. Exercisers should avoid excessive trunk extension during exercises such as push-ups and planks to prevent adding too much stress to the spine (lower back arch). Excessive instability, especially in suspension exercises that stress the shoulder joints, are also of concern. Fitness professionals should ensure that the exerciser is capable of safely performing each exercise through gradual progression in loads and the introduction of instability.

Bodyweight exercise is most appropriate during Phase 1 of the OPT model. During this phase, bodyweight exercises can assist in the development of muscular endurance, stability, mobility, and balance. Reactive exercises such as jumps and bounds can also be great exercises during Phase 5: Power. Bodyweight exercises performed at high speeds can be very beneficial when the training goal is to increase the rate of force development and stimulate the ability to move the body quickly through dynamic movements.

Suspension Training

Suspension training tools such as slings, straps, and ropes enable a greater variety in movement patterns, body positions, and joint angles than bodyweight training (**Figure 14.2**). These devices, sometimes referred to as *unstable resistance training*, generally involve two straps with handles, with an anchor at a central point generally about 8 feet off the ground, making them a portable and versatile tool. They enable the exerciser to add or reduce the amount of resistance through altering the amount of body weight that is suspended. This ability to unload and gradually progress is important in the initial stages of training.

The general consensus of the research associated with suspension training is that these devices can increase core muscle activation over standard versions of bodyweight exercises such as push-ups, prone iso-abs, and inverted rows by adding instability (Beach, Howarth, & Callaghan, 2008; Fenwick, Brown, & McGill, 2009; Snarr & Esco, 2014). Research also suggests that suspension

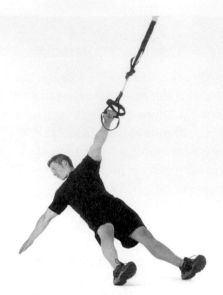

FIGURE 14.2 Suspension trainer.

training in the initial stages of an exercise program (first 7 weeks or so) may be just as effective as traditional resistance training for improving muscular strength and endurance, and may enhance the training benefits in the area of balance more than machine-based resistance training (Mate-Munoz, Monroy Anton, Jimenez, & Garnacho-Castano, 2014; Dannelly et al., 2011).

Free Weights and Implements

Free weights is a term that includes modalities such as barbells and weight plates, dumbbells, kettlebells, medicine balls, and sandbags. This modality involves the use of resistance that is not fixed to a set path or movement pattern, thus requiring the lifter to stabilize and direct the movement. These modalities are versatile and economical compared to exercise machines. The ability to perform the same exercises in slightly different ways, based on individual movement capabilities and strength levels, makes them a good option for fitness professionals. Free weight exercises have been studied extensively and have been shown to increase all aspects of muscular fitness, improve balance, promote muscle hypertrophy, reduce the risk of injury, improve bone density, and decrease physiological stress (Barbieri & Zaccagni, 2013; Stone, Plisk, & Collins, 2002). Many free weight exercises involve working large muscle groups, and some work multiple large muscles. Such exercises increase the metabolic demand of resistance training, burning more calories than single-joint, small muscle–group exercises (Scala, McMillan, Blessing, Rozenek, & Stone, 1987; Stone, Wilson, Blessing, & Rozenek, 1983). These benefits can be of value to all populations.

Some of the limitations or challenges with free weight training include the need to teach and master complex lifting techniques, the need for a spotter to prevent serious injury, and the lack of variations in the direction of resistance. Because free weights do not have set movement patterns (as with some resistance training machines), the lifters must control the movement path, stabilize the bar or **implement** themselves, and maintain proper lifting technique to avoid injury. However, once proper lifting technique is taught and mastered—and as long as training loads are kept within proper ranges—there is no evidence that greater risk of injury exists when training with free weights compared to other training modalities.

Free weights
Unrestricted objects of various weights that can be used as resistance for exercise movements.

Implement
A unique, free-standing object that can be used as resistance.

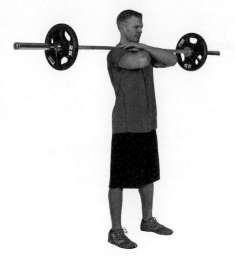

FIGURE 14.3 Barbell.

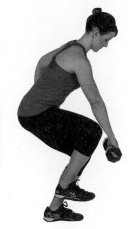

FIGURE 14.4 Dumbbell.

The need for a spotter, and the training of that spotter, is a potential limitation for the use of free weights. The spotter must be able to lift the amount of weight being attempted, in order to protect the lifter should an injury occur or if he or she is unable to complete the lift. This might mean that multiple spotters are needed at the same time.

An additional consideration when selecting free weight exercises is the source of resistance. Gravity represents the source of resistance for these exercises, meaning that there is only one line of pull (perpendicular to the ground). This limits the exercises that can be done while standing. The use of benches has allowed for some alterations in body positioning to change the line of resistance (e.g., incline and decline bench press benches). However, utilizing an external form of support decreases the requirements of the body to stabilize while exerting force.

MEMORY TIPS

When training with free weights, exercisers' movement patterns are unrestricted, and thus they are able to move freely.

Barbells and Dumbbells

Barbells, weight plates, and **dumbbells** are common free weight modalities and are found in most gyms. Barbells allow for greater amounts of resistance through the addition of plates, making them quite useful for high-load training in exercises such as squats, deadlifts, and bench presses (**Figure 14.3**). However, by fixing both hands on a bar (or in some cases placing the bar on the shoulders), stability and coordination requirements are diminished. It also prevents unilateral exercise completion. Dumbbells overcome these limitations, and are quite beneficial when coordination and mobility are desired during an exercise (**Figure 14.4**).

Barbells

Common free weight modality found in most gyms. Allows for greater amounts of resistance through the addition of plates. Useful for high-load training in exercises such as squats, deadlifts, and bench presses.

CHECK IT OUT

Compared to the dumbbell bench press, the barbell bench press can be completed at fairly high loads. However, the need to balance and coordinate the movement of two dumbbells is a greater challenge to stability. In addition, single-arm presses can be done with dumbbells to add to the neuromuscular component of this exercise.

Dumbbells

Common handheld free weight modality found in most gyms. Beneficial when coordination and mobility are desired during an exercise.

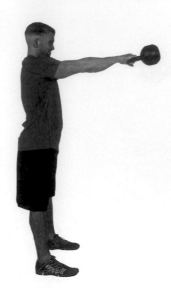

FIGURE 14.5 Kettlebell.

Kettlebells

Kettlebells have gained popularity in the United States in the last decade, making them a more accessible and common training tool (**Figure 14.5**). Their use dates back centuries in Eastern Europe, and Russia in particular. Although kettlebells can be used with exercises similar to those that use dumbbells (e.g, walking lunges, squats, side shoulder raises), their primary use is for various swings. The kettlebell serves as an implement during swings that incorporate ankle, knee, and hip flexion/extension. Most kettlebell exercises are total body, dynamic movements performed at a relatively fast pace.

Studies examining kettlebell training are fairly sparse; however, it was determined in a recent review that sufficient research evidence exists to support the use of kettlebells to improve power (Beardsley & Contreras, 2014). Kettlebell training may also be a promising tool for improving lumbo-pelvic-hip complex patterning and posterior chain power during horizontal movements (Beardsley & Contreras, 2014; Jay et al., 2011, 2013; Lake & Lauder, 2012a, 2012b; Otto, Coburn, Brown, & Spiering, 2012; Zebis et al., 2013).

The primary risks involved with kettlebell exercises, specifically swings, are the shear and compressive forces on the spine. However, when proper loading and technique are maintained, it appears that these exercises may actually help to diminish low back pain (Jay et al., 2011). That said, unique loading patterns and lumbar spine forces during kettlebell swings have been identified and are worthy of note. Greater posterior shear in relation to compression forces of the lumbar vertebrae have been measured during kettlebell swings compared to other exercises such as deadlifts and squats. Sufficient spine stability is required to ensure that the kettlebell swing is a beneficial exercise without causing lumbar issues. Progression in appropriate loads and the teaching of proper technique to stabilize the spine are vital roles of the fitness professional when prescribing the use of kettlebells among any population (McGill & Marshall, 2012).

Medicine Balls

Medicine balls have been used in exercise programs for many years as both an implement to add external resistance to bodyweight exercises, and for reactive exercises such as rotational throws (**Figure 14.6**). Because of their low cost, low space requirements, and the great variety of movement patterns and exercises that can be performed, medicine balls are an efficient choice.

Kettlebell

A cast-iron, cannonball-like weight with a handle used to perform ballistic exercises.

Medicine ball

An implement used to add external resistance to bodyweight exercises (similar to dumbbells and kettlebells) and for reactive exercises such as rotational throws.

TRAINER TIPS ⚊🏋⚊

When having your clients perform kettlebell exercises, aside from posture and form, be conscious of their surroundings to ensure that there is enough space to execute the exercise properly without risk of injuring another client or damaging equipment.

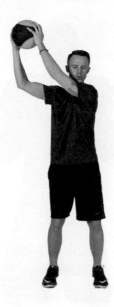

FIGURE 14.6 Medicine ball.

Many different types of medicine balls have been developed, and each has a different use. Leather and non-bounce rubber medicine balls are well suited for exercises where the ball is released with high power, and a rebound or bounce could be dangerous to the exerciser or bystanders. Medicine balls that bounce can be useful for throws against a wall or the ground, where a rebound is used to initiate stress for the next repetition. Some manufacturers now produce medicine balls with various handles, making for even greater variety in exercise choices.

Medicine balls offer several benefits. They allow for free movement in various patterns, making them a good choice for **functional movements**. They can also be used to add resistance to exercises. The greatest value of the medicine ball comes in the ability to produce very high speeds with some resistance throughout the entire movement. Exercisers can release the medicine ball and learn to exert force throughout the entire motion. This benefit has made medicine ball exercises popular among athletes, but anyone seeking high force and power development can benefit from these exercises.

Medicine ball training does have a few risks that should be considered. Bouncing balls or balls traveling through the air present a potential risk to the exerciser and bystanders. Fitness professionals must ensure that the exercise area is clear, and that bystanders are out of range. All exercisers should be properly trained on exercise technique, including catching technique. They must be allowed to practice and develop the necessary skill before being placed in high-stress, dynamic drills. Another risk, particularly during rotational movements, is the potential risk of low back injury. Clients should possess a high degree of strength and stability before being introduced to rotational medicine ball exercises. Selection of an appropriate medicine ball weight is also important to ensure safety. If the exerciser cannot perform each exercise with perfect technique, a lighter ball should be used.

Medicine ball use during various exercises may provide some value in the early phases of the OPT model to contribute to the development of stabilization and strength. However, their greatest value is in the development of power. Therefore, their use in Phase 5 of the OPT model is certainly recommended. Medicine balls may also add value in Phase 4: Maximal Strength, by presenting the neuromuscular system with a dynamic stress requiring rapid muscle activation.

Functional movements

Movements based on real-world biomechanics and activities.

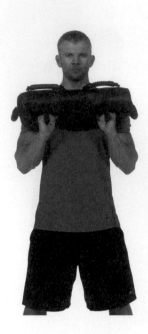

FIGURE 14.7 Sandbag.

Sandbags

Another unique free weight modality is sandbags. Sandbags, which are available in different sizes and weights, and with various handles, can serve as a distinctive form of external resistance (**Figure 14.7**). The flexibility of the bag requires the body to stabilize the implement while working. Sandbag exercises have the same value as other free weight implements, allowing for freestanding, free-moving exercises. By placing a sandbag on one shoulder or in one hand, core stabilization can be challenged and developed through the unequal weight placed on the body. As the sand moves slightly in the bag, the implement may contour itself to the body, making it a soft and somewhat comfortable form of dynamic resistance.

The incorporation of sandbag exercises into a resistance training program has been shown to help improve lean mass and bone integrity among youth, and to improve gait performance in rehabilitation settings (Teixeira-Salmela, Nadeau, McBride, & Olney, 2001; Yu et al., 2005).

As with other implements, appropriate loads and exercise technique are important to ensure safety and effectiveness. Because the sandbag is unstable and dynamic, exercisers must be prepared to adjust to the movement of the bag throughout the exercise. When bags are used to provide unequal loads to the body, the exerciser must have sufficient core strength to perform the exercise without harm.

Other Free Weight Implements

Other free weight implements have gained in popularity and represent unique training tools. Variation in training stress is a positive thing from both a physiological and psychological perspective. Therefore, unique implements can be introduced to vary training and increase the enjoyment of resistance exercise. Various "strongman" implements or exercises are becoming more common due to the unique challenges they provide. The farmer's walk, tire flip, overhead log press, sled pulls and pushes, and water-filled keg lifts and throws are just a few examples of these novel implements and exercises.

In the framework of the OPT model, strongman-style implements are best suited for use in Phases 4 and 5 where maximal strength and power are the desired outcomes. However, these implements, as well as all of the free weight modalities, may have value in all of the phases of

CHECK IT OUT

Personal trainers must be competent and skilled in various spotting techniques to ensure that all resistance training sessions are safe and effective for their clients. Research has shown that strength training–related injuries can be reduced through greater education, equipment warnings, and proper spotting technique. The following is a checklist for proper spotting technique:

- Determine how many repetitions the client is going to perform before the initiation of the set.
- Never take the weight away from the client (unless the client is in immediate danger of dropping or losing control of the weight). A proficient spotter provides just enough assistance for the client to successfully complete the lift.
- Spot at the client's wrists instead of the elbows, especially if the client is using dumbbells. Spotting at the elbows does not prevent the elbows from flexing and caving inward (particularly during the dumbbell chest press, incline dumbbell chest press, and dumbbell overhead press).
- Provide enough assistance for the client to successfully complete a lift through the "sticking point."
- Never spot a machine-based exercise by placing your hands underneath the weight stack.

the OPT model. Exercise selection, loads, and movements should be strategically directed towards the muscular goal of each phase.

Resistance Training Machines

Resistance training machines grew in popularity in the 1950s and 1960s as strength training began to be more accepted and promoted among the general population. Equipment manufacturers sought to develop machines that were more self-explanatory and less intimidating for the general population than free weights. These early machines enabled novice exercisers to engage in resistance training without the need to be experts in lifting techniques. It was also deemed safer for novices to use machines than to be required to stabilize resistance in free weight exercises. Helping more people in the general population participate in resistance training was a great success, and resistance training machines are still very common and popular in the fitness industry. Fitness professionals must be familiar with the various types of machines, and be prepared to make educated selections when prescribing exercises for their clients.

Fixed-Isolated Machines

The first generation of resistance machines included **fixed-isolated machines**. These machines provide a fixed range of motion with resistance provided by a weight stack (**Figure 14.8**). Fixed-isolated machines provide stability for the exerciser. A variety of fixed-isolated machines are available that are targeted at different muscle groups. The primary benefit of fixed-isolated machines is the protection they offer the exerciser from injury caused by weight falling during the exercise. These machines also allow for the resistance to be changed quickly and easily, usually through the simple change of a peg in the weight stack.

Although they have great value, fixed-isolated machines present less proprioceptive stimuli to the body and do not allow for individual variation in movement patterns. While slight

Resistance training machines

Machines that enable novice exercisers to engage in resistance training without needing to be, or become, experts in lifting techniques.

Fixed-isolated machines

Resistance training machines that provide a fixed range of motion.

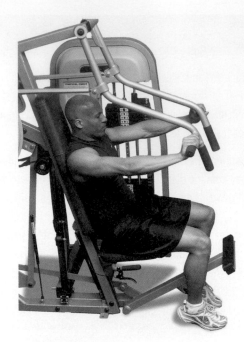

FIGURE 14.8 Fixed-isolated machines.

Cable resistance machines

Machine that offers protection and ease of load adjustments without a fixed movement path through the use of a cable.

adjustments to some machines are possible, some individuals may not fit perfectly in the range of adjustment. This could result in inappropriate movement patterns or ranges of motion for such clients. Additionally, the stability provided by the machine could be a limitation as well. Generally, in real life the body is required to stabilize itself while performing activities such as lifting, bending, squatting, and reaching. Due to the lack of proprioceptive challenge, individuals may not develop needed balance, muscle coordination, or mobility when using this type of equipment (Santana, Vera-Garcia, & McGill, 2007; Spennewyn, 2008). Research has demonstrated that exercisers who train with resistance machines, but are then tested for strength with free weights, do not perform as well as those who train with free weights (Stone et al., 2002). This demonstrates the importance of modality selection and application for assessments and functionality. There appears to be significant specificity in the strength developed, which should be a consideration when a determining the best modality for a client.

Fixed-isolated machines represent a good modality in various phases of the OPT model for individuals who need improvements in fitness but lack the balance or stability to perform other modalities at challenging loads. They also represent good choices when an individual has a weakness in a specific muscle group. Because of the lack of proprioceptive challenge, their use during Phase 1 of the OPT model may be less appropriate, as other modalities can promote stability more effectively (Spennewyn, 2008; Stone et al., 2002).

Cable Resistance Machines

Cable resistance machines provide a unique form of resistance that offers the protection and ease of load adjustments without a fixed movement path (**Figure 14.9**). This allows for individual variations in movement path and range of motion. In addition, the instability of the cable places a proprioceptive challenge to the neuromuscular system, requiring the body to balance and coordinate movement. However, exercisers must learn specific exercises and practice proper movement technique to safely and effectively perform such exercises. Thus, as with all modalities, the strengths and limitations of cable resistance machines must be considered when designing a training program.

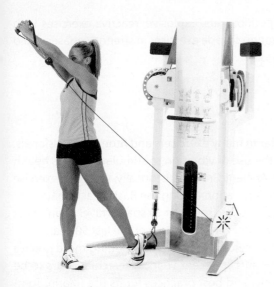

FIGURE 14.9 Cable resistance machines.

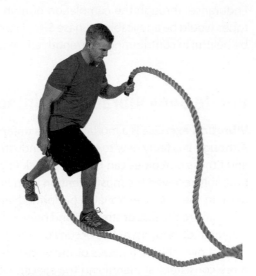

FIGURE 14.10 Battling rope exercise.

Cable resistance machines can present significant demands on muscular fitness as well as coordination, balance, muscle synchronization, and muscle activation. Therefore, their use can be valuable in all phases of the OPT model. Progressions can also be employed that increase the stabilization demand, muscle activation, and force requirement, making cable machines a very useful tool in functional fitness development.

Ropes

Ropes are quickly becoming a popular training modality because of the muscular and metabolic challenges they provide as well as the many variations of exercises that can be performed. Sometimes referred to as *battling ropes*, these exercises involve the use of large ropes (0.5–2.5 inches in diameter and 30–60 feet in length) anchored by a weight, tree, or post (**Figure 14.10**). Exercises are performed at very high speeds, with the arms often performing some type of whip or smash. The dynamic nature of the action requires great core and lower body stabilization, upper body strength, power, and muscular endurance. The ropes are relatively inexpensive, highly versatile, and portable, making them a reasonable training modality for many different settings and exercisers.

Studies examining the metabolic demands of rope exercises found that high-intensity rope exercise for approximately 10 minutes elicited high metabolic demands in terms of total energy consumption, oxygen consumption, and heart rate (Fountaine & Schmidt, 2015; Ratamess et al., 2015). Based on the weight of the rope, the number of repetitions performed, and the muscular actions required to perform the various movements, it can be expected that this modality would influence stability and muscular endurance. In addition, the ballistic nature of some smash rope exercises could be expected to contribute to power development. However, future research will be needed to verify these expectations.

Risks associated with rope training include the risk of being struck by the rope during training and perhaps muscle injury from the ballistic nature of the movements. With adequate preparation and training, these risks of injury should not exceed those of any other modality. Rope exercises fit very well within Phase 1 of the OPT model given their high demand on full-body stabilization during dynamic motions. This modality may also be of value during Phase 2: Strength

TRAINER TIPS

Your client may feel that the use of ropes is self-explanatory but will soon find that proper rope training is a skill that must be learned. One common mistake that clients make is using their elbow joints to conduct the waves in each rope. The waves should be created by the client's shoulders.

Endurance, through the completion of high-repetition sets. Explosive, reactive exercises with ropes would be applicable in Phase 5, and integration of rope exercises in strength phases could be helpful in contributing to strength adaptations.

Whole Body Vibration Training

Vibration exercise

The use of rapid oscillations of a platform or implement to stimulate and challenge the neuromuscular system.

Vibration exercise is a modality that is unfamiliar to many exercisers and fitness professionals. Although it is fairly new to the fitness industry, the use of vibration to stimulate various health and fitness outcomes can be traced back to the Ancient Greeks. Historically, vibration exercise probably received the most attention from its incorporation among the Russian astronaut program in the 1960s. Astronauts performed vibration exercises prior to space travel in an effort to minimize the loss of strength and bone mass during zero gravity. Over the last 50 years, considerable development has occurred in vibration exercise equipment, including more precise control over the parameters of the vibration stimulus. In recent years, research appears to be more consistent at identifying the specific benefits and best practices for its use (Marin, Tumminello, & Rhea, 2010). Fitness professionals can serve as valuable sources of education as this technology develops and becomes more accessible to the general public.

Vibration exercise imposes unique stresses on the body through oscillations delivered most frequently through platforms using motors to generate the vibration (**Figure 14.11**). As the platform moves vertically and then drops, various physiological responses occur. Muscle activation has been shown to increase with the application of vibration through these platforms (Perchthaler, Horstmass, & Grau, 2013). This activation theoretically occurs in an attempt to control or dampen the vibration as a protective mechanism. It also occurs as a response to the acceleration of the platform.

Traditionally, resistance training has used mass to increase force application. Vibration exercise increases acceleration, not mass, to elicit increased force production. The velocity of

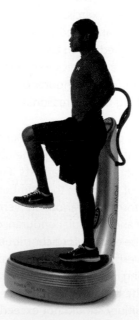

FIGURE 14.11 Vibration training exercise.

movement of the platform presents a challenge to the muscular system to maintain body positioning, and adaptations can occur in similar ways to traditional resistance training (Marin & Rhea, 2010b). For some, the use of moderate to heavy loads in resistance training is not feasible due to functional or orthopedic issues. In those cases, vibration exercise can be a valuable alternative to improving and sustaining muscular fitness.

Consistent use of vibration exercise has been shown to increase muscular power, strength, some measures of balance and mobility, flexibility, and blood flow (Bunker, Rhea, Simons, & Marin, 2011; Lohman, Petrofsky, Maloney-Hinds, Betts-Schwaub, & Thorpe, 2007; Luo, McNamara, & Morton, 2005; Maloney-Hinds, Petrofsky, & Zimmerman, 2008; Marin & Rhea, 2010a, 2010b; Orr, 2015; Rhea & Kenn, 2009). Some positive effects on bone density have been noted, but additional research is needed to clarify the effect of vibration exercise on bone mass in different populations (Lau et al., 2011; Liu, Zhou, Ye, & Bai, 2008; Totosy de Zepetnek, Giangregoria, & Craven, 2009). Other proposed benefits of vibration exercise include improved recovery from strenuous exercise and improved muscular performance during traditional resistance exercises (Marin et al., 2010; Rhea, Bunker, Marin, & Lunt, 2009).

Risks and side effects to vibration exercise are still being investigated. However, its use among many populations without the report of serious side effects or injury is promising. Based on the current research, it appears that vibration exercise can be performed safely with benefits. At minimum, it appears that vibration exercise is certainly no more risky than other training modalities. Particular caution is warranted among people with the following conditions (Marin et al., 2010):

- Pregnancy
- Recent operative wounds
- Joint implants
- Pacemakers
- Active cancer
- Circulatory conditions
- Gallstones
- Kidney stones
- Acute severe migraine headaches
- Infections
- Epilepsy
- Nephrolithiasis
- Cardiorespiratory disease
- Severe diabetes

Parameters that are important for the fitness professional to understand regarding vibration exercise include:

- Frequency: A measure of the number of oscillations per second in Hertz (Hz)
- Amplitude: Total vertical displacement, often measured in millimeters
- Time: Length of time that an exerciser experiences vibration in seconds

Research on the use of vibration exercise for balance, strength, and power supports the use of this modality in numerous phases of the OPT model. The proprioceptive demand of vibration exercise makes it a good tool during Phase 1: Stabilization, and the incorporation of vibration in Phases 4: Maximal Strength, and Phase 5: Maximal Power, is certainly warranted. The greatest benefits of vibration exercise appear to be when it is used in conjunction with other training modalities, making its use appropriate throughout the OPT model (Marin et al., 2010).

TRAINER TIPS

You should have an indication after you have fully assessed your client as to whether he or she is a candidate for vibration exercise. However, all exercisers should consult their physician to ensure that vibration exercise will not result in harm or exacerbate any health condition.

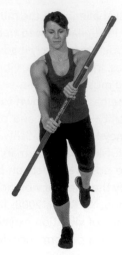

FIGURE 14.12 Rolling active resistance exercise.

Rolling Active Resistance Training

Rolling active resistance training works to train the body in the ways that it is truly challenged every day—with variation and unpredictability. Rolling active resistance implements are tubes filled with balls that roll as the bar is shifted (**Figure 14.12**). This pulls the exerciser off balance. The exerciser then engages stabilizing muscles to maintain balance. Because the active resistance shifts as the body moves, the individual is able to facilitate greater muscle activation, mind–muscle awareness, and reactive capabilities in order to stabilize the load based on what is felt during a given movement pattern. The movement patterns used with this modality can be used to build movement quality, balance, coordination, and core strength through the three progressive levels of the OPT model.

Group Training and the OPT Model

The role of the fitness professional is always to direct clients towards optimal health and fitness. Although workout locations may change, fitness professionals can have a profound impact on their clients through correct program design and skilled coaching. Opportunities for fitness professionals to guide clients along the path to optimal health and fitness have evolved significantly over the past 50 years. For decades, personal training (i.e., one-on-one interaction between the fitness professional and a client) has been a valuable setting for fitness professionals to influence their clients' exercise habits. In recent years, **group personal training** has become more common, allowing one fitness professional to provide individual direction to more than one client at a time. This form of training offers various benefits to the fitness professional, the client, and the facility offering this service. Although both personal and group training involve a fitness professional directing exercise clients, the training environment differs. It is important that the fitness professional understand the differences between these training settings, consider the advantages and challenges of each, and be capable of implementing the OPT model in small group settings to ensure success and enjoyment.

Group personal training
Exercise setting in which one trainer provides tailored exercise guidance to two or more individuals simultaneously.

Group personal training is a hybrid exercise setting, combining the focused attention of a fitness professional with the social atmosphere of a fitness class. The cost of the professional is shared among the group, making the service more feasible for those who are unable to afford personal training. Although it is a group setting, the fitness professional still provides individualized direction regarding exercise loads, techniques, and alternatives. Social interaction is achieved within the session as exercisers work in close proximity, and even potentially in tandem, making the workout environment motivating and challenging for all exercisers.

The fitness professional must be able to identify and respond to the needs of each client, offering exercise adaptations when necessary. The skill of the fitness professional will influence the number of clients that can be trained simultaneously, and little research exists to identify the optimal number of clients per session. Because the fitness professional must be able to address the individual needs of each member of the group, the size of the group should be kept small enough to enable such individual attention.

Group personal training presents a number of challenges, including coaching more than one person at a time, assessing multiple participants, ensuring that space and equipment are available, and successfully moving the entire group through a coordinated exercise plan. Despite the challenges, group personal training has become a valuable service and a growing trend in the fitness industry.

Determining Program Needs in Group Personal Training

Fitness professionals develop training programs that are tailored to their clients' individual needs. Information about each exerciser is vital in developing exercise prescription. In personal training sessions, where one-on-one interaction allows for focused attention on a single client, gathering this information is fairly easy. In group personal training settings, it becomes more challenging, simply due to the number of participants. Despite that challenge, it is the responsibility of the group fitness professional to ensure that individual alterations to the exercise regimen are made based on the needs of individual participants. To do so, the fitness professional must employ unique methods of information gathering.

CAUTION

The number of participants in a group personal training session greatly impacts the amount of individualized attention that can be given to each participant. Fitness professionals should be cognizant of their ability to provide individual attention to all members of the group and avoid creating groups with numbers that do not allow for adequate individual focus.

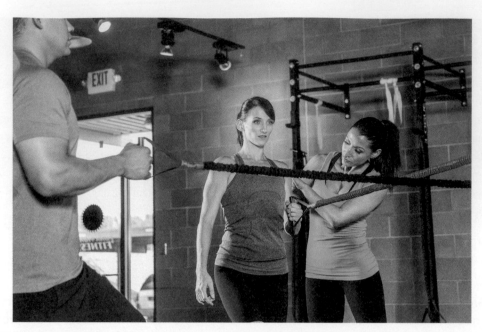

FIGURE 14.13 Group personal trainer conducting an assessment.

During each session, the fitness professional should observe each participant in every exercise. Observations of performance, including mechanics, load, pace, and exertion, will help the professional understand the current fitness capacity of each individual, and ensure that proper guidance is given.

Assessments are just as important in group personal training as in one-on-one training. Information regarding movement compensations, alterations to common exercises that may be needed, and equipment considerations must be factored in to ensure that group sessions effectively address individual needs. Health risk appraisals, static postural assessments, the overhead squat assessment, and other fitness tests should be conducted with each participant (**Figure 14.13**).

Movement assessments can be performed in a group setting with relative ease by an experienced fitness professional, providing vital evaluation of functional movement limitations. Both the warm-up (movement preparation) at the beginning of each session, and the cool-down at the end, represent useful times for information gathering. The fitness professional should use these parts of the workout to evaluate each participant. Tracking of information over time through the use of notes and assessment sheets will enable the professional to monitor change and adapt each training session to suit the needs of the participants.

Because individual needs will vary widely across even a small group of exercisers, the fitness professional must become adept at quickly identifying each participant's needs and determining the appropriate course of action. Conducting individual assessment appointments may be helpful to ensure familiarity with each client. Creating separate training groups with a specific focus (e.g, stabilization, strength, power) and encouraging clients to migrate to those groups that share a common goal may help the professional to better meet the needs of each client. However, this may not be feasible due to scheduling, or the desire of a client to exercise with a specific group of friends. Therefore, the group fitness professional must be skilled at gathering information quickly from a variety of assessments and observations, interpreting that information rapidly, and then quickly adjusting the workout for each individual client.

Methods for Implementing the OPT Model in Group Personal Training

Implementing the OPT model effectively in a group personal training setting requires planning, creativity, and flexibility. The fitness professional should plan out each workout and session to address every minor detail but also be prepared to alter the plan based on unforeseen circumstances. A variety of methods can be used, with specific exercises, training loads, and volume being altered depending on the particular phase of the OPT model being addressed.

Stations can be used—individually or as a group—to progress participants through a training session. If group stations are to be used, sufficient equipment must be available to allow all participants in the group to perform the exercise simultaneously. Each exercise within a given workout should also be able to be progressed, regressed, or adjusted to different phases in order to meet the different needs of each participant. Individual stations are more cost-efficient because only one piece of equipment is needed and participants simply rotate its use. The number of stations must meet or exceed the number of participants in the group to avoid periods of inactivity. If insufficient equipment is available, dynamic bodyweight exercises can be inserted into the workout.

Circuit training is also an effective method for group personal training sessions. This style of training was originally designed to combine full-body resistance and cardiorespiratory exercise into one routine. Traditionally, this is done by intermixing stations on resistance machines with assorted cardio exercises. The circuit training method has demonstrated effectiveness at improving health, increasing cardiorespiratory fitness, and enhancing muscular fitness (Gettman, Ayres, Polluck, & Jackson, 1978; Gettman, Ward, & Hagan, 1982; Messier & Dill, 1985). Circuits can be constructed with stations based on time, or the number of repetitions to be completed. Due to the transitional nature of the workouts, with exercisers moving quickly from one station to the next, this setup can accommodate groups of participants based on the availability of equipment; making them highly adaptable for group personal training sessions under the direction of a skilled fitness professional.

Variations of circuit routines have become popular in recent years, including boot camps, sport-specific programs, mixed martial arts workouts, and **metabolic resistance training**. Each involves a coordinated rotation or progression through a series of exercises, and all have the potential to be adapted to include a variety of exercises to target stability, strength, and power. For instance, a boot camp setup might include 8–10 participants who progress through a series of stabilization exercises. The group fitness professional observes and coaches each participant to ensure proper exercise technique, and to provide alternative challenges based on individual capabilities. A sport-specific circuit might include a combination of stability, strength, and power exercises with individual prescriptions to repeat specific exercises based on needed areas of improvement and different phases for each athlete.

In each method of training, the group fitness professional designs group workouts based on the available equipment, space, and number of participants. However, the primary focus should be to address specific needs within the OPT model, among multiple exercisers at the same time. This requires some flexibility in the structure and flow of the workout, rather than a strict sequence of exercises performed by all participants. The group fitness professional must balance the needs of the individual within the group setting. In each of these methods, exercise selection or modification, training loads, intensity, and volume can be adjusted based on the particular phase of the OPT model.

Metabolic resistance training
The use of high work-rate resistance activities with few or no recovery intervals.

Cueing

Verbal and nonverbal communication used to evoke an action response from participants.

Common Mistakes Fitness Professionals Make in Group Personal Training

The skillset of a successful group fitness professional will differ from that of a traditional one-on-one professional. Good communication skills are key to the effectiveness of every fitness professional. Fitness professionals should learn to gather information, use verbal and nonverbal **cueing** with participants, and practice active listening skills. This becomes especially more important for the fitness professional working with groups. Because one-on-one communication is limited in a group setting, the fitness professional needs to become very observant in the assessment of nonverbal communication, and be able to communicate to more than one person at a time. Maintaining a professional appearance, providing direct and clear instructions at the group and individual levels, and speaking clearly and loud enough to be heard in various group environments will enhance the fitness professional's reputation and effectiveness. A common mistake regarding communication in group personal training is failure to maintain proper volume when providing instruction. The group setting can become noisy, requiring the professional to speak in a louder voice to be heard.

Another common communication mistake is failing to adjust a coaching cue or message as needed. The "Tell, Show, Do" technique is vital within the group training setting. If further instruction or multiple cues are needed, the group fitness professional should be able to quickly alter the message and the mode of delivery. With familiarity, the fitness professional can learn which clients respond to specific forms of communication, and tailor cues to that style of learning; adjusting information delivery based on the receptiveness of the participant. If a message does not seem to alter the client's action in the desired manner, the message should be delivered in a different way.

With many participants working simultaneously, the fitness professional must be focused enough to catch important teaching opportunities, and recognize needed alterations or cueing, for each participant. However, the professional cannot be overly focused on one participant and neglect others in the group. Professional positioning is important to allow for broad observation of the group, while also being in a position to pinpoint small technique errors. Fitness professionals should reposition themselves frequently to adjust their field of vision, in order to avoid missing instructional opportunities that may be out of their line of sight. Failure to keep the group progressing through the session in a timely fashion may result from excessive focus on coaching or motivating. The use of devices to signal movement times may be helpful in ensuring proper timing.

Although planning and session design are vital to success in the group personal training setting, the fitness professional must be flexible enough to make needed changes before or within a workout session. Often times, even the best plans will require adjustments based on unforeseen circumstances. Alternative plans should be considered in the preparation phase, and the professional should be comfortable making quick decisions at any point.

Another challenge that should be considered in the planning and execution of group sessions is the proper management of volume, intensity, load, and recovery periods. Creating the sequence of exercises and planning traffic flow is just a portion of program design. To help clients meet their needs and progress through the OPT model effectively, the fitness professional must ensure that the acute training variables are kept within the recommended ranges. Failure to do so will result in a lack of progress in fitness adaptations toward the intended goal. Requiring every participant (regardless of training status) to perform the same exercises, at the same load, for the same amount of time, removes the individual value for the participants. Rather, group fitness professionals must be prepared to alter the training session for each participant based on his or her individual needs.

Through proper planning, flexible improvisation, effective communication skills, and maintaining the proper focus throughout the session, fitness professionals can effectively guide groups of individuals through the OPT model in group exercise settings, avoiding some of the common mistakes that often occur in this setting.

Populations with Special Considerations

Exercise has been shown to result in improved health and fitness in most populations (Williamson, 2012). In the past exercise was often considered a contraindication for special populations, but today researchers continue to demonstrate that appropriate exercise interventions can result in life-improving gains in fitness, reduced health risks, and enhanced well-being. That said, the appropriate exercise for special populations continues to be a focus of intervention research, and fitness professionals must be aware of the evolving body of literature on exercise in special populations.

A **special population** represents a group of people with similar conditions or characteristics that require unique alterations to an exercise program to ensure health, safety, and effectiveness. **Table 14.1** describes a number of the special populations that fitness professionals may encounter. The individualized approach to exercise prescription, as conducted through the

> **CAUTION**
>
> When using circuit-style group training, the group fitness professional should avoid simply processing each participant through the circuit without providing individual alterations or instructions along the way.

Special population

A group of people who have similar conditions or characteristics that require alterations to the general exercise plan.

TABLE 14.1 Special Populations	
Special Population	**Definition**
Youth	Children and adolescents between the ages of 5 and 18 years.
Older adults	Individuals aged 65 years or older.
Prenatal	Individuals who are pregnant.
Postnatal	Individuals who have recently given birth.
Obese	Individuals with a BMI of 30 or above.
Hypertension	Chronically high blood pressure as defined by a systolic pressure above 140 mm Hg and/or a diastolic blood pressure above 90 mm Hg.
Coronary heart disease	The coronary arteries of the heart become narrowed due to fatty build up along the walls of the arteries.
Congestive heart failure	A complex condition that is defined by impairment of the heart.
Atherosclerosis	Narrowing of the arteries due to a buildup of plaque along their walls.
Peripheral artery disease	Condition in which blood flow to the extremities is reduced due to the narrowing of arteries.
Stroke	Condition in which blood supply to the brain or areas of the brain is greatly reduced or interrupted.
Cancer	Condition in which there is uncontrollable abnormal growth of cells within the body.
Osteoporosis	Condition in which the bones become fragile and brittle due to reduced bone mass.

implementation of the OPT model, lends itself well to work with special populations. In order to make the necessary adjustments to training guidelines for implementation among different populations, the fitness professional must consider the capacity of the individual for exercise, the risks associated with certain exercises or loads, and how exercise might exacerbate specific health conditions. This requires a sound understanding of the research that has examined exercise among different populations, as well as the ability to make appropriate alterations to a training plan based on a particular client's needs.

Fitness professionals are not qualified to diagnose or treat any medical condition and must remain within their scope of training and practice when working with special populations. All clients must be cleared by their primary care physician before beginning an exercise regimen, and regular check-ups should be schedule to ensure that continued participation in exercise is appropriate. The fitness professional must never encourage or approve alterations in the directions given by the physician regarding medications or health practices. Communication between the physician and the fitness professional, with written approval from the client, can help ensure that the exercise prescription does not exacerbate the health condition, nor influence other treatments or medications that the physician has prescribed. Clients should openly discuss their exercise habits, training regimen, and goals with their physician, and the fitness professional should be prepared to share detailed information about the training plan with both parties.

In some instances, the primary care physician may be unsure of current exercise recommendations for specific conditions, or be unaware of the fitness guidelines for special populations. The fitness professional should be prepared to share this information with the client's physician as a valuable member of the client's health-fitness team. Fitness professionals can gain the confidence of those in the medical professions by remaining within their scope of practice, staying current in research on exercise in special populations, and being confident in their interactions with both clients and healthcare professionals.

Fitness and healthcare professionals share a common goal to "first do no harm" (Herndon, 2013). A thorough evaluation of the risks and benefits of exercise should be a continuous process, with the goal of achieving the greatest benefit with the least amount of risk. The information provided in this section is designed not to create fitness professionals who are "experts" in working with special populations, but rather to provide foundational information for fitness professionals as they begin working with clients who are members of special populations. The fitness professional can have a tremendous impact on the life of these clients when the exercise plan is designed and executed properly.

Age

Most general exercise guidelines are designed specifically for healthy individuals between 18 and 65 years of age. Ample evidence exists on the benefits of exercise for youths and older adults, but clients in these populations may require some adaptations in training to maintain safety and ensure effectiveness. Specific research examining the safety and effectiveness of resistance training programs in these populations provides the fitness professional with solid evidence upon which to build a training plan.

Youth

Multiple studies on youth resistance training have concluded that resistance training results in improved muscular fitness, body composition, power, and motor coordination among children and adolescents, and have shown a relatively low risk of injury with age-appropriate, supervised resistance training among younger populations (Buranarugsa, Oliveira, & Maia, 2012;

Behringer et al., 2010; Schranz, Tomkinson, & Olds, 2013; Peltier, Strand, & Christensen, 2008; Falk & Tenenbaum, 1996; Payne et al., 1997). An evaluation of different resistance training programs suggested the following resistance training prescription to safely improve muscular fitness among youth (Buranarugsa, Oliveira, & Maia, 2012; Behringer, Vom Heede, Yue, & Mester, 2010; Schranz, Tomkinson, & Olds, 2013; Peltier, Strand, & Christensen, 2008; Falk & Tenenbaum, 1996; Payne, Morrow, Johnson, & Dalton, 1997):

- ◆ Frequency: 2–3 days per week
- ◆ Volume: 1–5 sets
- ◆ Repetitions: 3–30 per set
- ◆ Intensity: 45–85% of the one-repetition maximum (1RM)

Reactive training programs in the following ranges were also shown to be effective at improving power, speed, and agility among youth:

- ◆ Frequency: 2–3 days per week
- ◆ Repetitions: 20–300 per session

Figure 14.14 shows basic exercise guidelines for youth training.

The most significant risk for youth performing resistance and reactive exercises appears to be the risk of falling objects in the training area. This and other risks, including muscle and joint strains/sprains, appear to be similar to those of any other population (Malina, 2006). Concerns regarding the effect of resistance training on growth among children appear to be widely exaggerated; as training protocols using free weights and machines have been found to be safe, with no negative impact on growth and maturation (Malina, 2006). The positive outcomes and the low risk of injury are a result of proper management of the stresses placed on the musculoskeletal system. Inappropriate supervision, excessive loads, improper lifting technique, excessive rate of progression in volume and intensity, and inappropriate rest between workouts may greatly increase risk of injury, as it would in any population (Abernathy & Bleakly, 2007; Micheli, 2006; Smith, Andrish, & Micheli, 1993). Fitness professionals must teach and ensure proper exercise technique and start at volumes and intensities at the lower range of accepted parameters. Slowly, over time, volume and intensity can be increased within acceptable ranges to progress in muscular fitness adaptation.

Fitness professionals should also keep in mind that most exercise equipment is designed for adults, and many children will not fit properly in such equipment. If the equipment cannot be

Mode	Walking, jogging, running, games, sports, resistance training
Frequency	5–7 days of the week or cardiorespiratory training
Intensity	Moderate to vigorous cardiorespiratory training
Duration	60 minutes per day of cardiorespiratory training
Flexibility	Follow the flexibility continuum specific for each level of training
Resistance Training	• Frequency: 2–3 days per week • Sets: 1–5 sets • Repetitions: 3–30 per set • Intensity: 45%–85% of 1RM • Levels 2 and 3 should be reserved for mature adolescents on the basis of dynamic postural control and licensed physician's recommendation
Special Considerations	Progression for the youth population should be based on postural control and not on the amount of weight that can be used. Make exercising fun!

FIGURE 14.14 Basic exercise guidelines for youth training.

WORKOUT				
Exercise	**Sets by Rep**	**Tempo**	**Rest**	**Coaching Tip**
Bench DB chest press	2 × 12	2/0/2	0 s	80% Superset 1
Push-ups	2 × 12	4/2/1	60 s	80% Superset 1
DB shoulder press	2 × 12	2/0/2	0 s	80% Superset 2
Assisted Pull-ups	2 × 12	4/2/1	60 s	80% Superset 2
Body weight squats	2 × 12	2/0/2	0 s	80% Superset 3
Transverse plane lunges	2 × 12	4/2/1	60 s	80% Superset 3

Notes and Observations:
Focus on technique. No rest between exercises.

FIGURE 14.15 Sample youth Phase 2 program.

adjusted sufficiently for a child, other modalities should be utilized to ensure proper lifting technique. Bodyweight exercises are a good starting point, allowing the child to build muscular fitness before progressing to the use of added training loads, with the use of a variety of different movements recommended. **Figure 14.15** provides a sample Phase 2 program for a youth client.

Older Adults

Older adults (65 years and older) can achieve life-altering improvements in muscular fitness through participation in a well-designed resistance training program. A significant body of research supports the use of resistance training among older adults for improving muscle mass, increasing muscle mass and strength, enhancing power, increasing function and balance, and either improving bone mineral density or preventing bone mass decline (Baechle & Westcott, 2010; Cadore, Pinto, Bottaro, & Izquierdo, 2014; Gomez-Cabello, Ara, Gonzalez-Aguero, Casajus, & Vicente-Rodriguez, 2012; Peterson, Sen, & Gordon, 2011; Stewart, Saunders, & Greig, 2014; Tschopp, Sattelmayer, & Hilfiker, 2011). Resistance training is a valuable tool for improving the health, fitness, and independence of older adults. Resistance training among older adults is highly productive, and the incidence of injury is extremely low (Baechle & Westcott, 2010). The following training parameters have been found safe and effective in older adults:

- ◆ Frequency: 1–3 days per week
- ◆ Volume: 1–5 sets
- ◆ Repetitions: 6–20 per set
- ◆ Intensity: 30–85% of 1RM

Figure 14.16 shows basic exercise guidelines for older adult training.

As with other populations, gradual progression from lower to higher training ranges over time is important to allow the client to become accustomed to training without excessive overload. Fitness professionals should begin with caution to ensure proper lifting techniques at very light loads and low volume. As the client becomes accustomed to training, masters proper lifting technique, and responds positively to low-volume, low-intensity training, loads can gradually increase to promote increased gains.

Due to the potential presence of numerous health conditions that accompany the aging process, the fitness professional must ensure that older adults have clearance from their primary care physician for participation in an exercise program. Special caution should be taken

Mode	Stationary or recumbent cycling, aquatic exercise, or treadmill with handrail support
Frequency	3–5 days per week of moderate cardiorespiratory activities or 3 days per week of vigorous cardiorespiratory activities
Intensity	40–85% of $\dot{V}O_2$ Peak
Duration	30–60 minutes per day or 8–10-minute bouts
Flexibility	Self-myofascial release and static stretching
Resistance Training	• Frequency: 1–3 days per week • Sets: 1–5 sets • Repetitions: 6–20 per set • Intensity: 30–85% of 1RM • Levels 2 and 3 should be progressed to based upon dynamic postural control and a licensed physician's recommendation
Special Considerations	Progression should be slow and well monitored. Exercises should be progressed toward free sitting (no support) or standing. Clients should breath in a normal manner and avoid holding their breathe as in a Valsalva maneuver. If a client cannot tolerate SMR or static stretches due to other conditions, perform slow rhythmic active or dynamic stretches. Standing up from sitting in a chair can be utilized as a special assessment.

FIGURE 14.16 Basic exercise guidelines for older adult training.

to ensure that medications and medical conditions will not be effected by physical exertion. If certain exercises and/or loads create pain or excessive discomfort in muscles, immediate alterations should be made to avoid injury. Pain or discomfort in the joints should also be avoided. Significant effort is warranted to find exercise strategies that do not exacerbate joint problems that may exist. Bodyweight exercises with the support of a chair or other device is a good starting point for many older adults. However, for those who lack the strength and stability to perform bodyweight exercises, low load exercise machines may allow for improvements in muscle fitness, which may be the cause of their instability and poor functional movement. Figure 14.17 provides an example of a Phase 3 program for an older adult client.

Pregnancy

Regular exercise before, during, and after pregnancy has been shown to have a wide range of benefits for both the mother and the baby (Fieril, Glantz, & Olsen, 2014; Hopkins & Cutfield, 2011; Larson-Meyer, 2002; O'Connor, Poudevigne, Cress, Motl, & Clapp, 2011; Schoenfeld, 2011; White, Pivarnik, & Pfeiffer, 2014). These benefits include:

- Improved weight management
- Reduced incidence of gestational diabetes
- Decreased hypertension
- Enhanced body image
- Improved psychological well-being
- Decreased risk of premature labor
- Shorter delivery and hospitalization

WORKOUT				
Exercise	Sets by Rep	Tempo	Rest	Coaching Tip
Chest press machine	4 × 12	2/0/2	60 s	80%
DB bench fly	4 × 12	2/0/2	60 s	80%
Leg press machine	4 × 12	2/0/2	60 s	80%
DB deadlift	4 × 12	2/0/2	60 s	80%

Notes and Observations:
Ensure everything is stable due to balance concerns

FIGURE 14.17 Sample older adult Phase 3 program.

♦ Improved fetal development
♦ Decreased risk of obesity in both the mother and child

These benefits appear to be achievable with relatively low risk to both the mother and the child when specific training guidelines are followed. Therefore, in the absence of serious health complications or contraindications, exercise is recommended before, during, and after pregnancy.

The body of research examining the risks and benefits continues to grow, and the fitness professional must ensure familiarity with this evolving body of literature. The design and implementation of an exercise program during and after pregnancy should be a close collaboration between the fitness professional and the woman's healthcare provider to ensure safety and effectiveness. The optimal route to fitness during pregnancy begins well before a woman becomes pregnant. The observance of a physically active lifestyle and the development of overall fitness prior to pregnancy will have a positive impact on the health of the woman and enable her to safely sustain an exercise regimen throughout her pregnancy. If little or no exercise has been performed prior to the pregnancy, caution is warranted when beginning an exercise routine during pregnancy to avoid overexertion and excessive soreness.

CHECK IT OUT

The health and safety of both the mother and the fetus is the primary concern when dealing with exercise programming for pregnant women. In a thorough review of the literature, Schoenfeld (2011) provided absolute and relative contraindications to exercise during pregnancy. Heart disease, lung disease, incompetent cervix, multiple gestation at risk for premature labor, persistent vaginal bleeding, placenta previa after 26 weeks, premature labor during the current pregnancy, ruptured membranes, and preeclampsia or pregnancy-induced hypertension are among the absolute contraindications to exercise during pregnancy. Other conditions, including anemia, chronic bronchitis, poorly controlled type 1 diabetes, morbid obesity, orthopedic limitations, seizure disorder, and poorly controlled hyperthyroidism, represent relative contraindications requiring either cessation of exercise for a period of time or significant alterations in the training regimen. The fitness professional should work closely with the pregnant client's physician to ensure that all exercise is safe and will not result in harm to either the mother or the fetus.

Increased blood pressure and excessive increases in body temperature are two concerns that are often discussed as challenges for exercise during pregnancy. Increased blood pressure may result in cardiorespiratory stress for both the mother and fetus; however, resistance training of appropriate loads, with the avoidance of the **Valsalva maneuver** can be beneficial without significant increases in blood pressure. Excessively high body temperature has been feared to increase complications in fetal development; however, research has shown that appropriate exercise does not result in excessive body temperature, nor any negative effects on the fetus (Schoenfeld, 2011). Miscarriage has also not been associated with levels of physical activity or exercise habits among pregnant women (Schoenfeld, 2011).

The fitness professional should modify the exercise routine to account for the increased secretion of the hormone relaxin during pregnancy. Relaxin relaxes the joints. As the joints become less stable, loads must be controlled and proper exercise technique strictly adhered to. High impact, ballistic exercises should be replaced with exercises that present less stress on the joints. The use of machines and benches may be helpful in providing external stability during exercises and reduce the risk of injury due to joint instability.

To ensure health and safety during and following pregnancy, the fitness professional should exhibit caution in exercise prescription. The focus throughout pregnancy should be to maintain fitness, not to maximize it. Aerobic training of light to moderate intensity lasting 30 minutes on most, if not all, days of the week appears safe and effective throughout pregnancy (Hopkins & Cutfield, 2011). Special attention should be paid to controlling body temperature during exercise, thus exercising in hot/humid environments should be limited.

The resistance exercises selected should promote total-body fitness, with special emphasis on the core musculature to reduce low back pain and maintain posture. Resistance training should be performed in moderate quantities and limited to the following parameters:

- Frequency: 1–3 days per week
- Volume: 1–3 sets per exercise
- Repetitions: 12–20 per set
- Intensity: Less than 70% of 1RM through the first and second trimesters
- Rest interval: At least 2 minutes to ensure ample recovery and reduction in heart rate and blood pressure

Fitness professionals should monitor their clients closely during exercise and alter volume, intensity, and training loads based on individual responses or needs. Especially during the first trimester, exercise may need to be adjusted based on nausea and excessive fatigue. During the third trimester, changes to the body may result in greater instability, difficulty in breathing, and decreased range of motion, requiring alterations in exercise selection and training loads. Olympic lifts and overhead lifting should be avoided after the first trimester due to the excessive stress and postural changes that occur throughout pregnancy (Schoenfeld, 2011). Unless complications arise during the pregnancy, little evidence exists to suggest that exercise cannot continue well into the third trimester.

Postpartum exercise has garnered a great deal of attention in the research literature as well, showing significant benefits to both the mother and child (Larson-Meyer, 2002). Benefits include:

- Body fat loss
- Improved cardiorespiratory and muscular fitness
- Improved bone health
- Enhanced mood

The timing of return to exercise following delivery should be at the discretion of the client's primary care physician, but suggestions include a range of 24 hours to 8 weeks (Larson-Meyer,

Valsalva maneuver

Movement in which a person tries to exhale forcibly with a closed glottis (windpipe) so that no air exits through the mouth or nose as, for example, in lifting a heavy weight. The Valsalva maneuver impedes the return of venous blood to the heart.

Mode	Low impact movements that avoid jarring motions such a treadmill walking, stationary cycling, and water activity
Frequency	5–7 days per week of cardiorespiratory activities
Intensity	Light to moderate intensity, 13–14 on the Borg scale
Duration	20–30 minutes of cardiorespiratory activity
Flexibility	Self-myofascial release, static stretching, and active stretching
Resistance Training	• Frequency: 1–3 days per week • Sets: 1–3 sets per exercise • Repetitions: 12–20 per set • Intensity: Less than 70% of 1RM through the first and second trimesters • Rest interval: At least 2 minutes to ensure ample recovery and reduction in heart rate and blood pressure • Levels 1 and 2 of the OPT model advised • Only Level 1 after the first trimester
Special Considerations	Avoid exercises in a prone or supine position after 12 weeks of pregnancy. Avoid SMR on varicose veins and areas of swelling. Reactive training is not advised in the second and third trimesters.

FIGURE 14.18 Basic exercise guidelines for pregnancy training.

2002). Once cleared for exercise by the physician, the goal of the initial training period following delivery should be a gradual progression through 3–6 days per week of low-intensity aerobic exercise for 25–60 minutes (Larson-Meyer, 2002). Low-intensity resistance training can be added to focus on core and total-body muscular endurance, within the following guidelines:

- Frequency: 2–3 days per week
- Volume: 1–3 sets per exercise (no more than 8–10 exercises per session)
- Repetitions: 10–15 per set
- Intensity: Less than 50% of 1RM

Figure 14.18 shows basic exercise guidelines for pregnancy training.

Bodyweight exercises, combined with exercises performed while holding the baby, can be excellent choices to produce improvements in muscular fitness, stability, and muscle coordination immediately following pregnancy. A sample Phase 1 program for pregnant clients is provided in Figure 14.19.

Obesity

Obesity is a rising concern among youth and adults in the United States. The various health issues that accompany excess body fat can be reversed with exercise and physical activity (Balsalobre-Fernandez & Tejero-Gonzalez, 2015; Strasser, Siebert, & Schobersberger, 2010). However, individuals who are overweight or obese may face unique challenges when beginning and sustaining long-term exercise. Fitness professionals can have a profound impact on the health and fitness of clients facing these challenges by designing and implementing effective exercise strategies and motivating them toward an active and healthy lifestyle.

Overweight and obese clients may require a few alterations to general exercise programming, especially those suffering from medical conditions that often coexist with overweight and obesity, including hypertension, hyperlipidemia, type 2 diabetes, and osteoarthritis (Balsalobre-Fernandez & Tejero-Gonzalez, 2015; Barnes, Elder, & Pujol, 2004; Strasser et al., 2010;

WORKOUT				
Exercise	**Sets by Rep**	**Tempo**	**Rest**	**Coaching Tip**
SL DB deadlift to overhead press	1 × 20	4/2/1	0 s	65%
Push-ups	1 × 20	4/2/1	0 s	65%
SL cable row	1 × 20	4/2/1	0 s	65%
SL scaption	1 × 20	4/2/1	0 s	65%
SL DB biceps curls	1 × 20	4/2/1	0 s	65%
SL triceps pushdowns	1 × 20	4/2/1	0 s	65%
Transverse plane lunge	1 × 20	4/2/1	60 s	65%

Notes and Observations:
First Trimester. Focus on building balance for late stages of pregnancy. Focus on technique and continue breathing (no Valsalva maneuver).

FIGURE 14.19 Sample pregnancy Phase 1 program.

Vincent, Raiser, & Vincent, 2012). As with all special populations, fitness professionals should consult with the client's primary care physician to ensure that exercise does not exacerbate other medical conditions. Clients should be monitored closely and exercise stopped or altered, as needed.

Obesity-related physical limitations may restrict individuals from participation in certain activities and excess body weight may contribute to chronic or activity-induced musculoskeletal pain, especially in the low back and lower body. Exercise programs should be designed to avoid adding excessive amounts of stress. The lack of physical activity due to pain is one of the primary factors leading to decreased muscular fitness and weight gain. Therefore, the fitness professional must employ various methods to alter exercise routines in an effort to find strategies that will promote activity and fitness without aggravating muscle and joint problems that may already exist. The use of resistance machines in a seated position and aerobic exercise in water are two examples of training strategies that can reduce muscle and joint impact. Fitness professionals should keep in mind that pain is a psychosocial factor that may result in avoidance of exercise in obese individuals, and methods to avoid or minimize pain during and following exercise should be implemented (Lamb et al., 2000).

Aerobic exercise is an important component of exercise programs for obese clients because it can contribute to decreased risk of cardiorespiratory disease and increase caloric expenditure (Ismail et al., 2012). Weight-bearing cardiorespiratory exercise may cause soreness and pain in the lower body, decreasing adherence to an exercise plan. Low-impact forms of cardiorespiratory exercise such as cycling, water aerobics, and swimming are a great option for many obese clients. For activities such as walking or jogging, footwear with ample cushioning and support is important to prevent overuse injuries. Aerobic training programs for this population should adhere to the following parameters to ensure safety and effectiveness (Ismail, Keating, Baker, & Johnson, 2012):

- Frequency: At least 5 days per week
- Intensity: 40–80% of maximum heart rate
- Duration: 20–60 minutes per session

Resistance training serves as a valuable training method to improve function, increase metabolic rate, and prevent musculoskeletal injuries. The following training parameters have

Mode	Low-impact activities such as treadmill walking, rowing, stationary cycling, and water activity
Frequency	5–7 days per week of cardiorespiratory activities
Intensity	60–80% of maximum heart rate; if needed the ranges for training can be adjusted to 40–70% maximal heart rate
Duration	40–60 minute per day or 20–30 minute sessions twice each day of cardiorespiratory training
Flexibility	Self-myofascial release if the client can tolerate it
Resistance Training	• Frequency: 1–3 days per week • Sets: 1–4 sets per exercise • Repetitions: 8–15 per set • Intensity: 40–80% of 1RM • Circuit style training advised if the client can tolerate it
Special Considerations	Make sure the client is comfortable. Always be aware of positions and locations in the facility your client is in. Exercise should be performed in a standing or seated position when possible. The client may have other chronic diseases. In these cases a medical release should be obtained from the individual's physician.

FIGURE 14.20 Basic exercise guidelines for obesity training.

been shown to be safe and effective for obese clients (Alexander, 2002; Balsalobre-Fernandez & Tejero-Gonzalez, 2015; Barnes et al., 2004; Strasser et al., 2010; Vincent et al., 2012):

- Frequency: 1–3 days per week
- Volume: 1–4 sets per exercise
- Repetitions: 8–15 per set
- Intensity: 40–80% of 1RM

Figure 14.20 shows basic exercise guidelines for obesity training.

The goal of exercise with obese clients is to improve physical function in order to support an active lifestyle. Exercise should not introduce significant risk of injury or excessive physical stress, especially at the onset of a training program, and the workout regimen should be sustainable over a long period of time. Overly aggressive, excessively demanding exercise regimens increase the likelihood of injury or the cessation of exercise due to pain. A well-designed, gradually progressive plan will foster improved fitness, decreased body fat, and long-term well-being. A sample Phase 2 program for an obese client is displayed in **Figure 14.21**.

High Blood Pressure

Exercise is now an acceptable and recommended strategy for preventing and reducing high blood pressure (Cornelissen & Fagard, 2005; Fagard, 2001; Kelley & Kelley, 2000; Li et al., 2015; Wallace, 2003; Whelton, Chin, Xin, & He, 2002). Exercise mode, intensity, and volume are important to ensure a positive impact while avoiding possible contraindications. With proper guidance and monitoring by the fitness professional, clients with or at risk for hypertension can achieve positive improvements in health with a reduction in heart disease risk.

Cardiorespiratory exercise should be the primary mode of activity to reduce blood pressure and risk of hypertension. Cardio requires the body to provide necessary oxygen to working muscles through an increase in stroke volume and heart rate (Vy-Van, Mitiku, Sungar, Myers, & Froelicher, 2008). This results in an increase in mean arterial pressure of about 40%. Among

WORKOUT				
Exercise	Sets by Rep	Tempo	Rest	Coaching Tip
DB chest press	1 × 8	2/0/2	0 s	70%
SL MB chest pass	1 × 8	4/2/1	0 s	70%
Seated lat pull down	1 × 8	2/0/2	0 s	70%
SL cable row	1 × 8	4/2/1	0 s	70%
Leg press	1 × 8	2/0/2	0 s	70%
Lateral lunge	1 × 8	4/2/1	60 s	70%

Notes and Observations:
Work in circuit fashion for maximal energy expenditure. First week, ensure that client can perform the exercises correctly and at the acute variables selected.

FIGURE 14.21 Sample Phase 2 obesity program.

healthy adults, this increase is of little danger; however, among those with chronic high blood pressure, caution is warranted to avoid excessive increases above the already elevated arterial pressure. A post-exercise drop in blood pressure (~5–8 mm Hg) for 6–11 hours following a single bout of aerobic activity has been reported (Pescatello, Fargo, Leach, & Scherzer, 1991; Wallace, Bogle, King, Krasnoff, & Jastremski, 1999). Average reductions in blood pressure of 11 mm Hg systolic, 8 mm Hg diastolic have been reported over time with consistent exercise (Hagberg, Park, & Brown, 2000).

The optimal prescription of aerobic exercise has been a topic of much research (Wallace, 2003). Current evidence suggests the following prescription:

- Frequency: 3–7 days per week
- Duration: 20–60 minutes
- Intensity: 40–85% of HR_{max}

Whereas higher intensities have been shown to provide little or no additional benefit, gradual increases in volume and frequency over time may result in even greater reductions in blood pressure. However, fitness professionals must ensure that the client does not experience excessive exercise-induced increases in blood pressure when progressing to vigorous exercise.

Resistance training was once considered a contraindication for hypertensive patients due to fear of excessive blood pressure during exercise and possible increased arterial stiffness (Li et al., 2015; Wallace, 2003). However, current evidence suggests that resistance training does not exacerbate high blood pressure. It can be used as a supplement to cardiorespiratory exercise to improve functional capacity, and that when intensity is low to moderate, weight training may contribute slightly to reductions in blood pressure and decreased arterial stiffness (Li et al., 2015; Wallace, 2003). Note that high-intensity resistance training is not recommended due to evidence that such intensities are associated with increased arterial stiffness and potentially unsafe increases in blood pressure (Li et al., 2015; McDougall, Tuxen, Moroz, & Sutton, 1985).

A recommended approach to implementing resistance training among those with hypertension begins with the following initial training prescription (Wallace, 2003):

- Volume: 1 set
- Repetitions: 12–15 for the set
- Intensity: 60% of 1RM

Mode	Stationary cycling, treadmill walking, rowers
Frequency	3–7 days per week of cardiorespiratory activities
Intensity	50–85% of maximum heart rate; if needed the ranges for training can be adjusted to 40–70% maximal heart rate
Duration	30–60 minute per day of cardiorespiratory training
Flexibility	Static and active stretching in a standing or seated position
Resistance Training	• Sets: 1 set • Repetitions: 12–15 for the set • Intensity: 60% of 1RM • Tempo should not exceed 1 second for isometric and concentric portions (4/1/1, 4/2/1) • Use circuit or PHA weight training as an option, with appropriate rest intervals
Special Considerations	Avoid heavy lifting and Valsalva maneuvers—make sure the client breathes normally. Do not let the client overgrip the weights or clench their fists when training. Modify tempo to avoid extended isometric and concentric muscle action. Perform exercises in a standing or seated position. Allow clients to stand up slowly to avoid possible dizziness.

FIGURE 14.22 Basic exercise guidelines for hypertension training.

WORKOUT				
Exercise	Sets by Rep	Tempo	Rest	Coaching Tip
DB Step-up to Balance to Overhead Press	1 × 15	4/2/1	0 s	50%
Push-up on bench	1 × 15	4/2/1	0 s	50%
Standing cable row	1 × 15	4/2/1	0 s	50%
Standing DB overhead press	1 × 15	4/2/1	0 s	50%
Standing alternating DB biceps curl	1 × 15	4/2/1	0 s	50%
Standing cable triceps press down	1 × 15	4/2/1	0 s	50%
Lateral lunge	1 × 15	4/2/1	0 s	50%

Notes and Observations:
Client has small proprioceptive threshold. Have standing. Needs heavy work on balance training before progressing to SL exercises. Monitor breathing. NO BREATH HOLDING!!

FIGURE14.23 Sample Phase 1 hypertension program.

Both upper and lower body exercises are used to promote total body fitness. These acute variables can be adjusted as the client becomes more accustomed to exercise. **Figure 14.22** shows basic exercise guidelines for hypertension training.

A sample Phase 1 program for a hypertensive client can be reviewed in **Figure 14.23**.

Cardiorespiratory Disease

Coronary heart disease, congestive heart failure, atherosclerosis, and peripheral arterial disease are conditions that impair physical function and increase risk of mortality. Exercise, in the proper doses, can improve cardiorespiratory and muscular fitness, decrease morbidity and mortality, positively influence risk factors such as obesity and hypertension, and enhance overall quality of life (LaFontaine, 2003; Parmenter, Dieberg, & Smart, 2015; Roitman & LaFontaine, 2006; Tran, 2005). Despite the benefits of exercise among these clients, fitness professionals must ensure safety and take all necessary steps to avoid adverse events. Due to the risks and potential danger, those suffering from any of these medical conditions should work with healthcare providers in a medical setting with proper supervision for 6 months following diagnosis or a cardiac episode. Cardiac rehabilitation is a specialized process that should be overseen by highly trained medical personnel. Upon completion of a rehabilitation program, and with medical clearance, fitness professionals may be of valuable service in helping individuals improve health and fitness through a post-rehabilitation exercise plan.

Light to moderately intense aerobic exercise can provide an appropriate level of stress to the cardiorespiratory system, resulting in improved function (Roitman & LaFontaine, 2006). Recommended safe and effective parameters for this population are as follows:

- Frequency: 5–7 days per week
- Duration: 20–45 minutes

Even short bouts a few minutes in duration spread throughout the day can have a positive impact. In some cases (specifically in cases of chronic heart failure), exercise tolerance and fatigue may be limiting, thus gradual progression based on tolerance is recommended.

Resistance training can complement aerobic exercise, because improved muscular fitness contributes to the ability to perform and eventually to sustain aerobic exercise. Studies among patients with heart disease have found that the following guidelines ensure safety and effectiveness with low-to moderate-intensity resistance training (Roitman & LaFontaine, 2006):

- Frequency: 2–3 days per week
- Volume: 2–3 sets
- Intensity: 40–80% of 1RM

Figure 14.24 shows basic exercise guidelines for respiratory disease training.

Several important safety considerations should be considered when monitoring clients with heart disease during exercise. A client who exhibits **dyspnea** (i.e., difficulty or troubled breathing)

Dyspnea
Difficulty or troubled breathing.

Mode	Stationary cycling, treadmill walking, steppers, and elliptical trainers
Frequency	3–5 days per week of cardiorespiratory activities
Intensity	40–60% of peak work capacity for cardiorespiratory activities
Duration	Work up to 20–45 minutes
Flexibility	Static and active stretching and self-myofascial release
Resistance Training	• Frequency: 2–3 days per week • Sets: 2–3 sets • Repetitions: 8–15 per set • Intensity: 40–80% of 1RM • Level 1 of the OPT model is advised • PHA training system recommended
Special Considerations	Upper body exercises cause increased dyspnea and must be monitored. Allow for sufficient rest between sets.

FIGURE 14.24 Basic exercise guidelines for respiratory disease training.

WORKOUT				
Exercise	Sets by Rep	Tempo	Rest	Coaching Tip
DB Step-up to Balance to Overhead Press	1 × 15	4/2/1	30 s	50%
MB Push-up	1 × 15	4/2/1	30 s	50%
SL DB bent row	1 × 15	4/2/1	30 s	50%
SL alternating DB overhead press	1 × 15	4/2/1	30 s	50%
SL DB biceps curl on Foam Pad	1 × 15	4/2/1	30 s	50%
SL cable triceps press down on Foam Pad	1 × 15	4/2/1	30 s	50%
Suspension trainer suspended lunge	1 × 15	4/2/1	30 s	50%

Notes and Observations:
Strong balance skills. Need to push the proprioceptively enriched environment. Needs a bit of recovery time to catch breath. NO BREATH HOLDING!!

FIGURE 14.25 Sample Phase 1 cardiorespiratory program.

Heart palpitations

Heart flutters or rapid beating of the heart.

during exercise should take longer rest breaks and train with reduced loads. Monitoring heart rate and blood pressure consistently throughout training sessions will provide valuable information and enable reductions in training volume or intensity if increases are excessive. Exercise must be ceased immediately if chest pain, nausea, dizziness, or **heart palpitations** result. The fitness professional should evaluate exercise tolerance and responses to training and progress gradually to ensure safety and effectiveness. **Figure 14.25** shows a sample Phase 1 program for a client who has cardiorespiratory disease.

Stroke

Stroke often leads to a sedentary lifestyle, physical inactivity, low fitness levels, and post-stroke functional limitations (Brogardh & Lexell, 2012). Muscle weakness after stroke has an impact on the ability to perform daily activities and restricts participation in society (Brogardh & Lexell, 2012; Morris, Dodd, & Morris, 2004). Post-stroke rehabilitation, lasting 6–12 months, should be completed in a medically based rehabilitation program supervised by a physician (LaFontaine, 2001). After rehabilitation, stroke survivors can see further fitness gains and functional improvements if exercise therapy is reinstituted (Tangemann, Banaitis, & Williams, 1990). Fitness professionals can assist during this period by prescribing appropriate exercise regimens designed to improve aerobic fitness, motor function, strength, and endurance (Ammann, Knols, Baschung, Bie, & Bruin, 2014; Dean, Richards, & Malouin, 2000; Weiss, Sazuki, Bean, & Fielding, 2000).

The American Heart Association recommends the following training guidelines for exercise and strength training after stroke (Gordon et al., 2004):

- ◆ Aerobic exercise
  - Frequency: 3–7 days per week
  - Mode: Large muscle group activities
  - Intensity: 50–80% of maximum heart rate
  - Duration: 20–60 minutes per session
- ◆ Resistance training
  - Frequency: 2–3 days per week

Mode	Stationary cycling, treadmill walking with support bars, recumbent cycling
Frequency	3–7 days per week of cardiorespiratory activities
Intensity	50–80% of maximum heart rate for cardiorespiratory activities
Duration	20–60 minutes per session for cardiorespiratory activities
Flexibility	Static and active stretching and self-myofascial release
Resistance Training	• Frequency: 2–3 days per week • Sets: 1–3 sets • Repetitions: 10–15 • Intensity: 40–80% of 1RM • Level 1 of the OPT model is advised • PHA training system recommended
Special Considerations	Be sure that the client can balance OK for the appropriate exercise. Standing or seated exercises are advised. Movement patterns should be progressed before weight.

FIGURE 14.26 Basic exercise guidelines for stroke training.

WORKOUT

Exercise	Sets by Rep	Tempo	Rest	Coaching Tip
DB chair squat to overhead press	1 × 15	4/2/1	60 s	50%
Standing cable chest press	1 × 15	4/2/1	60 s	50%
Standing cable row	1 × 15	4/2/1	60 s	50%
Standing scaption	1 × 15	4/2/1	60 s	50%
Standing tubing Biceps curl	1 × 15	4/2/1	60 s	50%
Standing tubing triceps press down	1 × 15	4/2/1	60 s	50%
Supported squat	1 × 15	4/2/1	60 s	50%

Notes and Observations:
Recently cleared for activity. Minimal balance. Provide support when possible. Longer rest periods. Maintain normal breathing pattern. NO BREATH HOLDING!!

FIGURE 14.27 Sample Phase 1 stroke program.

• Mode: Weight machines, circuit training, free weights, isometrics
• Volume: 1–3 sets of 10–15 repetitions

Figure 14.26 shows basic exercise guidelines for stroke training.

There is currently no evidence that strength training increases **spasticity** or reduces range of motion among post-stroke patients (Morris et al., 2004). Few negative effects of strength training have been reported in the literature; the most common complaint is minor joint pain (Morris et al., 2004). However, continuous monitoring and regular check-ups with the primary care physician are appropriate to ensure proper exercise progressions. Due to the decrease in physical function and motor skills that often accompany stroke, fitness professionals must ensure that proper exercise technique is possible and adhered to throughout training. The use of resistance exercise machines, at light loads, may be the appropriate initial modality to provide stability while improved balance and coordination are achieved. A sample Phase 1 program for a client recovering from a stroke can be reviewed in **Figure 14.27**.

Spasticity
An increase in muscle tone or stiffness that impairs movement.

Cancer

Cancer-related fatigue commonly interferes with normal functioning and contributes to muscle wasting, declines in aerobic fitness, negative changes in body composition, and depression (Dimeo, 2001; Strasser, Steindorf, Wiskemann, & Ulrich, 2013). Research has shown that aerobic exercise and resistance training may counteract many of the side effects of cancer treatments (Cramp, James, & Lambert, 2010; Hayes, Spence, Galvao, & Newton, 2009; Lonbro, 2014; Meneses-Echavez, Gonzalez-Jimenez, & Ramirez-Velez, 2015; Puetz & Herring, 2012; Singh Paramanandam, & Roberts, 2014; Strasser et al., 2013). A review of a large number of exercise intervention studies among cancer patients determined that exercise during and/or following treatments prevents decline or improves cardiorespiratory function; improves body composition; enhances immune function; increases strength and flexibility; improves body image and mood; and reduces the number and severity of side effects including nausea, fatigue, and pain (Hayes et al., 2009).

The majority of cancer-related exercise research has been conducted with women with breast cancer, although many different types of cancer in both men and women have been studied. It appears that exercise can bring about positive effects while not presenting harm to the patient or cancer survivor (Singh Paramanandam & Roberts, 2014). Individual responses to cancer treatments, as well as to exercise, requires flexibility in exercise programming. The fitness professional should keep extensive records regarding exercise intensity and volume, along with information detailing changes in symptoms or side effects throughout training. This enables the fitness professional, along with the primary care physician or treatment team, to make adjustments in training to minimize any negative effects (Hayes et al., 2009). Additionally, exercise should be avoided during periods of increased infection, **ataxia**, dizziness, or during wound recovery from surgery (Hayes et al., 2009). **Figure 14.28** displays a sample Phase 1 program for a client with cancer.

Aerobic exercise is important to maintain or improve cardiorespiratory health and fitness both during and after cancer treatment. The recommendations that have been shown to achieve a positive outcome in these individuals are as follows (Hayes et al., 2009):

◆ Frequency: 1–5 days per week
◆ Duration: 20–30 minutes
◆ Intensity: 60–80% of $\dot{V}O_{2max}$

Ataxia
The loss of control of body movements.

WORKOUT				
Exercise	Sets by Rep	Tempo	Rest	Coaching Tip
Lateral DB step-up to balance	1 × 15	4/2/1	60 s	60%
Standing SL cable chest press	1 × 15	4/2/1	60 s	60%
SL DB bent over row	1 × 15	4/2/1	60 s	60%
Standing tubing ITAs	1 × 15	4/2/1	60 s	60%
SL DB Biceps curl	1 × 15	4/2/1	60 s	60%
SL DB overhead triceps press	1 × 15	4/2/1	60 s	60%
Transverse plane lunge	1 × 15	4/2/1	60 s	60%

Notes and Observations:
Previously very active. Recently cleared for activity after completing chemo treatments. Dr. notes state focus of exercise should be on building movement patterns and developing muscular stabilization. Client has shown good level of balance. Longer rest periods to adjust for reduced endurance.

FIGURE 14.28 Sample Phase 1 cancer program.

Mode	Treadmill walking, stationary cycling, rowers
Frequency	1–5 days per week of cardiorespiratory activities
Intensity	60–80% of maximum heart rate for cardiorespiratory activities
Duration	20–30 minutes per session for cardiorespiratory activities
Flexibility	Static and active stretching and self-myofascial release
Resistance Training	• Frequency: 1–3 days per week • Volume: 1–4 sets • Repetitions: 6–10 exercises per session • Intensity: 50–80% of 1RM • Levels 1 and 2 of the OPT model • PHA or circuit training system recommended
Special Considerations	Avoid heavy lifting in initial stages of training. Allow for adequate rest intervals and progress the client slowly. Only use SMR if tolerated by the client. Avoid SMR for clients undergoing chemotherapy or radiation treatments. There may be a need to start with only 5 minutes of exercise and progressively increase, depending on the severity of conditions and fatigue.

FIGURE 14.29 Basic exercise guidelines for cancer training.

Gradual progression to avoid excessive fatigue is warranted. Resistance training can also be added to promote improvements in muscular fitness and prevent atrophy (Hayes et al., 2009; Lonbro, 2013; Strasser et al., 2013). Prescription recommendations for resistance training are as follows:

◆ Frequency: 1–3 days per week
◆ Volume: 1–4 sets (6–10 exercises per session)
◆ Intensity: 50–80% of 1RM

Figure 14.29 shows basic exercise guidelines for cancer training.

Many resistance training programs simply involve progressive resistance, where the load is the only variable altered over time. When the exerciser can perform more repetitions with the same weight, the weight is increased. It is expected that cancer patients, similar to healthy populations, will experience even greater gains in fitness with periodized training. Although exercise has not been shown to exacerbate cancer-related fatigue, and may even decrease this fatigue, fitness professionals should monitor exercise tolerance and avoid applying excessive stress through the exercise program. This will ensure proper balance of stress and optimal benefits from the exercise regimen.

Osteoporosis

Osteoporosis is a skeletal condition of decreased bone mass, which increases the risk of fracture (Wilhelm et al., 2012). Exercise has been shown to aid in the prevention of bone mass loss and has been found to increase bone mineral density (Petranick & Berg, 1997; Zhao, Zhao, & Xu, 2015). For those suffering from osteoporosis, exercise can be a valuable tool for improving physical function, decreasing risk of fall and fracture, and improving quality of life (Wilhelm et al., 2012). With proper guidance, those at risk for or suffering from osteoporosis can safely participate in an exercise regimen and gain these valuable benefits. Medical experts now strongly recommend that people with, or at risk for, osteoporosis engage in multicomponent exercise, including resistance and balance training (Giangregorio et al., 2014).

The greatest exercise risk for those suffering from osteoporosis is bone fracture, either caused by excessive training loads or falls during exercise sessions. Both are rare; however, fitness professionals should do all they can to help prevent a fracture from occurring. The exercise environment must be clean and free of clutter or objects that might increase risk of falls, and exercise in wet conditions is not recommended due to the risk of slipping (Giangregorio et al., 2014). Training progressions should be gradual, with focus on quality of exercise, rather than on quantity or intensity. Over time, bone strength will increase and the risk of adverse events will diminish, allowing for progression in training to achieve greater results. Muscle soreness and joint pain are also reported among those suffering from osteoporosis (Giangregorio et al., 2014). Exercises should be performed in a slow, controlled fashion, and movements between exercises should allow sufficient time to avoid rushing. Twisting motions should be done very slowly (if at all) to avoid excessive skeletal stress.

Resistance training should include gradual progression at a tolerance tailored to the individual, while targeting all major muscle groups. The following prescription has been shown to result in positive improvements in health and fitness among this population (Petranick & Berg, 1997; Wilhelm et al., 2012; Zhao et al., 2015):

- Frequency: 2–4 days per week
- Volume: 1–6 sets per exercise
- Repetitions: 5–25 per set
- Intensity: 40–70% of 1RM

Figure 14.30 shows basic exercise guidelines for older adult training.

Resistance machines may be difficult for some individuals to use safely depending on whether they can be adjusted to the specific to the size of the individual. Other modalities may be preferred as long as correct exercise technique can be sustained at all times. With any modality, slow and controlled movements are recommended.

Balance training, in addition to resistance exercise, may provide additional health and fitness benefits; with several sessions of balance exercises, beginning with static exercises and

Mode	Treadmill with hand rail support
Frequency	2–5 days per week of cardiorespiratory activities
Intensity	50–90% of maximum heart rate for cardiorespiratory activities
Duration	20–60 minutes per session for cardiorespiratory activities or 8–10 minute bouts
Flexibility	Static and active stretching
Resistance Training	• Frequency: 2–4 days per week • Sets: 1–6 sets per exercise • Repetitions: 5–25 per set • Intensity: 40–70% of 1RM
Special Considerations	Progression should be slow, well monitored, and based on postural control. Exercises should be progressed if possible toward free sitting or standing. Focus the exercises on the hips, thighs, back, and arms. Avoid excessive spinal loading on squat and leg press exercises. Make sure the client is breathing in a normal manner and avoid holding the breath as in a Valasalva maneuver.

FIGURE 14.30 Basic exercise guidelines for older adults training.

WORKOUT				
Exercise	Sets by Rep	Tempo	Rest	Coaching Tip
DB overhead Press	2 × 12	2/0/2	0 s	70%
SL DB scaption	2 × 12	4/2/1	15 s	70%
Machine row	2 × 12	2/0/2	0 s	70%
SL DB bent row	2 × 12	4/2/1	15 s	70%
DB squat	2 × 12	2/0/2	0 s	70%
SL squat	2 × 12	4/2/1	15 s	70%

Notes and Observations:
Working on development of bone mass while increasing endurance. Dr. cleared client for balance training. Noted that it is important to keep area clear to prevent falls.

FIGURE 14.31 Sample Phase 2 for older adults program.

gradually progressing to dynamic movements, being shown to help improve function and decrease the risk of falls (Giangregorio et al., 2014). Weight-bearing aerobic exercise such as walking can contribute to the maintenance of bone mineral density, as well as contribute to improved health outcomes such as decreased risk of heart disease. Resistance and balance training may lead to increased comfort and sustainable aerobic exercise over time. The fitness professional should monitor exercise tolerance, strength, and stability throughout the training program to ensure proper progression and effectiveness of the training program. A sample Phase 2 program for someone with osteoporosis can be reviewed in **Figure 14.31**.

Programming for Specific Populations

Designing specific workouts for various special populations begins with consulting the training recommendations that have been identified as safe and effective. Individual circumstances may require alterations to those recommendations and the fitness professional must be prepared to adjust daily training plans based on health and exercise preparedness. Health conditions alter exercise readiness on a daily basis; therefore, training plans must be flexible. The fitness professional should be ready to provide alternative exercises and make adjustments to training loads.

Working with Extended Healthcare Providers

The positive health effects of physical activity and exercise have become widely accepted in the medical community. Exercise is now viewed as an important tool for preventing or recovering from many chronic health conditions including cardiorespiratory disease, diabetes, cancer, hypertension, stroke, pulmonary disease, and mental illness (Robroek, Lenthe, Empelen, & Burdoff, 2009; Lakka & Bouchard, 2005; Williams, 2008). With the growing emphasis on the use of exercise to improve health, fitness professionals have a growing number of opportunities to work with **extended healthcare providers**, providing valuable direction to patients in need of individualized exercise programming.

Physicians often recommend increased physical activity and exercise to their patients. With little training and education in this area, physicians are limited in their knowledge and ability to prescribe safe and effective exercise programs, much like fitness professionals are not trained

Extended healthcare providers
Professionals in the healthcare system such as physicians, physical therapists, and cardiac rehabilitation therapists who provide specialized guidance to patients suffering from various physical illnesses or impairments.

in the area of disease diagnosis and treatment. However, fitness professionals can serve a valuable role in exercise program design for patients who have been referred by their primary care physician. To do so safely and effectively, fitness professionals must be aware of issues that can affect exercise risk and understand exercise programming for special populations and create an effective line of communication with the referring physician. Because medications may alter how the body responds to exercise, the fitness professional must ensure that training is altered when necessary. To do so, direction from the physician is necessary. The physician should provide recommendations for contraindicated exercises or limitations to the exercise plan that will reduce the risk of a negative response to exercise participation.

Post rehab

A period of time following general physical therapy before a patient returns to full fitness and function following an injury or surgery.

Post rehab is another healthcare setting where fitness professionals can provide a valuable service. Insurance limitations on physical therapy visits are significantly decreasing the number of treatment sessions that many people can access (Onks & Wawrzyniak, 2014; Sandstrom, Lehmen, Hahn, & Ballard, 2013). This results in individuals who have made significant progress following injury or surgery, but who are not fully prepared to return to full activity. Strategic exercise programs have been shown to lead to improvements in function for 1 year after knee surgery, yet most patients receive only 12–18 physical therapy visits before insurance companies cease coverage (Osteras, 2014). A meta-analysis of 11 studies examining extended exercise rehabilitation after hip fracture concluded that extended exercise programs have a significant impact on various functional abilities (Auais, Eilayyan, & Mayo, 2012).

The fitness professional, in consultation with a client's physical therapist, can provide important direction to ensure safety and effectiveness in returning to full functional capacity. Knowledge of, and experience in, corrective exercise is valuable for fitness professionals desiring to work in the post-rehab environment. Deep understanding of functional movement limitations, corrective strategies, and strategic functional training will enable the fitness professional to design appropriate post-rehab exercise programs.

As with physicians, physical therapists can provide much needed information about a client to ensure proper exercise selection, progression in training volume and intensity, and possible things to avoid. If pain is experienced among a post-rehab client at any time during exercise, the fitness professional should consult with the physical therapist to find alternative approaches to progressing. Post-rehab clients may suffer from poor stability, muscle atrophy, low levels of strength, decreased power, and poor neuromuscular coordination. Thus, the OPT model is a perfect framework for addressing these limitations in a strategic and effective progression.

Cardiac rehabilitation

A specialized medical process that helps individuals suffering from various cardiac conditions to return to full function and fitness.

Cardiac rehabilitation is a four-phase process, separate from the OPT model, that is an important part of the recovery for those who have experienced a heart attack, heart valve repair, artery bypass, angioplasty, or those who suffer from chronic chest pain.

◆ *Phase one*: Cardiac rehabilitation conducted at a medical facility that generally involves 36 outpatient visits over 12 weeks. Includes directly supervised exercise and lifestyle modification education.
◆ *Phase two*: Prescribed by a physician if continued improvement under direct supervision is needed. May last up to another 12 weeks and is also conducted in a cardiac rehabilitation setting.
◆ *Phases three and four*: Self-paced programs that involve exercise direction and motivation to sustain lifestyle changes and healthy behaviors. These phases may be conducted outside of a medical facility but require interaction between the physician and the health promotion team to ensure safety.

Research has shown that completion of a cardiac rehabilitation program is an important part of the recovery process, providing improved long-term control of risk factors associated with future heart disease or complications (Toms, O'Neil, & Gardner, 2003).

Fitness professionals can serve an important role during phases three and four of cardiac rehabilitation, as well as during the post-cardiac-rehab exercise period. Once again, the OPT model represents a valuable tool in that it enables individualized programming and a progressive structure for individuals to regain fitness and improve function. Exercise tolerance, based on individual fitness and cardiorespiratory health, must be monitored by the fitness professional to ensure safety throughout the process. Cardiac recovery generally involves numerous medications, which can influence cardiorespiratory response to exercise and tolerance. The fitness professional must seek the guidance of the cardiac physician to ensure that exercise mode, intensity, volume, and so on do not pose a risk to the patient and will not interfere with prescribed medications. Many cardiac rehab patients will lack the strength and stamina needed to perform even basic activities of daily living, requiring progression through the Stabilization and Strength Levels of the OPT model as they progress back to full fitness and function. Fitness professionals may assist clients in phases three and four of cardiac rehabilitation, but they must rely on cardiac physicians and cardiac rehabilitation specialists to ensure safety throughout those steps. As fitness professionals interact with these various extended healthcare providers, it is important that they remain within the scope of practice and are knowledgeable and current in their professional responsibilities.

Interacting with members of the extended healthcare community is a valuable opportunity to demonstrate the level of thought and planning that goes into the implementation of the OPT model. This model will help the fitness professional gain the confidence and credibility needed to secure more referrals and provide better service to patients in need of quality exercise guidance. Keep in mind that many healthcare providers will only refer their clients to those fitness professionals who have earned their trust in providing exercise guidance to their patients.

Corporate Health, Fitness, and Wellness

Corporate fitness is a well-established niche with promising growth potential (Archer, 2011). With many corporations now recognizing the value and benefits of offering structured health, fitness, and wellness programs, the corporate environment offers many opportunities for fitness professionals who enjoy working with a wide range of clients. Over the past decade, companies have begun to view health and fitness programs as a necessity rather than a luxury, and have elevated their expectations for fitness professionals who they recruit to serve their workforce (Williams, 2008). Fitness professionals can prepare themselves to secure corporate fitness opportunities, and to effectively guide the fitness programs in this environment through the use of the OPT model.

A growing body of research has demonstrated the great value offered by workplace health and fitness programs (Baicker, Cutler, & Song, 2010; Gates, Succop, Brehm, Gillespie, & Sommers, 2008; Kuoppala, Lamminpaa, & Paivi, 2008; Loyle, 2012; Parks & Steelman, 2008; Powell, 1997; Robroek et al., 2009; Rongon, Robroek, Lenthe, & Burdof, 2013; Okada, 1991). In general, this research has demonstrated the following benefits of well-designed corporate fitness and wellness programs:

- Medical cost savings for the company ranging from $2–$4 for every $1 spent on workplace fitness and wellness
- Decreased healthcare usage by fitter employees
- Decreased absenteeism
- Increased work productivity
- Increased job satisfaction

Corporate fitness
Implementation of health and fitness programming by a fitness professional within a company structure.

- Lower job-related injury rates
- Fewer workers' compensation claims

The quality of the fitness program greatly influences the benefits achieved (Rongen et al., 2013). Well-designed fitness programs, focusing on multiple fitness components in a progressive and organized fashion, with increased personal contact and regular encouragement, have higher participation rates and greater influences on positive outcomes. This has led companies to seek out highly qualified and well-organized fitness professionals, who understand the business aspects of worksite health promotion and offer services beyond basic exercise programming. Fitness professionals with NASM credentials, and who use the OPT model, will be well positioned to seek work opportunities with these companies.

The following qualities can increase a fitness professional's marketability and effectiveness in corporate fitness venues:

- Willingness to work with clients from a wide range of fitness and motivation levels
- Ability to modify exercise programming to each individual's needs
- Ability to motivate a variety of individuals toward better health and consistent exercise participation
- Flexibility in programming and implementation based on individual circumstances and the company's needs

The OPT model offers fitness professionals the perfect framework for working in the corporate fitness environment. The individual assessments that guide programming allow the fitness professional to demonstrate individualization, and to track client progress. The structure of the OPT model shows employers and participants that this is a long-term plan for promoting health and wellness, which will help in achieving buy-in. Fitness professionals can demonstrate how assessments and observations of each participant will result in individual modifications, to ensure that each participant starts at the proper level of exertion, and progresses at the appropriate pace over time. Finally, the amount of personal contact involved in this process ensures that each client will have close contact on a weekly basis with a fitness professional. These points of contact enable information sharing but also represent optimal times for motivation and encouragement from the professional.

Implementing the OPT model in the worksite fitness environment requires extensive record keeping and planning on the part of the fitness professional. Information about assessments, needs, fitness goals, limitations, and participation will enable the fitness professional to modify training plans based on individual circumstances. These records also serve as valuable documents to demonstrate progress and establish the effectiveness of the program. Effective fitness professionals in the corporate environment conduct daily planning sessions, including alternative plans and potential modifications to workouts based on equipment availability, attendance rates, and variety in participant needs. Planning will ensure quality implementation of the training plan.

Lifestyle Considerations

Each client presents lifestyle challenges to long-term adherence to an exercise program. Fitness professionals can be a valuable service provider in helping to implement the OPT model in consideration of these lifestyle challenges. Long-term exercise adherence requires a training plan that is flexible and adaptive, based on client's changing schedules, life demands, and time constraints. The OPT model is very adaptive and remains a proven tool for program design for clients in many different professional and personal circumstances.

Many clients may struggle to sustain a consistent workout regimen, and may feel that the inability to workout at the same times and days each week will diminish the value of their exercise routine. The fitness professional should stress the value of regular exercise participation over time, and reassure the client that sticking to a perfect schedule or training routine is not necessary to achieve the fitness improvements and health benefits of exercise. Although long gaps between workouts (e.g., 5–7 days) can hopefully be avoided, progress through the OPT model can be achieved even if workout participation varies from week to week. A common error among fitness professionals and clients, when exercise participation is inconsistent, is to add significant extra work into a training session with the hope of making up for missed training. Professionals should stick to the OPT plan, making slight alterations in workouts to ensure total body training without adding significantly to the volume or intensity of the individual training sessions. Adding volume and intensity to a single workout when participation is sporadic will only increase soreness and fatigue, possibly decreasing a client's motivation to attend workouts.

For clients who struggle to find significant amounts of time during the week for exercise, the fitness professional should prepare short, effective workouts that can be done in less than 30 minutes. These workouts will not involve a great deal of volume because time is very limited. The use of a wide variety of exercises, performed fairly quickly in succession, aids in total body fitness and provides some health benefits.

Business or personal travel is also a challenge for many when attempting to stick to a regular training routine. Fitness professionals can help frequent travelers by suggesting exercises that can be done without equipment in just about any environment. Providing OPT template sheets can provide guidance for traveling clients and help prevent long gaps between training sessions. Movement preparation exercises are often good choices for travelers addressing specific movement issues with minor equipment requirements. Providing exercise guidance for clients while traveling will help increase the likelihood of exercise adherence over time, avoiding the common habit among exercisers of failing to resume a training routine after a long gap between workouts.

Fitness professionals often encounter clients who are considered **weekend warriors**. These clients have busy professional or personal lives during the week but desire to be active, and often very aggressive, in their sport or recreational activities on the weekends. Many may work in sedentary jobs but wish to pursue vigorous activities outside of work. The lengthy amounts of time spent in inactivity followed by aggressive activities appears to be a significant health and injury risk (Lopez, 2014; Psoinos, Emhoff, Sweeney, Tseng, & Santry, 2012; Roberts et al., 2014). Examples of weekend warriors include clients who wish to participate in endurance events such as 10Ks, half-marathons, or relay events, but lack the time to effectively train for them. Others participate in softball leagues or community recreational sports but do little to prepare themselves for the physical demands of athletics. Even those who simply wish to participate in golf, tennis, mountain biking, and other activities for personal enjoyment will benefit from an exercise regimen that promotes functional movement and muscular fitness.

Fitness professionals should consider the activities and hobbies of their clients and mold their training plan to prepare them for these demands. For example, many recreational runners suffer from lower body overuse injuries, which can prevent them from running, or decrease their enjoyment of the activity. A lack of stability in the lower body and trunk increases the risk of these overuse injuries and can be addressed effectively with Phase 1: Stabilization, in the OPT model. Weekend golfers may experience low back pain caused by their lack of preparation for explosive rotational movements. Following the OPT phases will prepare recreational athletes for the demands of the sport and enable them to both participate without pain and increase performance. Even activities of daily living, such as yard work, place significant demands

Weekend warriors
Clients who work busy jobs or live sedentary lifestyles during the week but try to maintain participation in moderate to aggressive weekend recreational activities.

on the body and can result in injury (Psoinos et al., 2012). The increased stability and strength developed through the OPT model will serve as protection from overexertion or injuries from lifting, pushing, or pulling during common weekly chores.

Common Fitness Technologies and Trends

Many technological tools have been developed that fitness professionals can use to track and guide their clients, both inside and out of the gym. Emerging technologies will continue to shape personal training services and extend professionals' reach to more clients in much deeper and more impactful ways. Fitness professionals must consider how fitness apps, activity trackers, and social media can influence their practice and improve the health and fitness of their clients (**Figure 14.32**). They must also be prepared to evolve and adapt as new technologies emerge, perhaps even playing a role in the development of new technologies that will reshape how fitness leadership is implemented.

Smartphone Apps

Fitness professionals can use activity-related smartphone apps in a variety of ways, including providing direction to their clients, monitoring client progress, and tracking and evaluating nutritional habits. Incorporating these apps into a personal training services offers a number of advantages:

- More opportunities to interact with clients outside of the gym
- Increased chances to motivate clients throughout the day
- Assistance in tracking and evaluating clients' nutritional habits
- Ability to provide reminders to clients about healthy habits, at-home training assignments, and appointments

Workout design apps can be used to provide guidance to clients while they are traveling, or through remote personal training, allowing the fitness professional to create workouts that can be accessed through the Internet or smartphones. Exercise order (with visual demonstrations of exercise technique), sets, reps, and even rest periods can be prescribed through an app, allowing clients to complete the workouts on their own while on vacation, traveling for business,

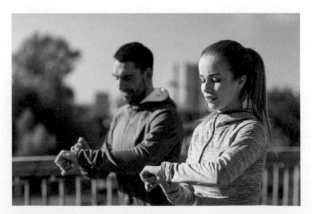

FIGURE 14.32 Tracking fitness with mobile technology.
© Syda Productions/Shutterstock

or away from the gym. Fitness professionals can use these apps to monitor workload, whether the workout is performed in person or remote. These apps are a great way to collect data and can be used to create visual displays of fitness progress and increased workloads, showing the client how the OPT model is changing their prescription over time.

Another valuable feature of fitness apps is their use in providing encouragement and motivation from the fitness professional and surrounding community. By monitoring progress and performance, the fitness professional can pinpoint areas of success to highlight in motivational messages. Needed areas of improvement or points in time where performance falters can be identified, and serve as a cue for a fitness professional to increase the number of motivational messages. The combination of social networking and exercise monitoring allows clients to compare their work and progress to others in their communities, providing motivation through social support and the desire to excel. Fitness professionals can help their clients interpret this comparative data to ensure that it is a positive motivation, rather than a negative indictment of poor fitness or effort. In this case, the role of the fitness professional extends beyond the gym to help clients achieve higher levels of performance and fitness through greater commitment to an active lifestyle.

Nutrition apps can also provide valuable information and assistance to the fitness professional. Nutritional habits throughout the day/week will have a profound impact on the success achieved through exercise, yet it is very difficult to track and evaluate nutrition data. Many fitness professionals do not have training in nutrition evaluation, and clients often struggle to remember to write down all of the foods they eat. A number of apps are available that allow for immediate input of food intake and provide an evaluation of eating habits based on current nutritional recommendations, thus offering valuable assistance in tracking and evaluating nutritional habits. As the professional accesses this information, additional opportunities for motivation and guidance beyond the gym setting arise, facilitating successful adoption and adherence to a healthy and fit lifestyle.

Activity Trackers

A growing segment in the fitness technology field that is very popular and beneficial to fitness professionals and their clients alike is activity trackers. These apps or devices can track movement and provide information regarding physical activity patterns. Although the time spent in the gym with a fitness professional is incredibly valuable for meeting health and fitness goals, physical activity patterns throughout the day can help or hinder a client's progress. By monitoring their clients' physical activity throughout the day, fitness professionals can help guide clients toward greater activity and facilitate faster results.

Some activity trackers allow for the monitoring of heart rate, which can be valuable data for a fitness professional. Lower heart rate during work and rest signifies a more efficient and fit cardiorespiratory system. Over time, resting heart rate should decrease as a client becomes more fit; higher resting heart rates are closely linked to cardiorespiratory disease and all-cause mortality (Donath, Faude, Roth, & Zahner, 2014; Purwanto, Wigati, & Elysana Asnar, 2014; Quan et al., 2013; Saxena et al., 2013). An increase in resting heart rate, or alterations in **heart rate variability**, may signify overtraining or increased life stress (Dressendorfer, Wade, & Scaff, 1985; Jeukendrup & VanDiemen, 1998; Uusitalo, Uusitalo, & Rusko, 1998; Vriz et al., 2015). If a client shows an increase in resting heart rate, the fitness professional should reduce training stress and examine the client's nutrition intake, sleep patterns, and stress management skills. Heart rate recovery following workouts or stressful events during the day can also help the professional identify effective recovery, or suggest improved methods for dealing with stress

Heart rate variability
Variations in the time interval between heartbeats.

or recovering from a workout. Heart rate data can be very useful and enable a higher level of service by the fitness professional.

Some activity trackers are able to track sleep patterns, enabling the fitness professional to evaluate the client's sleep quality and alter training plans as needed. Fitness professionals should explain to their clients how the various apps will be utilized and why their use is beneficial. Clients should understand that nutrition, physical activity, and sleep monitoring will contribute to the adoption of healthy habits as well as enable the professional to observe behaviors that can have a dramatic impact on fitness adaption and exercise readiness. Through prompts and messages, fitness professionals can have a greater impact on these habits and assist their clients in improvements as needed.

Social Media

Social media has changed the way many people interact, both with their social groups and with business services. The ability to use electronic means to connect to others is replacing many other means of social interaction, both personal and professional (Biscontini, 2012). Many different social media outlets exist and more are sure to be developed each year. Fitness professionals should consider the different audiences that each outlet can help them access and utilize each in strategic ways. Social media outlets are a powerful method of inexpensive promotion of personal training services, offering a unique opportunity for a fitness professional to position him or herself as an expert for those seeking guidance in their health and fitness efforts. They also offer opportunities for fitness professionals to connect with their clients outside of the gym in a more personal way and to develop a following of potential clients. Social media is instrumental in helping fitness professionals develop relationships with their clients.

The following are the primary ways that fitness professionals can use social media to further their personal training business:

- ◆ To connect with current and potential clients outside of the gym
- ◆ To establish a position of expertise and leadership
- ◆ To share information about services, events, and training opportunities

Fitness professionals must consider the audience they are seeking and determine what messages each different population might respond to. Fitness professionals who continuously post personal photos to social media sites are suggesting that they are more concerned with their own body and less about their clients'. However, using social media to share and congratulate client successes, through the use of client photos and experiences, is a great way for fitness professionals to document their clients' success, as well as the role the professional has had in helping them reach their goals.

Social media is a useful tool for providing educational messages, updates on developments in exercise science, studies examining different training methods, and reliable information related to exercise and diet fads. These posts demonstrate knowledge of current training practices, show an understanding of the many challenges that clients face, and establish credibility. These messages also establish the fitness professional as a source of information on fitness topics, and aid in the building of confidence among those seeking a professional. Credibility comes from a combination of education and professional experience. Social media can demonstrate both. Sharing photos of a fitness conference attended, a book that was recently read, or a new research article that supports a certain training style can demonstrate knowledge and commitment to continuous education. Equally important are photos and descriptions of workouts performed with clients of different backgrounds and with different needs, highlighting success in a wide range of fitness goals. The combination of educational messages and demonstrations of professional experience and success contributes to the fitness professional's reputation and leads to a larger social network. The following are examples of educational posts that can help the fitness professional gain credibility:

- Short videos discussing exercise techniques for various modalities
- Blog posts discussing recent research articles
- Suggestions for creative ways of overcoming barriers to fitness
- Recommendations of training strategies for specific populations, such as weight loss or older adults
- Examples of training plans for a variety of clients
- Philosophical statements that describe the fitness professional's approach to program design, along with examples of how programs are altered based on individual needs
- A fitness tip of the day

Promoting events and services becomes easier and more effective through social media. Social media is a great way to keep clients updated on upcoming events or changes to training services. Posting notices of changes to schedules is an easy way to keep clients informed. Although fitness events remain a great place to interact with potential clients who may desire some personal interaction before signing up for services, creating fliers and spending hours handing out promotional items at such events has now been largely replaced by more time and cost-efficient social media campaigns, which can reach many people with a single click.

When using social media accounts for business purposes, it is important to avoid unprofessional posts that can diminish one's reputation or credibility. Fitness professionals should avoid potentially polarizing statements that have little connection to their fitness business. Political statements, religious remarks, or opinionated statements about different lifestyles may drive potential clients away from one's social network and should be replaced by professional posts focused on fitness topics. Rather than taking credit for positive outcomes, effective professionals allow clients to post testimonial statements, discussing their experiences and demonstrating how their training plan assisted them in reaching their goals. Excessive posting should be avoided, as it may turn clients off and cause them to disregard all posts. Four to six messages a day is generally appropriate, but fitness professionals should ensure that their clients are not inundated with unnecessary posts. Copyrighted photos or material should not be used without permission, and permission must always be obtained from clients before posting photos that include them or that identify them by name.

Emerging Technologies

Fitness professionals must understand how current technologies can enhance their current services, but they also need to look to the future in order to anticipate how emerging technologies might change the industry. Determining what fitness trends are simply fads and what technologies will develop and thrive is helpful in planning ahead in the fitness industry. Unfortunately, it is difficult to really know what consumers will gravitate towards in coming years. However, there is no doubt that fitness technology will continue to influence exercisers in the future, and fitness professionals must consider their role in assisting clients in their use of fitness technology.

Wearable technology appears to be an area that will continue to see the greatest interest and development in fitness technology (Suciu, 2013; Vogel, 2015). Devices that can be synched to smartphones to track and display exercise habits in real time will be an area of rapid growth,

---

TRAINER TIPS　⊲▯—▯⊳

Posting new ideas or innovative strategies to training demonstrates creativity and ingenuity. This helps clients differentiate fitness professionals. Sharing a post about a new exercise that was included in a workout with positive results or showing a video of how an exercise was altered for a client provides opportunities for clients to see passion and excitement from the fitness professional and may increase their commitment.

Wearable technology
Devices that are worn during exercise and collect/transmit information regarding performance and physiological variables relating to the workout.

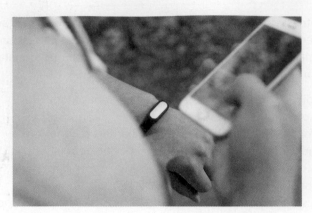

FIGURE 14.33 Wearable fitness tracker.
© Rasstock/Shutterstock

as will the development of new apps and devices that will monitor a larger number of physiological variables (**Figure 14.33**). The development of fitness apps is projected to continue, especially now that app developers are becoming more accessible to fitness professionals.

As these devices become more advanced and potentially more accessible, fitness professionals should consider their business goals and their target demographic. They should also identify any technology constraints that they, or their clients, might have (Kuan, 2015). Younger, more affluent populations are often early adopters of fitness technology; whereas lower-income, older adults may be less likely to embrace it. Online training or remote personal training may be a venue where greater reliance on emerging technologies can enhance personal training services. In the end, financial constraints may limit how many clients will have access to these technologies. However, fitness professionals should remain current in their awareness of fitness technology and consider its impact on this evolving industry.

Conclusion

Trends and technologies have given fitness professionals additional tools to connect and work with their clients, allowing for valuable data gathering and personal connection. When combined with an understanding of the various modalities appropriate for different levels of the OPT model, as well as considerations for groups and various special populations, the fitness professional can begin to review instructing and cueing techniques to produce results in his or her clientele.

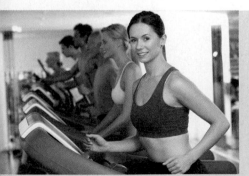
© Monkey Business Images/Shutterstock

Case in Review

Think back to your five clients who had approached you with the goal of losing weight together. It is apparent that they use each other for both motivation and support. Because they can only meet offsite and during times that are not conducive to space and time availability at the gym, you think of alternatives to ensure you are meeting the individual needs of all five clients. You have addressed the following considerations to ensure your clients' workouts are just as effective as if they were in the gym with you.

Modalities

Mobile equipment may be important for this group because accommodations at the gym may not be available. Body weight exercises, suspension trainers, medicine balls, kettlebells, jump ropes, battling ropes, ladders, cones, and other equipment that can be easily moved will be the core of the program design for this group. Accordingly, exercises should be selected that can easily be modified with different modalities for the benefit of each client. The exercises will also need to be selected in a manner so that clients in different phases of the OPT model can accomplish the same thing (e.g., a dumbbell chest press for a stable strength exercise for one client can be an unstable push-up for another client). This group is going to require creativity and planning to ensure that exercise modifications for each client are fully planned before the workout begins.

Individual vs. Group Personal Training

With group personal training, clients benefit from the companionship of working out together and paying a lower individual rate. The fitness professional is, in turn, able to maximize pay with several clients at once, as well as gain a broader reach through word-of-mouth recommendations. If the trainer plans appropriately for each client, the sessions can meet each client's needs by modifying exercises or changing acute variables on an individual basis. Some of the participants may need more one-on-one attention than others, and this may require a private discussion about the need for supplemental one-on-one training sessions.

Programming Challenges

Similar to a one-on-one client, group clients will require the same kind of background understanding from the trainer to ensure that the designed program is going to best meet their needs. In the group setting, all of your clients may be looking for core stability but some of the clients may require a modification or a more advanced exercise. For example, consider the following with regards to the utilization of the prone iso-abs exercise:

- Client with no issues: Prone iso-abs

- Client who can hold position well for the given length of time: Prone iso-abs with one leg elevated

- Client who does not have the stability to hold the position: Prone iso-abs with hands on bench

- Client who cannot hold the position with hands on bench: Quadruped with drawing-in maneuver

References

Abernathy, L., & Bleakley, C. (2007). Strategies to prevent injury in adolescent sport: A systematic review. *Sports Medicine, 41,* 627–639.

Alexander, J. L. (2002). The role of resistance exercise in weight loss. *Strength Conditioning Journal, 24,* 65–69.

Ammann, B. C., Knols, R. H., Baschung, P., Bie, R. A., & Bruin, E. D. (2014). Application of principles of exercise training in sub-acute and chronic stroke survivors: A systematic review. *BMC Neurology, 14,* 167.

Archer, S. (2011). How to become a corporate fitness professional. Available at: http://www.ideafit.com/fitness-expert/shirley-archer.

Auais, M. A., Eilayyan, O., & Mayo, N. E. (2012). Extended exercise rehabilitation after hip fracture improves patients' physical function: A systematic review and meta-analysis. *Physical Therapy, 92,* 1437–1451.

Baechle, T. R., & Westcott, W. (2010). *Fitness professional's guide to strength training older adults* (2nd ed.). Champaign, IL: Human Kinetics.

Baicker, K., Cutler, D., & Song, Z. (2010). Workplace programs can generate savings. *Health Affairs, 29,* 1–8.

Balsalobre-Fernandez, C., & Tejero-Gonzalez, C. M. (2015). Effects of resistance training on the body fat in obese people. *Revista Internacional de Medicina y Ciencias de la Actividad Fisica y el Deporte, 15,* 371–386.

Barbieri, D., & Zaccagni, L. (2013). Strength training for children and adolescents: Benefits and risks. *Collegium Antropologicum, 37*(2), 219–225.

Barnes, J. T., Elder, C. L., & Pujol, T. J. (2004). Overweight and obese adults: Exercise intervention. *Strength and Conditioning Journal, 26,* 31–33.

Barnett, A., Smith, B., Lord, S. R, Williams, M., & Baumand, A. (2003). Community-based group exercise improves balance and reduces falls in at-risk older people: A randomized controlled trial. *Age and Aging, 32*(4), 407–414.

Beach, T. A., Howarth, S. J., & Callaghan, J. P. (2008). Muscular contributions to low-back loading and stiffness during standard and suspended push-ups. *Human Movement Science, 27,* 457–472.

Beardsley, C., & Contreras, B. (2014). The role of kettlebells in strength and conditioning: A review of the literature. *Strength and Conditioning Journal, 36*(3), 64–70.

Behringer, M., Vom Heede, A., Yue, Z., & Mester, J. (2010). Effects of resistance training in children and adolescents: A meta-analysis. *Pediatrics,* 126, 1199–1210.

Biscontini, L. (2012). The encyclopedia of social media. *American Fitness,* May/June, 12–14.

Brogardh, C., & Lexell, J. (2012). Effects of cardiorespiratory fitness and muscle-resistance training after stroke. *Physical Medicine and Rehabilitation, 4,* 901–907.

Bunker, D. J., Rhea, M. R., Simons, T., & Marin, P. J. (2011). The use of whole-body vibration as a golf warm-up. *Journal of Strength and Conditioning Research, 25,* 293–297.

Buranarugsa, R., Oliveira, J., & Maia, J. (2012). Strength training in youth. An evidence-based review. *Revista Portuguesa de Ciencias do Desport, 12,* 87–116.

Cadore, E. L., Pinto, R. S., Bottaro, M., & Izquierdo, M. (2014). Strength and endurance training prescription in health and frail elderly. *Aging and Disease, 5,* 183–195.

Cornelissen, V. A., & Fagard, R. A. (2005). Effect of resistance training on resting blood pressure: A meta-analysis of randomized controlled trials. *Journal of Hypertension, 23,* 251–259.

Cramp, F., & James, A., & Lambert, J. (2010). The effects of resistance training on quality of life in cancer: A systematic literature review and meta-analysis. *Supportive Care in Cancer, 18,* 1367–1376.

Daneshjoo, A., Mokhtar, A. H., Rahnama, N., & Yusof, A. 2012. The effects of comprehensive warm-up programs on proprioception, static and dynamic balance on male soccer players. *PLOS One, 7*(12), e51568, 1–10.

Dannelly, B. D., Otey, S. C., Croy, T., Harrison, B., Rynders, C. A., Hertel, J. N., & Weltman, A. (2011). The effectiveness of traditional and sling exercise strength training in women. *Journal of Strength and Conditioning Research,* 25(2), 464–471.

Dean, C. M., Richards, C. L., & Malouin, F. (2000). Task-related circuit training improves performance of locomotor tasks in chronic stroke: A randomized controlled pilot trial. *Archives of Physical Medicine and Rehabilitation, 81*, 409–417.

Dimeo, F. (2001). Effects of exercise on cancer-related fatigue. *Cancer, 92*, 1689–1693.

Donath, L., Faude, O., Roth, R., & Zahner, L. (2014). Effects of stair-climbing on balance, gait, strength, resting heart rate, and submaximal endurance in healthy seniors. *Scandinavian Journal of Medicine and Science in Sports, 24*, 92–102.

Dressendorfer, R. H., Wade, C. E., & Scaff, J. H. (1985). Increased morning heart rate in runners: A valid sign of overtraining? *Physician and Sportsmedicine, 13*, 77–81.

Fagard, R. H. (2001). Exercise characteristics and the blood pressure response to dynamic physical training. *Medicine & Science in Sports and Exercise, 33*, S484–S492.

Falk, B., & Tenenbaum, G. (1996). The effectiveness of resistance training in children: A meta-analysis. *Sports Medicine, 22*, 176–186.

Fenwick, C. M., Brown, S. H., & McGill, S. M. 2009. Comparison of different rowing exercises: Trunk muscle activation and lumbar spine motion, load, and stiffness. *Journal of Strength and Conditioning Research, 23*(5), 1409–1417.

Fieril, K. P., Glantz, A., & Olsen, M. F. (2014). The efficacy of moderate-to-vigorous resistance exercise during pregnancy: A randomized controlled trial. *Acta Obstetricia et Gynecologica Scandinavica, 94*, 35–42.

Fountaine, C., & Schmidt, B. (2015). Metabolic cost of rope training. *Journal of Strength and Conditioning Research, 29*(4), 889–893.

Gates, D. M., Succop, P., Brehm, B. J., Gillespie, G. L., & Sommers, B. D. (2008). Obesity and presenteeism: The impact of body mass index on work-place productivity. *Journal of Occupational and Environmental Medicine, 50*, 39–45.

Gettman, L. R., Ayres, J. J., Pollock, M. L., & Jackson, A. (1978). The effect of circuit weight training on strength, cardiorespiratory function, and body composition of adult men. *Medicine and Science in Sports and Exercise, 10*, 171–176.

Gettman, L. R., Ward, P., & Hagan, R. D. (1982). A comparison of combined running and weight training with circuit weight training. *Medicine and Science in Sports and Exercise, 14*, 229–234.

Giangregorio, L. M., Papaioannou, A., MacIntyre, N. J., Ashe, M. C., Heinonen, A., . . . Cheung, A. M. (2014). Too fit to fracture: Exercise recommendations for individuals with osteoporosis or osteoporotic vertebral fracture. *Osteoporosis, 25*, 821–835.

Gomez-Cabello, A., Ara, I., Gonzalez-Aguero, A., Casajus, J. A., & Vicente-Rodriguez, G. (2012). Effects of training on bone mass in older adults: A systematic review. *Sports Medicine, 42*, 301–325.

Gordon, N. F., Gulanick, M., Costa, F., Fletcher, B. A., Roth, E. J., & Shephard, T. (2004). Physical activity and exercise recommendations for stroke survivors: An American Heart Association Scientific Statement from the Council on Clinical Cardiology. *Circulation, 109*, 2031–2041.

Hagberg, J. M., Park, J. J., & Brown, M. D. (2000). The role of exercise training in the treatment of hypertension: An update. *Sports Medicine, 30*, 193–206.

Hayes, S. C., Spence, R. R., Galvao, D. A., & Newton, R. U. (2009). Australian association for exercise and sport science position stand: optimizing cancer outcomes through exercise. *Journal of Science and Medicine in Sport, 12*, 428–434.

Herndon, J. H. (2013). The patient first. Above all do no harm (primum non nocere). *Journal of Bone and Joint Surgery, 95*, 289–291.

Hopkins, S. A., & Cutfield, W. S. (2011). Exercise in pregnancy: Weighing up the long-term impact on the next generation. *Exercise and Sport Sciences Reviews, 39*, 120–127.

Ismail, I., Keating, S. E., Baker, M. K., & Johnson, N. A. (2012). A systematic review and meta-analysis of the effect of aerobic vs. resistance exercise training on visceral fat. *Obesity Reviews, 13*, 68–91.

Jay, K., Frisch, D., Hansen, K., Zebis, M., Andersen, C., Mortensen, O., & Andersen, L. (2011). Kettlebell training for musculoskeletal and cardiorespiratory health: A randomized controlled trial. *Scandinavian Journal of Work, Environment, & Health, 37*, 196–203.

Jay, K., Jakobsen, M., Sundstrup, E., Skotte, J., Jorgensen, M., Andersen, C., . . . Andersen, L. L. (2013). Effects of kettlebell training on postural coordination and jump performance: A randomized controlled trial. *Journal of Strength and Conditioning Research, 27*, 1202–1209.

Jeukendrup, A., & VanDiemen, A. (1998). Heart rate monitoring during training and competition in cyclists. *Journal of Sports Science, 16*, S91–S99.

Kelley, G. A., & Kelley, K. S. (2000). Progressive resistance exercise and resting blood pressure: A meta-analysis of randomized, controlled trials. *Hypertension, 35*, 838–843.

Kuan, J. (2015). Taking an investor's perspective to leveraging fitness technology. *IDEA Fitness Journal*, January, 80–81.

Kuoppala, J., Lamminpaa, A., & Paivi, H. (2008). Work health promotion, job well-being, and sickness absences—a systematic review and meta-analysis. *Journal of Occupational and Environmental Medicine, 50*, 1216–1227.

LaFontaine, T. (2001). Strength and conditioning in the prevention and management of cerebrovascular accident (stroke). *Strength and Conditioning Journal, 23*, 49–52.

LaFontaine, T. (2003). Resistance exercise for persons with coronary heart disease. *Strength and Conditioning Journal, 25*, 17–21.

Lake, J., & Lauder, M. (2012a). Kettlebell swing training improves maximal and explosive strength. *Journal of Strength and Conditioning Research, 26*, 2228–2233.

Lake, J., & Lauder, M. (2012b). Mechanical demands of kettlebell swing exercises. *Journal of Strength and Conditioning Research, 26*, 3209–3216.

Lakka, T. A., & Bouchard, C. (2005). Physical activity, obesity, and cardiovascular disease. *Handbook of Experimental Pharmacology, 170*, 137–165.

Lamb, S. E., Guralnik, J. M., Buchner, D. M., Ferrucci, L. M., Hochberg, M. C., . . . Fried, L. P. (2000). Factors that modify the association between knee pain and mobility limitation in older women: The Women's Health and Aging Study. *Annals of the Rheumatic Diseases, 59*, 331–337.

Larson-Meyer, D. E. (2002). The effects of regular postpartum exercise on mother and child. *International SportMed Journal, 4*, 1–14.

Lau, R., Liao, L., Yu, F., Teo, T., Chung, R., & Pang, M. (2011). The effects of whole body vibration therapy on bone mineral density and leg muscle strength in older adults: A systematic review and meta-analysis. *Clinical Rehabilitation, 25*(11), 975–988.

Li, Y., Hanssen, H., Cordes, M., Rossmeissi, A., Endes, S., & Schmidt-Trucksass, A. (2015). Aerobic, resistance and combined exercise training on arterial stiffness in normotensive and hypertensive adults: a review. *European Journal of Sport Science, 15*, 443–457.

Liu, Y., Zhou, J., Ye, C. Q., & Bai, G. C. (2008). Osteogenetic effect of mechanical vibration on bone. *Zhongguo Gu Shang, 21*, 400–402.

Lohman, E. B., Petrofsky, J. S., Maloney-Hinds, C., Betts-Schwab, H., & Thorpe, D. (2007). The effect of whole body vibration on lower extremity skin blood flow in normal subjects. *Medical Science Monitor, 13*, CR71–CR76.

Lonbro, S. (2014). The effect of progressive resistance training on lean body mass in post-treatment cancer patients—a systematic review. *Radiotherapy and Oncology, 110*, 71–80.

Lopez, J. D. (2014). Protecting the weekend warrior from injury. *Interdisciplinary Journal of Rehabilitation, 27*, 30–32.

Loprinzi, P. D., Cardinal, B. J., Karp, J. R., & Brodowicz, G. R. (2011). Group training in adolescent runners: Influence on VO2max and 5-km race performance. *Journal of Strength and Conditioning Research, 25*(10), 2696–2703.

Loyle, D. (2012). The business of corporate fitness. Club Industry.com, May 26–34. Available at: http://clubindustry.com/corporate/business-corporate-fitness.

Luo, J., McNamara, B., & Moran, K. (2005). The use of vibration training to enhance muscle strength and power. *Sports Medicine, 35*, 23–41.

Malina, R. M. (2006). Weight training youth-growth, maturation, and safety: An evidence-based review. *Clinical Journal of Sports Medicine, 16*, 478–487.

Maloney-Hinds, C., Petrofsky, J. S., & Zimmerman, G. (2008). The effect of 30 Hz vs. 50 Hz passive vibration and duration of vibration on skin blood flow in the arm. *Medical Science Monitor, 14*, CR112–CR116.

Marin, P. J., Herrero, A. J., Sáinz, N., Rhea, M. R., & García-López, D. (2010). Effects of different magnitudes of whole-body vibration on arm muscular performance. *Journal of Strength and Conditioning Research, 24*, 2506–2511.

Marin, P. J., & Rhea, M. R. (2010a). Effects of vibration training on muscle power: A meta-analysis. *Journal of Strength and Conditioning Research, 24,* 871–878.

Marin, P. J., & Rhea, M. R. (2010b). Effects of vibration training on muscle strength: A meta-analysis. *Journal of Strength and Conditioning Research, 24,* 548–556.

Marin, P. J., Tumminello, L., & Rhea, M. (2010). *Vibration exercise.* Nibley, UT: Race Rx Publishing.

Mate-Munoz, J. L., Monroy Anton, A. J., Jimenez, P. J., & Garnacho-Castano, M. V. (2014). Effects of instability versus traditional resistance training on strength, power, and velocity in untrained men. *Journal of Sports Science and Medicine, 13,* 460–468.

McDougall, J. D., Tuxen, D. S., Moroz, J. R., & Sutton, J. R. (1985). Arterial blood pressure response to heavy resistance exercise. *Journal of Applied Physiology, 58,* 785–790.

McGill, S., & Marshall, L. (2012). Kettle swing, snatch, and bottoms-up carry: Back and hip muscle activation, motion, and low back loads. *Journal of Strength and Conditioning Research, 26*(1), 16–27.

Meneses-Echavez, J. F., Gonzalez-Jimenez, E., & Ramirez-Velez, R. (2015). Supervised exercise reduces cancer-related fatigue: A systematic review. *Journal of Physiotherapy, 61,* 3–10.

Messier, S. P., & Dill, M. E. (1985). Alterations in strength and maximal oxygen uptake consequent to Nautilus circuit weight training. *Research Quarterly for Exercise and Sport, 56,* 345–351.

Micheli, L. (2006). Preventing injuries in sports: What the team physician needs to know. In: Chan et al. (Eds.), *FIMS Team Physician Manual* (2nd ed., pp. 555–572). Hong Kong: CD Concept.

Morris, S. L., Dodd, K. J., & Morris, M. E. (2004). Outcomes of progressive resistance strength training following stroke: A systematic review. *Clinical Rehabilitation, 18,* 27–39.

Mutrie, N., Campbell, A., Whyte, F., McConnachie, A., Emslie, C., Lee, L., . . . Ritchie, D. (2007). Benefits of supervised group exercise programme for women being treated for early stage breast cancer: Pragmatic randomized controlled trial. *BMJ, 334*(7592), 517.

O'Connor, P. J., Poudevigne, M. S., Cress, M. E., Motl, R. W., & Clapp, J. F. (2011). Safety and efficacy of supervised strength training adopted in pregnancy. *Journal of Physical Activity and Health, 8,* 309–320.

Okada, K. (1991). Effects of long-term corporate fitness program on employees' health. *Journal of Nutritional Science and Vitaminology, 37,* S131–S138.

Onks, C. A., & Wawrzyniak, J. (2014). The physical therapy prescription. *Medical Clinics of North America, 98,* 869–880.

Osteras, H. (2014). A 12-week medical exercise therapy program leads to significant improvement in knee function after degenerative meniscectomy: A randomized controlled trial with one year follow-up. *Journal of Bodywork and Movement Therapies, 18,* 374–382.

Otto, W., Coburn, J., Brown, L., & Spiering, B. (2012). Effects of weightlifting vs. kettlebell training on vertical jump, strength and body composition. *Journal of Strength and Conditioning Research, 26,* 1199–1202.

Orr, R. (2015). The effect of whole body vibration exposure on balance and functional mobility in older adults: A systematic review and meta-analysis. *Maturitas, 80,* 342–358.

Parks, K. M., & Steelman, L. A. (2008). Organizational wellness programs: A meta-analysis. *Journal of Occupational Health Psychology, 13,* 58–68.

Parmenter, B. J., Dieberg, G., & Smart, N. A. (2015). Exercise training for management of peripheral arterial disease: A systematic review and meta-analysis. *Sports Medicine, 45,* 231–244.

Payne, V., Morrow, J., Johnson, L., & Dalton, S. (1997). Resistance training in children and youth: A meta-analysis. *Research Quarterly for Exercise and Sports, 68,* 80–88.

Peltier, L., Strand, B., & Christnsen, B. (2008). Youth performing resistance training: A review. *Journal of Youth Sports, 4,* 18–23.

Perchthaler, D. , Horstmann, T., & Grau, S. (2013). Variations in neuromuscular activity of thigh muscles during whole-body vibration in consideration of different biomechanical variables. *Journal of Sports Science and Medicine, 12,* 439–446.

Pescatello, L. S., Fargo, A. E., Leach, C. N., & Scherzer, H. H. (1991). Short-term effect of dynamic exercise on arterial blood pressure. *Circulation, 83,* 1557–1561.

Peterson, M. D., Sen, A., & Gordon, P. M. (2011). Influence of resistance exercise on lean body mass in aging adults: A meta-analysis. *Medicine and Science in Sports and Exercise, 43,* 249–258.

Petranick, K., & Berg, K. (1997). The effects of weight training on bone density of premenopausal, postmenopausal, and elderly women: A review. *Journal of Strength and Conditioning Research, 11,* 200–208.

Powell, D. R. (1997). Implementing a self-care program: effect on employee health care utilization. *AAOHN Journal, 45,* 41–42.

Psoinos, C. M., Emhoff, T. A., Sweeney, B., Tseng, J. F., & Santry, H. P. (2012). The dangers of being a "weekend warrior": A new call for injury prevention efforts. *Journal of Trauma and Acute Care Surgery, 73,* 469–473.

Puetz, T. W., & Herring, M. P. (2012). Differential effects of exercise on cancer-related fatigue during and following treatment: A meta-analysis. *American Journal of Preventive Medicine, 43,* e1–e24.

Purwanto, B., Wigati, K. W., & Elysana Asnar, S. T. P. (2014). Age and resting heart rate are discriminators to predict endurance without physical test. *Folia Medica Indonesiana, 50,* 110–113.

Quan, H. L., Blizzard, C. L., Sharman, J. E., Magnussen, C. G., Dwyer, T., Raitakari, O, . . . Venn, A. J. (2013). Resting heart rate and the association of physical fitness with carotid artery stiffness. *American Journal of Hypertension, 27,* 65–71.

Ratamess, N. A., Rosenberg, J. G., Klei, S., Dougherty, B. M., Kang, J., Smith, C. R., . . . Faigenbaum, A. D. (2015). Comparison of the acute metabolic responses to traditional resistance, body-weight, and battling rope exercises. *Journal of Strength and Conditioning Research, 29*(1), 47–57.

Rhea, M. R., Bunker, D., Marin, P. J., & Lunt, K. (2009). Effect of iTonic whole-body vibration on delayed-onset muscle soreness among untrained individuals. *Journal of Strength and Conditioning Research, 23,* 1677–1682.

Rhea, M. R., & Kenn, J. G. (2009). The effect of acute applications of whole-body vibration on the iTonic platform on subsequent lower-body power output during the back squat. *Journal of Strength and Conditioning Research, 23,* 58–61.

Roberts, D. J., Ouellet, J. F., McBeth, P. B., Kirkpatrick, A. W., Dixon, E., & Ball, C. G. (2014). The "weekend warrior": Fact or fiction for major trauma? *Canadian Journal of Surgery, 57,* E62–E68.

Robroek, S. J. W., Lenthe, F. J., Empelen, P., & Burdoff, A. (2009). Determinants of participation in worksite health promotion programmes: A systematic review. *International Journal of Behavioral Nutrition and Physical Activity, 6,* 1–12.

Roitman, J. L., & LaFontaine, T. (2006). Exercise, atherosclerosis, and the endothelium: Where the action is (part II). *Strength and Conditioning Journal, 28,* 75–77.

Rongon, A., Robroek, S. J. W., Lenthe, F. J., & Burdof, A. (2013). Workplace health promotion: A meta-analysis of effectiveness. *American Journal of Preventive Medicine, 44,* 406–415.

Sandstrom, R. W., Lehman, J., Hahn, L., & Ballard, A. (2013). Structure of the physical therapy benefit in a typical Blue Cross Blue Shield preferred provider organization plan available in the individual insurance market in 2011. *Physical Therapy, 93,* 1342–1350.

Santana, J., Vera-Garcia, F., & McGill, S. (2007). A kinetic and electromyographic comparison of the standing cable press and bench press. *Journal of Strength and Conditioning Research, 21*(4), 1271–1279.

Saxena, A., Minton, D., Lee, D. C., Sui, X., Fayad, R., Lavie, C. J., & Blair, S. N. (2013). Protective role of resting heart rate on all-cause and cardiovascular disease mortality. *Mayo Clinic Proceedings, 88,* 1420–1426.

Scala, D., McMillan, J., Blessing, D., Rozenek, R., & Stone, M. (1987). Metabolic cost of a preparatory phase of training in weightlifting: A practical observation. *Journal of Applied Sports Science Research, 1*(3), 48–52.

Schoenfeld, B. (2011). Resistance training during pregnancy: Safe and effective program design. *Strength and Conditioning Journal, 5,* 67–75.

Schranz, N., Tomkinson, G., Olds, T. (2013). What is the effect of resistance training on the strength, body composition and psychosocial status of overweight and obese children and adolescents? A systematic review and meta-analysis. *Sports Medicine, 43,* 893–907.

Singh Paramanandam, V., & Roberts, D. (2014). Weight training is not harmful for women with breast cancer-related lymphoedema: A systematic review. *Journal of Physiotherapy, 60,* 136–143.

Smith, A., Andrish, J., & Micheli, L. (1993). The prevention of sports injuries in children and adolescents. *Medicine and Science in Sports and Exercise, 25,* 1–8.

Snarr, R. L., & Esco, M. R. (2014). Electromyographical comparison of plank variations performed with and without instability devices. *Journal of Strength and Conditioning Research, 28,* 3298–3305.

Spennewyn, K. (2008). Strength outcomes in fixed versus free-form resistance training. *Journal of Strength and Conditioning Research, 22,* 75–81.

Stewart, V. H., Saunders, D. H., & Greig, C. A. (2014). Responsiveness of muscle size and strength to physical training in very elderly people: A systematic review. *Scandinavian Journal of Medicine and Science in Sports, 24,* e1–e10.

Stone, M., Plisk, S., & Collins, D. (2002). Training principles: Evaluation of modes and methods of resistance training—a coaching perspective. *Sports Biomechanics, 1*(1), 79–103.

Stone, M., Wilson, G., Blessing, D., & Rozenek, R. (1983). Cardiovascular responses to short-term Olympic style weight-training in young men. *Canadian Journal of Applied Sports Science Research, 8*(3), 134–139.

Strasser, B., Siebert, U., & Schobersberger, W. (2010). Resistance training in the treatment of the metabolic syndrome. *Sports Medicine, 40,* 397–415.

Strasser, B., Steindorf, K., Wiskemann, J., & Ulrich, C. M. (2013). Impact of resistance training in cancer survivors: A meta-analysis. *Medicine and Science in Sports and Exercise, 45,* 2080–2090.

Suciu, P. (2013). The fitness tech explosion. Technewsworld. Available at: http://www .technewsworld.com/story/77064.html

Tangemann, P. T., Banaitis, D. A., & Williams, A. K. (1990). Rehabilitation of chronic stroke patients: Changes in functional performance. *Archives of Physical Medicine and Rehabilitation, 71,* 876–880.

Teixeira-Salmela, L., Nadeau, S., McBride, I., & Olney, S. (2001). Effects of muscle strengthening and physical conditioning training on temporal, kinematic and kinetic variables during gait in chronic stroke survivors. *Journal of Rehabilitation Medicine, 33,* 53–60.

Toms, L. V., O'Neil, M. E., & Gardner, A. (2003). Long-term risk factor control after a cardiac rehabilitation programme. *Australian Critical Care, 16,* 24–28.

Totosy de Zepetnek, J. O., Giangregorio, L. M., & Craven, B. C. (2009). Whole-body vibration as potential intervention for people with low bone mineral density and osteoporosis: A review. *Journal of Rehabilitation Research and Development, 46,* 529–542.

Tran, Q. T. (2005). Resistance training and safety considerations for chronic heart failure patients. *Strength and Conditioning Journal, 27,* 71–72.

Tschopp, M., Sattelmayer, M. K., & Hilfiker, R. (2011). Is power training or conventional resistance training better for function in elderly persons? A meta-analysis. *Age and Ageing, 40,* 549–556.

Uusitalo, A. L., Uusitalo, A. J., & Rusko, H. K. (1998). Endurance training, overtraining and baroflex sensitivity in female athletes. *Clinical Physiology, 18,* 510–520.

Vincent, H. K., Raiser, S. N., & Vincent, K. R. (2012). The aging musculoskeletal system and obesity-related considerations with exercise. *Ageing Research Reviews, 11,* 361–373.

Vogel, A. (2015). Fitness technology conundrum. *IDEA Fitness Journal,* July/August, 62–71.

Vriz, O., Argiento, P., D'Alto, M., Ferrar, F., Vanderpool, R., Naeije, R., & Bossone, E. (2015). Clinical research: Increased pulmonary vascular resistance in early stage systemic hypertension: A resting and exercise stress echocardiography study. *Canadian Journal of Cardiology, 31,* 537–543.

Vy-Van, L., Mitiku, T., Sungar, G., Myers, J., & Froelicher, V. (2008). The blood pressure response to dynamic exercise testing: A systematic review. *Progress in Cardiovascular Disease, 51,* 135–160.

Wallace, J. P. (2003). Exercise in hypertension: A clinical review. *Sports Medicine, 33,* 585–598.

Wallace, J. P., Bogle, P. G., King, B. A., Krasnoff, J. B., & Jastremski, C. A. (1999). The magnitude and duration of ambulatory blood pressure reduction following acute exercise. *Journal of Human Hypertension, 13,* 361–366.

Watanabe, Y., Tanimoto, M., Oba, N., Sanada, K., Miyachi, M., & Ishii, N. (2015). Effect of resistance training using bodyweight in the elderly: Comparison of resistance exercise movement between slow and normal speed movement. *Geriatrics Gerontology International, 15,* 1270–1277.

Weiss, A., Suzuki, T., Bean, J., & Fielding, R. A. (2000). High-intensity strength training improves strength and functional performance after stroke. *American Journal of Physical Medicine and Rehabilitation, 79,* 369–376.

Whelton, S. P., Chin, A., Xin, X., & He, J. (2002). Effect of aerobic exercise on blood pressure: A meta-analysis of randomized, controlled trials. *Annals of Internal Medicine, 136,* 493–503.

White, E., Pivarnik, J., & Pfeiffer, K. (2014). Resistance training during pregnancy and perinatal outcomes. *Journal of Physical Activity and Health*, *11*, 1141–1148.

Wilhelm, M., Roskovensky, G., Emery, K., Manno, C., Valek, K., & Cook, C. (2012). Effect of resistance exercises on function in older adults with osteoporosis or osteopenia: A systematic review. *Physiotherapy Canada*, *64*, 386–394.

Williams, A. (2008). Corporate wellness- programming for profit. *IDEA Fitness Journal*, May, 36–41.

Williamson, P. (2012). *Exercise for special populations*. Baltimore, MD: Lippincott Williams & Wilkins.

Yu, C., Sung, R., So, R., Lui, K., Lau, W., Lam, P., & Lau, E. (2005). Effects of strength training on body composition and bone mineral content in children who are obese. *Journal of Strength and Conditioning Research*, *19*, 667–672.

Zebis, M., Skotte, J., Andersen, C., Mortensen, P., Petersen, H., Viskaer, T., . . . Andersen, L. (2013). Kettlebell swing targets semitendinosus and supine leg curl targets biceps femoris: An EMG study with rehabilitation implications. *British Journal of Sports Medicine*, *47*(18), 1192–1198.

Zavanela, P. M. Crewther, B. T., Lodo, L., Florindo, A. A., Miyabara, E. H., & Aoiki, M. S. (2012). Health and fitness benefits of a resistance training intervention performed in the workplace. *Journal of Strength and Conditioning Research*, *26*(3), 811–817.

Zhao, R., Zhao, M., & Xu, Z. (2015). The effects of different resistance training modes on the preservation of bone mineral density in postmenopausal women: A meta-analysis. *Osteoporosis International*, *26*, 1605–1618.

15

EXERCISE TECHNIQUE

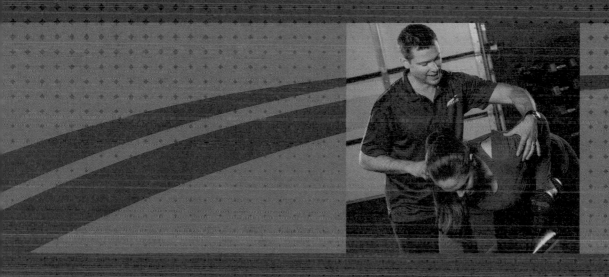

OBJECTIVES

After studying this chapter, you will be able to:

1 **Classify** flexibility and resistance training exercises.

2 **Identify** common exercise technique mistakes.

3 **Demonstrate** coaching and cueing strategies to correct exercise techniques on various fitness clients.

4 **Select** exercises for specific client populations and fitness goals.

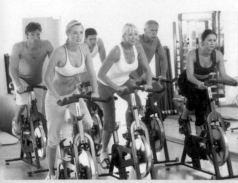
© Monkey Business Images/Shutterstock

Case Scenario

You have been working with a group of five clients who have the same underlying goal of losing weight. It is apparent that all five enjoy working out together, watching them challenge and motivate each other throughout each group personal training session. You have been working on ways to address the group as a whole while still providing a personal training focus for each client. One specific area you have been struggling with is using proficient coaching and cueing strategies to ensure proper exercise technique. Because your clients' abilities vary greatly within your group you feel it is necessary to coach and cue each client individually during the sessions. In order to coach and cue on a personal level you review each of the five women you are training to reflect on who they are, and identify what struggles each is having during the sessions.

- **Sally, age 46, the "comparer"**: Sally works out best when supporting others who are exercising with her, affirming her drive to make it to every workout session. You have noticed that Sally has struggled with the workout intensities in her last few sessions. It is evident that she continuously tries to keep up with her friends' progress. This often results in her executing exercises improperly, which could possibly lead to injury.

- **Holly, age 37, the "veteran"**: Holly is a motivator and natural leader. She has been pivotal in keeping the group together and holding everyone accountable. Because she is not new to these types of workout sessions, she shows few signs of being challenged during the exercises you have the group conduct. It is becoming increasingly clear that she is in need of learning something more to take her to the next level.

- **Jackie, age 52, the "experienced"**: Jackie has experience working in a gym, and finds herself gravitating toward the exercises she is most comfortable with and/or can execute with proper technique. Because of this, she finds herself only using a handful of common exercises, many of which do not properly isolate the specific muscle groups or joint actions brought up by her assessments.

- **Melanie, age 61, the "maintainer"**: Melanie has always taken her health seriously, and has been a frequent exerciser in hopes of maintaining mobility. Throughout the group personal trainings sessions, she has never shown signs of falling behind, nor has struggled to keep up with the programs. She requires little explanation on the exercises you have the group do.

- **Lisa, age 30, the "newbie"**: Lisa is new to working with a personal trainer, let alone in a manner that is structured with a purpose and goals. Because of her novice mindset she continuously asks you why you are instructing her to do things a certain way, but she is receptive to the information you give her. From what you have observed, she has shown little sign of struggling with the intensity levels you place on the group, but you notice that she needs more personal attention to execute the exercises properly.

Based on your observations of your group personal training class, you feel there are some crucial changes you should make in how you progress each client, while still maintaining everyone's underlying goal of losing weight together. Without making one or more of your clients potentially feel singled out, summarize a strategy while considering the following:

- What is one flexibility and one resistance training exercise you would have them conduct, and why?

- How would you explain to each client how to conduct the exercises, the movements involved, the joint actions that occur, and common mistakes or obstacles?

- How can you tailor coaching and cueing for each client?

- What would you do to regress and/or progress the exercises, and what would you need to know in order to make that decision for each client?

Introduction to Exercise Technique

Exercise technique is one of the most important aspects of an exercise regimen. Without proper technique, clients may fail to progress toward meeting their fitness goals, as well as increase their chance of injury during workout sessions. Continuous use of exercises with incorrect technique can also lead to kinetic chain dysfunction, creating postural and movement imbalances and increasing the risk of injury during daily activities. Therefore, it is vital for the fitness professional to be able to properly coach and cue correct technique during all aspects of an integrated training session. This requires a thorough understanding of the various components of exercises. In order to effectively develop a strategy for programming, the fitness professional must understand how each exercise is going to affect the kinetic chain. Understanding the agonist (i.e., prime mover) and synergist muscles activated during each exercise will show the fitness professional how they interact to generate force around the joints (i.e., force-couples). Understanding the planes of motion an exercise is occurring in will ensure the program is designed in a way that complements the 360-degree environment the client lives within. Further, knowing different modalities and similar exercises will allow for creativity and flexibility with program design, whereas *progressions and regressions* will provide the opportunity for a program to be adapted if an exercise seems too easy or too hard for the client to perform. Although by no means an exhaustive collection—as there are myriad ways for the fitness professional to be creative with programming and to utilize the various modalities available—this chapter will serve as a working guide for a wide variety of exercises to be used throughout all levels of the Optimum Performance Training (OPT) model.

Flexibility Exercises

Flexibility exercises should be incorporated into any integrated exercise program in order to correct muscle imbalances, increase joint range of motion (ROM), decrease muscle soreness, relieve joint stress, improve muscle extensibility, and maintain the functional length of all muscles. It is essential that muscles be stretched in all planes of motion with correct movement performance to ensure that these beneficial adaptations occur. Selection of self-myofascial release (SMR), static stretching, active-isolated stretching, or dynamic stretching should be made based on the client's individual needs and the stage of the progressive training program he or she may be in.

Self-Myofascial Release (SMR)

- *Progressions and regressions:*
  ‣ If the traditional foam roller is not dense enough, perform SMR on a smaller and denser object, such as a massage ball.
  ‣ If the traditional foam roller is too dense (i.e., too painful), perform SMR on a larger and/or less dense object. If a larger/less dense foam roller is not available, try using two foam rollers to increase the surface area of compression.

- *Common form mistakes:*
  ‣ Rolling too quickly.
  ‣ Not identifying the tender spot.
  ‣ Not holding static pressure on the tender spot. It is common for people to feel the desire to "knead" the tissue. This is incorrect. The first step is to hold with no movement to replicate trigger point release.
  ‣ Tensing the body in the presence of discomfort.

- *Cues to correct:*
  ‣ "The idea is to 'calm down' the muscle, and rolling fast will excite the muscle."
  ‣ "When the tender spot is found, just simply relax the muscle and focus on deep breathing."

- *Contraindications and special considerations:*
  ‣ *Varicose veins*: Excessive pressure may cause varicose veins to rupture. Avoid putting pressure directly on varicose veins.
  ‣ *High blood pressure*: Massage has been shown to decrease blood pressure; however, the positions and tenderness in SMR may be problematic. Controlled high blood pressure is not a contraindication.
  ‣ *Diabetes*: Poor circulation to the lower extremities may lead to the inability of the body to properly flush out the "waste" from breaking up adhesions and knots.
  ‣ *Pregnancy*: Miscarriage has been associated with massage in the first trimester. In the third trimester, pressure points in the calf and adductor may induce contractions.
  ‣ *Any time the trainer is unsure of a condition*: SMR is a great tool to integrate into a warm-up. However, if the fitness professional is unsure of whether a client has a condition, it is better to postpone SMR until speaking with the client's physician.

- **Kinetic chain checkpoints and movement dysfunctions affecting correct technique:**
  - ‣ Use SMR on the indicated muscles, as dysfunctions are observed during both static postural and dynamic movement assessments.

- **Myths and misconceptions:**
  - ‣ *"Foam-rolling feels good, but doesn't really do anything."* SMR is a proven method to help increase flexibility without a concurrent decrease in force production (MacDonald et al., 2012). In addition, it has been found that SMR before static stretching leads to increased ROM when compared to performing each modality separately (Mohr, Long, & Goad, 2014).
  - ‣ *"Foam-rolling is only beneficial after a workout."* Studies have shown that SMR before a workout helps to increase ROM (Sullivan et al., 2013). Increased ROM may help to reduce the potential for injury.
  - ‣ *"Before exercise you should roll fast to get the muscles ready for activity."* In most people, SMR should not be used as a method of activation before exercise. SMR is used as an inhibition technique, not an activation technique. The evidence does not support its use as a method of activation. Therefore, it should be used as part of an integrated warm-up.
  - ‣ *"Foam-rolling after a workout helps get the lactic acid out."* Performing SMR postexercise (as part of a cool-down) does not flush out "lactic acid." In fact, there is no such thing as lactic acid in the body (Robergs, Ghiasvand, & Parker, 2004). In addition, Robergs and colleagues (2004) provided evidence that the accumulation of hydrogen causes acidosis (the burning felt during a workout). Using a foam roller after exercise can help to "flush out" the accumulated hydrogen following a workout.
  - ‣ *"Foam-rolling after a workout will prevent soreness."* Performing SMR after a workout may reduce soreness. However, in one study participants who performed SMR after intense workouts had faster recovery but did not experience significantly decreased soreness compared to those who did not perform SMR. The participants who performed SMR experienced maximum soreness 24 hours after training, whereas those who did not perform SMR experienced maximum soreness 48 hours after training (MacDonald et al., 2013). If the recovery process is sped up, the client is able to train harder, longer, and more often.

SMR Gastrocnemius/Soleus (Calves)

- **Other name(s):** Foam-rolling posterior lower leg.

- **Muscle(s) inhibited:** Gastrocnemius/Soleus.

- **Performance technique:** Begin by sitting on a flat surface with the foam roller placed just above the ankle. Cross the nonworking leg over the working leg to increase compression, if needed. Place the hands near the hips with the fingertips pointing away from the body. Raise the hips and slowly begin to roll the body down (so the foam roller comes up) toward the knee.

Flexibility Exercises *continued*

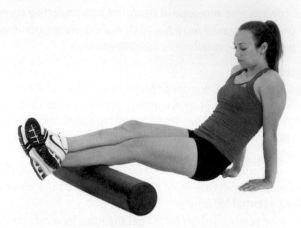

Roll at a pace of about 1 inch per second until a tender spot is identified. A tender spot is pain/discomfort that could be classified as 6–9 on a scale from 1–10. Hold this spot for 20–30 seconds or until the tenderness begins to decrease. Identify one or two of these spots in the calf before switching to the opposite leg.

SMR Quadriceps

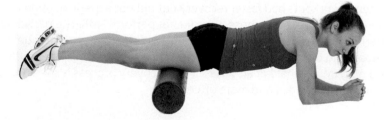

- *Other name(s):* Foam-rolling the front of the upper leg.

- *Muscle(s) inhibited:* Quadriceps muscle group.

- *Performance technique:* Begin by lying face down on a flat surface with the foam roller placed just below the hip. Both quadriceps can be rolled at the same time, or they can be rolled one at a time. If rolling one at a time, place the nonworking leg out to the side, so it is relaxed but providing light support. Place the arms in front of the body, with the elbows under the shoulders for support. The spine should be neutral. Do not place the hips on the ground, as this will increase compression into the low back. Slowly begin to roll up (so the foam roller goes down) toward the knee. Roll at a pace of about 1 inch per second until a tender spot is identified. A tender spot is pain/discomfort that could be classified as 6–9 on a scale from 1–10. Hold this spot for 20–30 seconds or until the tenderness begins to decrease. Identify one or two of these spots in the quadriceps before switching to the opposite leg.

SMR Adductors

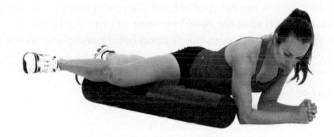

- **Other name(s):** Foam-rolling the inside of the upper leg.

- **Muscle(s) inhibited:** Adductors.

- **Performance technique:** Begin by lying face down on a flat surface with the foam roller placed on the inside of the leg, just above the knee. The leg being rolled should be placed with the hip close to 90 degrees, and the nonworking leg should be extended straight. Place the arms in front of the body, with the elbows under the shoulders for support. The spine should be neutral. Slowly begin to roll towards the roller (so the foam roller goes toward the hip). Roll at a pace of about 1 inch per second until a tender spot is identified. A tender spot is pain/discomfort that could be classified as 6–9 on a scale from 1–10. Hold this spot for 20–30 seconds or until the tenderness begins to decrease. Identify one or two of these spots in the adductors before switching to the opposite leg.

SMR Vastus Lateralis

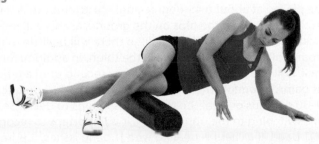

Flexibility Exercises *continued*

- *Other name(s):* Foam-rolling the IT band.

- *Muscle(s) inhibited:* Vastus Lateralis.

- *Performance technique:* Begin by lying on the side, with the roller placed just below the hips at a 45-degree angle of rotation. The nonworking leg should be placed in front of the body to offer additional support during rolling. The spine should be neutral. Do not place the hips on the ground, as this will increase compression into the lower back. Slowly begin to roll up (so the foam roller goes down) toward the knee. Roll at a pace of about 1 inch per second until a tender spot is identified. A tender spot is pain/discomfort that could be classified as 6–9 on a scale from 1–10. Hold this spot for 20–30 seconds or until the tenderness begins to decrease. Identify one or two of these spots in the IT band before switching to the opposite leg.

SMR Tensor Fasciae Latae (TFL)

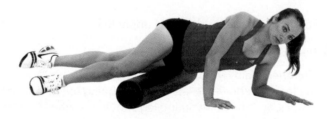

- *Other name(s):* Foam-rolling the hip flexor.

- *Muscle(s) inhibited:* Tensor fascia latae.

- *Performance technique:* Begin by lying face down on a flat surface with the foam roller placed just below the iliac crest of the hip, but above the greater trochanter (top of femur). The body will be placed at about a 45-degree angle to attempt to isolate the TFL. Spine should be neutral. Do not place the hips on the ground, as this will increase compression into the low back. The area of the TFL is small, so there will be little rolling. Slowly begin to roll up (so the foam roller goes down) toward the thigh. In addition, one can roll the body forward and back. Roll at a pace of about 1 inch per second until a tender spot is identified. A tender spot is pain/discomfort that could be classified as 6–9 on a scale from 1–10. Hold this spot for 20–30 seconds or until the tenderness begins to decrease. Identify one spot in the TFL before switching to the opposite leg. It is important to recognize that the TFL attaches to the IT band. If a client is dealing with IT band issues, it is important to also address the TFL.

SMR Piriformis

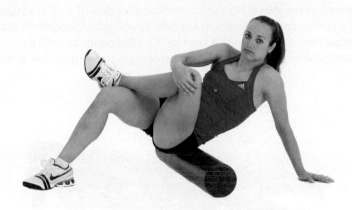

- **Other name(s):** Foam-rolling the piriformis.
- **Muscle(s) inhibited:** Piriformis.
- **Performance technique:** Begin by sitting with the glutes to be rolled in the center of the roller. Place the same-side hand on the ground and lean back slightly to relax the glutes. The leg on the side being rolled can be crossed over the opposing leg to open the hip. Slowly begin to roll up (so the foam roller goes down) toward the knee. Roll at a pace of about 1 inch per second until a tender spot is identified. A tender spot is pain/discomfort that could be classified as 6–9 on a scale from 1–10. Hold this spot for 20–30 seconds or until the tenderness begins to decrease. Identify one or two of these spots in the glutes before switching to the opposite leg.

SMR Latissimus Dorsi

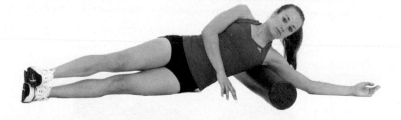

- **Other name(s):** Foam-rolling the side of the upper torso.
- **Muscle(s) inhibited:** Latissimus dorsi.
- **Performance technique:** Begin by lying on one side with the roller placed just below the armpit. The arm of the side being rolled should be relaxed on the ground above the head. The

Flexibility Exercises *continued*

area of the lat being rolled is small; therefore, it is a small, rolling motion. The spine should be neutral. Slowly begin to roll up (so the foam roller goes down). Roll at a pace of about 1 inch per second until a tender spot is identified. A tender spot is pain/discomfort that could be classified as 6–9 on a scale from 1–10. Hold this spot for 20–30 seconds or until the tenderness begins to decrease. Identify one spot in the lats before switching to the opposite arm.

SMR Peroneals

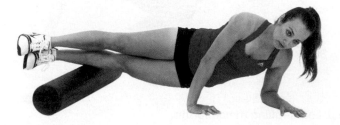

- *Other name(s):* Foam-rolling the outside of the leg.

- *Muscle(s) inhibited:* Peronials.

- *Performance technique:* Begin by lying on the side with the foam roller placed under the low leg at the inferior portion of the calf. Position the roller at an approximate 90-degree angle under the leg to be rolled. Do not perform a large rolling motion across the entire lower leg Do not roll onto a bone at the knee joint or the ankle joint. Roll at a pace of about 1 inch per second until a tender spot is identified. A tender spot is pain/discomfort that could be classified as 6–9 on a scale from 1–10. Hold this spot for 20–30 seconds or until the tenderness begins to decrease. Identify one tender spot in the leg before switching to the opposite leg.

SMR Thoracic Spine

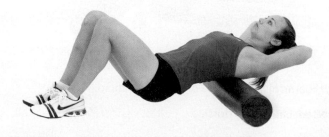

- **Other name(s):** Foam-rolling the upper back.

- **Muscle(s) inhibited:** Middle/lower trapezius.

- **Performance technique:** Begin by lying back on a flat surface with the roller placed just below the shoulder blades. Place the hands behind the head so the neck muscles can be relaxed. Keep the hips and knees bent, with feet flat on the floor. Raise the hips slightly off the ground and begin rolling down (so the roller rolls up toward the shoulder). Do not roll on the neck or the low back. Slowly roll at a pace of about 1 inch per second until a tender spot is identified. A tender spot is pain/discomfort that could be classified as 6–9 on a scale from 1–10. Hold this spot for 30–60 seconds or until the tenderness begins to decrease.

Static Stretching

- **General performance technique:** Hold the stretch for 30–60 seconds, depending on the client's flexibility and phase of the OPT model.

- **Contraindications and special considerations:**
  - Only perform static stretching on muscles that have been identified as being overactive in the overhead squat assessment.
  - Do not perform if experiencing joint instability.
  - Do not perform if diseases affecting the tissues to be stretched are present, such as rheumatoid arthritis or conditions that have altered the properties of the connective tissue.
  - Do not perform in the area of an acute injury. Consult a physician prior to beginning a stretching program after an injury.
  - Stop stretching immediately and consult a physician if excessive pain is experienced.
  - Do not force a joint beyond its normal ROM.
  - Take precaution with conditions such as osteoporosis.
  - Avoid aggressive stretching.
  - Do not stretch muscles that have apparent swelling and inflammation.
  - Make sure to continue to breathe during the stretch.

- **Myths and misconceptions:**
  - "Static stretching before working out is bad because it will decrease performance." This is both true and misunderstood. Static stretching for extended periods of time can decrease the ability of the muscle being stretched to contract. Kay and Blazevich (2012) found that continuous stretching of longer than 2 minutes resulted in decreased performance. However, durations of no longer than 30 seconds were found not to decrease the ability of the muscle to contract. Static stretching should be performed only for muscles identified as overactive by the overhead squat assessment. Therefore, decreasing the activity of these muscles will lead to increased performance in total body motion. In addition, research suggests that those who stretch before activity are able to better stabilize and control the center of pressure (Adelsberger & Troster, 2014).

Flexibility Exercises *continued*

> ▸ *"More is better."* More is never better. Muscles can only be stretched a small amount before tissue damage results. Only take a stretch to the first point of tension and then hold. Over time the ROM will increase.

Static Gastrocnemius/Soleus (Calves) Stretch

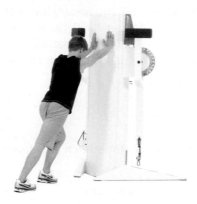

- **Other name(s):** Ankle stretch.

- **Muscle(s) lengthened:** Gastrocnemius and soleus.

- **Performance technique:** Begin by standing approximately arm-length away from a wall or stable object. The leg to be stretched should be extended at the hip and knee and slightly internally rotated. Place the hands on the wall, contract the glutes and quadriceps as the arms are bent, and lean into the wall. The leg being stretched should have the foot flat on the ground. Lean into the wall until the first point of tension is felt. Hold this for 20–30 seconds.

- **Progressions and regressions:**
  - ▸ If the stretch is uncomfortable, reduce the amount of forward lean.
  - ▸ If more stretch is needed, lean into the stretch more.

- **Common form of mistakes:**
  - ▸ *Foot is not straight*: The most common mistake is to rotate the foot out in an attempt to get more motion from the stretch.
  - ▸ *Allowing the foot to flatten*: In another attempt to force more motion out of the ankle, many will excessively flatten the foot.
  - ▸ *Leaning forward at the hip*: In order to stretch the calf, the motion needs to occur at the ankle. A common compensation is to lean forward at the hip.
  - ▸ *Letting the heel hang off a step*: A common misunderstanding is to let the heels hang off a step, or similar object, to use body weight to intensify the stretch. In this position the calves are supporting the body's weight, and therefore not able to relax. The heel needs to be secure on the ground.

- *Cues to correct:*
  - ▸ "Engage the core, glutes, and quadriceps, and then slowly lean forward at the ankle."
  - ▸ "Take to the first point of tension and hold."
  - ▸ "Stretches may be uncomfortable, but they are not intended to cause pain."

- *Plane of motion where movement occurs:* Sagittal.

- *Kinetic chain checkpoints and movement dysfunctions affecting correct technique:*
  - ▸ Static stretch the calves if the client has the following dysfunction during the overhead squat assessment:
    - • Feet turn out.
    - • Knees fall in.

Static Standing Adductor Stretch

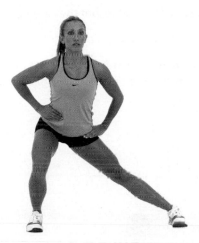

- *Other name(s):* Inner hip stretch.

- *Muscle(s) lengthened:* Adductors.

- *Performance technique:* Begin by standing with the legs spread far apart (normal adductor ROM is approximately 45 degrees). The majority of the adductors assist in hip flexion; therefore, a slight hip extension will be performed by stepping the nonstretching leg forward. A general rule of thumb is to line the heel of the nonstretching leg's foot up with the toes of the stretching leg's foot. Keep the feet parallel and face directly ahead. Place the hands on hips and, while keeping the torso upright, contract the glutes and quadriceps on the stretching leg and then shift the weight sideways toward the forward leg. The forward leg will bend at the hip, knee, and ankle; the rear leg (stretching leg) stays extended.

Flexibility Exercises *continued*

- *Progressions and regressions:*
  - ▸ If the stretch is uncomfortable, reduce the amount of forward lean.
  - ▸ If more stretch is needed, lean more or raise the arm on the opposite side from the stretch.
  - ▸ If the position is difficult to maintain, perform the stretch in a chair or on a stability ball.

- *Common form mistakes:*
  - ▸ *Foot not straight*: The most common mistake is to rotate the foot out in an attempt to get more motion from the stretch. This allows the adductors to shorten and may feel like a hamstring stretch. Both feet should point straight ahead.
  - ▸ *Leaning forward at the hip*: The torso needs to stay upright to keep the center of gravity over the hips. A forward lean allows the hips to flex, possibly shortening some of the adductors.

- *Cues to correct:*
  - ▸ "Engage the core, glutes, and quadriceps, and slowly shift the weight."
  - ▸ "Take to the first point of tension and hold."
  - ▸ "Stretches may be uncomfortable, but they are not intended to cause pain."

- *Plane of motion where movement occurs:* Frontal.

- *Kinetic chain checkpoints and movement dysfunctions affecting correct technique:*
  - ▸ Static stretch the calves if the client has the following dysfunctions during the overhead squat assessment:
    - • Knees go in.
    - • Anterior pelvic tilt.
    - • Feet turn out.

Static Biceps Femoris Stretch

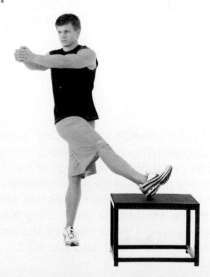

- *Other name(s):* Lateral hamstring stretch.

- *Muscle(s) lengthened:* Biceps femoris.

- *Performance technique:* Begin by standing near a small box or bench. Place the leg to be stretched on the box, with the leg adducted across the front of the body, the knee extended, and the toes pointing toward the sky. Then, contract the core and quadriceps on the stretching leg, and slowly lean forward at the hip until a stretch is felt.

- *Progressions and regressions:*
  - If the stretch is uncomfortable, reduce the amount of forward lean.
  - If more stretch is needed, lean forward more.
  - If a standing position cannot be maintained, perform the stretch in a seated or supine position.

- *Alternatives and related exercises:*
  - SMR of the hamstrings.
  - Hamstring stretch.

- *Common form mistakes:*
  - *Foot not straight*: The most common mistake is to rotate the foot out. Rotating the foot out in this position is an external hip rotation, which will shorten the biceps femoris.
  - *Rounded forward through the back and not in the hip*: When the biceps femoris is short, a stretch is often felt with no forward lean. Oftentimes this leads to excessive lumbar flexion, as opposed to hip flexion, which does not benefit the stretch and may predispose the individual to back pain.
  - *Performing stand-to-reach/sit-to-reach to stretch the hamstrings*: The sit-to-reach is a measurement of the extensibility of the muscles, tendons, and ligaments all through the posterior aspect of the body. It also stretches the hamstrings. Also, do not confuse medial hamstring stretches with lateral hamstring stretches. Oftentimes the medial hamstrings are overstretched.

- *Cues to correct:*
  - "Engage the core and quadriceps, and slowly lean forward at the hips with the toes up and leg across the front of the body."
  - "Take to the first point of tension and hold."
  - "Stretches may be uncomfortable, but they are not intended to cause pain."

- *Plane of motion where movement occurs:* Sagittal.

- *Kinetic chain checkpoints and movement dysfunctions affecting correct technique:*
  - Static stretch the biceps femoris if the client has the following dysfunctions during the overhead squat assessment:
    - Toes turn out.
    - Knees go in.

Flexibility Exercises *continued*

Static Sternocleidomastoid Stretch

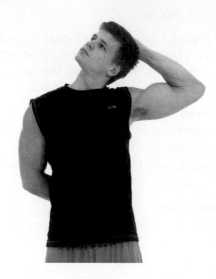

- *Other name(s):* Front neck stretch.

- *Muscle(s) lengthened:* Sternocleidomastoid.

- *Performance technique:* Begin by standing in a neutral position, with feet parallel, hips neutral, and hands at sides. To stretch the right sternocleidomastoid, tilt the head to the left as far as possible while allowing no rotation. Once in this position, begin slowly rotating the head towards the sky by looking up. Attempt to look directly to the sky and not over the right shoulder. Take to the first point of tension.

- *Progressions and regressions:*
  - If the stretch is uncomfortable, reduce the amount of rotation and look up.
  - If more stretch is needed, rotate more.
  - If the position is difficult to achieve or maintain, perform a simple scalene stretch.

- *Common form mistakes:*
  - *Not laterally tilting to tension*: The sternocleidomastoid is a same-side tilter, opposite-side rotator, and neck flexor. In order to stretch, the opposing motions must be performed. Begin with the lateral flexion or opposite side tilt until the sternocleidomastoid is stretched, then rotate.
  - *Attempting to look over the shoulder and not toward the sky:* A simple rotation of the head to look over the shoulder does not put the neck into the necessary extension to stretch the muscle.

- ***Cues to correct:***
    - ▸ "Tilt the head to the side, and raise your chin up to look to the sky."
    - ▸ "Take to the first point of tension and hold."
    - ▸ "Stretches may be uncomfortable, but they are not intended to cause pain."

- ***Plane of motion where movement occurs:*** Frontal.

- ***Kinetic chain checkpoints and movement dysfunctions affecting correct technique:***
    - ▸ Static stretch the SCM if the client has the following dysfunction during the overhead squat assessment:
        - • Forward head.

Static Upper Trapezius/Scalenes Stretch

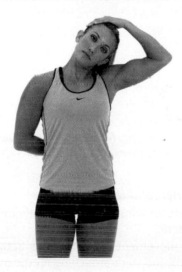

- ***Other name(s):*** Rear neck stretch.

- ***Muscle(s) lengthened:*** Upper trapezius and scalenes.

- ***Performance technique:*** Begin by standing in a neutral position, with feet parallel, hips neutral, and hands at sides. To stretch the right upper trapezius and scalenes, tilt the head to the left as far as possible while allowing no rotation. Once in this position, reach the same side arm (right) toward the ground to assist in depressing the scapula. Take to the first point of tension.

- ***Progressions and regressions:***
    - ▸ If the stretch is uncomfortable, reduce the amount of lateral tilt.
    - ▸ If more stretch is needed, tilt more.
    - ▸ If the position cannot be maintained, it should not be performed.

Flexibility Exercises *continued*

- ***Common form mistakes:***
  - ▸ *Elevating the shoulder*: Shoulder elevation allows the muscle to shorten.

- ***Cues to correct:***
  - ▸ "Keep the head neutral in rotation and only flex laterally, or tilt the head away from the stretch."
  - ▸ "Reach the arm toward the floor."
  - ▸ "Take to the first point of tension and hold."
  - ▸ "Stretches may be uncomfortable, but they are not intended to cause pain."

- ***Plane of motion where movement occurs:*** Frontal.

- ***Kinetic chain checkpoints and movement dysfunctions affecting correct technique:***
  - ▸ Static stretch the upper trapezius and scalenes if the client has the following dysfunctions during the overhead squat assessment:
    - • Arms fall forward.
    - • Forward head.

Active-Isolated Stretching

- ***General active-isolated stretching performance technique:*** For all active-isolated stretches, take the stretch to the first point of tension and hold for 1–2 seconds. Repeat this for 5–10 repetitions per set.

- ***Contraindications and special considerations:***
  - ▸ Active-isolated stretches are suggested for preactivity warm-up, as long as no postural distortions are present.
  - ▸ If an individual has movement compensations, active-isolated stretching should be performed after SMR and static stretching for the overactive muscles.
  - ▸ Do not perform if experiencing joint instability.
  - ▸ Do not perform with diseases affecting the tissues to be stretched, such as rheumatoid arthritis or conditions that have altered connective tissue properties.
  - ▸ Do not perform in the area of an acute injury. Consult a physician prior to beginning a stretching program after an injury.
  - ▸ Stop stretching immediately and consult a physician if excessive pain is experienced.
  - ▸ Do not force a joint beyond its normal ROM.
  - ▸ Take precautions with clients who have been diagnosed with osteoporosis.
  - ▸ Avoid aggressive stretching.
  - ▸ Do not stretch muscles that have apparent swelling and inflammation.
  - ▸ Make sure to continue to breathe during the stretch.

- ***General active-isolated stretching myths and misconceptions:***
  - ▸ *"Active stretching is better for warm-up."* Active stretching is great for warm-up because it uses surrounding muscles to assist in the stretch. However, it should only be performed alone if the client does not have movement compensations. In the presence of movement compensations, begin with SMR and static stretching on the muscles identified as being overactive.
  - ▸ *"More is better."* More is never better. Muscles can only be stretched a small amount before tissue damage results. Only take to the first point of tension and hold. Over time, the motion will increase.

Active Kneeling Hip Flexor Stretch

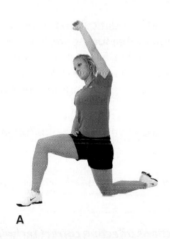

A

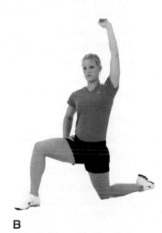

B

- ***Other name(s):*** Knee stretch, front hip stretch.

- ***Muscle(s) lengthened:*** Quadriceps.

- ***Performance technique:*** Begin by getting into a half-kneeling position, with the hip to be stretched on the down leg and the free leg at 90 degrees with the foot flat on the ground. Internally rotate the back hip to target the psoas muscle or maintain a neutral position to target the rectus femoris. Raise the arm aligned with the down knee overhead. Contract the glutes on the down leg to posteriorly tilt the hips (imagine the hips are a bowl of water and try to "pour the water out the back"). Once this is achieved, shift the hips forward until the first point of tension is felt. Side bend and rotate the body posteriorly. Hold the stretch for 1-2 seconds and repeat for 5-10 repetitions.

Flexibility Exercises *continued*

- ***Progressions and regressions:***
  - ▸ If the stretch is uncomfortable, reduce the amount of forward lean.
  - ▸ If more stretch is needed, elevate the rear foot on a foam roller and/or add in an arm reach toward the sky.
  - ▸ If the position is difficult to maintain, the hip flexor stretch can be performed in the standing position.

- ***Common form mistakes:***
  - ▸ *Hips not posteriorly tilted*: The most common mistake is for the hips to dip forward, thereby allowing the hip flexor muscles to stay shortened. The efficacy of this stretch relies on the posterior tilt.
  - ▸ *Stretching too far*: It is common for individuals to feel the need to overstretch this area. This is often done with the half-kneeling position, while no posterior tilt is performed via shifting the hips a far distance forward. This incorrectly stretches ligaments in the hip and compresses the lower back.
  - ▸ *Standing quadriceps stretch*: The standing stretch is difficult to perform correctly. First, balance is an issue for many people. Remember that for the stretch to work it needs to be held for 30 seconds while standing on one leg. Second, the position of the knee in the stretching leg, when the foot is held back against the glutes, far exceeds the recommended 120–130 degrees of flexion necessary to lengthen the quadriceps.

- ***Cues to correct:***
  - ▸ "Engage the core and glutes to tilt the hips and then shift the hips forward to the first point of tension."
  - ▸ "Take to the first point of tension and hold."
  - ▸ "Stretches may be uncomfortable, but they are not intended to cause pain."

- ***Plane of motion where movement occurs:*** Sagittal.

- ***Kinetic chain checkpoints and movement dysfunctions affecting correct technique:***
  - ▸ Active-isolated stretch the quadriceps/hip flexors, after static stretching and SMR, if the client has the following dysfunctions during the overhead squat assessment:
    - • Excessive forward lean.
    - • Anterior pelvic tilt.
    - • Feet turn out.
    - • Knees go in.

Active Ball Piriformis Stretch

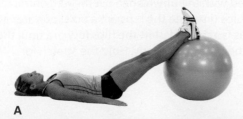
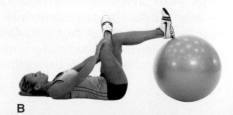

A   B

- **Other name(s):** Rear hip stretch.

- **Muscle(s) lengthened:** Piriformis.

- **Performance technique:** Begin by lying on a flat surface with both legs extended and heels resting on a ball. The spine must remain in a neutral position. Place the heel of the leg to be stretched on the mid-thigh of the nonstretching leg. Use the opposite hand to grab the ankle and hold the foot from slipping. Place the same-side hand on the knee of the stretching leg and pull toward the opposite shoulder keeping the heel on the ball. Take until the first point of tension is felt. Hold the stretch for 1-2 seconds and repeat for 5-10 repetitions.

- **Progressions and regressions:**
  - If the stretch is uncomfortable, reduce the amount of pull.
  - If more stretch is needed, pull more.
  - If the position on the floor cannot be maintained, then perform the stretch while standing with the leg on a table or chair.

- **Common form mistakes:**
  - *Performing the stretch when not needed*: The overhead squat assessment should indicate whether these muscles are short. In the majority of the population the knees fall in, which means the abductor and external rotator (piriformis) are not short and do not need to be stretched. Corrective stretching is indicated only if the knees go out; however, brief active-isolated performance of this stretch can be quite beneficial for general warm-up and movement prep.
  - *Performing with the leg crossed over the opposing leg*: This stretch is not incorrect, but it is not the most advantageous position to stretch the intended muscle due to common tightness in the posterior hip capsule.
  - *Not feeling the stretch when performed correctly*: If the stretch is performed correctly and is not felt, then revisit the overhead squat assessment to verify that the area needs to be stretched.

- **Cues to correct:**
  - "Stabilize the foot and slowly pull the knee toward the opposite shoulder."
  - "Take to the first point of tension and hold."
  - "Stretches may be uncomfortable, but they are not intended to cause pain."

- **Plane of motion where movement occurs:** Sagittal.

- **Kinetic chain checkpoints (plus movement dysfunctions affecting correct technique):**
  - Active-isolated stretch the piriformis, after static stretching and SMR, if the client has the following dysfunction during the overhead squat assessment:
    - Knees bow out.

Flexibility Exercises *continued*

Active Supine Biceps Femoris Stretch

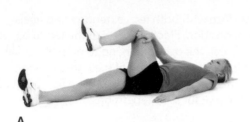

A

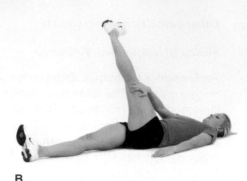

B

- *Other name(s):* Lateral hamstring stretch.

- *Muscle(s) lengthened:* Biceps femoris, short head.

- *Performance technique:* Begin by lying on the back on a flat surface. Bring the leg to be stretched toward the chest so the hip is flexed greater than 90 degrees, while slightly adducting the leg across the body. Use the opposite hand to stabilize the leg by placing it behind the knee. Place the fingers on the short head of the biceps femoris. Engage the core and extend the knee until the first point of tension is felt. Hold the stretch for 1-2 seconds and repeat for 5-10 repetitions.

- *Progressions and regressions:*
  - ‣ If the stretch is uncomfortable, reduce the amount of knee extension.
  - ‣ If more stretch is needed, extend more.

- *Common form mistakes:*
  - ‣ *Foot not straight*: A common mistake is to rotate the foot out. Rotating the foot out in this position is external hip rotation, which will shorten the biceps femoris.
  - ‣ *Letting the hip extend*: The hip should remain flexed past 90 degrees. If the hip begins to extend, the stretch is reduced from the biceps femoris.

- *Cues to correct:*
  - ‣ "Engage the core and quadriceps, and slowly lean forward at the hip with toes up and leg across front of body."
  - ‣ "Take to the first point of tension and hold."
  - ‣ "Stretches may be uncomfortable, but they are not intended to cause pain."

- *Plane of motion where movement occurs:* Sagittal.

- *Kinetic chain checkpoints and movement dysfunctions affecting correct technique:*
  - ‣ Active-isolated stretch the biceps femoris, after static stretching and SMR, if the client has the following dysfunctions during the overhead squat assessment:
    - • Feet turn out.
    - • Knees go in.

Active Latissimus Dorsi Stretch

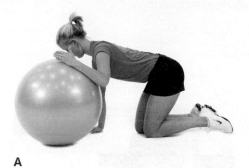

A

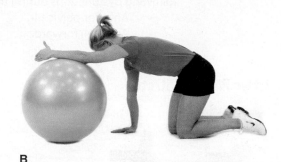

B

- *Other name(s):* Shoulder stretch.

- *Muscle(s) lengthened:* Latissimus dorsi.

- *Performance technique:* Begin by kneeling near a stability ball, box, or chair. Place the arm to be stretched on the ball and support the upper body with nonstretching arm by placing it under the shoulder. Rotate the thumb of the stretching arm up, reaching forward with the arm and shifting the hips back toward the heels. This position should be similar to the yoga position "child's pose," with the low back slightly flexed to further increase the stretch. Hold the stretch for 1-2 seconds and repeat for 5-10 repetitions.

- *Progressions and regressions:*
  - If the stretch is uncomfortable, shift the body forward or turn the palm flat to reduce the stretch.
  - If more stretch is needed, flex the back more or externally rotate the shoulder.
  - If kneeling position cannot be maintained, perform the stretch standing with the arm on a wall.

- *Common form mistakes:*
  - *Arching of the low back*: It is common for the low back arch with this stretch, essentially allowing the latissimus dorsi to shorten. Encourage a flexed or neutral lumbar spine.
  - *Bending the elbow*: The arm should be fully outstretched over the head.
  - *Not supporting the head*: The cervical spine should remain neutral.

- *Cues to correct:*
  - "Rotate the thumb to the sky, reach forward to engage the shoulder, and shift the hips toward the heels."
  - "Take to the first point of tension and hold."
  - "Stretches may be uncomfortable, but they are not intended to cause pain."

- *Plane of motion where movement occurs:* Sagittal.

Flexibility Exercises *continued*

- ***Kinetic chain checkpoints and movement dysfunctions affecting correct technique:***
  - ▸ Active-isolated stretch the lats, after static stretching and SMR, if the client has the following dysfunctions during the overhead squat assessment:
    - • Anterior pelvic tilt.
    - • Arms fall forward.

Active Pectoral Stretch

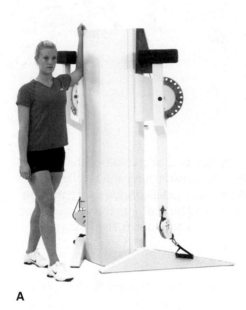

A

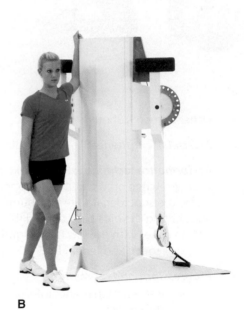

B

- ***Other name(s):*** Shoulder stretch.

- ***Muscle(s) stretched:*** Pectoralis major.

- ***Performance technique:*** Begin by standing near a corner or doorway. Place the stretching arm on the corner with the elbow at approximately shoulder height and bent to 90 degrees. The doorway will ensure that the arm is at 90 degrees. Engage the core, squeeze the shoulder blades, and then step the body forward about a half step or until tension is felt. Hold the stretch for 1-2 seconds and repeat for 5-10 repetitions.

- ***Progressions and regressions:***
  - ▸ If the stretch is uncomfortable, reduce the amount of lean forward.
  - ▸ If more stretch is needed, lean more or turn the head away from the stretching arm.
  - ▸ If the position cannot be maintained due to shoulder pain, perform with elbow extended, similar to the bicep stretch.

- ***Common form mistakes:***
  - ▸ *Proper standing posture not maintained*: Stand with the core engaged, and the hips and shoulders facing square and ahead.
  - ▸ *Not squeezing the shoulder blades*: To squeeze the shoulder blades the rhomboids must be engaged, leading to a better pectoral stretch.

- ***Cues to correct:***
  - ▸ "Engage the core and glutes, and slowly lean forward."
  - ▸ "Take to the first point of tension and hold."
  - ▸ "Stretches may be uncomfortable, but they are not intended to cause pain."

- ***Plane of motion where movement occurs:*** Sagittal.

- ***Kinetic chain checkpoints and movement dysfunctions affecting correct technique:***
  - ▸ Active-isolated stretch the pectorals, after static stretching and SMR, if the client has the following dysfunction during the overhead squat assessment:
    - • Arms fall forward.

Dynamic Stretching

- ***General performance technique:*** Dynamic stretching should be performed at a smooth, controlled speed to simulate normal, functional movement. Perform dynamic stretches for up to 10 repetitions per set.

- ***Contraindications and special considerations:***
  - ▸ Do not perform dynamic stretching alone in the presence of movement compensations or muscle imbalances. If muscle imbalances are present, perform SMR and static stretching prior to dynamic stretching.
  - ▸ The chosen exercise should complement the daily training session.
  - ▸ No movement dysfunction should be apparent when using dynamic flexibility.
  - ▸ Dynamic stretches use available ROM.

- ***Myths and misconceptions:***
  - ▸ *"Ballistic stretching is better."* Ballistic stretching is a type of stretching that involves rapid, repetitive bouncing movements. This is not the preferred method of stretching within the OPT model. Movements should be smooth and controlled. Oftentimes, ballistic stretching forces a joint past its ideal ROM, increasing the chance of injury.

Flexibility Exercises *continued*

Prisoner Squat

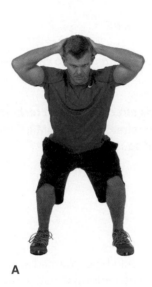

A

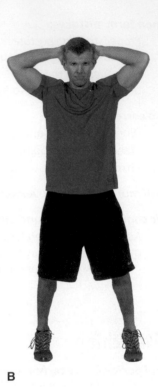

B

- *Performance technique:* Stand in a shoulder-width stance with toes pointed straight ahead. Keeping an upright torso, place the hands behind the head while pulling the shoulders and elbows back. Lower into a squat position by pushing the hips back and bending the knees. Lower as far as can be controlled with proper form and then extend the hips, knees, and ankles to return to a standing position.

- *Progressions and regressions:*
  - To increase the stretch, attempt to squat lower and then stand up to toes (triple extension) before repeating.
  - To decrease the stretch, do not squat as low or hold arms in front of the body to offset the center of gravity.

- *Common form mistakes:*
  - Performing the exercise in a fast, more ballistic pattern.
  - Allowing the feet to turn out or the knees to fall inward.

- *Cues to correct:*
  - "Use the muscles to take the joints through the full ROM."
  - "Do not use a bouncing motion."
  - "Sit back into the heels."
  - "Draw in the core to keep the back in neutral alignment."

- ***Plane of motion where movement occurs:*** Sagittal.

- ***Kinetic chain checkpoints:***
  - ‣ Feet shoulder-width apart pointed straight ahead.
  - ‣ Knees in line with the feet.
  - ‣ Lumbo-pelvic-hip complex (LPHC) in neutral position with back parallel to shins through the squat.
  - ‣ Shoulders pulled back and elbows in line with neck and trunk.
  - ‣ Chin tucked to keep head and neck in neutral alignment.

Multiplanar Lunge with Reach

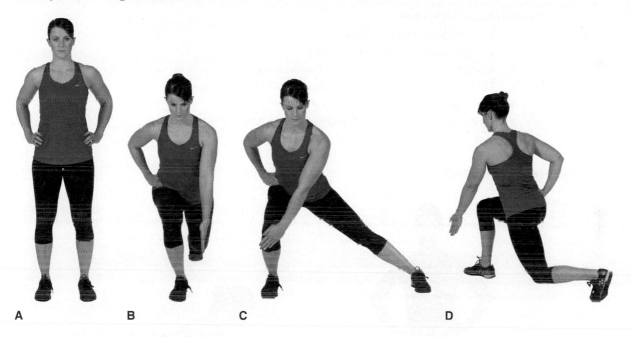

A   B   C   D

- ***Performance technique:*** Stand in proper alignment with hands on hips and feet straight ahead. Engage the core. While maintaining total body alignment, step forward (sagittal plane), and descend into a lunge position while reaching the opposite hand toward the forward toe. Use the hips and thigh muscles to push back up into standing position. Then, perform the lunge by stepping to the side (frontal plane), reaching the opposite hand toward the toe, and return to standing position. Next, perform a turning lunge (transverse plane), with the opposite hand reaching toward the toe, and return to standing. All three motions make for one repetition.

Flexibility Exercises *continued*

- *Progressions and regressions:*
  - ‣ To increase the stretch, increase the range of motion.
  - ‣ To decrease the stretch, perform it in only one or two planes of motion.

- *Common form mistakes:*
  - ‣ Performing the exercise in a quicker, more ballistic pattern or with improper form.

- *Cues to correct:*
  - ‣ "Use the muscles to take the joints through the full ROM."
  - ‣ "Do not perform in a bouncing motion."
  - ‣ "Reach for the ground."

- *Plane of motion where movement occurs:* Multiplanar.

- *Kinetic chain checkpoints:*
  - ‣ Feet pointed straight ahead.
  - ‣ Lunging knee in line with the foot.
  - ‣ Nonlunging leg straight and in line with torso.
  - ‣ LPHC in neutral position with back parallel to lunging shin.
  - ‣ Shoulders in line with neck and trunk.
  - ‣ Chin tucked to keep head and neck in neutral alignment.

Single-Leg Squat Touchdown

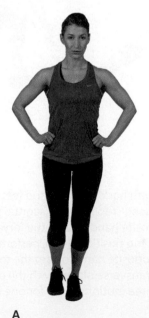

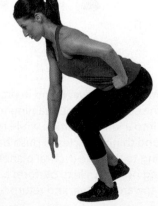

A   B

- **Performance technique:** Begin in a single-leg standing posture with optimal form. Keeping the raised leg parallel to the standing leg, engage the core and squat in a controlled manner. Bend the ankle, knee, and hip while reaching the opposite hand toward the stance leg's toes. Return to the standing position by extending the hip, knee, and ankle. Complete one set for each leg.

- **Progressions and regressions:**
  - To increase the stretch, squat lower or add a small weight to the reaching arm.
  - To decrease the stretch, do not squat as low.

- **Common form mistakes:**
  - Performing the exercise in a quicker, more ballistic pattern or with improper form.

- **Cues to correct:**
  - "Pick a spot on the floor 10 feet in front of you and keep your eyes on it."
  - "Tuck the chin."
  - "Sit back like you're in a chair."

- **Plane of motion where movement occurs:** Sagittal.

- **Kinetic chain checkpoints:**
  - Foot pointed straight ahead.
  - Knee in line with the foot.
  - LPHC in neutral position with back parallel to the shin through the squat.
  - Shoulders in line with neck and trunk.
  - Chin tucked to keep head and neck in neutral alignment.

Lateral Tube Walking

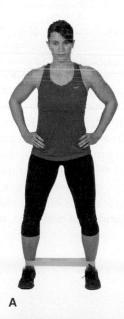
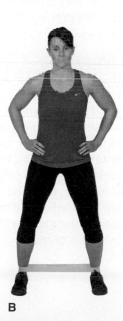

A   B

Flexibility Exercises *continued*

- **Performance technique:** Stand with feet hip-width apart, knees slightly bent, and feet straight ahead. Place a small band around both legs near the knees. Engage the core, keep the feet straight ahead, and take small steps sideways without allowing the knees to cave inward. Complete a full set for both the left and right directions.

- **Progressions and regressions:**
    - To increase the stretch, keep the feet further apart.
    - If the position cannot be maintained, perform the stretch without the band.

- **Common form mistakes:**
    - Using too strong a band.
    - Taking too large of steps.
    - Turning the feet out.
    - Allowing the knees to cave inward.

- **Cues to correct:**
    - "Begin light and work up over time."
    - "Take small steps. Begin at hip width and step to shoulder width, no wider."
    - "Keep the feet parallel, as if on a pair of skis."
    - "Keep the knees pulled out to maximize the use of the glutes."

- **Plane of motion where movement occurs:** Frontal.

- **Kinetic chain checkpoints:**
    - Feet pointed straight ahead.
    - Knees in line with the feet and slightly bent.
    - LPHC in neutral position to ensure a straight back.
    - Shoulders in line with neck and hips.
    - Chin tucked so the head and neck are in proper cervical alignment.

- **Myths and misconceptions:**
    - *"Around the feet is harder, and therefore better."* The band around the feet or ankles may be harder, but it is often associated with poor form and reduced effectiveness. When the band is around the feet/ankles it is further away from the pivot point (hip), and therefore has a longer lever arm, requiring more muscular effort than when the band is around the knees. This additional resistance makes it harder to move, and can lead to compensations from other unintended muscles. In addition, when both feet are on the ground, then the hip abductor muscles are able to relax with the band around the feet/ankles. To maximize the effects of this exercise, the band should small enough to where the knees must be held together to put it on. Then, when the knees get in proper alignment the glutes are already engaged. In this instance, the glutes will be engaged during the entire set, which is usually close to 90 seconds or more.

Push-Up with Rotation

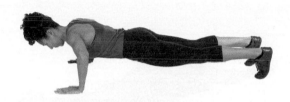

A

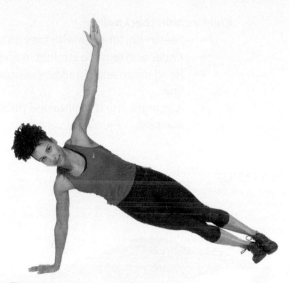

B

- *Performance technique:* Begin in a push-up position with the feet together and toes on the floor. Hands should be placed slightly wider than shoulder-width apart. Engage the core, while keeping the spine neutral, and lower the chest to the floor. Push back to starting position, then rotate the body 90 degrees from the floor and fully extend one arm toward the sky. Reverse the movement of rotation and return to the starting position. Perform the next push-up with rotation to the opposite side to complete one repetition.

- *Progressions and regressions:* If full push-ups are too difficult, the exercise can be performed with knees on the ground. Leave only one knee on the ground during the rotation.

- *Common form mistakes:*
  - Performing the exercise in a quicker, more ballistic pattern.
  - Allowing the hips to drop when rotated.
  - Excessive arching or rounding of the back during the push-up.

- *Cues to correct:*
  - "Squeeze the quads and glutes, and engage the core to straighten the back and legs."
  - "Point the tip of your nose straight down at the floor."
  - "Rotate and reach up to the sky."
  - "Form a sideways T."

- *Plane of motion where movement occurs:* Sagittal, transverse.

Flexibility Exercises *continued*

- *Kinetic chain checkpoints:*
    - ‣ Feet in dorsiflexion with toes on the ground.
    - ‣ Knees and legs are straight in line with the back.
    - ‣ Head down and shoulders neutral, so that the neck, back, hips, and legs form a straight line.
    - ‣ A straight line is maintained through the body during the rotational portion of the exercise.

Iron Cross

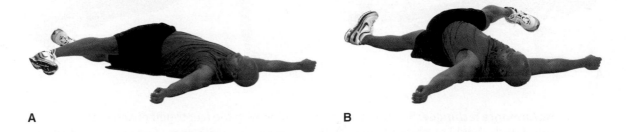

A   B

- *Performance technique:* Lie flat on the back with arms outstretched to the sides. Begin by kicking one leg up to approximately 90 degrees of hip flexion with the knee extended. Lower the leg back to ground and repeat on the other side to complete one repetition.

- *Progressions and regressions:*
    - ‣ To increase the stretch, attempt to kick the leg higher.
    - ‣ To decrease the stretch, do not kick as high.

- *Common form mistakes:*
    - ‣ The back comes off the floor. Do not strain or excessively reach to touch the toes.
    - ‣ The leg does not stay fully extended.

- *Cues to correct:*
    - ‣ "Push your back to the floor to stay flat."
    - ‣ "Aim for toes to fingers."

- *Plane of motion where movement occurs:* Tranverse.

- *Kinetic chain checkpoints:*
    - ‣ Body lies flat on the ground.
    - ‣ Stretching leg and arm are fully extended through the movement.

Scorpion

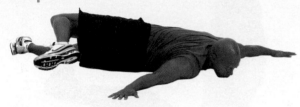

A

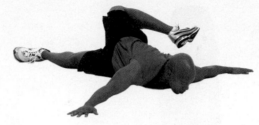

B

- *Performance technique:* Lie on the stomach, with the arms outstretched and feet flexed so that only the toes are touching the ground. Rotate at the hips and kick the right foot over the body toward the left arm, while keeping the arms, shoulders, and trunk in contact with the floor, and lower it back to the starting position. Then repeat with the left foot toward the right arm. Perform as a slow, controlled motion.

- *Progressions and regressions:*
    - To increase the stretch, attempt to kick the leg higher toward the hand.
    - To decrease the stretch, do not kick as high.

- *Common form mistakes:*
    - Not keeping core, arms, and shoulders in contact with the ground.
    - Forcing the stretch in a ballistic manner, moving too fast.

- *Cues to correct:*
    - "Push your stomach into the floor."
    - "Push your fingers into the ground."

- *Plane of motion where movement occurs:* Sagittal, transverse.

- *Kinetic chain checkpoints:*
    - Arms, shoulders, and nonmoving side stay in contact with the ground at all times.
    - Arms and nonmoving leg fully extended (body forms a "T").

Straight-Leg March

- *Other name(s):* Walking kick.

- *Performance technique:* In a forward walking motion, kick one leg straight out in front with the toes flexed toward the sky. Attempt to kick the outstretched hand. Drop the leg and repeat with the opposite side to complete one repetition. Maintain an upright neutral spine throughout the exercise.

Flexibility Exercises *continued*

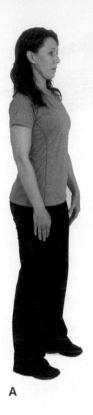

A

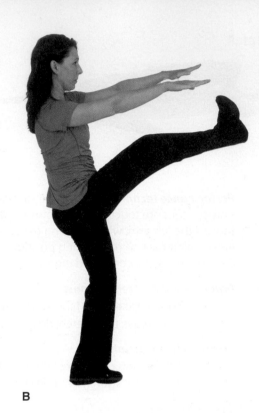

B

- • *Progressions and regressions:*
  - ‣ To increase the stretch, attempt to kick the foot higher toward the hand.
  - ‣ To decrease the stretch, do not kick as high in an attempt to touch the toe.

- • *Common form mistakes:*
  - ‣ Bending at the hips or back.
  - ‣ Dropping the hands to allow the toes to touch the fingers.

- • *Cues to correct:*
  - ‣ "Balance a glass of water on the back of your hand."
  - ‣ "Tuck your chin and engage your core to keep your back straight."
  - ‣ "Kick up to the hand."

- • *Plane of motion where movement occurs:* Sagittal.

- • *Kinetic chain checkpoints:*
  - ‣ Feet pointed straight ahead and parallel.
  - ‣ Knees in line with feet.
  - ‣ Hips, back, shoulders, and neck in straight alignment.

Inchworms

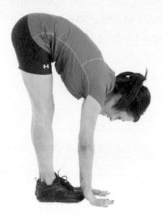

A

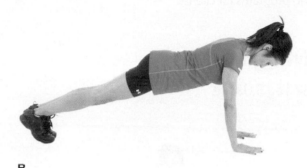

B

- *Other name(s):* Handwalks.

- *Performance technique:* Stand straight with optimal posture, legs together, and toes pointing straight ahead. Bend over at the hip until both hands are on the ground, then walk the hands forward until the back is straight (push-up position). Keeping the legs straight, then walk the hands back toward the feet. Complete this sequence for one repetition.

- *Progressions: and regressions:*
  ‣ For an added strength element, perform a push-up at the bottom of the exercise.
  ‣ For additional challenge to shoulder stabilizers, walk hands out with arms straight past pushup position.

- *Common form mistakes:*
  ‣ Sagging the back.
  ‣ Bending the knees or elbows.
  ‣ Not maintaining a neutral spine.

- *Cues to correct:*
  ‣ "Walk hands in only as far as is comfortable while keeping the legs straight, then slowly curl up to standing."
  ‣ "Tuck your chin and engage your core to keep your back in neutral alignment."

- *Plane of motion where movement occurs:* Sagittal.

- *Kinetic chain checkpoints:*
  ‣ Feet pointed straight ahead and parallel.
  ‣ Knees in line with feet with legs straight.
  ‣ Hinge at the hips.
  ‣ Back, shoulders, and neck in neutral alignment.

Resistance Training

Resistance training is the core of the OPT model. In order to progress through the levels, numerous and varied exercises are needed to gain the adaptations of increased balance, strength, and power. Given the ever-changing fitness environment, a number of modalities will be discussed here in order to provide the fitness professional with a comprehensive base from which to develop creative and dynamic progressive training programs for clients.

Bodyweight Exercise

Single-Leg Balance

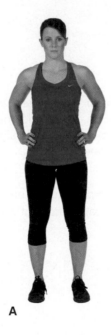
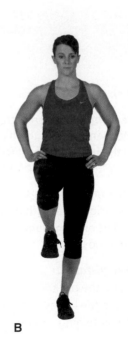

A B

- **Other name(s):** N/A.
- **Exercise classification:** Balance Stabilization.
- **Joint(s) where motion occurs:**
  - Knee.
  - LPHC.
- **Performance technique:** With hands on the hips raise one leg, bending at the knee, to a 90-degree position and hold for the required amount of time. Lower the foot and alternate legs for the recommended repetitions.

- *Force-couples:*
  - ‣ *Agonists*: Gluteus maximus/medius, quadriceps, hip flexors.
  - ‣ *Synergists*: Hamstrings complex, gastrocnemius.

- *Alternatives and related exercises:* N/A.

- *Progressions:*
  - ‣ Perform the exercise on a balance pad.
  - ‣ Lunge to balance—frontal plane.

- *Regression:* Two-leg standing on a balance pad.

- *Common form mistakes:*
  - ‣ Removing hands from hips to balance.
  - ‣ Foot not pointing straight ahead.

- *Cues to correct:* "Engage the core to maintain balance and stability."

- *Contraindications and special considerations:* N/A.

- *Plane of motion where movement occurs:* N/A

- *Kinetic chain checkpoints:*
  - ‣ Ankles, knees, and hips align at starting position.
  - ‣ Maintain neutral spine throughout.

Prone Iso-Abs

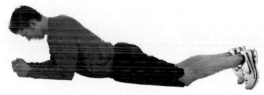

A

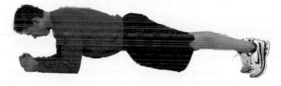

B

- *Other name(s):* Front plank.

- *Exercise classification:* Core Stabilization.

- *Joint(s) where motion occurs:* N/A.

- *Performance technique:* Place both elbows on the ground with hands parallel, straight ahead, and shoulder-width apart. Have the feet in dorsiflexion with toes on the ground. Engage the abs, glutes, and quadriceps to raise the hips off the ground and form a straight line from the shoulders to the ankles. Hold in position for the desired amount of time.

Resistance Training *continued*

- *Force-couples:*
  - ‣ *Agonists*: Rectus abdominus, quadriceps, anterior deltoids.
  - ‣ *Synergists*: Gluteus maximus/medius, pectorals, latissimus dorsi.

- *Alternatives and related exercises:* Side plank.

- *Progression:* Single-leg front plank.

- *Regressions:*
  - ‣ Quadruped drawing in.
  - ‣ Quadruped arm and opposite leg raise.

- *Common form mistakes:*
  - ‣ Arching or rounding back; dropping or raising hips.
  - ‣ Elevating shoulders.
  - ‣ Head falling or cervical spine extension.

- *Cues to correct:*
  - ‣ "Squeeze the core, glutes, and quads to form a straight line."
  - ‣ "Don't allow the butt to drop or to stick up in the air."

- *Contraindications and special considerations:*
  - ‣ Do not perform with clients who are pregnant, as it is recommended to avoid supine and prone exercises, particularly after the first trimester.

- *Plane of motion where movement occurs:* N/A.

- *Kinetic chain checkpoints:*
  - ‣ Ankles, knees, hips, and shoulders all aligned.
  - ‣ Elbows bent, but static.

Floor Cobra

- *Other name(s):* Palms-down superman.

- *Exercise classification:* Core Stabilization.

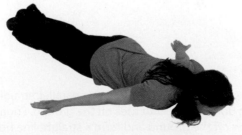
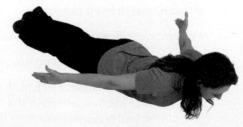

A   B

- **Joint(s) where motion occurs:**
  - Shoulders.
  - LPHC.

- **Performance technique:** Start by lying face down (prone) on the floor with arms at a reverse angle to the sides and palms up. Toes should remain touching the floor throughout the exercise. Engage the glutes, squeeze the shoulder blades together as if trying to hold a pencil between them, and lift the shoulders off the floor. The thumbs will be pointed up and arms externally rotated. The head should stay in line with the spine in a neutral position (do not look up or down). Hold this position and then slowly lower the shoulders back to the ground. Repeat for the desired number of repetitions.

- **Force-couples:**
  - *Agonists:* Latissimus dorsi, lower trapezius.
  - *Synergists:* Middle trapezius, erector spinae.

- **Alternatives and related exercises:** N/A.

- **Progression:** Stability ball cobra.

- **Regression:** Floor cobra with hands remaining on the floor.

- **Common form mistakes:**
  - Putting feet too far apart.
  - Arching back too far on the upward motion.
  - Fully extending shoulders to where the arms are above the head.
  - Rocking in a ballistic manner.

- **Cues to correct:**
  - "Squeeze a pencil between the shoulder blades."
  - "Keep your chin tucked and head still."
  - "Engage the glutes."

- **Contraindications and special considerations:**
  - Should not be performed with clients who exhibit excessive curvature of the spine during the overhead squat assessment.
  - Do not perform with clients who are pregnant, as it is recommended to avoid supine and prone exercises, particularly after the first trimester.

- **Plane of motion where movement occurs:** Sagittal.

- **Kinetic chain checkpoints:**
  - Toes remain on floor pointed straight down.
  - Legs fully extended with hips in line with spine.
  - Shoulders pull back and elevate off the floor during motion.
  - Head should be neutral with chin tucked to maintain optimal cervical alignment.

Resistance Training *continued*

Floor Bridge

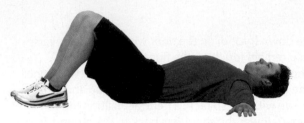

A

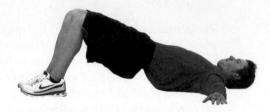

B

- *Other name(s):* N/A.

- *Exercise classification:* Core Stabilization.

- *Joint(s) where motion occurs:* LPHC.

- *Performance technique:* Start by lying on the back with feet flat on the floor and shoulder-width apart, with knees bent. Then lift hips off the floor until the knees, hips, and shoulders are all in alignment and hold for 3–5 seconds. Lower the hips slowly back to the floor and repeat for the desired number of repetitions.

- *Force-couples:*
    ‣ *Agonist*: Gluteus maximus.
    ‣ *Synergist*: Hamstrings complex, erector spinae.

- *Alternatives and related exercises:*
    ‣ Stability ball bridge.
    ‣ Bench bridge.

- *Progression:* Single-leg floor bridge.

- *Regression:* Supine marching.

- *Common form mistakes:*
    ‣ Raising hips too far off the floor and hyperextending the lower back.
    ‣ Performing the movement too quickly; not holding to stabilize.

- *Cues to correct:*
    ‣ "Drive through the heels."
    ‣ "Engage the core and squeeze the glutes to keep the back straight."

- *Contraindications and special considerations:*
    ‣ Do not perform with clients who are pregnant, as it is recommended to avoid supine and prone exercises, particularly after the first trimester.

- *Plane of motion where movement occurs:* Sagittal.

- ***Kinetic chain checkpoints:***
    - ‣ Feet pointed straight ahead and flat on the floor.
    - ‣ Knees hip- to shoulder-width apart and above heels.
    - ‣ Shoulders flat and relaxed on the floor.
    - ‣ Head rested on the floor with chin tucked to maintain cervical alignment.

Single-Leg Floor Bridge

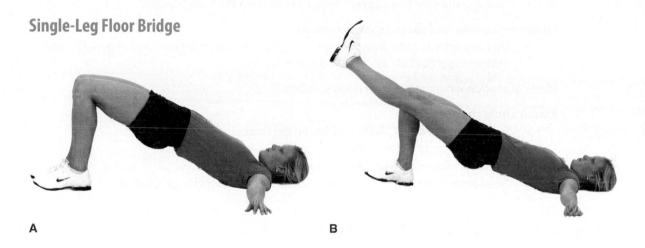

A   B

- ***Other name(s):*** N/A.
- ***Exercise classification:*** Core Stabilization.
- ***Joint(s) where motion occurs:*** LPHC.
- ***Performance technique:*** Start by lying on the back with feet flat on the floor and shoulder-width apart, with knees bent. Extend one leg fully, then lift hips off the floor until the knees, hips, and shoulders are all in alignment and hold for 3–5 seconds. Lower the hips slowly back to the floor and repeat with the other leg extended.
- ***Force-couples:***
    - ‣ *Agonist*: Gluteus maximus.
    - ‣ *Synergists*: Hamstrings complex, erector spinae.
- ***Alternatives and related exercises:***
    - ‣ Stability ball bridge.
    - ‣ Bench bridge.
- ***Progressions:***
    - ‣ Single-leg floor bridge with foot on unstable surface.
    - ‣ Bridge with feet in suspension trainer.
- ***Regression:*** Floor bridge.

Resistance Training *continued*

- *Common form mistakes:*
  - ‣ Raising hips too far off the floor and hyperextending the lower back.
  - ‣ Performing too fast; not holding to stabilize.

- *Cues to correct:*
  - ‣ "Drive through the heels."
  - ‣ "Engage the core and squeeze the glutes to keep the back straight."

- *Contraindications and special considerations:*
  - ‣ Do not perform with clients who are pregnant, as it is recommended to avoid supine exercises, particularly after the first trimester.

- *Plane of motion where movement occurs:* Sagittal.

- *Kinetic chain checkpoints:*
  - ‣ Feet pointed straight ahead and flat on the floor.
  - ‣ Knees hip- to shoulder-width apart and above heels.
  - ‣ Shoulders flat and relaxed on the floor.
  - ‣ Head rested on the floor with chin tucked to maintain cervical alignment.

Quadruped Opposite Arm and Opposite Leg Raise

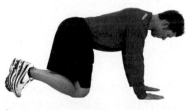
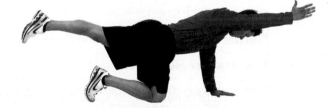

A   B

- *Other name(s):* Bird dogs.

- *Exercise classification:* Core Stabilization.

- *Joint(s) where motion occurs:*
  - ‣ Knee.
  - ‣ LPHC.
  - ‣ Shoulder.

- *Performance technique:* Start on hands and knees. Draw in the core and keep the chin tucked. Raise the arm straight ahead with the thumb pointed up, and fully extend the opposite leg behind while keeping the back flat, so a straight line can be drawn across the body. Hold for 3–5 seconds and repeat with the other side to complete one repetition. Repeat the sequence for the desired number of repetitions.

- **Force-couples:**
  - *Agonists*: Anterior deltoid, gluteus maximus.
  - *Synergists*: Upper/middle trapezius, quadriceps.

- **Alternatives and related exercises:**
  - Prone iso-abs.
  - Side iso-abs.

- **Progressions:**
  - Perform on an unstable surface, such as a foam pad.
  - Perform holding dumbbells.

- **Regression:** Perform prone arm and leg raises separately.

- **Common form mistakes:**
  - Arching low back.
  - Performing the exercise too quickly and not pausing at the top of the motion.

- **Cues to correct:**
  - "Draw in the core and squeeze the glutes to maintain a straight back."
  - "Legs and arms fully extended."
  - "Hold at the top for 2–3 seconds."

- **Contraindications and special considerations:**
  - Do not perform if client has excessive lower back arch.

- **Plane of motion where movement occurs:** Sagittal.

- **Kinetic chain checkpoints:**
  - Feet in dorsiflexion rested on toes.
  - Hips in neutral position with back straight.
  - Shoulders in neutral alignment with hips and neck.
  - Chin tucked so the neck is in straight alignment with the back.

- **Myths and misconceptions:**
  - *"Not a difficult core exercise."* This is a core stabilization exercise, and is meant to directly challenge the local musculature of the body. It should be used with clients in the Stabilization Endurance Phase of the OPT model to develop total body stability and balance.

Floor Crunch

- **Other name(s):** Crunches.

- **Exercise classification:** Core Strength.

Resistance Training *continued*

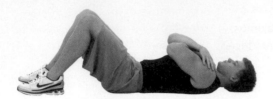
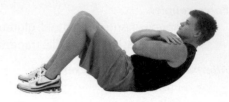

A   B

▸ ***Joint(s) where motion occurs:*** LPHC.
▸ ***Performance technique:*** Start by lying on the back with knees bent to 90 degrees and feet flat on the ground shoulder-width apart. Keep arms crossed over the chest throughout the exercise. Raise the upper back and shoulders off the ground by bending the thoracic spine. Hold the up position for approximately 1–2 seconds, then relax and return to the starting rest position. Repeat for the desired number of repetitions.

- ***Force-couples:***
    ▸ *Agonist*: Rectus abdominus.
    ▸ *Synergist*: Transverse abdominus, internal/external obliques.

- ***Alternatives and related exercises:***
    ▸ Sit-up.
    ▸ Reverse crunch.

- ***Progressions:***
    ▸ Stability ball crunch.
    ▸ Knee-up.

- ***Regressions:***
    ▸ Prone iso-abs.
    ▸ Supine marching.

- ***Common form mistakes:***
    ▸ Putting feet too close together.
    ▸ Hips coming off the floor.
    ▸ Hands coming off the chest.

- ***Cues to correct:***
    ▸ "Push heels into the ground, and pull up with the core, not the legs and hips."
    ▸ "Keep the feet planted and arms crossed over the chest."

- ***Contraindications and special considerations:***
    ▸ Do not perform if client has low back pain during flexion.

- ▸ Do not perform if client has posterior pelvic tilt or excessive rounding through the upper back.
- ▸ Do not perform with clients who are pregnant, as it is recommended to avoid supine and prone exercises, particularly after the first trimester.

- *Plane of motion where movement occurs:* Sagittal.

- *Kinetic chain checkpoints:*
  - ▸ Feet flat on floor.
  - ▸ Shoulders remain still but lift off the floor in a controlled manner.
  - ▸ Head should be neutral with cervical spine in straight alignment.

Reverse Crunch

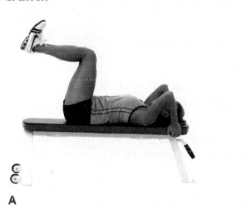

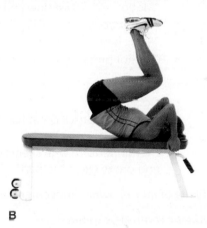

A   B

- *Other name(s):* N/A.

- *Exercise classification:* Core Strength.

- *Joint(s) where motion occurs:* LPHC.

- *Performance technique:* Start by lying on the back with knees bent at a 90-degree angle and feet flat on the floor. Position the arms a few inches away from the body, palms down. Focusing on the abdominal muscles for movement, slowly elevate the hips from the floor, rolling them back toward the upper body. At the peak of the movement the hips should be raised off the floor, while maintaining contact of the upper back, shoulder blades, head, and arms. Do not allow any movement or momentum from the legs. Gently lower the hips back to the floor and repeat for the desired number of repetitions and sets.

- *Force-couples:*
  - ▸ *Agonist.* Rectus abdominus.
  - ▸ *Synergists*: Transverse abdominus, internal/external obliques.

Resistance Training *continued*

- *Alternatives and related exercises:*
  - ‣ Sit-up.
  - ‣ Stability ball crunch.

- *Progression:* Incline reverse crunch.

- *Regression:* Prone iso-abs.

- *Common form mistakes:*
  - ‣ Using quads and hips to raise the legs instead of the core.
  - ‣ Curling knees too far up to the chest.
  - ‣ Rocking to force legs off the floor.

- *Cues to correct:*
  - ‣ "Motion should be slow and controlled, not rocking body forward and back."
  - ‣ "Upper body remains firmly on the ground."
  - ‣ "Relax hands and arms as much as possible."
  - ‣ "Do not press stomach out during crunching motion."

- *Contraindications and special considerations:*
  - ‣ Do not perform if client has low back pain during flexion.
  - ‣ Do not perform if client has posterior pelvic tilt or excessive rounding through the upper back.
  - ‣ Do not perform with clients who are pregnant, as it is recommended to avoid supine and prone exercises, particularly after the first trimester.

- *Plane of motion where movement occurs:* Sagittal.

- *Kinetic chain checkpoints:*
  - ‣ Feet and knees should remain aligned.
  - ‣ Hips should be stable through the movement.

- *Myths and misconceptions:*
  - ‣ *"The crunch and reverse crunch are used to stabilize your core."* Stabilization of the core requires exercise with no movement of the LPHC/spine during recruitment of the intrinsic core stabilization system. The floor crunch recruits the rectus abdominus as the prime mover, with the obliques as synergists to flex the spine, classifying the movement as a Strength movement.

Knee-Up

- *Other name(s):* Reverse crunch with straight legs.

- *Exercise classification:* Core Strength.

- *Joint(s) where motion occurs:* LPHC.

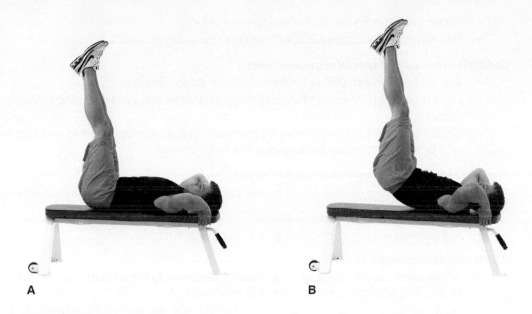

A   B

- **Performance technique:** Lie with the back on a bench or flat surface with the hips bent at a 90-degree angle and legs fully extended in the air, with hands grabbing a stable object above the shoulders for support. Draw the navel in, lift the hips off the bench, and press the feet toward the ceiling. Breathe out during the motion and slowly return to the starting position. Repeat for the desired number of repetitions.

- **Force-couples:**
  - *Agonists:* Rectus abdominus.
  - *Synergists:* Transverse abdominus, internal/external obliques.

- **Alternatives and related exercises:**
  - Sit-up.
  - Balance ball crunch.

- **Progression:** Increase incline.

- **Regressions:**
  - Decrease incline.
  - Incline reverse crunch.

- **Common form mistakes:**
  - Using momentum to rock the lower body up.
  - Using the lats too much.

- **Cues to correct:**
  - "Motion should be slow and controlled, not kicking legs forward and back."
  - "Keep the legs straight and feet pointed straight up."

Resistance Training *continued*

> ▸ "Relax your hands and arms as much as possible."
> ▸ "Do not press your stomach out during the crunching motion."

- **Contraindications and special considerations:**
  - ▸ Do not perform if the client has low back pain during flexion.
  - ▸ Do not perform if the client has posterior pelvic tilt or excessive rounding through the upper back.
  - ▸ Do not perform with clients who are pregnant, as it is recommended to avoid supine and prone exercises, particularly after the first trimester.

- **Plane of motion where movement occurs:** Sagittal.

- **Kinetic chain checkpoints:**
  - ▸ Feet and knees should remain aligned.
  - ▸ Hips should remain stable throughout the movement.

- **Myths and misconceptions:**
  - ▸ *"Crunches are bad for the back."* If a crunch is performed after a client has been taught to properly stabilize the spine, it will be much safer.
  - ▸ *"Abs should only be worked after the workout to prevent fatigue."* Abs can be worked after a workout, especially if the goal is to fatigue the core. However, performing some abdominal work near the beginning of the workout can help to increase activation of the core, resulting in more stability throughout the workout.
  - ▸ *"More crunches leads to better-defined abs."* Crunches should be used in moderation to help activate and engage the core. This results in better control of the spine over time. However, definition of the abdominal region is in large part due to nutrition, body fat, and genetics.
  - ▸ *"Incline knee-ups target the lower abs."* Due to the line of pull from gravity it may feel as though the lower abs are working more. However, when a muscle is used the entire muscle fiber will contract. This means that the rectus abdominus will always contract over its full length. In addition, with the hips in a flexed position the hip flexors (most notably) and the psoas will be engaging to stabilize the body, potentially causing an increased sensation in the "lower abs."

Push-Up with Plus

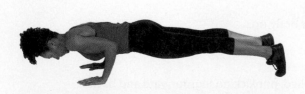

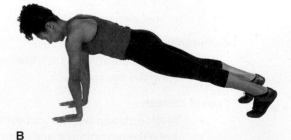

A   B

- *Other name(s):* Push-up with shoulder raise.

- *Exercise classification:* Chest Stabilization.

- *Joint(s) where motion occurs:*
  - Shoulder.
  - Elbow.

- *Performance technique:* Begin from a standard push-up position with hands at chest level and slightly wider than shoulder-width apart, arms fully extended, hips neutral, and back straight. Perform a standard push-up, then, as the elbows reach full extension, further engage the pectorals and continue past the standard end range by opening the shoulder blades as wide across the back as possible (i.e., continuing to push the spine towards the ceiling). As much as possible, avoid dropping the head, rounding through the mid-spine, or elevating the shoulder blades toward the ears.

- *Force-couples:*
  - *Agonists:* Pectoralis major, triceps.
  - *Synergists:* Anterior deltoids, pectoralis minor.

- *Alternatives and related exercises:* Bench press with plus.

- *Progressions:*
  - Stability ball push-up with plus.
  - Suspension push-up with plus.

- *Regressions:*
  - Cable chest press with plus.
  - Quadruped push-up with plus.

- *Common form mistakes:*
  - Dropping the head or shrugging the shoulders toward the ears during the plus movement.
  - Arching or rounding the back.
  - Not keeping the knees fully extended.

- *Cues to correct:*
  - "Squeeze the quads and glutes, and engage the core to straighten the back and legs."
  - "Make sure the hips and shoulders travel to the floor together; don't let the hips lead the way."
  - "Point the tip of your nose straight down at the floor."
  - "Engage the pectorals and open your shoulder blades."

- *Contraindications and special considerations:*
  - Do not perform unless the Stabilization Level has been completed.
  - Do not perform if experiencing or recovering from a wrist or an elbow injury.

Resistance Training *continued*

- *Plane of motion where movement occurs:* Sagittal.

- *Kinetic chain checkpoints:*
    ‣ Feet in dorsiflexion with toes on the ground.
    ‣ Knees and legs are straight in line with the back.
    ‣ Head down and shoulders neutral, so that the neck, back, hips, and legs form a straight line.
    ‣ Shoulders should not elevate toward the ears during the plus motion.

Stability Ball Hamstring Curl

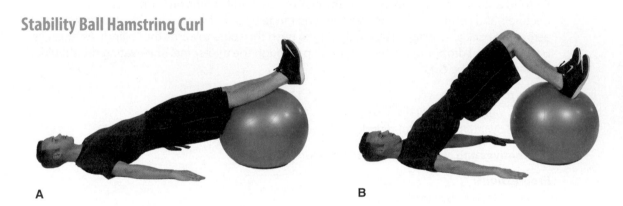

A   B

- *Other name(s):* Balance ball leg curls, balance ball bridge.

- *Exercise classification:* Legs Stabilization.

- *Joint(s) where motion occurs:* LPHC.

- *Performance technique:* Start by lying with shoulders on the mat, with legs fully extended and feet parallel, hip width apart. A straight line should be drawn from the shoulders to the feet. Then brace the core, and flex the knees to a 90-degree angle while driving the heels in to the stability ball, while maintaining a straight line from the shoulders to the knees. Extend the legs and lower the hips slowly back to the starting position and repeat for the desired number of repetitions.

- *Force-couples:*
    ‣ *Agonist*: Hamstrings complex.
    ‣ *Synergist*: Gluteus medius/minimus, anterior tibialis.

- *Alternatives and related exercises:*
    ‣ Hamstring curl machine.

- *Progression:* Single-leg stability ball hamstring curl.

- *Regression:* Floor bridge.

- *Common form mistakes:*
  - ‣ Not keeping the back and LPHC straight, allowing them to overextend or sag.
  - ‣ Allowing knees to fall in and feet to turn out.

- *Cues to correct:*
  - ‣ "Drive through the heels."
  - ‣ "Engage the core and squeeze the glutes to keep the back straight."

- *Contraindications and special considerations:*
  - ‣ Do not perform with clients who are pregnant, as it is recommended to avoid supine and prone exercises, particularly after the first trimester.

- *Plane of motion where movement occurs:* Sagittal.

- *Kinetic chain checkpoints:*
  - ‣ Feet parallel and hip width apart.
  - ‣ Knees hip-width apart.
  - ‣ Shoulders flat and relaxed on the floor.
  - ‣ Head rested on the floor with chin tucked to maintain cervical alignment.

Multiplanar Lunge to Balance

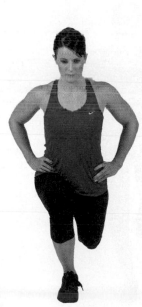

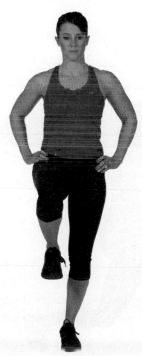

A   B

Resistance Training *continued*

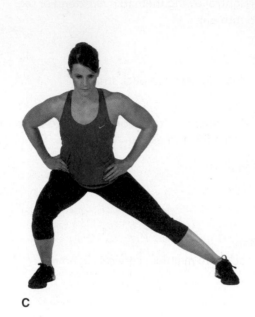

C

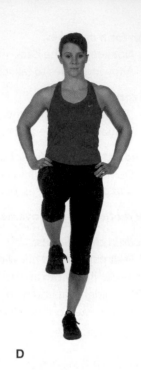

D

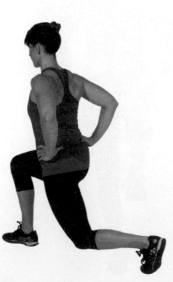

E

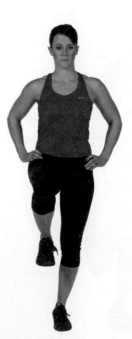

F

- **Other name(s):** Front, side, and turning lunge to balance. Lunge to balance in all planes of motion.

- **Exercise classification:** Balance Strength.

- **Joint(s) where motion occurs:**
  - Knee.
  - LPHC.

- **Performance technique:** Begin in a standing position with feet hip- to shoulder-width apart. Draw in the core and step forward into the lunge to form a 90-degree angle at the knee. The trunk and lunging shin should be parallel through the movement. The opposite leg should naturally bend at the knee, allowing the foot to roll up to the ball/toe. Squeeze the glutes, push off the lunging foot through the heel to a single-leg balance on the nonlunging leg, hold for 3–5 seconds, and then drop back into the lunge. Repeat for 3–5 repetitions, then perform on the other leg. Once performed on both legs, step out to the side with opposite leg about 2–3 feet with the foot pointed straight ahead. Keep the spine neutral and slowly bend the knee of the stepping leg, shifting the hips back and lowering the body toward the floor. Stop when the thigh is parallel to the floor. Keep the torso and shins parallel. Press back up to standing on a single leg, hold the balance for 3–5 seconds, and then step back out into a side lunge. Repeat for 3-5 repetitions, then perform on the other leg. Lastly, draw in the core and turn the body 135 degrees (i.e., start facing 12 o'clock and rotate the body to 4 o'clock) while stepping into a forward lunge. The trunk and lunging shin should be parallel through the movement. The opposite leg should naturally bend at the knee, allowing the foot to roll up to the ball/toe and rotate in place. Squeeze the glutes, and push off the lunging foot through the heel, while rotating back to a single-leg balance on the nonlunging leg, facing the original direction (i.e., rotate back to 12 o'clock). Hold the balance for 3–5 seconds, and then drop back into the lunge while again rotating 135 degrees. Repeat for 3–5 repetitions, then perform on the other leg to complete a full set.

- **Force-couples:**
  - *Agonists*: Gluteus maximus, quadriceps, gastrocnemius.
  - *Synergists*: Gluteus medius/minimus, soleus.

- **Alternatives and related exercises:** Step-up to balance, transverse plane.

- **Progressions:**
  - Perform with nonlunging foot on balance pad.
  - Perform holding dumbbells or medicine ball.

- **Regressions:**
  - Lunge to balance, frontal plane only.
  - Lunge to balance, sagittal plane only.
  - Side lunges.
  - Forward lunges.

Resistance Training *continued*

- *Common form mistakes:*
  - ▸ Putting too much weight in the front of the foot, not pushing through the heel.
  - ▸ Landing with foot turned out.
  - ▸ Internal/external rotation of nonlunging knee.
  - ▸ Excessive forward lean.
  - ▸ Back foot not rotating to keep feet parallel during lunge motion.

- *Cues to correct:*
  - ▸ "Push through the heel."
  - ▸ "Make sure the hip, knee, and ankle of the back leg stay in line."
  - ▸ "Keep torso parallel with the lunging shin."
  - ▸ "Pivot the back foot while turning the body from 12 to 4 o'clock."

- *Contraindications and special considerations:*
  - ▸ Do not perform unless the Stabilization Level has been completed.
  - ▸ Do not perform if experiencing or recovering from an ankle, a knee, or a hip injury.
  - ▸ Use caution performing with clients with severe knee valgus requiring corrective exercise.

- *Plane of motion where movement occurs:* Sagittal, frontal, transverse.

- *Kinetic chain checkpoints:*
  - ▸ Feet pointed straight ahead.
  - ▸ Lunging knee in line with the foot.
  - ▸ Nonlunging leg straight and in line with torso.
  - ▸ LPHC in neutral position with back parallel to lunging shin.
  - ▸ Shoulders in line with neck and trunk.
  - ▸ Chin tucked to keep head and neck in neutral alignment.

Sagittal Plane Hop with Stabilization

- *Other name(s):* Front-to-back hop with balance.

- *Exercise classification:* Balance Power.

- *Joint(s) where motion occurs:*
  - ▸ Ankle.
  - ▸ Knee.
  - ▸ LPHC.

- *Performance technique:* Stand with feet shoulder-width apart and pointing straight ahead with hands on the hips. Hips should be in neutral position. Lift one leg directly beside the balance leg. Hop forward, landing on the opposite foot, and hold for 3–5 seconds (use the time

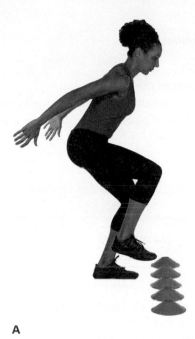

A

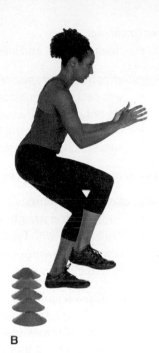

B

to reinforce proper alignment and control). Hop backward to the starting foot and hold for 3–5 seconds. Then switch the starting foot and perform again to complete one repetition. Repeat for the desired number of repetitions.

- ***Force-couples:***
  - ▸ *Agonists*: Gluteus maximus, quadriceps, gastrocnemius.
  - ▸ *Synergists*: Gluteus medius/minimus, soleus.

- ***Alternatives and Related Exercises:*** N/A.

- ***Progressions:***
  - ▸ Sagittal plane hop with stabilization.
  - ▸ Multiplanar hop with stabilization.
  - ▸ Single-leg box hop-up with stabilization.

- ***Regressions:*** Double-leg hop to single-leg landing with stabilization.

- ***Common form mistakes:***
  - ▸ Excessive forward lean.
  - ▸ Landing with foot externally rotated.
  - ▸ Landing with knee valgus.
  - ▸ Taking hands off hips for stabilization.

Resistance Training *continued*

- *Cues to correct:*
  - ‣ "Maintain feet and knee straight ahead with neutral hips."

- *Contraindications and special considerations:*
  - ‣ Use caution with older adults who have an increased risk of falling.
  - ‣ Do not perform if experiencing or recovering from an ankle, a knee, or a hip injury.
  - ‣ Do not perform if the Stabilization and Strength Level balance exercises have not been successfully completed.

- *Plane of motion where movement occurs:* Sagittal.

- *Kinetic chain checkpoints:*
  - ‣ Foot pointed straight ahead.
  - ‣ Knee in line with foot.
  - ‣ Hips in neutral position.
  - ‣ Chin tucked so neck, shoulders, back, and hips are aligned.

- *Myths and misconceptions:*
  - ‣ *"Jumping is bad for the knees."* Landing from a jump is a vital part of force reduction in functional movement. The majority of walking occurs on one leg; therefore, learning how to properly decelerate in all planes of motion may reduce the chance of noncontact injuries.

Horizontal Jump with Stabilization

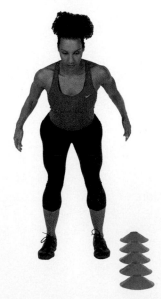

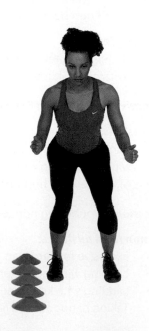

A

B

- **Other name(s):** Frontal plane jump with stabilization.

- **Exercise classification:** Reactive Balance.

- **Joint(s) where motion occurs:**
  - Ankle.
  - Knee.
  - LPHC.

- **Performance technique:** Stand with both feet shoulder-width apart and pointed straight ahead. Hips should be in a neutral position, and knees should be aligned over the mid-foot with arms at sides. Squat slightly as if sitting to a chair, then jump up and to the side, extending the arms overhead. Land softly, with ankles, knees, and hips slightly flexed. Maintain optimal alignment and returning arms to sides. Hold landing for 3–5 seconds and repeat in the opposite direction to complete one repetition. Repeat for the desired number of repetitions.

- **Force-couples:**
  - *Agonists*: Gluteus maximus, quadriceps, gastrocnemius.
  - *Synergists*: Gluteus medius/minimus, soleus.

- **Alternatives and related exercises:** Box jump up with stabilization.

- **Progressions:**
  - Transverse plane jump with stabilization.
  - Horizontal box jump-up with stabilization.

- **Regressions:**
  - Squat jump with stabilization in sagittal plane.
  - Squat to triple extension with stabilization.

- **Common form mistakes:**
  - Feet turning out on landing.
  - Not extending the hips at the top of the jump.
  - Landing with too much force.
  - Landing with knees locked.

- **Cues to correct:**
  - "Hold landing position."
  - "Fully extend the body at the top of the jump."
  - "Focus on the landing rather than on getting height."
  - "Land softly."

- **Contraindications and special considerations:**
  - Use caution with older adults who are at increased risk of falling.
  - Do not perform if experiencing or recovering from an ankle, a knee, or a hip injury.
  - Do not perform if the Stabilization and Strength Level balance exercises have not been successfully completed.

Resistance Training *continued*

- *Plane of motion where movement occurs:* Frontal.

- *Kinetic chain checkpoints:*
  - ‣ Feet pointed straight ahead.
  - ‣ Knees in line with foot.
  - ‣ Hips in neutral position.
  - ‣ Chin tucked so neck, shoulders, back, and hips are aligned.

- *Myths and misconceptions:*
  - ‣ *"Jumping is bad for the knees."* Landing from a jump is a vital part of force reduction in functional movement. Learning how to properly decelerate in all planes of motion may reduce the risk of noncontact injuries.

Multiplanar Jump

- *Exercise classification:* Reactive Strength.

- *Joint(s) where motion occurs:*
  - ‣ Ankle.
  - ‣ Knee.
  - ‣ LPHC.

- *Performance technique:* Stand with both feet shoulder-width apart and pointed straight ahead. Hips should be in a neutral position, and knees should be aligned over the mid-foot with arms at sides. Squat slightly as if sitting to a chair, then jump up and forward in the sagittal plane while extending arms overhead. Land softly, with ankles, knees, and hips slightly flexed. Maintain optimal alignment and return arms to sides. Repeat to the rear, left and right sides

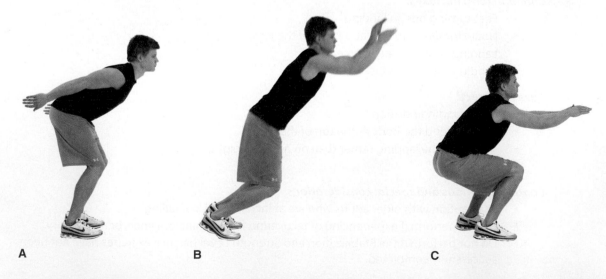

A   B   C

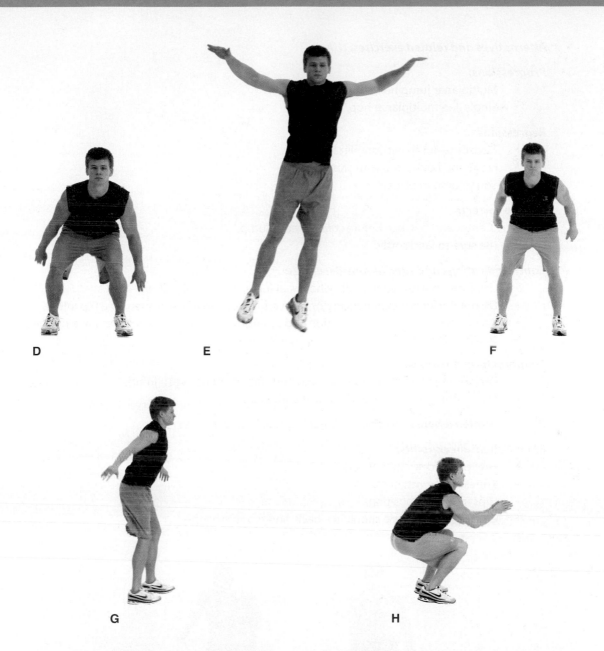

D

E

F

G

H

in the frontal plane, and again with left and right 90-degree twists in the transverse plane to complete one repetition. Repeat sequence for the desired number of repetitions.

- *Force-couples:*
  - ▸ *Agonists*: Gluteus maximus, quadriceps, gastrocnemius
  - ▸ *Synergists*: Gluteus medius/minimus, soleus.

Resistance Training *continued*

- *Alternatives and related exercises:* N/A.

- *Progressions:*
  - ▸ Multiplanar jump holding medicine ball.
  - ▸ Single-leg multiplanar hop.

- *Regressions:*
  - ▸ Horizontal jump with stabilization.
  - ▸ Front and back jump with stabilization.
  - ▸ Squat jump in place.

- *Cues to correct:*
  - ▸ "Center and balance before starting each jump."
  - ▸ "Be sure to land softly."

- *Contraindications and special considerations:*
  - ▸ Use caution with older adults who are at increased risk of falling.
  - ▸ Do not perform if experiencing or recovering from an ankle, a knee, or a hip injury.
  - ▸ Do not perform if the Stabilization and Strength Level balance exercises have not been successfully completed.

- *Common form mistakes:*
  - ▸ Performing too fast without pausing and stabilizing between jumps.
  - ▸ Not bending knees on landing to absorb impact.

- *Plane of motion where movement occurs:* Sagittal, frontal, transverse.

- *Kinetic chain checkpoints:*
  - ▸ Feet pointed straight ahead.
  - ▸ Knees in line with feet.
  - ▸ Hips in neutral position.
  - ▸ Chin tucked so neck, shoulders, back, and hips are aligned.

Ice Skaters

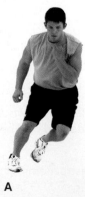 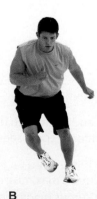

A   B

- *Other name(s):* N/A.

- *Exercise classification:* Reactive Power.

- *Joint(s) where motion occurs:*
  - Ankle.
  - Knee.
  - Shoulder.

- *Performance technique:* Begin standing on one leg. Hop from side to side, switching legs as if you were hoping over a puddle of water or speed skating. Swing your arms side to side, reaching toward or touching the opposite hand to the opposite standing leg. Keep the body low, going as fast as can be controlled. Repeat for the desired number of repetitions.

- *Force-couples:*
  - *Agonists*: Gluteus maximus, quadriceps, gastrocnemius.
  - *Synergists*: Gluteus medius/minimus, soleus.

- *Alternatives and related exercises:* N/A.

- *Progressions:*
  - Increase speed.
  - Increase depth of squat.
  - Increase distance jumped.

- *Regressions:*
  - Decrease speed.
  - Decrease depth of squat.
  - Decrease distance jumped.

- *Common form mistakes:*
  - Feet not pointing straight ahead.
  - Excessive forward lean.
  - Rotation of the trunk.

- *Cues to correct:*
  - "Keep feet, chest, and face pointed straight ahead."
  - "Engage the core to stabilize the spine and avoid rotation."

- *Contraindications and special considerations:*
  - Do not perform unless the Stabilization Level has been completed.
  - Do not perform if experiencing or recovering from an ankle, a knee, or a hip injury.
  - Use caution when performing with clients with severe knee valgus requiring corrective exercise.
  - Perform at functional speed of actual ice skating for optimal transfer effect.

- *Plane of motion where movement occurs:* Frontal, transverse.

Resistance Training *continued*

- *Kinetic chain checkpoints:*
    ‣ Foot pointed straight ahead.
    ‣ Knee in line with foot.
    ‣ Hips in neutral position.
    ‣ Chin tucked so the neck, shoulders, back, and hips are aligned.

- *Myths and misconceptions:*
    ‣ "My client is not participating in a sport; therefore, this type of exercise has little benefit." Reactive power relies on the body's ability to react to movement, decelerating and accelerating force in a highly functional amount of time. This is a useful skill for the general population client for activities of daily living, because many injuries are due to the inability to properly decelerate force. Reactive Power training will help teach that skill.

Sagittal Plane Proprioceptive Reactives

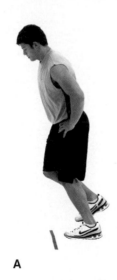

A

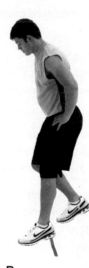

B

- *Other name(s):* Single-leg front-back hops.

- *Exercise classification:* Reactive Power.

- *Joint(s) where motion occurs:*
    ‣ Ankle.
    ‣ Knee.
    ‣ LPHC.

- **Performance technique:** Stand with feet shoulder-width apart and pointing straight ahead with hands on the hips. Hips should be in the neutral position. Lift one leg directly beside the balance leg. Hop forward and then back to the starting position, repeating as fast as possible while maintaining optimal form, for as many repetitions as desired. Then perform with the other leg.

- **Force-couples:**
  - *Agonists*: Gluteus maximus, quadriceps, gastrocnemius.
  - *Synergists*: Gluteus medius/minimus, soleus.

- **Alternatives and related exercises:** Single-leg box jump-up.

- **Progressions:**
  - Perform with eyes closed.
  - Multiplanar proprioceptive reactives.

- **Regressions:** Single-leg front-back hop with stabilization.

- **Common form mistakes:**
  - Excessive forward lean.
  - Landing with foot externally rotated.
  - Landing with knee valgus.
  - Taking hands off hips for stabilization.

- **Cues to correct:** "Maintain feet and knee straight ahead with neutral hips."

- **Contraindications and special considerations:**
  - Use caution with older adults who are at increased risk of falling.
  - Do not perform if experiencing or recovering from an ankle, a knee, or a hip injury.
  - Do not perform if the Stabilization and Strength Level balance exercises have not been successfully completed.

- **Plane of motion where movement occurs:** Sagittal.

- **Kinetic chain checkpoints:**
  - Foot pointed straight ahead.
  - Knee in line with foot.
  - Hips in neutral position.
  - Chin tucked so the neck, shoulders, back, and hips are aligned.

Free Weights

Standing Two-Arm Hammer Curl

- **Other name(s):** N/A.

- **Exercise classification:** Biceps Strength.

Resistance Training *continued*

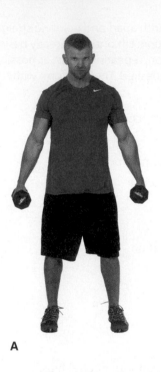

A

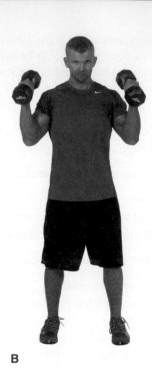

B

- *Joint(s) where motion occurs:* Elbow.

- *Performance technique:* Stand with feet hip- to shoulder-width apart and pointed straight with knees slightly bent. Arms begin extended at the side of the body with dumbbells in each hand. Draw in the core and curl both dumbbells, keeping thumbs up and palms facing the body, toward the shoulders as if swinging a hammer. Reverse the movement and return to the starting position. Repeat for the desired number of repetitions.

- *Force-couples:*
  - *Agonist*: Biceps brachii.
  - *Synergist*: Brachialis, brachioradialis.

- *Alternatives and related exercises:* Preacher hammer curl.

- *Progression:* Single-leg standing two-arm hammer curl.

- *Regressions:*
  - Seated two-arm hammer curl.
  - Standing barbell curl.

- *Common form mistakes:*
  - Using too much weight.
  - Rocking hips for momentum and arching the back.
  - Swinging arms for momentum.

- ***Cues to correct:***
  - ▸ "Keep the motion smooth and under control."
  - ▸ "Keep the core braced and back still and straight."

- ***Contraindications and special considerations:***
  - ▸ Do not perform if the Stabilization and Strength Level balance exercises have not been successfully completed.

- ***Plane of motion where movement occurs:*** Sagittal.

- ***Modality substitutions:***
  - ▸ Resistance bands.
  - ▸ Kettlebells.

- ***Kinetic chain checkpoints:***
  - ▸ Feet pointed straight ahead.
  - ▸ Knees in line with the feet and slightly bent.
  - ▸ LPHC in neutral position to ensure a straight back.
  - ▸ Shoulders in line with neck and hips.
  - ▸ Chin tucked so the head and neck are in proper cervical alignment.

Barbell Russian Deadlift

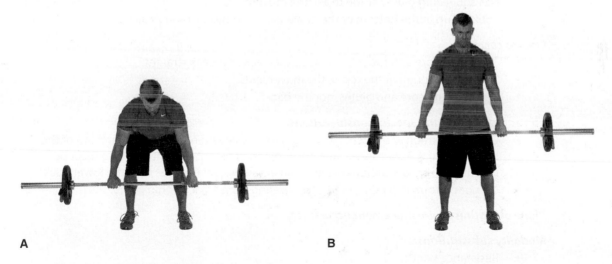

A   B

- ***Other name(s):*** Straight-leg deadlift.

- ***Exercise classification:*** Legs Strength.

- ***Joint(s) where motion occurs:*** LPHC.

Resistance Training *continued*

- *Performance technique:* Stand with feet straight and shoulder-width apart, knees slightly bent. Remove barbell from rack and hold in front of thighs gripped wider than shoulder-width apart. Support the core with abdominal bracing, and slowly bend at the waist by pushing the glutes back, lowering the barbell toward the floor and keeping the back flat. Lift with the glutes to return to the starting position, taking care to not strain the lower back. Keep the chin tucked to maintain cervical alignment throughout the entire motion.

- *Force-couples:*
  - *Agonist*: Gluteus maximus, hamstrings.
  - *Synergists*: Quadriceps.

- *Alternatives and related exercises:* Dumbbell Russian deadlift.

- *Progressions:*
  - Increase resistance.
  - Perform standing on elevated blocks to increase distance traveled.

- *Regressions:*
  - Decrease resistance.
  - Single-leg floor bridge.
  - Floor bridge.

- *Common form mistakes:*
  - Arching of lower back.
  - Not squeezing glutes at the top of the movement.
  - Looking up at the bottom of the movement to move into cervical extension.

- *Cues to correct:*
  - "Brace the core and tuck chin to keep the back and neck straight."
  - "Pull hips through at the top of the movement."
  - "Lift with the core and glutes, not the back."

- *Contraindications and special considerations:*
  - Use with caution with clients who show excessive anterior pelvic tilt (arching of the back) during the overhead squat assessment. Proper abdominal bracing must be practiced to ensure preferred activation of the gluteal muscles over the lower back.
  - Do not perform if experiencing or recovering from a back or hip injury.

- *Plane of motion where movement occurs:* Sagittal.

- *Modality substitutions:*
  - Resistance bands.
  - Kettlebells.
  - Smith machine.

- *Kinetic chain checkpoints:*
  - Feet pointed straight ahead.

- ▸ Knees in line with the feet and slightly bent.
- ▸ LPHC in neutral position to ensure a straight back.
- ▸ Shoulders in line with neck and hips.
- ▸ Chin tucked so the head and neck are in proper cervical alignment.

- *Myths and misconceptions:*
  - ▸ *"Deadlifts are bad for the back."* It is true that when performed incorrectly, by lifting with the muscles of the mid and lower back, deadlifts can be detrimental and potentially cause injury to the spinal structure. However, when the core is properly braced, hips are in neutral alignment with knees slightly bent, and the back and neck are straight with the chin tucked, the exercise primarily targets the glutes and hamstrings, leading to beneficial adaptations to potentially reduce instances of lower back pain and injury.

Stationary Dumbbell Lunge

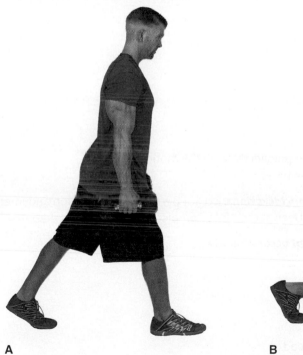
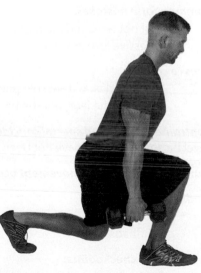

A   B

- *Other name(s):* N/A.
- *Exercise classification:* Legs Strength.

Resistance Training *continued*

- *Joint(s) where motion occurs:*
  - ‣ Knee.
  - ‣ LPHC.

- *Performance technique:* Start standing, feet together, holding a dumbbell in each hand. Take a big step behind you with one leg, with the heel off of the floor, keeping most of the weight on the nonstepping leg. Slowly bend both knees, lowering the body straight down until both knees are at 90-degree angles. Keep the back and front shin parallel through the lunging movement. Push through the front heel and slowly return to standing. Perform for the desired number of repetitions, and repeat with the other leg forward.

- *Force-couples:*
  - ‣ *Agonists*: Gluteus maximus, quadriceps, gastrocnemius.
  - ‣ *Synergists*: Gluteus medius/minimus, soleus.

- *Alternatives and related exercises:* Transverse plane jumping lunges.

- *Progression:* Stationary dumbbell lunge on balance pad.

- *Regressions:*
  - ‣ Stationary bodyweight lunge.
  - ‣ Squat with hands on hips.

- *Common form mistakes:*
  - ‣ Feet not remaining parallel.
  - ‣ Excessive forward lean.

- *Cues to correct:*
  - ‣ "Keep back and front shin parallel through the motion."
  - ‣ "Lift with the legs, not the back."

- *Contraindications and special considerations:* Do not perform if Stabilization and Strength Level balance exercises have not been successfully completed.

- *Plane of motion where movement occurs:* Sagittal.

- *Modality substitutions:*
  - ‣ Kettlebells.
  - ‣ Sandbags.

- *Kinetic chain checkpoints:*
  - ‣ Feet pointed straight ahead.
  - ‣ Lunging knee in line with the foot.
  - ‣ Nonlunging leg straight and in line with torso.
  - ‣ LPHC in neutral position with back parallel to lunging shin.
  - ‣ Shoulders in line with neck and trunk.
  - ‣ Chin tucked to keep head and neck in neutral alignment.

Barbell Squat

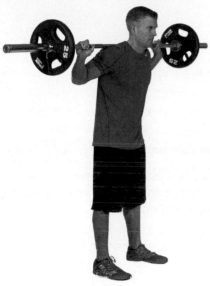

A

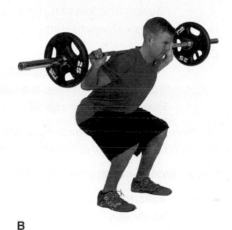

B

- *Other name(s):* N/A

- *Exercise classification:* Legs Strength.

- *Joint(s) where motion occurs:*
    - Knee.
    - LPHC.

- *Performance technique:* Stand in a shoulder-width stance with toes pointed straight ahead. Keeping an upright torso, step under the barbell in the squat rack, rest the bar on the shoulders and upper traps just below the base of the neck, and place the hands on the bar to form a 90-degree angle at the elbows. Lift slightly up to remove the bar from the rack, take one small step back, and return to standing with feet shoulder width apart and knees soft. Brace the core, and lower into a squat position by pushing the hips back and bending the knees. Keep the LPHC neutral and back straight throughout the entire movement. Lower as far as can be controlled with proper form and then drive through the heels, lifting with the glutes to return to a standing position.

- *Force-couples:*
    - *Agonists*: Gluteus maximus, quadriceps, gastrocnemius.
    - *Synergists*: Gluteus medius/minimus, soleus, hamstrings.

- *Alternatives and related exercises:*
    - Stability ball wall squat.
    - Leg press machine.

Resistance Training *continued*

- *Progression:* Perform standing on a balance pad.

- *Regression:* Hanging arm dumbbell squat.

- *Common form mistakes:*
  ‣ Arching the lower back.
  ‣ Allowing the feet to turn out or the knees to fall inward.
  ‣ Excessive forward lean.

- *Cues to correct:*
  ‣ "Sit back into the heels and lift with the glutes."
  ‣ "Brace the core to keep the back in neutral alignment."
  ‣ "Do not lift with the back!"

- *Contraindications and special considerations:* Do not perform if the Stabilization and Strength Level balance exercises have not been successfully completed.

- *Plane of motion where movement occurs:* Sagittal.

- *Modality substitutions:*
  ‣ Dumbbells.
  ‣ Sandbags.
  ‣ Smith machine.
  ‣ Resistance bands.

- *Kinetic chain checkpoints:*
  ‣ Feet shoulder-width apart pointed straight ahead.
  ‣ Knees in line with the feet.
  ‣ LPHC in neutral position with back parallel to shins through the squat.
  ‣ Shoulders pulled back and elbows in line with neck and trunk.
  ‣ Chin tucked to keep head and neck in neutral alignment.

Ball Dumbbell Chest Press

- *Other name(s):* Balance ball dumbbell press.

- *Classification of exercise:* Stabilization Strength.

- *Joint(s) where motion occurs:*
  ‣ Shoulder.
  ‣ Elbow.

- *Performance technique:* Begin with feet flat on the ground shoulder width apart, knees at a 90-degree angle, and seated on a stability ball. Pick up a dumbbell in each hand, hold them in

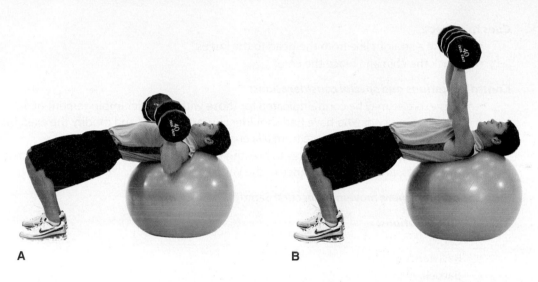

A   **B**

the start position tucked near the shoulders, and roll back on to the ball so the body weight is supported near the lower shoulder blades. Head, neck, LPHC, and legs should form a straight line to the knees. Keeping the core tight, fully extend the arms and elbows. Do not lock out the elbows at the end ROM. Return to starting position in a controlled manner and repeat for the desired number of repetitions.

- **Force-couples:**
  - *Agonists*: Pectoralis major, anterior deltoid, triceps brachii.
  - *Synergist*: Pectoralis minor.

- **Alternatives and related exercises:**
  - Push-up.
  - Standing cable chest press.
  - Supine kettlebell chest press.
  - Dumbbell incline chest press.
  - Dumbbell decline chest press.
  - Medicine ball chest pass.
  - Suspension trainer chest press.

- **Progression:** Alternating arm stability ball chest press.

- **Regression:** Bench dumbbell chest press.

- **Common form mistakes:**
  - Arching the low back.
  - Moving the head forward.
  - Elevating the shoulders.

Resistance Training *continued*

- *Cues to correct:*
  - ▸ "Make a straight line from the head to the knees."
  - ▸ "Tuck the chin and brace the core."

- *Contraindications and special considerations:*
  - ▸ This exercise may be contraindicated for those with shoulder impingement or a shoulder injury or who have had shoulder surgery. Regress and modify the exercise for these individuals if clearance from a licensed professional is not secured.
  - ▸ Ensure that the client continues to breathe throughout the exercise to avoid increased blood pressure and performance of the Valsalva maneuver.

- *Plane of motion where movement occurs:* Sagittal.

- *Modality substitutions:*
  - ▸ Cable.
  - ▸ Resistance bands.
  - ▸ Barbell.

- *Kinetic chain checkpoints:*
  - ▸ Feet flat on floor, pointed straight ahead and hip-width apart.
  - ▸ Knees in line with the second and third toes bent to 90 degrees.
  - ▸ LPHC in neutral position, forming a straight line from knees to shoulders.
  - ▸ Shoulder blades flat against the ball in a neutral position.
  - ▸ Chin tucked so head is in neutral alignment with cervical spine.

Squat, Curl to One-Arm Overhead Press

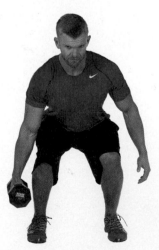

A

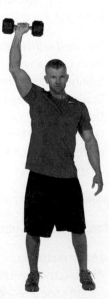

B

- **Other name(s):** Single-arm squat, curl to military press.

- **Exercise classification:** Total Body Strength.

- **Joint(s) where motion occurs:**
  - ‣ Ankle.
  - ‣ Knee.
  - ‣ LPHC.
  - ‣ Elbow.
  - ‣ Shoulder.

- **Performance technique:** Hold a dumbbell in one hand at the side of the body (palm facing body) with the feet straight and shoulder-width apart. Brace the core, squeeze the glutes, and perform a squat, keeping the back parallel to the shins. Return to standing and immediately curl the dumbbell. From the curl-up position, press the dumbbell overhead, fully extending and rotating the arm so the palm faces away. Reverse the motion and return the dumbbell to the side of the body to complete one repetition. Perform the desired number of repetitions, and then repeat with the other arm.

- **Force-couples:**
  - ‣ *Agonists:*
    - • *Squat:* Gluteus maximus, quadriceps, gastrocnemius.
    - • *Curl:* Biceps.
    - • *Overhead press:* Deltoids, triceps.
  - ‣ *Synergists:*
    - • *Squat:* Gluteus medius/minimus, soleus.
    - • *Curl:* Brachialis, brachioradialis.
    - • *Overhead press:* Upper trapezius, pectoralis minor.

- **Alternatives and related exercises:** N/A.

- **Progression:** Perform standing on balance pad.

- **Regressions:**
  - ‣ Squat, curl to two-arm overhead press.
  - ‣ Standing curl to one-arm overhead press.

- **Common form mistakes:**
  - ‣ Not completing each movement fully before starting the next.
  - ‣ Swinging hips for momentum and straining the back.

- **Cues to correct:**
  - ‣ "Keep the chest tall and above the hips, with the back parallel to the shins."
  - ‣ "Don't swing the weight during the curl."
  - ‣ "Focus on form over the amount of weight lifted."
  - ‣ "Complete each movement individually before starting the next."

Resistance Training *continued*

- *Contraindications and special considerations:* Do not perform unless the Stabilization and early Strength Level exercises have been successfully completed.

- *Plane of motion where movement occurs:* Sagittal, transverse.

- *Modality substitutions:*
    - ‣ Resistance bands.
    - ‣ Kettlebells.

- *Kinetic chain checkpoints:*
    - ‣ Feet shoulder-width apart pointed straight ahead.
    - ‣ Knees in line with the feet.
    - ‣ LPHC in neutral position with back parallel to shins through the squat.
    - ‣ Shoulders pulled back and elbows in line with neck and trunk.
    - ‣ Chin tucked to keep head and neck in neutral alignment.

Sagittal Plane Step-Up, Balance, Curl to One-Arm Overhead Press

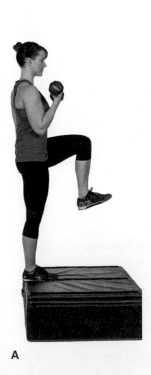

A

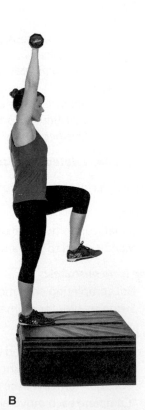

B

- **Other name(s):** N/A.

- **Exercise classification:** Total Body Stabilization.

- **Joint(s) where motion occurs:**
  - Ankle.
  - Knee.
  - LPHC.
  - Elbow.
  - Shoulder.

- **Performance technique:** Hold a dumbbell in one hand at the side of the body (palm facing body), with the feet straight and shoulder-width apart. Brace the core, and step up onto an elevated box to a single-leg balance. While balanced on one leg, immediately curl the dumbbell. From the curl-up position, press the dumbbells overhead, fully extending and rotating the arm so the palm faces away. Reverse the motion and return the dumbbell to the side of the body, and then step down off the box with the nonbalance leg to complete one repetition. Perform the desired number of repetitions, and repeat with the other arm.

- **Force-couples:**
  - *Agonists:*
    - *Step-up:* Gluteus maximus, quadriceps, gastrocnemius.
    - *Curl:* Biceps.
    - *Overhead press:* Deltoids, triceps.
  - *Synergists:*
    - *Step-up:* Gluteus medius/minimus, soleus.
    - *Curl:* Brachialis, brachioradialis.
    - *Overhead press:* Upper trapezius, pectoralis minor.

- **Alternatives and related exercises:** N/A.

- **Progression:** Increase height of step-up box.

- **Regressions:**
  - Step-up, balance, curl to two-arm overhead press.
  - Standing one-leg curl to overhead press.

- **Common form mistakes:**
  - Not completing each movement fully before starting the next.
  - Swinging hips for momentum and straining the back.
  - Dropping nonbalance foot to the box.

- **Cues to correct:**
  - "Keep chest tall and above the hips, with the back parallel to the shins."
  - "Don't swing the weight during the curl."
  - "Focus on form over the amount of weight lifted."
  - "Complete each movement individually before starting the next."

Resistance Training *continued*

- *Contraindications and special considerations:* Do not perform unless the Stabilization and early Strength Level exercises have been successfully completed.

- *Plane of motion where movement occurs:* Sagittal, transverse.

- *Modality Substitutions:* N/A.

- *Kinetic chain checkpoints:*
    - ‣ Feet pointed straight ahead.
    - ‣ Knees in line with the feet and slightly bent.
    - ‣ LPHC in neutral position to ensure a straight back.
    - ‣ Shoulders in line with neck and hips.
    - ‣ Chin tucked so the head and neck are in proper cervical alignment.

Cable Machines

Cable Leg Extension

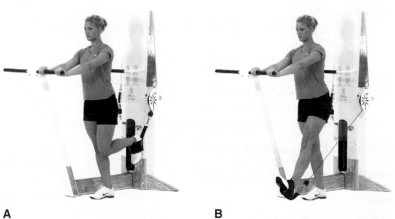

A   B

- *Other name(s):* Standing leg extension.

- *Exercise classification:* Legs Strength.

- *Joint(s) where motion occurs:*
    - ‣ Knee.
    - ‣ LPHC.

- *Performance technique:* Begin facing away from the machine with the cable position at its lowest setting. Place the foot into the ankle-cuff attachment. Balance on the opposite foot or use the support bar for stability. Allow the cable to pull the foot back in a controlled manner until the shin is parallel to the floor (the knee should be flexed to approximately 90 degrees). Extend the knee back to the starting position with a straight leg. Do not allow the foot to touch the ground. Keep the knee, hip, and foot pointed straight ahead.

- *Force-couples:*
  - *Agonists*: Quadriceps, gluteus maximus.
  - *Synergists*: Gluteus medius/minimus, anterior tibialis.

- *Alternatives and related exercises:*
  - Step-up.
  - Lunge.
  - Single-leg squat.

- *Progression:* Barbell squat.

- *Regression:* Machine leg extension.

- *Common form mistakes:*
  - Not fully extending the knee.
  - Anterior pelvic tilt.
  - Externally rotating the hip or knee.

- *Cues to correct:*
  - "Squeeze the quads at the end ROM."
  - "Remember to keep the water in the LPHC bucket!"
  - "Heel up at the back, toe up at the front."

- *Contraindications and special considerations:*
  - Note that although this exercise does not have a true synergist, other muscles are activated while performing this exercise. The hip flexor and ilipsoas muscle groups will help keep the foot elevated from the floor by elevating the hip.
  - The end ROM of the exercise (knee fully extended) should be avoided for those recently released from physical therapy of the knee. The end ROM produces the largest shearing forces and may cause reinjury to the affected knee (Signorile et al., 2014).

- *Plane of motion where movement occurs:* Sagittal.

- *Modality substitutions:*
  - Resistance bands.
  - Ankle weights.

- *Kinetic chain checkpoints:*
  - Feet pointed straight ahead.
  - Knees in line with the feet with stance leg slightly bent.

Resistance Training *continued*

> ▸ LPHC in neutral position to ensure a straight back.
> ▸ Shoulders in line with neck and hips.
> ▸ Chin tucked so the head and neck are in proper cervical alignment.

- **Myths and misconceptions:**
  - ▸ *"Turning the foot in or out will isolate specific muscles within the quadriceps muscle group."* When performing the leg extension, the entire quadriceps muscle group will be activated regardless of foot position. Specific muscles may be targeted more strongly based on the foot position (the vastus lateralis is activated more strongly with toes in, and the rectus femoris benefits more from toes out). However, it appears that the emphasis is also related to the ROM of the exercise as well, as the vastus lateralis is activated more at the top of the ROM when the foot is in neutral position (Signorile et al., 2014). Although the research seems to support a portion of the toe positioning, the professional also needs to consider the ROM.
  - ▸ *"Standing on an unstable surface is a progression."* This may be considered a progression, but first the goal of the exercise must be considered. If the goal of the leg extension is to develop strength within the quadriceps muscle group, then providing an unstable surface will not be the best choice, because the body will not have a stable point from which it can produce the most force. However, if the goal of the exercise is to work on balance and stability, performing this exercise in a proprioceptively enriched environment with lower weights would be acceptable.

Cable Pushdown

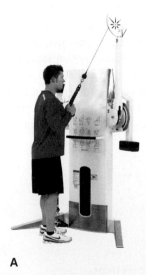

A

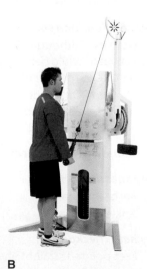

B

- ***Other name(s):*** Triceps pushdown, cable triceps extension.

- ***Exercise classification:*** Triceps Strength.

- ***Joint(s) where motion occurs:*** Elbow.

- ***Performance technique:*** Begin with the cable setting in a position that is at least above the head. Stand facing the cable with feet hip to shoulder-width apart and a slight bend in the knees. Grab the bent triceps pressdown bar in an overhand grip with the elbows bent fully flexed. The elbows should be close to the side of the body. The shoulder blades should be locked into a retracted and depressed position. Squeeze the triceps and pushdown, fully extending the arms. Return to the starting position in control of the weight.

- ***Force-couples:***
  - ▸ *Agonist*: Triceps brachii.
  - ▸ *Synergist*: N/A.

- ***Alternatives and related exercises:***
  - ▸ Supine stability ball dumbbell triceps extension.
  - ▸ Prone stability ball dumbbell triceps extension.
  - ▸ Supine bench barbell triceps extension.
  - ▸ Suspension trainer triceps extension.
  - ▸ Single-leg triceps pressdown.

- ***Progressions:***
  - ▸ Use a rope attachment.
  - ▸ Unilateral cable pushdown.

- ***Regressions:***
  - ▸ Perform on knees.
  - ▸ Perform seated.

- ***Common form mistakes:***
  - ▸ Allowing the elbows to move.
  - ▸ Not fully flexing or extending the elbows.
  - ▸ Not maintaining upright body posture.
  - ▸ Allowing the shoulders to perform the movement.

- ***Cues to correct:***
  - ▸ "Imagine you have tied your elbows to your sides."
  - ▸ "Use your elbow to crack a nut when you come back to starting position."
  - ▸ "Slap the wall behind you."
  - ▸ "Brace yourself and stand up tall."
  - ▸ "Lock your shoulders down."

Resistance Training *continued*

- **Contraindications and special considerations:**
  - ‣ Elbow pain or instability.
  - ‣ Recent elbow surgery.

- **Plane of motion where movement occurs:** Sagittal.

- **Modality substitutions:**
  - ‣ Resistance bands.

- **Kinetic chain checkpoints:**
  - ‣ Feet pointed straight ahead.
  - ‣ Knees in line with the feet and slightly bent.
  - ‣ LPHC in neutral position to ensure a straight back.
  - ‣ Shoulders in line with neck and hips.
  - ‣ Chin tucked so the head and neck are in proper cervical alignment.

- **Myths and misconceptions:**
  - ‣ *"Changing hand positions will target different aspects of the triceps muscle."* In order to extend the elbow, all three heads of the triceps must be activated in order to achieve movement. Because of this, different hand positions will not have an effect on the head of the triceps muscle that is targeted in order to perform the exercise.

Cable Rotation

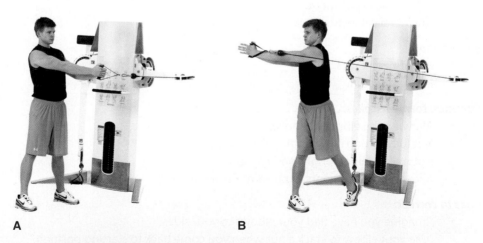

A   B

- **Other name(s):** Standing cable trunk rotation.

- **Classification of exercise:** Core Strength.

- **Joint(s) where motion occurs:**
  - ‣ Lumbar spine.

- ‣ Hips.
- ‣ Knees.
- ‣ Ankles.

- *Performance technique:* Begin with the cable set to shoulder height. Stand with feet shoulder-width apart, knees slightly flexed, and toes pointing straight ahead. Hold the cable handle with both hands directly in front of the chest, with arms extended and shoulder blades retraced and depressed. Rotate the body away from the machine using the abdominals and gluteal muscles. Allow the back foot to pivot to achieve triple extension. Return to the starting position in a controlled manner and repeat.

- *Force-couples:*
  - ‣ *Agonists*: Internal/external obliques, gluteus medius/minimus.
  - ‣ *Synergists*: Transverse abdominus, hip flexors.

- *Alternatives and related exercises:*
  - ‣ Cable lift.
  - ‣ Cable chop.
  - ‣ Russian twist.
  - ‣ Rotational medicine ball chest pass.

- *Progression:* Cable lift.

- *Regressions:*
  - ‣ Perform on knees.
  - ‣ Use resistance bands.

- *Common form mistakes:*
  - ‣ Allowing elbows to flex and bring the cable close to the body.
  - ‣ Not pivoting trailing leg into triple extension.
  - ‣ Shoulder elevation and protraction.
  - ‣ Cervical spine not staying in line with torso.

- *Cues to correct:*
  - ‣ "Push the cable away from your body."
  - ‣ "Drive your trailing hip forward as you rotate."
  - ‣ "Pull your shoulders away from your ears."
  - ‣ "Follow the cable with your eyes."

- *Contraindications and special considerations:*
  - ‣ It is important for the triple extension of the back leg to happen in order to decrease stress on the low back. This also ensures proper neuromuscular efficiency of the muscles that extend the lower extremities (i.e., gluteus maximus, quadriceps, gastrocnemius, and soleus).
  - ‣ Individuals with low back pain may need to avoid this exercise.

- *Plane of motion where movement occurs:* Transverse.

Resistance Training *continued*

- *Modality substitutions:*
  ‣ Resistance bands.
  ‣ Medicine ball.

- *Kinetic chain checkpoints:*
  ‣ Feet pointed straight ahead, slightly wider than hip-width apart.
  ‣ Knees in line with the feet and slightly bent.
  ‣ LPHC in neutral position to ensure a straight back.
  ‣ Shoulders in line with neck and hips, with arms pointed straight ahead.
  ‣ Chin tucked so the head and neck are in proper cervical alignment.

- *Myths and misconceptions:*
  ‣ *"Keep the feet planted in place."* Keeping the feet planted without rotation of the hips may produce shearing forces on the lumbar spine, leading to injury and/or low back pain. By rotating the hips with the exercise, the lumbar spine will be kept in alignment, reducing the forces produced on the low back.

Cable Chop

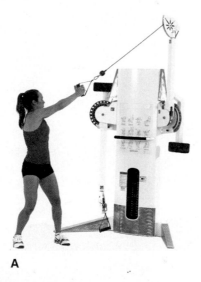

A

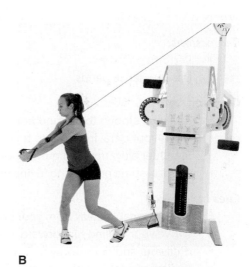

B

- *Other name(s):* Cable wood-chop.

- *Exercise classification:* Core Strength.

- *Joint(s) where motion occurs:*
  ‣ Thoracic spine.
  ‣ Lumbar spine.

- ‣ Shoulders.
- ‣ Hips.
- ‣ Knees.

- **Performance technique:** Begin by setting the cable arm to its highest setting. Grab the handle with both hands with the arms fully extended and with the right side closest to the machine. Knees should be soft with feet slightly wider than hip-width apart. The cervical spine should remain neutral and follow the torso for the duration of the exercise. Maintain tension on the cable through the duration of the exercise. Bring the cable handles down and across the body by squeezing the abdominal muscles, rotating the body, and driving the shoulders in a chopping motion. The hip closest to the machine should rotate so that the trailing toe is in line with the cable. Return to the starting position and repeat for the next repetition.

- **Force-couples:**
  - ‣ *Agonists*: Internal/external obliques, gluteus medius/minimus, latissimus dorsi.
  - ‣ *Synergists*: Transverse abdominus, rectus abdominus, hip flexors, posterior deltoids.

- **Alternatives and related exercises:**
  - ‣ Medicine ball lift and chop.
  - ‣ Cable rotation.
  - ‣ Cable lift.

- **Progression:** Cable chops on an unstable surface.

- **Regression:** Kneeling cable chop.

- **Common form mistakes:**
  - ‣ Not rotating trailing hip.
  - ‣ Shoulder elevation.
  - ‣ Elbow flexion.
  - ‣ Cervical spine not staying in line with the torso.

- **Cues to correct:**
  - ‣ "Squish the bug with your trailing foot."
  - ‣ "Pull your shoulders away from your ears."
  - ‣ "Push the cable away from your body."
  - ‣ "Follow the cable with your eyes."

- **Contraindications and special considerations:**
  - ‣ Client needs to have good strength and stability to perform this exercise.
  - ‣ Do not perform if client has low back pain.

- **Plane of motion where movement occurs:** Transverse sagittal.

- **Modality substitutions:**
  - ‣ Resistance bands.
  - ‣ Medicine ball.

Resistance Training *continued*

- **Kinetic chain checkpoints:**
  - ▸ Feet pointed straight ahead, slightly wider than hip-width apart.
  - ▸ Knees in line with the feet and slightly bent.
  - ▸ LPHC in neutral position to ensure a straight back.
  - ▸ Shoulders in line with neck and hips, with lead arm straight and following arm slightly bent.
  - ▸ Chin tucked so the head and neck are in proper cervical alignment.

- **Myths and misconceptions:**
  - ▸ *"The exercise finishes in a squat."* This exercise focuses on hip and core rotation. Finishing with a squat will interfere with hip rotation and will place a greater focus on developing leg strength as opposed to core strength.

Cable Lift

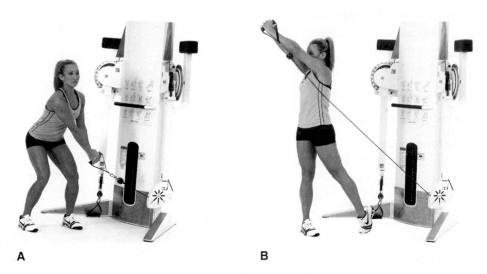

A   B

- **Other name(s):** Cable rotational lift, standing cable lift.

- **Classification of exercise:** Core Strength.

- **Joint(s) where motion occurs:**
  - ▸ Thoracic spine.
  - ▸ Lumbar spine.
  - ▸ Shoulders.
  - ▸ Hips.
  - ▸ Knees.

- **Performance technique:** Begin by setting the cable arm to its lowest setting. Grab the handle with both hands with the arms fully extended, with the right side closest to the machine. Drop into a semi-squat position with feet hip-width apart and parallel. The cervical spine should remain neutral and follow the torso for the duration of the exercise. Maintain tension on the cable through the duration of the exercise. Bring the cable handles up and across the body by squeezing the abdominal muscles, rotating the body, and driving the shoulders in an upward arcing motion. Drive the hips, knees, and ankles up. The hip closest to the machine should rotate so that the trailing toe is in line with the cable. This leg will finish in triple extension Return to the starting position and repeat for the next repetition.

- **Force-couples:**
  - *Agonists*: Internal/external obliques, gluteus medius/minimus, medial deltoids.
  - *Synergists*: Quadriceps, gluteus maximus, posterior deltoids.

- **Alternatives and related exercises:**
  - Medicine ball lift and chop.
  - Kettlebell lift and chop.

- **Progression:** Cable lift using rope attachment.

- **Regressions:**
  - Cable rotation.
  - Resistance band lift.
  - Kneeling cable lift.

- **Common form mistakes:**
  - Not performing triple extension through the trailing leg.
  - Not rotating the trailing hip.
  - Shoulder elevation.
  - Elbow flexion.
  - Cervical spine not staying in line with the torso.

- **Cues to correct:**
  - "Drive the cable up with your back leg."
  - "Squish the bug with your trailing foot."
  - "Pull your shoulders away from your ears."
  - "Push the cable away from your body."
  - "Explode through the core."
  - "Follow the cable with your eyes."

- **Contraindications and special considerations:**
  - Client needs to have good gluteus maximus activation to properly perform this exercise.
  - Client needs to have good strength and stability to perform this exercise.
  - Do not perform if client has low back pain.

- **Plane of motion where movement occurs:** Transverse, sagittal.

Resistance Training *continued*

- **Modality substitutions:**
    - ‣ Resistance bands.
    - ‣ Medicine ball.
    - ‣ Kettlebell.
    - ‣ Dumbbell.
    - ‣ Rope handles.
    - ‣ Battling ropes.

- **Kinetic chain checkpoints:**
    - ‣ Feet pointed straight ahead.
    - ‣ Knees in line with the feet and slightly bent.
    - ‣ LPHC in neutral position to ensure a straight back.
    - ‣ Shoulders in line with neck and hips, with arms extended and slightly bent.
    - ‣ Chin tucked so the head and neck are in proper cervical alignment.

- **Myths and misconceptions:**
    - ‣ *"The arms should perform the lift."* This exercise should focus on the ability of the core to drive the weight up in the transverse plane. The legs will play a part on assisting the drive of the weight up as will the arms. However, the main motion and force produced within the transverse plane will be performed by the core musculature within the LPHC.

Machines

Biceps Curl Cable Machine

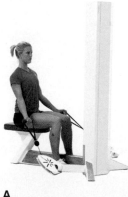
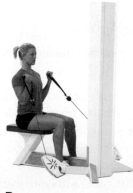

A   B

- **Other name(s):** N/A.
- **Exercise classification:** Biceps Strength.
- **Joint(s) where motion occurs:** Elbow.

- **Performance technique:** Sit tall on the machine's bench, with the core drawn in and hips in a neutral position. Pull the shoulder blades back, extend the arms, and keep the elbows in a fixed position on the machine. Perform a biceps curl, pulling the hands toward the shoulders and squeezing the biceps. Return the arms to the starting position by extending the elbows.

- **Force-couples:**
  - *Agonist*: Biceps brachii.
  - *Synergists*: Brachialis, brachioradialis.

- **Alternatives and related exercises:**
  - Suspension biceps curl.
  - Preacher curl.

- **Progressions:**
  - Standing barbell curl.
  - Seated dumbbell curl.

- **Regression:** Lower resistance of machine.

- **Common form mistakes:**
  - Allowing elbows to move forward.
  - Leaning torso back to use momentum.

- **Cues to correct:**
  - "Sit tall and keep the torso still."
  - "Keep totally still above the elbows."

- **Contraindications and special considerations:** Do not perform unless the Stabilization Level has been completed.

- **Plane of motion where movement occurs:** Sagittal.

- **Modality substitutions:**
  - Dumbbells.
  - Barbells.
  - Resistance bands.
  - Suspension trainer.
  - Kettlebells.

- **Kinetic chain checkpoints:**
  - Feet flat on floor pointed straight ahead.
  - Knees directly over ankles, bent at a 90-degree angle.
  - LPHC in neutral alignment.
  - Shoulders should be depressed and retracted.
  - Chin tucked so head and cervical spine are in alignment.

Resistance Training *continued*

Machine Pull-Down

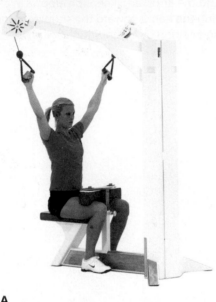

A

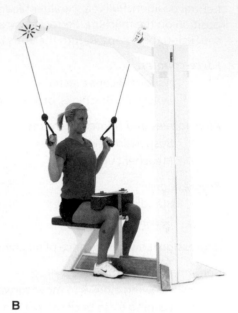

B

- *Other name(s):* Seated lat pull-down.

- *Classification of exercise:* Back Strength.

- *Joint(s) where motion occurs:*
    ‣ Shoulder.
    ‣ Elbow.

- *Performance technique:* Set the machine up to meet individual needs based on the manufacturer's guidelines. Sit upright with feet flat on the floor and pointing straight ahead. Grab the handles or bar and pull toward the body by flexing the elbows and depressing the shoulder blades. Maintain a neutral spine through the exercise. Bring the bar or handles down in front of the head. Upon reaching the end ROM, guide the handles or bar back to the starting position in a controlled manner.

- *Force-couples:*
    ‣ *Agonists*: Latissimus dorsi, teres major, biceps.
    ‣ *Synergists*: Brachialis, brachioradialis, middle/lower trapezius, rhomboid major/minor.

- *Alternatives and related exercises:*
    ‣ Seated cable row.
    ‣ Standing cable row.

- ‣ Stability ball dumbbell row.
- ‣ Inverted suspension row.
- ‣ Swimmer's pull.
- ‣ Lat sweep.

- *Progressions:*
  - ‣ Alternating arm pull-down.
  - ‣ Pull-up.

- *Regression:* Resistance band pull-down.

- *Common form mistakes:*
  - ‣ Pulling weight behind the head.
  - ‣ Elevating the shoulders.
  - ‣ Leaning the torso back to create movement.
  - ‣ Allowing the body to come off the seat during the eccentric phase.

- *Cues to correct:*
  - ‣ "Sweep your face with the bar."
  - ‣ "Squeeze your shoulder blades down and together."
  - ‣ "Squeeze your core and maintain an upright posture."
  - ‣ "Glue yourself to the seat."

- *Contraindications and special considerations:*
  - ‣ Scapular stability is required to properly perform a lat pull-down.
  - ‣ This exercise may be contraindicated for those with shoulder impingement or a shoulder injury or who have had shoulder surgery. Modify the exercise for these individuals if clearance from a licensed professional is not secured.

- *Plane of motion where movement occurs:* Frontal.

- *Modality substitutions:*
  - ‣ Resistance bands.
  - ‣ Barbell.

- *Kinetic chain checkpoints:*
  - ‣ Feet flat on floor pointed straight ahead.
  - ‣ Knees directly over ankles, bent at a 90-degree angle.
  - ‣ LPHC in neutral alignment.
  - ‣ Shoulders should be depressed and retracted.
  - ‣ Chin tucked so head and cervical spine are in alignment.
  - ‣ *"Behind-the-head lat pull-downs are better."* Not only do behind-the-neck lat pull-downs put the cervical spine in a dangerous position, but there is no evidence that more latissimus dorsi activation occurs by bringing the bar down behind the head.

Resistance Training *continued*

Alternate Arm Machine Row

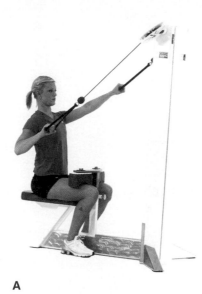

A

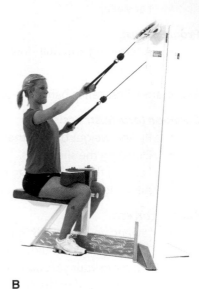

B

- ***Other name(s):*** Seated machine row, alternating machine row, single-arm machine row.

- ***Classification of exercise:*** Back Strength.

- ***Joint(s) where motion occurs:***
  - ‣ Shoulder.
  - ‣ Elbow.

- ***Performance technique:*** Sit facing the machine, with feet shoulder-width apart, pointing straight ahead and flat on the floor. Hold the machine handles with the arms fully extended. Pull the handle of one arm toward the torso by flexing the elbow and extending the shoulder. The movement should stop when the thumb reaches the armpit. Let the arm extend back to the starting position in a controlled manner. Repeat with the opposite arm. This is one repetition.

- ***Force-couples:***
  - ‣ *Agonists*: Posterior deltoids, middle/lower trapezius, biceps brachii.
  - ‣ *Synergists*: Rhomboid major/minor, latissimus dorsi.

- ***Alternatives and related exercises:***
  - ‣ Bent-over alternating dumbbell row.
  - ‣ Seated alternating tubing row.
  - ‣ Stability ball alternating dumbbell row.

- *Progression:* Standing alternating cable row.

- *Regression:* Two-arm machine row.

- *Common form mistakes:*
    - Jutting the head forward.
    - Rocking the torso, creating momentum.
    - Elevating the shoulders.

- *Cues to correct:*
    - "Pull your head back and gaze straight ahead."
    - "Sit up tall, engage the core, and lock your hips in place."
    - "Relax your shoulders and pull your shoulders away from your ears."

- *Contraindications and special considerations:*
    - This is an excellent exercise for individuals who need to strengthen the back but do not have the ability to perform standing or bent rows due to functional or stability issues.
    - For pregnancy, ensure that the client is not pressing her belly against the abdominal pad. This will better protect the fetus.

- *Plane of motion where movement occurs:* Sagittal.

- *Modality substitutions:*
    - Dumbbells.
    - Resistance bands.

- *Kinetic chain checkpoints:*
    - Feet flat on floor pointed straight ahead.
    - Knees directly over ankles, bent at a 90-degree angle.
    - LPHC in neutral alignment.
    - Shoulders should be depressed and retracted.
    - Chin tucked so head and cervical spine are in alignment.

- *Myths and misconceptions:*
    - *"Machine exercises develop movement dysfunction because they force the body into a single line of movement that is not natural."* Machines are designed to provide proper biomechanics when the machine is set up for the individual. Be sure to read the instructions on the different machines for proper setup procedures so the machine fits the client.
    - *"Machines are safer because the weight is contained and risk for falling is minimized."* Although some risk for injury is removed by utilizing machines, ensure that the client is performing the exercise correctly. Incorrect setup or improper use of a machine can lead to injury.

Resistance Training *continued*

Cable Machine Chest Press

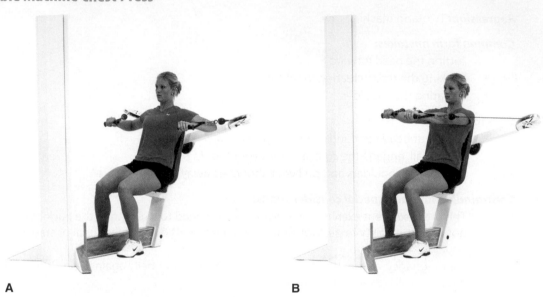

A   B

- ***Other name(s):*** Seated chest press.

- ***Classification of exercise:*** Chest Strength.

- ***Joint(s) where motion occurs:***
  - ‣ Shoulder.
  - ‣ Elbow.

- ***Performance technique:*** Begin seated with feet pointed straight ahead, back should be flat against the back rest along with the head. Ensure that the machine is set up for the client according to the manufacturer's directions. Draw in the belly button. Grab the handles with both hands. Fully extend the arms and elbows. Do not lock out the elbows at the end ROM. Return to starting position in a controlled manner.

- ***Force-couples:***
  - ‣ *Agonists*: Pectoralis major, anterior deltoid, triceps brachii.
  - ‣ *Synergist*: Pectoralis minor.

- ***Alternatives and related exercises:***
  - ‣ Push-up.
  - ‣ Standing cable chest press.
  - ‣ Supine kettlebell chest press.
  - ‣ Dumbbell incline chest press.
  - ‣ Bench press.
  - ‣ Dumbbell decline chest press.

- ▸ Stability ball dumbbell chest press.
- ▸ Medicine ball chest pass.
- ▸ Suspension trainer chest press.

- *Progression:* Alternating arm machine chest press.

- *Regression:* Seated resistance band chest press.

- *Common form mistakes:*
  - ▸ Arching the low back.
  - ▸ Moving the head forward.
  - ▸ Elevating the shoulders.

- *Cues to correct:*
  - ▸ "Glue your low back to the pad."
  - ▸ "Glue your head to the pad."
  - ▸ "Lock your shoulder blades down and keep them glued to the pad."

- *Contraindications and special considerations:*
  - ▸ This exercise may be contraindicated for those with shoulder impingement or a shoulder injury or who have had shoulder surgery. Modify the exercise for these individuals if clearance from a licensed professional is not secured.
  - ▸ Ensure that the client continues to breathe throughout the exercise to avoid increased blood pressure and performance of the Valsalva maneuver.

- *Plane of motion where movement occurs:* Sagittal.

- *Modality substitutions:*
  - ▸ Cable machine.
  - ▸ Resistance bands.

- *Kinetic chain checkpoints:*
  - ▸ Feet flat on floor, pointed straight ahead and hip-width apart.
  - ▸ Knees in line with the second and third toes.
  - ▸ Hips in neutral position and flat against the bench.
  - ▸ Shoulder blades flat against the pad in a neutral position.
  - ▸ Chin tucked so head is in neutral alignment with cervical spine, with head against the pad.

- *Myths and misconceptions:*
  - ▸ *"Machine exercises develop movement dysfunction because they force the body into a single line of movement that is not natural."* Machines are designed to provide proper biomechanics when the machine is set up for the individual. Be sure to read the instructions on the different machines for proper setup procedures so the machine fits the client.
  - ▸ *"Machines are safer because the weight is contained and risk for falling is minimized."* Although some risk for injury is removed by utilizing machines, ensure that the client is performing the exercise correctly. Incorrect setup or improper use of a machine can lead to injury.

Resistance Training *continued*

Leg Press Machine

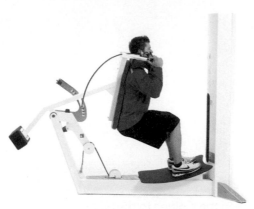

A

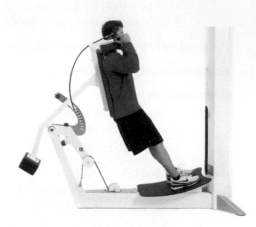

B

- **Other name(s):** N/A.

- **Classification of exercise:** Legs Strength.

- **Joint(s) where motion occurs:**
  - ‣ Hips.
  - ‣ Knee.
  - ‣ Ankle.

- **Performance technique:** Begin by adjusting the machine to fit the individual based on the manufacturer's instructions. Place feet on the platform hip- to shoulder-width apart with the toes pointed straight ahead. Knees should be straight ahead and in line with the second and third toes. The torso should be flat against back rest. Lower the weight into a squat position with the knees bent to 90 degrees or a ROM that can be effectively controlled. Squeeze the quadriceps and push through the midfoot, extending the legs to return to the start position.

- **Force-couples:**
  - ‣ *Agonists*: Quadriceps, gluteus maximus, gastrocnemius.
  - ‣ *Synergists*: Soleus, gluteus medius/minimus.

- **Alternatives and related exercises:**
  - ‣ Barbell squat.
  - ‣ Ball squat.
  - ‣ Step-up.
  - ‣ Lunge.

- **Progression:** Barbell squat.

- *Regression:* Ball squat.

- *Common form mistakes:*
  - Moving the feet in or out.
  - Moving the knees in or out.
  - Arching the low back.

- *Cues to correct:*
  - "Glue your feet in place."
  - "Push your knees out."
  - "Imagine you are holding a piece of paper against the pad with your low back."

- *Contraindications and special considerations:*
  - Some hip sleds may not allow for full hip extension, decreasing the ability to maximize gluteus maximus activation.
  - Depending on the type of machine available and body position required by the machine, this may be a bad choice for individuals who should avoid the prone position (pregnancy) or those who have a limited ROM. Look for alternatives in these cases.
  - Avoid locking out the knees.

- *Plane of motion where movement occurs:* Sagittal.

- *Modality substitutions:*
  - Barbell.
  - Dumbbell.
  - Kettlebell.
  - Sandbag.
  - Medicine ball.
  - Suspension trainer.

- *Kinetic chain checkpoints:*
  - Feet flat on floor, pointed straight ahead and hip-width apart.
  - Knees soft and in line with the feet.
  - Hips in neutral position and flat against bench.
  - Shoulder blades should be flat against pad in a neutral position.
  - Chin tucked so head is neutrally aligned with cervical spine, with head against the pad.

- *Myths and misconceptions:*
  - *"Turning your feet out will target different muscles and/or reduce stress upon the knee."* A 30-degree turnout has not been shown to activate different quadriceps muscles more or provide less forces upon the soft tissues of the knee (Escamilla et al., 2001).
  - *"Placing the feet higher or lower on the platform will emphasize different muscles of the quadriceps more than others."* A higher or lower foot placement, as well as a wider or narrower foot placement on the platform, has been shown to have very little effect on the muscular activation of the different quadriceps muscle groups (Escamilla et al., 2001).

Resistance Training *continued*

Medicine Ball

Medicine Ball Lift and Chop

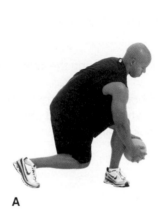

A

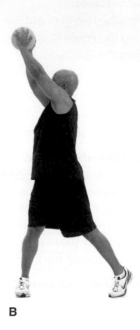

B

- *Other name(s):* N/A.

- *Classification of exercise:* Total Body Strength.

- *Joint(s) where motion occurs:*
  - ‣ Shoulder.
  - ‣ Hips.
  - ‣ Knees.

- *Performance technique:* Begin by standing with feet hip-width apart. Hold a medicine ball in both hands at the right hip. Drop into a quarter squat with the ball at the right foot. Extend the hips and knees to begin a motion to stand up. At the same time lift the medicine ball overhead diagonally. The end ROM should be standing straight up with the medicine ball over the left shoulder with arms fully extended. Return to the starting position in a controlled manner. Complete all repetitions for one side before moving to the other side.

- *Force-couples:*
  - ‣ *Agonists:* Internal/external obliques, gluteus medius/minimus, medial deltoids.
  - ‣ *Synergists:* Quadriceps, gluteus maximus, posterior deltoids.

- *Alternatives and related exercises:*
  - ▸ Cable lift.
  - ▸ Cable chop.
  - ▸ Resistance band lift.
  - ▸ Resistance band chop.

- *Progression:* Perform standing on one leg or a balance pad.

- *Regression:* Do not use medicine ball when performing motion.

- *Common form mistakes:*
  - ▸ Shoulders elevating.
  - ▸ Squatting too low.
  - ▸ Cervical spine extension.
  - ▸ Anterior pelvic tilt.
  - ▸ Feet turned out.

- *Cues to correct:*
  - ▸ "Lock your shoulders in place."
  - ▸ "Focus your eyes straight ahead."
  - ▸ "Draw belly in towards spine."
  - ▸ "Squeeze your glutes all the way to the top of the exercise."

- *Contraindications and special considerations:* This exercise may be contraindicated for those with shoulder impingement or a shoulder injury or who have had shoulder surgery. Modify the exercise for these individuals if clearance from a licensed professional is not secured.

- *Plane of motion where movement occurs:* Transverse, sagittal.

- *Modality substitutions:*
  - ▸ Dumbbell.
  - ▸ Kettlebell.
  - ▸ Sandbag.

- *Kinetic chain checkpoints:*
  - ▸ Feet shoulder-width apart and pointed straight ahead.
  - ▸ Knees slightly bent and in line with the feet.
  - ▸ LPHC in neutral alignment.
  - ▸ Shoulder blades retracted and depressed.
  - ▸ Head in neutral alignment.

- *Myths and misconceptions:*
  - ▸ *"This exercise needs to be performed explosively to be effective."* This is a strength exercise; therefore, it should not be performed explosively. If the medicine ball is too light or easy, modality substitutions can increase the stress of the movement pattern in order to continue developing strength.

Resistance Training *continued*

One-Hand Medicine Ball Push-Up

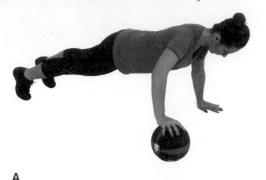

A

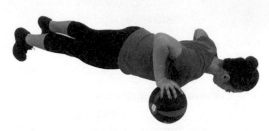

B

- *Other name(s):* N/A.

- *Classification of exercise:* Chest Stabilization.

- *Joint(s) where motion occurs:*
  ‣ Shoulder.
  ‣ Elbow.

- *Performance technique:* Start in a push position with one hand on a medicine ball. Draw in the navel and contract the gluteal muscles. Maintaining a neutral pelvis, slowly lower the body toward the ground by flexing the elbows and retracting and depressing the shoulder blades. The chest should come within 6 inches of the ground. Push back up to a starting position by extending the elbows and contracting the chest.

- *Force-couples:*
  ‣ *Agonists*: Pectoralis major, triceps.
  ‣ *Synergists*: Anterior deltoids, pectoralis minor.

- *Alternatives and related exercises:*
  ‣ Push-up with one leg elevated.
  ‣ Push-up with hands staggered.
  ‣ Push-up close grip.
  ‣ Push-up with rotation.
  ‣ Push-up with lateral hop.

- *Progressions:*
  ‣ Use a medicine ball with a larger diameter.
  ‣ Roll the medicine ball to the other hand between repetitions.

- ***Regressions:***
  - ‣ Push-up.
  - ‣ Use a medicine ball with a smaller diameter.

- ***Common form mistakes:***
  - ‣ Arching the low back.
  - ‣ Jutting the head forward.
  - ‣ Winging of the scapula.

- ***Cues to correct:***
  - ‣ "Pull your head away from the ground and keep your chin tucked."
  - ‣ "Squeeze your quads, glutes, and core."
  - ‣ "Push the ground away from you."
  - ‣ "Squish the ball."
  - ‣ "Dig your toes into the ground."

- ***Contraindications and special considerations:*** This may be a contraindicated exercise for those with shoulder stability or injury issues. The ball may also place added stress on the wrists, so clients who have weakness in the wrists should avoid this exercise.

- ***Plane of motion where movement occurs:*** Sagittal.

- ***Modality substitutions:***
  - ‣ Dumbbell.
  - ‣ Kettlebell.
  - ‣ Plyo box.
  - ‣ Aerobics step.

- ***Kinetic chain checkpoints:***
  - ‣ Feet in dorsiflexion with toes on the ground.
  - ‣ Knees and legs are straight in line with the back.
  - ‣ Head down and shoulders neutral, so that the neck, back, hips, and legs form a straight line.

- ***Myths and misconceptions:***
  - ‣ *"The feet should be together."* This position decreases the base of support for the exercise. This may be considered a progression to the exercise because it will increase the demand for stability of the exercise.
  - ‣ *"The elbows should be against the body."* This increases the demand of the triceps musculature and may make the exercise too difficult for some individuals to complete. The correct form will have the elbows positioned at a 45-degree angle from the body.

Resistance Training *continued*

Kneeling Medicine Ball Chest Pass

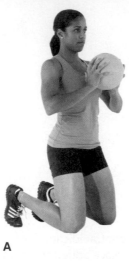

A

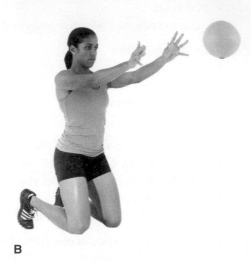

B

- *Other name(s):* N/A.

- *Classification of exercise:* Chest Power.

- *Joint(s) where motion occurs:*
  - ‣ Elbow.
  - ‣ Shoulder.

- *Performance technique:* Facing a wall or partner, kneel on the floor with knees hip-width apart, a 90-degree bend in the knees, and toes pointing straight back. Position the body squared up to a wall or partner. Hold a medicine ball (about 5–10% of body weight) with both hands, elbows flexed at chest level. As explosively as possible, push the ball forward and release by extending the elbows and contracting the chest. Do not allow shoulders to elevate. Catch the ball and repeat as quickly as possible.

- *Force-couples:*
  - ‣ *Agonists*: Pectoralis major, triceps brachii, anterior deltoid.
  - ‣ *Synergists*: Pectoralis minor.

- *Alternatives and related exercises:*
  - ‣ Rotation chest pass.
  - ‣ Standing medicine ball chest pass.

- *Progression:* Perform standing.

- *Regression:* Perform seated.

- *Common form mistakes:*
  - ▸ Lack of follow through with arms after releasing ball.
  - ▸ Elevating the shoulders.

- *Cues to correct:*
  - ▸ "Throw the ball through the wall."
  - ▸ "Follow through with arms."
  - ▸ "Lock the shoulders down."

- *Contraindications and special considerations:*
  - ▸ Use with caution with clients with previous knee, shoulder, elbow, neck, or wrist injuries and unstable shoulder, elbow, or wrist joints.
  - ▸ A pad may be needed to place the knees on for client comfort.

- *Plane of motion where movement occurs:* Sagittal.

- *Modality substitutions:* Balance pad.

- *Kinetic chain checkpoints:*
  - ▸ Feet shoulder-width apart and pointed straight ahead.
  - ▸ Knees bent at 90 degrees and in line with the feet.
  - ▸ LPHC in neutral alignment.
  - ▸ Shoulder blades retracted and depressed.
  - ▸ Head in neutral alignment.

Medicine Ball Rotation Chest Pass

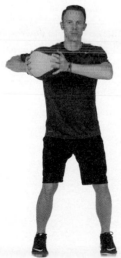
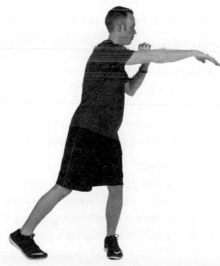

A   B

Resistance Training *continued*

- **Other name(s):** Twist pass.

- **Classification of exercise:** Core Power.

- **Joint(s) where motion occurs:**
  - Elbow.
  - Shoulder.
  - Hip.
  - Knee.
  - Ankle.

- **Performance technique:** Stand with the body turned at a 90-degree angle from a wall or partner. Hold a medicine ball with both hands and elbows flexed at chest level. Use the abdominal muscles, hips, and gluteal muscles to rotate the body quickly and explosively toward the wall or partner. As the body turns, pivot the back leg and allow it to go into triple extension. With the upper body, push the medicine ball using the back arm to extend and apply the force driving the ball forward. Catch the ball on the return and repeat as quickly as possible.

- **Force-couples:**
  - *Agonists*: Pectoralis major, triceps, anterior deltoid, internal and external obliques.
  - *Synergists*: Pectoralis minor, transverse abdominus, latissimus dorsi, gluteus medius/minimus.

- **Alternatives and related exercises:**
  - Kneeling medicine ball rotation chest pass.
  - Two-arm medicine ball chest pass.
  - Cable rotation.

- **Progression:** Perform standing on a balance pad.

- **Regression:** Kneeling medicine ball rotation chest pass.

- **Common form mistakes:**
  - Lack of follow through with arm after releasing ball.
  - Lack of triple extension.
  - Shoulder elevation and protraction.
  - Cervical spine not staying in line with torso.

- **Cues to correct:**
  - "Drive your trailing hip forward as you rotate."
  - "Pull your shoulders away from your ears."
  - "Follow the ball with your eyes."
  - "Explode through the ball."
  - "Throw the ball through the wall."

- *Contraindications and special considerations:* Use caution when performing this exercise with clients with potential back issues. A standing medicine ball chest pass may be a better option to avoid potential force issues due to the torque being placed on the spine.

- *Plane of motion where movement occurs:* Transverse, sagittal.

- *Modality substitutions:* Resistance bands.

- *Kinetic chain checkpoints:*
  - ‣ Feet shoulder-width apart and pointed straight ahead.
  - ‣ Knees slightly bent and in line with the feet.
  - ‣ LPHC in neutral alignment.
  - ‣ Shoulder blades retracted and depressed.
  - ‣ Head in neutral alignment.

Medicine Ball Pullover Throw

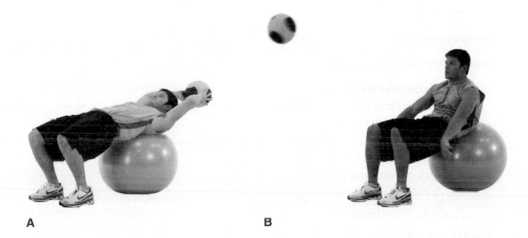

A   B

- *Other name(s):* Medicine ball power throw.

- *Classification of exercise:* Core Power.

- *Joint(s) where motion occurs:*
  - ‣ Shoulder.
  - ‣ Thoracic spine.

Resistance Training *continued*

- **Performance technique:** Place a stability ball under the low back, and bend the knees at a 90-degree angle. Keep the feet flat on the ground with the toes pointing straight forward. Hold a medicine ball that is approximately 5–10% of total body weight overhead in both hands with arms fully extended. Using the abdominals, quickly crunch forward. At the same time, throw the medicine ball forward while keeping the elbows fairly straight. As the ball is released, continue pulling the arms through to the sides of the body. Keep the chin tucked throughout the exercise. Repeat as quickly as possible, keeping the ball under control.

- **Force-couples:**
  - *Agonists*: Triceps brachii, rectus abdominus, teres major.
  - *Synergists*: Pectoralis major/minor, latissimus dorsi, anterior deltoids.

- **Alternatives and related exercises:**
  - Rotation chest pass.
  - Front oblique throw.
  - Overhead throw.
  - Overhead throw with rotation.
  - Side oblique throw.
  - Soccer throw.

- **Progression:** Heavier medicine ball.

- **Regression:** Perform on floor.

- **Common form mistakes:**
  - Stability ball placed too high on back causing hips to drop lower, leading to less core engagement.
  - Lack of follow through with arms after releasing ball.
  - Lack of overhead extension.
  - Lack of explosive power.
  - Feet turned out.
  - Feet not flat on floor.

- **Cues to correct:**
  - "Extend arms overhead."
  - "Crunch forward quickly—be explosive."
  - "Follow through with the arms."
  - "Exhale during the crunch."

- **Contraindications and special considerations:**
  - Use with caution in clients with previous shoulder, elbow, neck, or wrist injuries and unstable shoulder, elbow, or wrist joints.
  - It is imperative that the client be able to demonstrate proper core stabilization and strength. This greatly helps in reducing chances of movement compensation, muscle imbalances, and potential injury.

‣ It is important that the client have proper extensibility of the latissimus dorsi before performing this exercise to decrease stress to the low back and shoulders.

- *Plane of motion where movement occurs:* Sagittal.

- *Modality substitutions:*
  ‣ Throw to partner.
  ‣ Throw to wall.
  ‣ Throw to trampoline.

- *Kinetic chain checkpoints:*
  ‣ Feet flat on floor, pointed straight ahead.
  ‣ Knees bent at 90 degrees in line with feet.
  ‣ LPHC positioned neutrally on the ball.
  ‣ Keep shoulder blades depressed.
  ‣ Chin tucked to maintain a neutral cervical spine.

Side Medicine Ball Oblique Throw

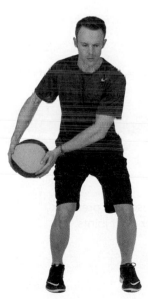

A

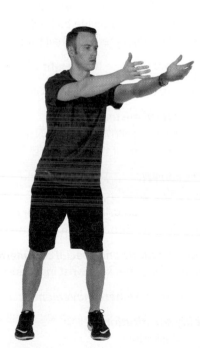

B

Resistance Training *continued*

- *Other name(s):* Side medicine ball toss.

- *Exercise classification:* Core Power.

- *Joint(s) where motion occurs:*
  - Shoulder.
  - Elbow.
  - Trunk.

- *Performance technique:* Stand perpendicular to a wall or partner with the knees slightly bent, hip-width apart, and feet pointing straight forward. Hold a medicine ball (about 5–10% of body weight) at the hip. Draw the belly inward toward the spine and as explosively as possible toss the ball against a wall or to a partner with an underhanded motion. Use a scooping motion to catch the ball. Repeat as quickly as can be controlled. Exercise may be performed continuously to one side or by alternating sides.

- *Force-couples:*
  - *Agonists:* Internal/external obliques, medial/posterior deltoids.
  - *Synergists:* Latissimus dorsi, gluteus medius/minimus.

- *Alternatives and related exercises:*
  - Kneeling medicine ball oblique throw.
  - Overhead medicine ball throw.

- *Progression:* Increase the weight of the ball.

- *Regression:* Kneeling medicine ball oblique throw.

- *Common form mistakes:*
  - Lack of follow through with arms after releasing ball.
  - Elevation of the shoulders.

- *Cues to correct:*
  - "Explode through the core."
  - "Focus on using the anterior deltoids."
  - "Follow through with the arms."

- *Contraindications and special considerations:* Use with caution in those with previous shoulder, elbow, neck, or wrist injuries and unstable shoulder, elbow, or wrist joints.

- *Plane of motion where movement occurs:* Transverse, sagittal.

- *Modality substitutions:*
  - Basketball.
  - Soccer ball.
  - Throw to trampoline.

- *Kinetic chain checkpoints:*
  - ‣ Feet shoulder-width apart and pointed straight ahead.
  - ‣ Knees slightly bent and in line with the feet.
  - ‣ LPHC in neutral alignment.
  - ‣ Shoulder blades retracted and depressed.
  - ‣ Head in neutral alignment.

Overhead Medicine Ball Throw

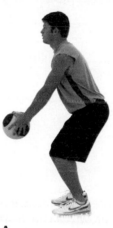

A

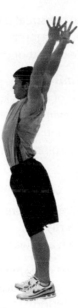

B

- *Other name(s):* Reverse ball throw.

- *Exercise classification:* Back Power.

- *Joint(s) where motion occurs:*
  - ‣ Shoulder.
  - ‣ Hips.
  - ‣ Knees.
  - ‣ Lumbar spine.

- *Performance technique:* Stand with the back facing a wall or in an open area. Hold the medicine ball with two hands between the knees in a semi-squat position. Jump off the ground explosively while driving the arms and medicine ball overhead. Release the ball before it reaches the ears, throwing behind. Land in a controlled and stable manner.

Resistance Training *continued*

- *Force-couples:*
  - *Agonists*: Anterior deltoids, quadriceps, gluteus maximus, gastrocnemius.
  - *Synergists*: Pectoralis major/minor, gluteus medius/minimus, medial deltoids, soleus.

- *Alternatives and related exercises:* Kettlebell swings.

- *Progression:* Increase weight of the medicine ball.

- *Regressions:*
  - Reduce the squat depth.
  - Take out the jump.
  - Reduce weight of the medicine ball.

- *Common form mistakes:*
  - Arching of the back.
  - Knees caving in.
  - Feet turning out.
  - Cervical spine extension.

- *Cues to correct:*
  - "Draw in your belly button."
  - "Squeeze your core."
  - "Land softly."
  - "Maintain a forward gaze."

- *Contraindications and special considerations:*
  - This exercise can also be utilized as a performance assessment. If there is an open area to perform this in, the distance the ball is thrown can be measured over three attempts. The furthest distance can then be recorded. Performing this again at a reassessment should show an increase in distance, indicating increased power development.
  - In order to perform this exercise the client needs to have displayed good landing mechanics as well as excellent core stability. Clients with low back pain or who are susceptible to back and/or knee injuries should not perform this exercise.

- *Plane of motion where movement occurs:* Sagittal.

- *Modality substitutions:* N/A.

- *Kinetic chain checkpoints:*
  - Feet shoulder-width apart and pointed straight ahead.
  - Knees slightly bent and in line with the feet.
  - LPHC in neutral alignment.
  - Shoulder blades retracted and depressed.
  - Head in neutral alignment.

Whole Body Vibration (WBV) Exercises

WBV Triceps Dips

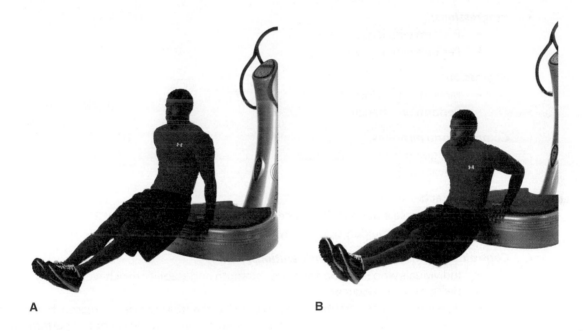

A   B

- *Other name(s):* Vibration plate dips.

- *Exercise classification:* Triceps Stabilization.

- *Joint(s) where motion occurs:*
  - Elbow.
  - Shoulder.

- *Performance technique:* Sit in front of the platform with knees bent at 90 degrees and facing away from the console. Place the hands on the edge of the platform and raise the body off the ground. Allow the body weight to drop straight toward the ground with the elbows flexing but remaining close to the side. Then push the body weight back to the starting position by extending the elbows.

- *Force-couples:*
  - *Agonist*: Triceps brachii.
  - *Synergists*: Pectoralis major/minor, teres major.

Resistance Training *continued*

- *Alternatives and related exercises:*
    - ‣ Supine ball dumbbell triceps extension.
    - ‣ Cable pushdown.
    - ‣ Bench triceps dip.

- *Progressions:*
    - ‣ Perform with legs straight.
    - ‣ Perform with legs elevated.

- *Regressions:*
    - ‣ Move the feet closer to the platform.
    - ‣ Perform on a bench.

- *Common form mistakes:*
    - ‣ Not going through a full ROM.
    - ‣ Elevating shoulders.

- *Cues to correct:*
    - ‣ "Bend those elbows to 90 degrees."
    - ‣ "Pull those shoulders down away from the ears."

- *Contraindications and special considerations:*
    - ‣ Individuals who lack good shoulder strength and stability may have difficulty performing this exercise.
    - ‣ If an individual has trouble with this exercise, the ROM can be decreased. However, the exercise should be attempted on a bench to ensure that the client can perform the technique appropriately.

- *Plane of motion where movement occurs:* Sagittal.

- *Modality substitutions:*
    - ‣ Bench.
    - ‣ Step to elevate feet.

- *Kinetic chain checkpoints:*
    - ‣ Feet pointed straight ahead.
    - ‣ Knees should be flexed, pointed straight ahead, aligned with the feet.
    - ‣ Hips in neutral alignment.
    - ‣ Shoulders in neutral position.
    - ‣ Chin tucked so cervical spine remains neutral.

- *Myths and misconceptions:*
    - ‣ *"This exercise is bad for the shoulders."* This exercise can provide added stress to the shoulder. However, if the individual has adequate shoulder strength and stability, this exercise will help develop more strength within the shoulder joint. It is important to ensure that the client has enough shoulder strength and stability prior to implementing this exercise.

WBV Straight Leg

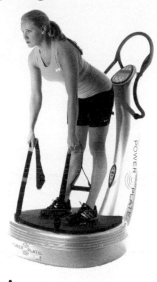

A

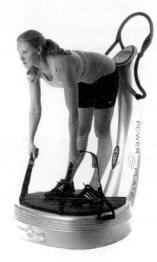

B

- *Other name(s):* Vibration plate deadlift.

- *Classification of exercise:* Legs Stabilization.

- *Joint(s) where motion occurs:* Hips.

- *Performance technique:* Stand with both feet shoulder-width apart and pointing straight ahead on the WBV platform. Grab the resistance band handles with soft knees. Retract the shoulder blades to avoid slumping at the shoulders. Bend at the waist and slowly allow the hands to go down toward the platform by performing a hip hinge. Once the end ROM is reached without compromising form, use the gluteal muscles to extend the hips and raise the torso back up to the starting position. Repeat as necessary.

- *Force-couples:*
  - ‣ *Agonist*: Gluteus maximus.
  - ‣ *Synergists*: Quadriceps, erector spinae.

- *Alternatives and related exercises:*
  - ‣ WBV dumbbell deadlift.
  - ‣ Squat.
  - ‣ Lunge.

- *Progression:* WBV single-leg deadlift.

Resistance Training *continued*

- *Regressions:*
  - ‣ Standing deadlift.
  - ‣ Dumbbell deadlift.

- *Common form mistakes:*
  - ‣ Rounding the back.
  - ‣ Flexion of the knees.
  - ‣ Moving head into cervical flexion.

- *Cues to correct:*
  - ‣ "Squeeze the core."
  - ‣ "Keep the knees soft, don't bend them."
  - ‣ "Find a spot on the floor 10 feet in front of you and keep your eyes there."
  - ‣ "Keep the chin tucked."
  - ‣ "Push the glutes back and hinge at the hips."

- *Contraindications and special considerations:*
  - ‣ Individuals with low back pain or injuries should be especially careful to not put stress on the low back with this exercise.
  - ‣ The ROM should be shortened so that form is not compromised when attempting to reach all the way to the floor. The client can reach to the knees, shins, or somewhere in between as long as stress is not placed on the lumbar spine.

- *Plane of motion where movement occurs:* Sagittal.

- *Modality substitutions:*
  - ‣ Dumbbells.
  - ‣ Kettlebells.
  - ‣ Barbells.

- *Kinetic chain checkpoints:*
  - ‣ Feet pointed straight ahead.
  - ‣ Knees in line with the feet and slightly bent.
  - ‣ LPHC in neutral position to ensure a straight back.
  - ‣ Shoulders in line with neck and hips.
  - ‣ Chin tucked so the head and neck are in proper cervical alignment.

- *Myths and misconceptions:*
  - ‣ *"This exercise is dangerous for the low back and increases risk of injury to the low back."* If the individual has enough strength and stability, as well as neuromuscular control, performing this exercise should present no issues.
  - ‣ *"You should look up during this exercise."* Looking up will engage the pelvo-occular reflex, which will ultimately put the pelvis in an anteriorly tilted position, leading to stress on the lumbar spine. In addition, the cervical flexion created by continuing to look up will produce stress on the cervical spine. The head should remain neutral with the gaze remaining forward.

WBV Two-Arm Bent-Over Row

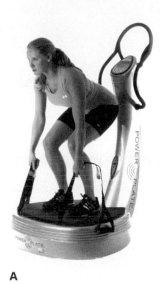

A

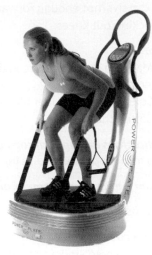

B

- **Other name(s):** N/A.

- **Exercise classification:** Back Stabilization.

- **Joint(s) where motion occurs:**
    - ▸ Elbow.
    - ▸ Shoulder.

- **Performance technique:** Stand on the vibration plate with feet pointed straight ahead and shoulder width apart. Bend slightly at the knees, with core tight, hips pulled back, and chin tucked so the neck and back form a straight line, and bend over slightly at the hip. Start with holding straps in each hand with arms extended, pull up while retracting the shoulder blades until the elbows are slightly past a 90-degree angle, and then return to the starting position.

- **Force-couples:**
    - ▸ *Agonists*: Rhomboid major/minor, latissimus dorsi.
    - ▸ *Synergists*: Posterior deltoids, middle/lower trapezius, biceps brachii.

- **Alternatives and related exercises:** Single-arm bent-over row.

- **Progression:** Increase weight being lifted.

- **Regression:** Standing two-arm bent-over row.

Resistance Training *continued*

- *Common form mistakes:*
  - ▸ Movement in the low back.
  - ▸ Excessive/not enough forward lean.
  - ▸ Locking out knees.

- *Cues to correct:*
  - ▸ "Maintain stable posture in the low back and avoid any movement except at the elbow and shoulder."
  - ▸ "Squeeze the shoulder blades together."
  - ▸ "Soften the knees."

- *Contraindications and special considerations:* Use caution with clients experiencing or recovering from upper body joint injuries.

- *Plane of motion where movement occurs:* Sagittal, frontal.

- *Modality substitutions:* Kettlebells.

- *Kinetic chain checkpoints:*
  - ▸ Feet pointed straight ahead.
  - ▸ Knees in line with the feet and slightly bent.
  - ▸ LPHC in neutral position to ensure a straight back.
  - ▸ Shoulders in line with neck and hips.
  - ▸ Elbows just past 90 degrees at top of row with shoulders pulled back. Shoulders held stable with slight rotational movement.

WBV Step-Up to Balance

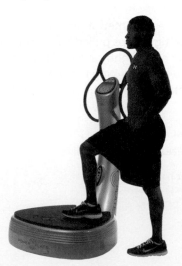

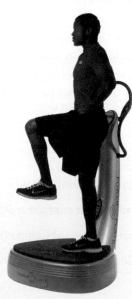

A   B

- *Other name(s):* N/A.

- *Classification of exercise:* Balance Stabilization.

- *Joint(s) where motion occurs:*
  - Ankles.
  - Knees.
  - Hips.
  - Shoulders.

- *Performance technique:* Stand in front of the WBV platform with feet pointed straight ahead. Step onto the platform with one leg, keeping the foot pointed straight ahead and the knee lined up over the mid-foot. Push through the heel and stand up straight, balancing on one leg. Flex the other leg at the hip and knee and dorsiflex the foot. Return the "floating" leg to the ground and step off the platform, maintaining optimal alignment. Repeat on the other leg.

- *Force-couples:*
  - *Agonists:* Gluteus maximus, quadriceps, gastrocnemius.
  - *Synergists:* Gluteus medius/minimus, soleus.

- *Alternatives and related exercises:*
  - Multiplanar step-up to balance.
  - Multiplanar step-up.

- *Progressions:*
  - WBV multiplanar step-up to balance.
  - Hold dumbbells.

- *Regressions:*
  - WBV step up to balance with arms supported on handlebars.
  - Step-up to balance.

- *Common form mistakes:*
  - Arching the low back.
  - Turning the foot out.
  - Not bringing leg up to top position.

- *Cues to correct:*
  - "Squeeze the glutes and core."
  - "Keep the water in the pelvic bucket."
  - "Point that toe straight ahead."
  - "Balance a glass of water on your knee."

- *Contraindications and special considerations:*
  - The client should be able to maintain stability while performing this exercise on a plyometric box before progressing to the WBV platform.

Resistance Training *continued*

> ▸ Many individuals lack the flexibility and stabilization requirements to execute a lunge properly. This exercise is a great way to regress the lunge until one develops proper flexibility and stabilization capabilities to perform it correctly.

- *Plane of motion where movement occurs:* Sagittal.

- *Modality substitutions:*
  - ▸ Plyometric box.
  - ▸ Dumbbell.

- *Kinetic chain checkpoints:*
  - ▸ Feet pointed straight ahead.
  - ▸ Knee slightly bent on stance leg, pointed straight ahead.
  - ▸ LPHC in neutral position to ensure a straight back.
  - ▸ Shoulders in line with neck and hips.
  - ▸ Chin tucked so the head and neck are in proper cervical alignment.

- *Myths and misconceptions:*
  - ▸ *"Ankle flexion does not matter during this exercise."* Maintaining good dorsiflexion on the floating leg will activate the anterior tibialis. This is a great way to work this generally underactive muscle to help balance out generally overactive calf musculature.

WBV Standing Cobra to Shoulder Scaption

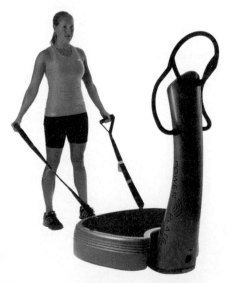
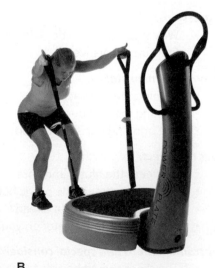

A   B

- *Other name(s):* N/A.

- *Exercise classification:* Shoulders Stabilization.

- *Joint(s) where motion occurs:* Shoulder.

- *Performance technique:* Stand facing the WBV platform with the straps held at the sides. Maintaining straight arms, pull the straps back by squeezing the scapulae together performing a standing cobra. Perform a quarter squat. Raise both arms, thumbs up, at a 45-degree ablgle in front of the body until the hands reach approximately eye level. Slowly return the arms back to the sides of the body while standing up in a controlled manner and repeat.

- *Force-couples:*
  - *Agonists*: Anterior/medial deltoids.
  - *Synergists*: Upper trapezius, teres minor, supraspinatus.

- *Alternatives and related exercises:*
  - Dumbbell shoulder scaption.
  - Resistance band shoulder scaption.
  - Seated shoulder scaption.

- *Progression:* WBV single-leg shoulder scaption alternating arms.

- *Regressions:*
  - WBV standing shoulder scaption.
  - Single-leg dumbbell shoulder scaption.

- *Common form mistakes:*
  - Bending at the elbow.
  - Thumbs not up.
  - Going too high with the raise.
  - Not staying at a 45-degree angle.

- *Cues to correct:*
  - "Give me a thumbs up."
  - "Keep the triangle for the 45-degree angles."

- *Contraindications and special considerations:*
  - If the client has shoulder joint instability, injuries, or surgeries, the ROM may need to be decreased. Make sure the client is moving within a pain-free ROM for performance of this exercise.
  - With appropriate clearance, this can be an excellent exercise for activation of the shoulder musculature in those who have shoulder impingement.

- *Plane of motion where movement occurs:* Frontal, sagittal.

- *Modality substitutions:*
  - Bands.
  - Body weight.
  - Weight plates.

Resistance Training *continued*

- *Kinetic chain checkpoints:*
    - Foot pointed straight ahead.
    - Knee in line with the foot and slightly bent on the balance leg.
    - LPHC in neutral position to ensure a straight back.
    - Shoulders in line with neck and hips, with arms in full extension through the movement.
    - Chin tucked so the head and neck are in proper cervical alignment.

- *Myths and misconceptions:*
    - *"It is better to perform lateral and front raises."* Performing shoulder exercises in the scapular plane (45-degree angle) decreases the risk of the supraspinatus muscle becoming impinged between the head of the humerus and the coracoacromial arch of the scapula. This makes this a safer and effective alternative to lateral and front shoulder raises.

Conclusion

It is essential to have as many resources available as possible in order to continuously progress clients through the OPT model, as well as to adjust to any changes or roadblocks that may come up during everyday training sessions. The exercises outlined in this chapter provide the fitness professional with a solid starting point to build a creative and dynamic exercise tool-kit to use with clients every day. By having a thorough understanding of the various aspects of each exercise and modality, and how to observe, coach, queue, progress, and regress each one, the fitness professional will be ready to build fun and challenging programs for clients of all ages and fitness levels.

Case in Review

You have identified individual training goals for each of your five clients as they seek to reach their weight loss targets. You realize the importance of coaching and motivating the group as a whole, while still providing personal attention to each client. Before your next group personal training session, you review the needs of your client Sally (age 46, the "comparer") as an example of how to best coach and cue the exercises you have selected.

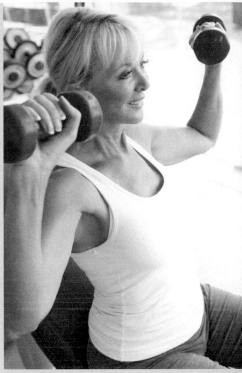

© Monkey Business Images/Shutterstock

You have observed that Sally is at her best when supporting others, affirming her motivation to make it to every session. However, it is evident that even though Sally has continued to struggle with the workout intensities, she still tries to keep up with her friends' progress. This often results in her executing the exercises incorrectly, which could lead to injury.

Using the questions you wrote down to analyze the group, you have developed the following strategy for exercise selection, coaching, and cueing considerations for Sally:

- What is one flexibility and one resistance training exercise you would have Sally conduct and why?

  - *SMR calves*: This is a tight muscle for most people. This exercise can also help address the needs of all members of the group, thus it can easily be worked into the group personal training session.

  - *Step-up, balance, curl to one-arm overhead press*: This is a full-body exercise with many components, that has a variety of modifications and does not focus on increasing resistance. It also assists with stabilization and balance.

- How would you explain to Sally how to conduct the exercise, the movements involved, joint actions that occur, and any mistakes or obstacles that are common?

  - *SMR calves*: "Begin by sitting on a flat surface with the foam roller placed just above the ankle. Cross your nonworking leg over the working leg to increase compression, if needed. Place your hands near your hips, with fingertips pointing away from the body. Raise your hips and very slowly begin to roll your body down (so the foam roll comes up) toward the knee. Roll at a pace of about 1 inch per second until a tender spot is identified. A tender spot is pain/discomfort that could be classified as 6–9 on a scale from 1–10. Remember to focus on deep breathing, and hold at this spot for 20–30 seconds, or until the tenderness begins to decrease. Identify one or two of these spots in the calf before switching to the opposite leg."

▸ *Step-up, balance, curl to one-arm overhead press:* "Hold a dumbbell in one hand at the side of your body, with feet straight and shoulder-width apart. Brace the core, and step up onto the elevated box to a single-leg balance. While balanced on one leg, immediately curl the dumbbell. From the curl-up position, press the dumbbell overhead, fully extending and rotating the arm so the palm faces away. Reverse the motion and return the dumbbell to the side of your body, then step down off the box with the nonbalance leg to complete one rep. Complete the set, then repeat with the other arm."

- How would you tailor coaching and cueing of the exercises selected for Sally?

    ▸ Continually encourage her through affirmations of her decision to be there. Tell her that she should not compare herself to her friends. Steer her focus to using workout journals to compare herself against how she was doing in previous weeks. She does not have to perform the same exercises at the same intensities as everyone else, but can be proud with personal gains week to week.

- What would you do to regress and/or progress the exercises, and what would you need to know in order to make that decision for Sally?

    ▸ *SMR calves:* The exercise can be regressed by using a less dense foam roller or by using two foam rollers to spread the pressure out more evenly. It can be progressed by utilizing a more dense foam roll or a smaller implement, such as an SMR ball, to get deeper into potential knots. You will have her regress if it is too painful for her, and progress once she becomes more experienced with SMR technique.

    ▸ *Step-up, balance, curl to one-arm overhead press.* Regressions would be to perform the exercise with two arms or to remove the step-up and perform a curl to overhead press standing in place on one leg. Progressions would include increasing the weight or raising the height of the box. Regressions will need to be made if she cannot maintain her balance or optimal form. Progressions can be made when her form is properly learned and additional strength challenges are desired.

References

Adelsberger, R., & Troster, G. (2014). Effects of stretching and warm-up on stability and balance during weight-lifting: A pilot investigation. *BioMed Central*, 1005–1024.

Escamilla, R. F., Fleisig, G. S., Zheng, N., Lander, J. E., Barrentine, S. W., Andrews, J. R., Moorman, C. T. III. (2001). Effects of technique variations on knee biomechanics during the squat and leg press. *Medicine and Science in Sports and Exercise, 33*(9), 1552–1566.

Kay, A. D., & Blazevich, A. J. (2012). Effect of acute static stretching on maximal performance: A systematic review. *Medicine and Science in Sports and Exercise, 44*(1), 154–165.

MacDonald, G. Z., Button, D. C., Drinkwater, E. J., & Behm, D. G. (2013). Foam rolling as a recovery tool after an intense bout of physical activity. *Medicine and Science in Sports and Exercise*, 131–142.

MacDonald, G. Z., Penney, M., Mullaley, M., Cuconato, A., Drake, C., Behm, D. G., & Button, D. C. (2012). An acute bout of self-myofascial release increases range of motion without a subsequent decrease in muscle activation or force. *Journal of Strength and Conditioning Research, 27*, 812–821.

Mohr, A. R., Long, B. C., & Goad, C. L. (2014). Foam rolling and static stretching on passive hip flexion range of motion. *Journal of Sport Rehabilitation, 23*(4), 296–299.

Robergs, R. A., Ghiasvand, F., & Parker, D. (2004). Biochemistry of exercise-induced metabolic acidosis. *American Journal of Physiology: Regulatory, Integrative, and Comparative Physiology, 287*, 502–516.

Sarhmann, S. A. (2002). *Diagnosis and treatment of movement impairment syndromes.* St. Louis, MO: Mosby.

Signorile, J. F., Lew, K. M., Stoutenberg, M., Pluchingo, A., Lewis, J. E., & Jinrun, G. (2014). Range of motion and leg rotation affect electromyography activation levels of the superficial quadriceps muscles during leg extension. *Journal of Strength and Conditioning Research, 28*(9), 2536–2545.

Sullivan, K. M., Silvey, D. B. J., Button, D., & Behm, D. G. (2013). Roller-massager application to the hamstrings increases sit-and-reach range of motion without performance impairments. *International Journal of Sports Physical Therapy, 8*(3), 228–236.

CHAPTER 16

BEHAVIOR CHANGE STRATEGIES FOR CLIENT RESULTS

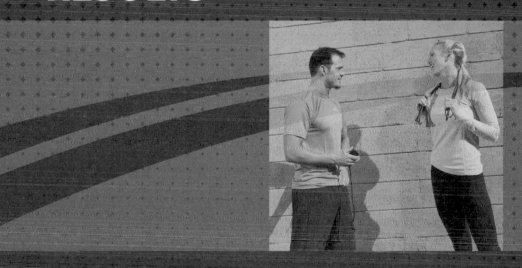

OBJECTIVES

After studying this chapter, you will be able to:

1. **Explain** the Transtheoretical Model (Stages of Change).

2. **Explain** various influences on human behavior.

3. **Apply** coaching and communication strategies.

4. **Identify** behavior change strategies.

5. **Identify** goal-setting practices and principles.

6. **Implement** progress evaluation practices.

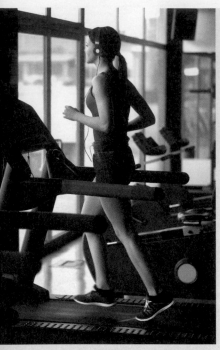

© fotoinfot/Shutterstock

Case Scenario

By now, you feel as though you are a natural at leading your clients down the path to success, coming up with solutions based on their fitness needs. You have discovered that it can be relatively easy to obtain new clients, but that it can be challenging to help those who struggle with adhering to their workouts, getting in daily physical activity, and eating healthy—all requirements to turn actions into long-term behaviors. Although you feel that you are helping your clients in changing their behaviors, you have never really looked deep into the strategies that could be integrated into your services to assist in that change.

Mary was one of your initial clients and has been with you throughout your growth and transformation in becoming a NASM Certified Personal Trainer. She came to you with the goal of losing 20 pounds. Over the past month, she has shown little progress towards her goal, losing only 3.5 pounds. Mary is in her early 40s and has been very vocal about losing weight. Her purchase of your services was the first step she took toward making her goal a reality. Over the past month, however, she has been struggling with eating healthy. Because of her minimal successes, she is finding it harder and harder to stick with the program you have designed her. Consider the following with regard to how you can help Mary reach her goals:

- Explain to Mary which stage she is currently in with regards to the Transtheoretical Model. Provide examples of behaviors she might exhibit as she progresses through each of the stages.

- How would you educate Mary about the specific influences she may encounter as she strives to lose 20 pounds?

- Use goal-setting principles to create an action plan for Mary that provides strategies she can use to foster behavior change, and identify measurable goals that can be used to evaluate her success. Also, how would you incorporate Mary throughout this process to ensure buy-in and commitment?

An Introduction to Behavior Change Strategies

In addition to knowing exercises and methods that can be used to help clients achieve their fitness goals, fitness professionals must also know how to coach and communicate with clients in order to help them stay motivated. The most successful trainers are typically able to apply behavior change techniques, whether strategically or intuitively (**Figure 16.1**). This chapter reviews strategies for fostering productive communication and positively influencing client behavior.

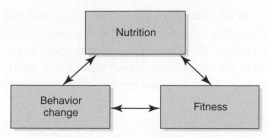

FIGURE 16.1 Three elements necessary for creating long-lasting healthy lifestyle changes.

The Transtheoretical Model (Stages of Change)

For many years, models and programs designed to change behavior focused predominantly on the extinction or control of negative behaviors, such as smoking, substance abuse, and overeating, rather than on the promotion of positive behaviors such as exercise and healthy eating. In much of the early research on behavior change, it was found to be extremely difficult to change behaviors that had become habitual. In fact, researchers discovered that people in behavior change programs had similar experiences as they struggled to change their longtime behaviors (Prochaska & DiClemente, 1983). Behavior change came to be seen as a process that occurred over time. These observations led to the development of the Transtheoretical Model (Stages of Change) (Prochaska & DiClemente, 1983).

Stages of Change

The **Transtheoretical Model (TTM)** states that individuals progress through a series of stages of change, and that movement through these stages is cyclical—not linear—because many do not succeed in their efforts at establishing and maintaining lifestyle changes. The cyclical pattern of the TTM is shown in Figure 16.2 and is comprised of six stages: precontemplation, contemplation, preparation, action, maintenance, and termination.

It is important to understand how the stages relate to personality traits and states. Specifically, a **trait** is part of a person's behavior and shapes the person's personality. Traits are typically viewed as stable and not open to change. In contrast, a **state** is temporary change in

Transtheoretical Model (TTM)

States that individuals progress through a series of stages of behavior change and that movement through these stages is cyclical, not linear, because many do not succeed in their efforts at establishing and maintaining lifestyle changes.

Trait

A part of an individual's behavior that shapes his or her personality.

State

A temporary change in one's personality, such as an emotion.

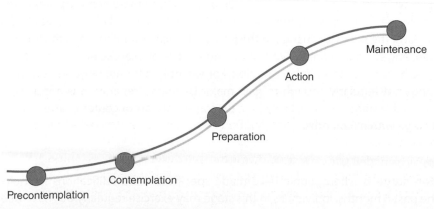

FIGURE 16.2 Transtheoretical Model.

Stable

A trait that does not change over time.

Dynamic

A trait that changes over time.

Precontemplation stage

Stage of change in the TTM where individuals do not intend to change their high-risk behaviors in the foreseeable future.

Contemplation stage

The stage of change in the TTM where individuals are contemplating making a change within the next 6 months.

Chronic contemplation

Individuals who constantly weigh the pros and cons of changing a particular behavior (e.g., exercising).

Preparation stage

The stage of change in the TTM where individuals intend to take action in the near future, usually within the next month.

Action stage

The stage of change in the TTM where individuals have made specific, overt modifications in their lifestyle within the past 6 months.

one's personality, such as an emotion. States are readily changed and typically lack stability. Stages can be **stable**, in that they may last a considerable length of time, as well as **dynamic**, in that they are open to change. The fitness professional needs to understand that the TTM seeks to change the states of the individual, not their traits. Being able to discern the difference between the place someone is in and personality traits will help to apply the Model effectively.

Precontemplation

In the **precontemplation stage** of the TTM, individuals do not intend to change their high-risk behaviors in the foreseeable future. In relation to exercise, this usually means the individual is not anticipating starting an exercise regimen in the next 6 months. Essentially, these individuals are non-exercisers. They may be at this stage for a variety of reasons. For example, they may be uninformed or misinformed about the consequences (especially long term) of their behavior, or they may have tried to change their behavior a number of times, and have become demoralized about their ability to change. Finally, these individuals may be defensive due to social pressures to change. They may even dislike the exercise experience itself. People in this stage tend to avoid reading, talking, or thinking about the behavior that needs to be changed (Prochaska & Velicer, 1997).

Contemplation

Individuals in the **contemplation stage** are contemplating making a behavior change within the next 6 months. They are typically aware of the pros of changing their behavior (here, the positive effects of exercise), but they are also acutely aware of the cons of this behavior change (e.g., more time away from the family). Say that a person is contemplating a weight loss nutrition plan; she is aware that it would be beneficial to lose weight, but she also recognizes that it would be difficult and make life less enjoyable. This delicate balance between the costs and benefits of changing behavior can produce profound uncertainty that can keep people "stuck" in this stage for long periods. Being stuck in this stage of the TTM has been characterized as **chronic contemplation**, meaning that the individual is constantly weighing the pros and cons of the behavior change. Despite their good intentions, these individuals may stay in this stage for months or years. For example, a non-exerciser might have a fleeting thought about starting to exercise, but is still unlikely to act on that thought. Individuals in this stage are generally not ready for traditional action-oriented programs.

Preparation

In the **preparation stage** of the TTM, individuals usually intend to take action in the near future, usually within the next month (e.g., "I plan on exercising three or more times a week for 20 minutes or longer"). In addition, these individuals usually have taken some significant action toward making the behavior change in the past year, such as joining a health club, contacting a physician, engaging in more activity, or buying a piece of exercise equipment. Most people in this stage have some sort of plan of action. For example, a former nonexerciser may actually exercise, but not regularly enough to gain major benefits. Preparation is not a stable stage; individuals in this stage are more likely than precontemplators or contemplators to progress to the next stage within 6 months.

Action

The **action stage** is when people have made specific overt modifications in their lifestyle within the past 6 months. Individuals in this stage may exercise regularly but have been doing so for less than 6 months. Change in this phase is not stable, and it tends to correspond with the highest risk for relapse. Because action is observable, behavior change is often mistakenly equated with taking a particular action. The difficulty is coming to a consensus on what really represents action. Generally speaking, with regards to exercise, individuals must attain a criterion that health professionals agree is sufficient to reduce risk for disease.

Maintenance

The **maintenance stage** of the TTM is the period from 6 months after the criterion has been reached, until such time that the risk of returning to the old behavior has been terminated. For example, individuals in this stage have been exercising regularly and have done so for more than 6 months. Once they stay in this stage for 5 years, it is likely they will continue to maintain regular exercise throughout their life span, except in the event of injury or other health-related problems. In this stage, people are working to prevent relapse, but they do not need to apply change processes as frequently as in the action stage. Although relapse (i.e., moving from the action or maintenance stage to an earlier stage) is always a problem when talking about behavior change, in exercise it is rare for people to regress all the way back to the precontemplation stage (Marcus, Banspach, et al., 1992). Most people will return to the contemplation or preparation stage for another serious attempt at action. At this stage, one is truly a regular exerciser—probably for a lifetime.

Termination

The **termination stage** is the point where individuals have zero temptation to engage in the old behavior and exhibit 100% **self-efficacy** in all previously tempting situations. No matter whether they are depressed, anxious, bored, lonely, or angry, they are sure they will not return to their old unhealthy habit as a way of coping. In the area of exercise, it might be an ideal goal to expect a lifetime of maintenance without ever really reaching termination because there always may be temptations to not exercise. The former nonexerciser may never reach the termination stage, but staying in maintenance might be sufficient because the individual is engaging in regular physical activity.

Applications of the TTM to Physical Activity

The initial application of the TTM to exercise was conducted at the University of Rhode Island (Sonstroem, 1988). However, the majority of work done with this model, as applied to exercise,

Maintenance stage
The stage of change in the TTM that begins 6 months after the criterion has been reached until such time that the risk of returning to the old behavior has been terminated.

Termination stage
The stage of change in the TTM in which individuals have zero temptation to engage in the old behavior and exhibit 100% self-efficacy in all previously tempting situations.

Self-efficacy
Belief regarding one's ability to succeed or perform in a specific situation.

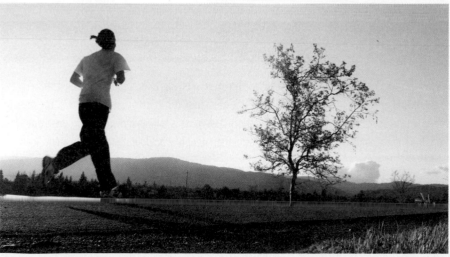

© Galina Barskaya/Shutterstock

CHECK IT OUT

Participants in the preparation stage used more behavioral processes such as putting things around the house to remind them to exercise than did people in other stages. In addition, although there were many similarities between the findings in this study and those for smoking cessation, there were important differences. Specifically, the use of behavioral processes declines from the action to maintenance stage in smoking cessation, but there is no such decline in exercise (Marcus, Rossi, Selby, Niaura, & Abrams, 1992).

has been conducted by Bess H. Marcus, PhD, and her colleagues. For example, they conducted a study as part of a large worksite exercise-promotion project. Participants were classified into the following categories: precontemplation, contemplation, preparation, action, and maintenance. They found that participants in different stages of the model used different behavior change processes (Marcus, Rossi, Selby, Niaura, & Abrams, 1992).

Research has demonstrated that when there is a mismatch between the stage of change and the intervention strategy, attrition is high (Marcus, Rossi, et al., 1992). For example, if an individual is in the contemplation stage, and the intervention focuses on maintenance strategies (e.g., refining specific types of exercise behavior) rather than on motivational strategies for the contemplators, the risk of dropout increases. Individuals with a precontemplation profile cannot be treated as if they are ready for action intervention and then be expected to stay with the program. Therefore, matching strategies to an individual's stage of change is one strategy to improve adherence and reduce attrition.

The underlying theme of the TTM is that people are at different levels of readiness to change their behavior, and therefore different strategies or interventions are needed to bring about the desired change (Prochaska, DiClemente, & Norcross, 1992). Marcus and colleagues examined this matching approach as part of the program **Imagine Action**, which was designed to help people through the different stages of change (Marcus, Banspach, et al.,1992). The participants were separated into groups based on the stage they were in: contemplation, preparation, or action. The participants were then provided with specific strategies that matched the stage they were in. Results of this matching approach revealed that the intervention successfully got people close to exercise, if not exercising. These findings demonstrate that a low-cost, relatively low-intensity intervention can produce significant improvements in stage of exercise adoption.

Imagine Action

Program designed to help people through the different stages of change.

CHECK IT OUT

Early research using smokers (and later research using exercisers) has indicated that the best strategy to promote retention is matching interventions to the stage of change (Prochaska & Velicer, 1997). The research has indicated that a reasonable goal for any therapeutic intervention is to help individuals progress one stage, which makes them about two-thirds more successful than people who do not progress to any stage.

Influences of Human Behavior

Human behavior is extremely complex, and myriad factors influence the way individuals behave. Influences include, but are not limited to, cognitive influences (e.g., self-confidence, self-talk), affective influences (e.g., positive and negative emotions), interpersonal influences (e.g., walking groups, group fitness classes, eating in groups), behavior influences (e.g., positive reinforcement, self-monitoring), and sensation influences (e.g., pain associated with working out, feelings of hunger). Fitness professionals need to be aware of these influences, because they may make the difference between a client staying with a program or dropping out. In addition, fitness professionals can use this information to design programs to maximize adherence.

Cognitive Influences

What individuals think about and how they think can have a large influence on their behavior. Two important cognitive factors that influence behavior are **confidence** and **self-talk**.

Confidence

Probably the most consistent finding with regard to exercise behavior is the positive relationship between **self-confidence** (often called *self-efficacy* in the scientific literature) and exercise adherence. In fact, research has found it to be the strongest predictor of physical activity across gender, ethnicity, and body mass index; supporting the generalized positive effects of self-efficacy on physical activity (Rovinak et al., 2010). Simply stated, self-efficacy is the belief in one's ability to execute a certain behavior. Getting started in an exercise program, for example, is likely affected by the confidence a person has in his or her ability to perform the desired behavior (e.g., walking, running), and to keep up the behavior. Besides initiating an exercise program, fitness professionals will typically be interested in their clients' belief that they can successfully complete and stay with a training regimen. Or, for a more specific behavior, it might be a person's belief that he can successfully run a 5K in less than 25 minutes, or that he can adhere to a nutrition plan. Self-efficacy is task specific; for example, a client may have confidence in riding a bike for an hour, but not in running for 30 minutes.

Confidence stems from several different sources (Bandura, 1997). Fitness professionals can tap into these sources to increase their clients' confidence:

- *Performance accomplishments:* This is the strongest source of self-confidence. It focuses on personal task improvement and success, rather than on comparisons with others.
- *Modeling:* Watching other, similar individuals successfully perform the desired task can increase a person's confidence in his or her ability to complete the task, too.
- *Verbal persuasion:* Being persuaded by someone else (e.g., fitness professional, coach, friend) that he or she can perform the task successfully.
- *Imagery:* When people imagine themselves performing a task, it increases their confidence that they will actually be able to perform it.

It is important to understand that confidence can be both a determinant of exercise as well as a consequence of exercise. More specifically, in terms of exercise or nutrition plans, confidence can enhance adherence to a program. Conversely, adherence to regular exercise or keeping to one's nutrition plan can also work in return to enhance a person's confidence. In essence, it is like a continuous circle, in that confidence can lead to greater exercise adherence, which, in turn, results in more confidence, which leads to increased exercise, and so on and so on. Therefore, fitness professionals should try to build their clients' confidence, so they can initiate and maintain a commitment to exercise, or at the very least help them to begin engaging

Confidence
Feeling or belief of certainty.

Self-talk
One's internal dialogue.

Self-confidence
The belief in one's ability to execute a certain behavior.

in fitness activities. This should increase their confidence that they can, in fact, maintain (or at least start) an exercise program.

Fitness professionals should make use of the sources of confidence (e.g., performance accomplishments, modeling, verbal persuasion, imagery) to help build confidence in their clients. For example, fitness professionals could try to persuade their clients verbally by saying, "You have been able to stick to your meal plan during the holidays before, so I know you can do it again" or "This workout is tough, but I know you are going to be able to push through it", in order to help them with their program. Similarly, because the strongest sense of confidence comes from performance accomplishments, helping clients achieve a level of performance success will help build their confidence that they can in fact perform certain behaviors. This reinforces why progress tracking in various forms and through multiple assessments is so important for the client.

Self-Talk

What individuals say to themselves (internally or aloud) can have a large influence on their behavior. Sometimes this self-talk is positive and motivational (e.g., "I'm good at this new exercise," "I like eating healthy"), and sometimes it can be negative and self-defeating (e.g., "You're never going to lose the weight," "You don't have time to go to the gym"). Rather than the situation itself causing an individual to feel either good or bad, it is usually the person's internal dialogue that determines the emotional reaction. By changing clients' thoughts and self-statements, the fitness professional can keep them motivated, even when things are not going as planned. This is very important for fitness professionals, because most clients have setbacks that cause them to stop exercising or to deviate from a nutrition plan. Most of the time it is a person's inner dialogue that turns a temporary situation into a catastrophe; in the client's mind she will never be successful at maintaining a nutrition or exercise regimen.

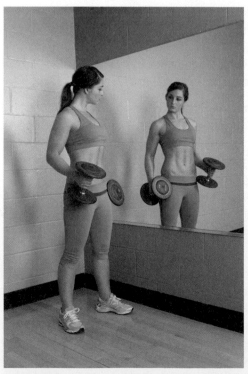

© Carl Stewart/Shutterstock

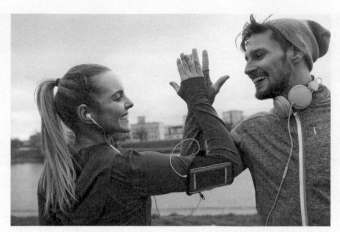

© gpointstudio/Shutterstock

Interpersonal Influences

Eating and exercise, as well other behaviors, are influenced by a client's social network. Social support includes companionship, encouragement, assistance, or information from friends, family members, and others; tangible aid and service from the community; and advice, suggestions, and information from professionals. These people can have a large influence on an individual's motivation and actual behaviors. Specifically, significant others can cue exercise through verbal reminders (e.g., "Did you put your exercise clothes in your car?"), as well as through modeling physical activity and reinforcing it by their companionship during exercise. In addition, friends and family can give practical assistance, providing transportation, measuring exercise routes, or lending exercise clothing or equipment. This is why one of the most consistent and successful factors influencing exercise adherence is the individual's social environment. Specifically, social support, or **interpersonal influences**, is a key aspect of one's social environment, and support from friends, family, and others has consistently been linked to physical activity and adherence to structured exercise programs among adults (U.S. Department of Health and Human Services, 1996).

Many group-oriented programs are effective because they offer enjoyment, social support, an increased sense of personal commitment to continue, and an opportunity to compare progress and fitness with others. If an individual typically jogs for 30 minutes with a partner at 7:00 AM, but one morning doesn't particularly feel like getting up and working out, he won't want to let down his partner so he will show up and exercise anyway. Also, being part of a group also fulfills the need for affiliation, which is one of the main reasons people give for why they exercise. Fitness professionals can use the positive effect of significant others on exercise adherence by making sure to include them (especially spouses) in the program, whenever possible, as well setting up small groups and buddy systems.

Interpersonal influences
Influences from those individuals or groups one interacts with regularly.

Affective Influences

Another important influence on behavior in exercise and eating situations is the participant's emotions. These are known as **affective influences**. Positive or negative emotions may make it more or less likely for a person to adhere to an exercise program or nutrition plan. Conversely, the effects of exercising and eating on emotions can be just as important. With regard to exercise, the close relationship between exercise and mood has been studied in various settings, and considerable experimental and experiential evidence supports that positive mood states are related to exercise (Berger & Tobar, 2011). Along these same lines, psychologists and

Affective influence
Influence resulting from emotions.

CHECK IT OUT

The following studies provide empirical evidence regarding the importance of social support and the social climate of exercise on exercise adherence:

- A spouse's attitude can exert even more influence than the exerciser's own attitude. Raglin (2001) found that the dropout rate for married singles (only one spouse from a married couple exercising) was higher than for married pairs (both spouses were in the exercise program). Thus, actually taking part in an exercise program together provides a great deal of mutual support for spouses.
- A study by Estabrooks and colleagues (2011) applied principles of group dynamics (e.g., group structure, group environment, group processes) to a physical activity intervention called the Move More program in a large corporate setting. Compared with a traditional physical activity program, the "Move More" group exhibited increased physical activity along with positive changes in self-efficacy, satisfaction, goals, and social support. Studies comparing exercising alone versus exercising with a partner have found increased adherence when working out with a partner (Trost, Owen, Bauman, Sallis, & Brown, 2002).
- Wankel (1984) developed a program to enhance social support that included a leader, a class, a buddy (partner), and family members. The leader regularly encouraged the participants to establish and maintain their home and buddy support systems, attempted to develop a positive class atmosphere, and ensured that class attendance and social support charts were systematically marked. Results indicated that participants receiving these various aspects of social support had better attendance and adherence than the control condition.

psychiatrists rate exercise as the most effective technique for changing a bad mood, and they are more likely to use exercise than other techniques to energize themselves (Thayer, Newman, & McClain, 1994). As fitness professionals train their clients, they might be helping to enhance their clients' mood. However, specifically using exercise to enhance mood should be left to trained health professionals and psychologists.

A great deal has been written on the relationship between emotions and eating. Emotional eating means turning to food for comfort, not because of appetite. Individuals, especially those

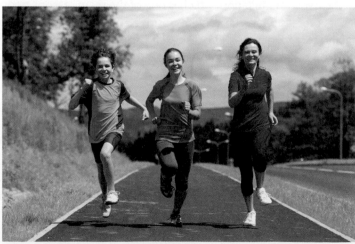

© gbh007/iStockphoto.com

with weight problems, often eat based on negative emotions (e.g., depression, anxiety) rather than simply because they are hungry. Licensed psychologists who were surveyed on how they dealt with patients' weight and weight loss challenges in their practice repeatedly identified emotions as not only an important factor affecting their clients' weight problems, but also the major barrier to overcoming them (*Consumer Reports*, 2013). Specifically, when asked which strategies were essential to losing weight and keeping it off, the psychologists cited understanding and managing the behaviors and emotions related to weight management as essential for addressing weight loss with their clients. In addition, psychologists cited emotional eating as a barrier to weight loss. In general, gaining self-control over behaviors and emotions related to eating were both important, indicating that the two go together. Fitness professionals need to be aware of this close relationship between eating and emotions and follow appropriate referral procedures to healthcare providers.

Sensation Influences

Exercisers and individuals on nutrition plans are typically very sensitive to different physical sensations associated with exercise and nutrition. **Sensation influences** are physical feelings an individual experiences as it relates to behaviors involved in establishing a healthy lifestyle. For example, beginners who are starting a workout and training regimen almost assuredly will feel some physical discomfort following the first few workouts. Therefore, fitness professionals should try to ensure that they do not overload new clients with too much exercise too early, as the pain may turn them off to continuing to exercise. In addition to specific emotions (e.g., anxiety, depression), feelings of hunger also are very prevalent for people trying to decrease calories on a nutrition plan. Some report always feeling hungry, and sometimes hunger is the dominating feeling throughout the day.

People who are overweight often feel it physically, and their weight can be a central part of their feelings and thoughts throughout the day. Fitness professionals need to be sensitive to these feelings of hunger and heaviness for those clients who are overweight and/or are on diets. These feelings can be very strong and provide a barrier for adhering to an exercise program.

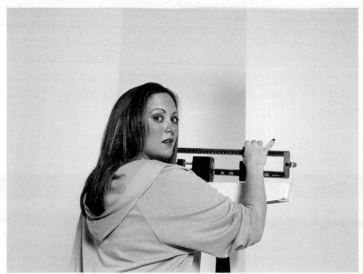

© Creatas/Thinkstock

TRAINER TIPS

If emotions (e.g., anxiety, depression) become debilitating to a client, the fitness professional should refer the client to a licensed psychologist or healthcare professional.

Sensation influences

Physical feelings an individual experiences as it relates to behaviors involved in establishing a healthy lifestyle.

TRAINER TIPS

Fitness professionals could point out to their clients that many people start out in not so great shape and that they should focus more on what they want to become, and not what they are right now. In essence, the focus should be on what behaviors are necessary to improve their fitness, health, or wellness.

Behavior Influences

Behavior influences are those influences that are created as a result of an individual's own behavior. Clients experience a number of behavioral influences; our focus here will be on positive reinforcement and journaling.

Positive Reinforcement

Positive reinforcement focuses on providing individuals with some sort of reward for exhibiting a specific type of behavior. The goal is to increase the likelihood of the desirable behavior being repeated in the future. Sport psychologists agree that the predominant approach with sport and physical activity participants should be positive reinforcement, although criticism is sometimes necessary (Smith, 2006). A 5:1 ratio of positive to negative feedback is recommended (Positive Coaching Alliance, 2013).

Rewards can come from many sources. They may be: nonverbal, such as a pat on the back or a big smile; verbal, such as positive statements like "Way to go!" or "Nice job today!"; material reward incentives, such as money; or an activity, such as playing a game instead of running on the treadmill. It is important for fitness professionals to find out what types of reinforcements work with different clients, because people will react differently to the same reinforcement. With new exercisers, fitness professionals should focus on providing positive reinforcement and positive feedback. Because these individuals typically experience more pain, discomfort, and failure than more experienced exercisers, they may need more positive reinforcement to keep them going.

Journaling

Another behavioral practice that can help clients keep up with their exercise and nutrition programs is **journaling**. Journaling is a type of self-monitoring, and is a practical way to collect information about behavior patterns that can be used to identify cues and barriers to exercise and nutrition plans (**Figure 16.3**). Information from journaling can help identify the best times in a person's schedule for an exercise routine, and any accommodations that may be necessary, such as having dinner an hour later to accommodate exercising after work. Journaling can also help individuals on a nutrition plan understand the situations that make them more likely to eat inappropriately, and then establish strategies to avoid or successfully cope with these situations. Journaling has traditionally been a writing activity, but today people are turning to various computer programs and smartphone apps that can be used to record daily or weekly progress. Fitness professionals can periodically evaluate clients' journals and offer meaningful positive feedback to help them reach their goals. If clients know that professionals will be periodically looking at their journals, they are more apt to exhibit positive behaviors throughout their exercise regimen.

TRAINER TIPS

When working with new clients, you should use low- to moderate-intensity activities, because these do not put as much stress on the body and do not cause the discomfort that often causes people who are starting to exercise to stop exercising.

Behavior influences

Influences that are created as a result of an individual's own behavior.

Positive reinforcement

The practice of offering a reward following a desired behavior to encourage repetition of the behavior.

Journaling

A type of self-monitoring and a practical way to collect information about behavior patterns that can be used to identify cues and barriers to exercise and nutrition plans.

Date: 4/11

I was really hoping this would be a great day—and that's how it started. Hard to know where to begin. Good 10,000-step walk, but then I added high-fat cheese to my egg-white omelet. Why did I do that? I don't even know why I keep that crap in the house. Time to get a big garbage bag and dump the junk. That's it: DUMP THE JUNK!!! I don't know that I can do this but maybe, just maybe, we'll see.

FIGURE 16.3 Journal example.

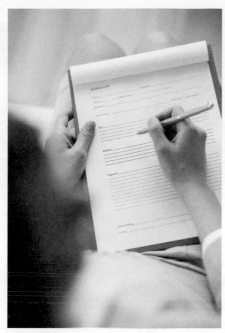

© shironosov/iStockphoto.com

Human behavior is extremely complex, and is affected by many different factors. Physical activity and eating are no different. There are several types of influences on behavior, including cognitive influences, interpersonal influences, affective influences, sensation influences, and behavioral influences. Fitness professionals need to be sensitive to all these different influences and how they may affect their clients.

Coaching and Communication Strategies

Being an effective fitness professional requires knowledge of physiology, anatomy, biomechanics, and training methods to provide clients with proper information to enhance their flexibility, speed, endurance, and strength, and to meet their personal goals. Fitness professionals with good communication skills are much more likely to make positive connections with their clients.

Motivational Interviewing

Motivational interviewing has been defined as a collaborative person-centered form of guiding to elicit and strengthen motivation for change. More specifically, it is a brief psychotherapeutic intervention designed to increase the likelihood that a client will consider, initiate, and maintain specific strategies for reducing a harmful behavior. Although it was developed to enhance motivation in a variety of health contexts, it has been applied to adherence to exercise behavior. The foundation of this technique is an empathetic, person-centered style, emphasizing evoking and strengthening the client's own motivation for healthy change. Motivational interviewing involves knowledge and skills in four areas (Rollnick, Miller, and Butler, 2007):

1. Expressing empathy
2. Helping the client realize the gap between values and problematic behavior (developing discrepancy)

Motivational interviewing
A collaborative person-centered form of guiding to elicit and strengthen motivation for change.

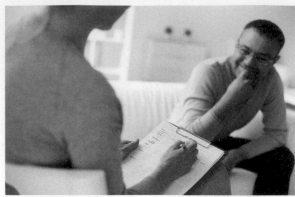

© shironosov/iStock/Thinkstock

3. Respecting the client's resistance as being normal
4. Supporting the client's self-efficacy

The spirit of motivational interviewing can be captured in the following fitness-related principles (Breckon, 2002):

◆ It is the client's task, not the fitness professional's, to articulate the client's ambivalence (exercise vs. not exercising).
◆ Motivation to change is elicited from the client.
◆ Readiness to change is not a client trait, but rather a fluctuating product of interpersonal interaction (the fitness professional might be assuming a greater readiness for change than is the case).

A fitness professional may or may not be skilled in motivational interviewing. If the fitness professional lacks this skill, oftentimes a staff member at a fitness center will know this technique and can help in conducting the interview. If the fitness professional is knowledgeable about this technique, then he or she can use it when dealing with clients who might be ambivalent about exercising.

Verbal Communication

Good communication skills are among the most important ingredients contributing to the performance and personal growth of exercise participants. For example, studies of coaches have shown that athletes look to their coaches' social competence relative to communication, even before their technical skills (Phillippe & Seiler, 2006). The following guidelines are helpful for sending effective messages.

Be Direct
Fitness professionals should tell their clients exactly what they mean, and not assume that their clients know what they want or feel. This means straightforward communication in the spirit of promoting positive change.

Be Clear and Consistent
Avoid double messages like "I think you are doing well and trying hard but I need you to be more consistent in your effort." The client might think, "If you think I am doing well and trying hard, then why do I need to be more consistent in my effort?" If clients need improvement,

just tell them what they need to improve upon. For example, a fitness professional might say, "you only give effort occasionally; you need to be consistent in your effort in order to reach your goals."

Own Your Message

Use "I" and "my" and not "the club" or "most professionals believe." Fitness professionals disown their messages when they do not take personal responsibility for them. When professionals say what they believe, they are expressing ownership in the statement and not relying on what others might think or feel.

Deliver Messages Immediately

When professionals see clients doing a movement or lift incorrectly, feedback should be provided immediately with specific information about how to perform the movement or lift correctly. Similarly, if the fitness professional notices the client is falling into old and unhealthy habits, this should be addressed at the time of observation.

Be Supportive

If fitness professionals want their clients to listen to their messages, then they should not be delivered with threats, negative comparisons, sarcasm, or judgment. Be positive, but when corrections are necessary be sure to provide information regarding how to correct the error.

Be Consistent with Nonverbal Messages

Because a lot of information is conveyed nonverbally through gestures, facial expressions, and body posture, fitness professionals should make sure that their verbal messages match their nonverbal ones. For example, fitness professionals may tell their clients that it is okay to make mistakes when doing different lifts, but if their expression (frown) and posture (hands across the chest) contradict their words, then the client may be receiving two different messages.

Look for Feedback That the Message Was Actually Received and Interpreted

Watch for verbal and nonverbal signals that clients have received the message, such as nodding of the head or simply saying "OK." If no signal is given, the fitness professional should ask questions to solicit the feedback, such as "Do you understand what I am telling you?" or "Are you clear about what you should do?"

Active Listening

When people communicate, they typically think about what they want to say or how they want to say it. But sometimes it is more important as a fitness professional to listen carefully to clients and to what they have to say (which includes being sensitive to their body language, as well as the actual words they speak). The best way to listen better is to listen actively. **Active listening** involves the following:

- ◆ Attending to the main and supporting ideas
- ◆ Acknowledging and responding
- ◆ Giving appropriate feedback
- ◆ Paying attention to the client's total communication

Active listening

A listening technique that requires the listener to provide feedback to the speaker by restating what the listener heard in his or her own words.

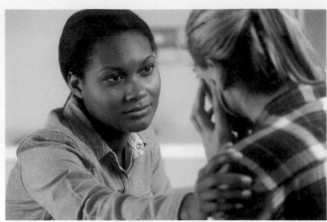
© monkeybusinessimages/iStock/Thinkstock

Active listening also involves nonverbal communication, such as making direct eye contact and nodding to confirm understanding of what has been said. In essence, the listener (in this case, the fitness professional) shows concern for the content and the intent of the message and for the client's feelings (**Table 16.1**).

Of all the things that can make a client feel accepted, significant, and worthwhile, none is more vital than being listened to. If fitness professionals want clients to confide in them, they should make a concerted effort to listen to them. In essence, good listening shows sensitivity and encourages an open exchange of ideas and feelings.

An active listener often paraphrases what the speaker has said. The following are some typical lead-ins for a paraphrase:

- "What I hear you saying is . . ."
- "Let me see if I've got this right. You said . . ."
- "What you're telling me is . . ."

Asking specific questions to allow a client to express his or her feelings is also part of active listening, as demonstrated by the following example:

Statement: "I am thinking about increasing my exercise times from 3 days a week to 5 days a week, but I'm not sure this is the best thing to do right now."
Question: "What do you gain or lose by increasing your exercise time?"
Paraphrase: "It sounds as though you're struggling with trying to balance getting fit with other demands in your life."

By paraphrasing their clients' thoughts and feelings, fitness professionals let their clients know that they are listening and that they care. Often times, this leads to more open communication and exchange, because the client senses that the fitness professional is interested. When asking questions, the fitness professional should avoid using the interrogative "why," as this can sound judgmental. Reference the following information on active listening skills (Rosenfeld and Wilder, 1990):

- Hearing should not be mistaken for listening.
- Hearing is simply receiving sounds, whereas listening is an active process.
- Hearing someone is not the same as listening to the meaning of the message.
- It is frustrating to the speaker when a receiver hears but does not listen.
- Someone who finds herself not listening should practice focusing her concentration on the speaker.

TABLE 16.1　Strategies for Active Listening	
Listen attentively	Show that you are listening attentively by making consistent eye contact, nodding, and possibly taking notes.
Focus completely on the client	Avoid multitasking or checking text messages or emails when with a client.
Filter out internal chatter	Avoid thinking about topics that are irrelevant to the client. Do not try responding to what the client is saying in your head before the person has finished speaking. Do not think about what you need to do later in the day.
Ask probing questions	Avoid using too many questions that require only a "yes" or "no" response. Ask open-ended questions. For example, use a question like "How did that make you feel?" instead of "Did that make you feel bad?"
Hold silences	Do not try to fill silences by talking. Let the silence continue to prompt the client to talk.
Use the client's language	Use similar language to the client if it feels authentic and natural. Avoid using unfamiliar terminology that is specific to a particular industry in which the client is not familiar.

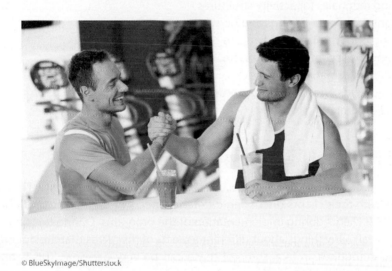

© BlueSkyImage/Shutterstock

Coaching Styles

Fitness professionals often spend a great deal of time with their clients, and the climate that they create is important in fostering motivation. Although there are a number of coaching styles, the one recommended by sport and exercise psychologists is an autonomy-supportive style.

Autonomy-Supportive Style

The **autonomy-supportive style** of coaching focuses on creating an environment that empha-sizes self-improvement, rather than beating others (i.e., direct competition). In addition, clients are engaged in the decision-making process, and fitness professionals help them feel that they "own" their workouts and have had choice in program selection. In essence, individuals feel that their behavior originates from and expresses their true selves, rather than being a response to external sources. This is not to say that clients simply determine their own workout programs.

Autonomy-supportive style

A coaching style that focuses on creating an environment that emphasizes self-improvement, rather than competing against others.

Rather, fitness professionals should solicit input from clients, as to the exercises they prefer and the environments that make them feel most comfortable.

Research has revealed that individuals who perceived that their coaches supported their autonomy, and better met their autonomy, relatedness, and competence needs, were more autonomy motivated (Ntoumanis & Standage, 2009). In addition, in exercise environments, autonomy support has been positively linked to self-determined motivation, exercise intentions, effort expenditure, persistence, and enrollment in physical activity classes (Wilson & Rodgers, 2004). What this means for fitness professionals is that increasing autonomy is important, because when clients feel autonomous, they are typically more intrinsically motivated. In turn, when individuals are intrinsically motivated, they tend to exhibit greater adherence to exercise programs than those who are motivated primarily from external sources (i.e., rewards). Therefore, fitness professionals should try to devise programs for clients that are interesting and intrinsically motivating, while still providing support along the way. For example, some clients might enjoy running in groups, whereas others might like the solitude of running alone. Some people may enjoy the competition offered by sport, whereas others do not like the competitive environment. Fitness professionals can support their clients' autonomy by:

- Providing choices within limits
- Offering rationales for activity structures
- Recognizing clients' feelings and perspectives
- Creating opportunities for clients to demonstrate initiative
- Avoiding overt control and criticism
- Providing informational feedback
- Limiting clients' ego involvement throughout their program (i.e., focus on self-improvement instead of comparing to others)

Level of Personal Disclosure

Many fitness professionals develop close relationships with their clients. They often spend many hours with their clients discussing different aspects of their exercise programs and are often with their clients during implementation of the programs. During this time together, clients often reveal many things about different aspects of their lives that are not directly related to the exercise routines. In fact, some of these can be very personal. This is not unlike athletic professionals who often deal with injured athletes several times a week and hear many personal stories. Because the clients are revealing a great deal of personal information about themselves, fitness professionals often feel at ease telling clients about their own personal life. Although this might be tempting, fitness professionals should be very careful about how much they share with their clients. Despite often-close relationships with clients, fitness professionals need to remember that they are still professional relationships, and should be treated as such. This does not mean that fitness professionals need to be stiff and rigid, and never offer up any personal information; rather, they simply need to remember their status as a professional, and that personal boundaries should always be honored.

The relationship between fitness professionals and clients is critical for client success. Just like in counseling, the quality of the relationship is just as (or even more) important as the skill of the counselor or professional. Knowing how to effectively give verbal messages and listen actively are two ways in which to solidify this relationship. Along these lines, creating the proper environment for clients helps them to feel comfortable and stay motivated. Specifically, an autonomously supportive professional, who creates an environment in which clients feel empowered and engaged in decision making, will foster positive relationships as well as enhance performance.

TRAINER TIPS

As you build your relationships with your clients, you may want to add them to your social media pages and feeds. However, keep in mind that you are your brand. The pictures you share on social media may conflict with a client's values. To avoid this conflict, create a social media page or feed, separate from your personal web presence, that depicts you as a personal trainer; posting articles, images, and insights that are only health and fitness related.

Behavior Change Strategies

One of the most difficult things to do is to change someone's behavior, or for someone to change their own behavior. This is, in part, one reason for the growing problem of overweight and obesity around the world. Sport and exercise psychologists have used information regarding the determinants of physical activity, along with behavior change theories, to develop and test the effectiveness of different strategies to enhance exercise adherence.

It is important to note that any **intervention** should always attempt to match the individuals in the program, and the situational/environmental factors surrounding the program. Consistent with the Transtheoretical Model, fitness professionals should always be sensitive to the stage of behavior change that their clients are in and, as much as possible, design a program that matches that stage (Prochaska & DiClemente, 1983). A quantitative review of studies examining the efficacy of interventions for increasing physical activity among people in community, school, work, home, and healthcare settings, found that interventions, on average, increased adherence (Dishman & Buckworth, 1997). Note, however, that there was a wide range of effectiveness in the interventions studied, based on the number of individuals in a particular study and environmental factors. For example, larger effects were found for interventions that sought to increase participation in low- to moderate-intensity activities than for strength training activities, and effects are greater when supported or delivered through audio or visual media (Gauvin, Levesque, & Richard, 2001). The main point is that interventions to enhance exercise adherence can work. The key for the fitness professional is to find the best intervention for the particular setting, and the client in that setting.

Here we will discuss seven different classifications of intervention strategies: behavior modification approaches, cognitive-behavioral approaches, social support approaches, self-monitoring, cognitive restructuring, coping strategies, and intrinsic approaches.

Behavior Modification Approaches

A review of different behavior modification approaches was performed, in regards to improving exercise adherence, through which multiple methods were shown to consistently produce positive results. The fitness professional can utilize these same methods to help clients modify their behaviors. By effectively applying these tools, the client will be better equipped to make the modifications for long term behavior change. The following approaches and techniques were shown to be successful in behavior modification. (Dishman and Buckworth, 1997).

Prompting

One technique for establishing a behavior is the use of prompts, or **prompting**. A prompt is a cue that initiates a behavior. Prompts can be verbal, physical, or symbolic. For example, a verbal prompt may be a simple statement, such as "Okay, let's get going," or a slogan that is meaningful to the individual, such as "Time to get more steps in!" A physical prompt might be helping someone get over a "sticking point" in a strenuous activity. A symbolic prompt generally reminds a person to begin or continue a behavior, such as leaving out one's workout gear the night before to promote physical activity, or placing a sticky note on the refrigerator. The goal is to increase cues for the desired behavior and decrease cues for competing behaviors.

Contracting

Another way to change exercise behavior is to have participants enter into a contract with the fitness professional or a peer. Written statements that outline specific behaviors and establish

Intervention
Strategies within a fitness professional's scope of practice that are aimed at disrupting unhealthy habits and/or promoting healthy behaviors.

Prompting
Promoting an action through encouragement, persuasion, or reminding.

CHECK IT OUT

Vanden Auweele, Boen, Schapendonk, and Dornez (2005) conducted a worksite study where they placed a sign linking stair use to health and fitness at a junction between the staircase and an elevator. They found that stair use increased significantly from baseline to intervention. A second intervention involved an additional email sent a week later by the worksite's doctor, pointing out the health benefits of regular stair use. Results revealed an increase in stair use. However, once the sign was removed stair use declined to around baseline levels. This is a good demonstration of how effective just a sign can be, but it also shows that people easily go back to their old behavior if the new behavior has not been internalized.

Contracts

Agreements between two or more parties that specify expectations, responsibilities, and contingencies for behavior change.

consequences for fulfillment (or lack thereof) are known as contracts. In essence, **contracts** typically specify expectations, responsibilities, and contingencies for behavioral change. Usually, the purpose of these contracts is to maintain or enhance an individual's motivation to continue exercising. More specifically, the purpose of contracts is to help the client take action, establishing criteria for meeting goals, and providing a means for clarifying consequences (Kanfer and Gaelick, 1986). In essence, contracts increase the individual's public commitment and foster a sense of self-control.

Charting Attendance and Participation

Public reporting of attendance and performance is another way to increase the motivation of participants in exercise programs. A performance or attendance graph usually represents data in a form that is easily understood by everyone involved. The chart is helpful and motivational, in that it shows at a glance what changes are taking place, and if the client is on target for the behavior involved. The visual representation of progress by a chart is extremely helpful because a client can note even small changes in behavior and performance. This may be important in maintaining a client's interest, especially later in a program when the individual reaches the point where improvements are often small and occur less frequently. This public information also allows fitness professionals, as well as other clients, to offer praise and encouragement to the client on the chart. For instance, a professional could use a graph to track a client's progress and share it with the client once a week (or month), keeping motivation high because the client clearly sees improvements (even if they are small). With smartphone apps, activity tracking devices, and social media, fitness professionals and clients have many opportunities to chart progress.

Providing Feedback on Progress

An important motivational technique that capitalizes on individuals' inherent interest to reach certain outcomes is to provide periodic, positive feedback on the progress that has been made. Providing feedback regarding various fitness tests, such as submaximal exercise tests, resting/recovery pulse rate, and body composition measures can be very motivational to clients in exercise programs. A fitness professional praising a client for finishing an especially hard workout would be an example of positive reinforcement or feedback, which is meant to increase motivation and eventual participation.

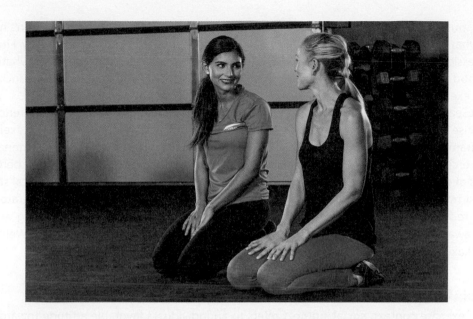

Fitness professionals need to provide feedback that provides specific information on performing the behavior in question. A study was created which established two groups to examine the effectiveness of feedback: (1) a feedback-only group that received feedback on their motives for participation in exercise and barriers for participation; and (2) a group that received the same feedback but was also provided information on how to adhere to exercise, as well as how to overcome barriers. Results revealed that participants receiving specific information regarding how to adhere to exercise, as well as how to overcome barriers to exercise, exhibited the highest levels of adherence and participation (Ortís et al., 2007).

Cognitive-Behavioral Approaches

Cognitive-behavioral approaches to behavior change and therapy evolved out of the operant conditioning theories that dominated psychology from the 1940s to the 1960s. This approach focuses on ways to help someone solve current issues. Ultimately, the focus will rely upon addressing thoughts and behaviors that are detrimental to the growth of the individual. In one form or another, these approaches all assume that private or internal events have an important role in behavior change. Applying simple strategies to address the thoughts and behaviors that provide barriers to fitness can help the client reach their goals.

Association and Dissociation

Association and **dissociation** strategies predominantly involve thoughts, which will eventually affect behavior. In essence, what clients think about and focus their attention on while exercising is important. When the focus is on internal body feedback (e.g., how their muscles feel or their breathing feels), it is called association; when the focus is on the external environment (e.g., noticing how pretty the scenery is or listening to music while exercising), it is called dissociation. Dissociation can act as a distraction, allowing the person to shift his or her focus from the pain and fatigue that often accompany vigorous physical activity. Exercising

Association

Focus on internal body feedback (e.g., how muscles or breathing feels).

Disassociation

Focus on the external environment (e.g., noticing the scenery or listening to music).

Social support

An individual's favorable attitude toward another person's involvement in an exercise program.

with music is a great example of using a dissociative technique, as it takes the person's mind off what he or she is doing, and usually makes the time appear to pass more quickly. Fitness professionals should encourage their clients (especially beginning exercisers) to use whatever method they can to take their mind off the potential monotony and fatigue often associated with exercise.

Research has revealed that people who dissociate have significantly better adherence to exercise than do those who associate. In one study, the dissociative subjects in an exercise program were more likely than associative subjects to demonstrate long-term maintenance of exercise (Martin et al., 1984). Specifically, when beginning an exercise program, perceptions of exertion, affective responses of displeasure and discomfort, and physiological stress could make the exercise experience especially aversive. The use of dissociative strategies may reduce these negative psychological and physiological feelings, by directing attention away from the pain and discomfort that first-time exercisers often feel (Lind, Welch, & Ekkekakis, 2009).

Social Support

In an exercise context, **social support** refers to an individual's favorable attitude toward another person's involvement in an exercise program. Most people think of social support as coming from significant others in the environment, such as spouses, family members, and close friends. This is indeed the case, as a review of studies investigating the relationship between social support and adherence to exercise revealed that family and friends exert a strong influence on compliance with exercise programs (Carron, Hausenblas, & Mack, 1996).

In addition to the social support offered by significant others, the support that occurs inside a fitness program, especially the behavior of the fitness professional, is crucial for adherence to exercise. By establishing a warm and nonthreatening relationship with the client, the fitness professional may influence the individual's level of motivation. The fitness professional should create an expectation of participation that is challenging, yet still attainable to the exerciser. Then, the fitness professional should reward these positive behaviors. Rewards could simply be verbal reinforcement such as, "Your techniques are improving" or "It's great to see you come here regularly." When a fitness professional gives personalized, immediate feedback,

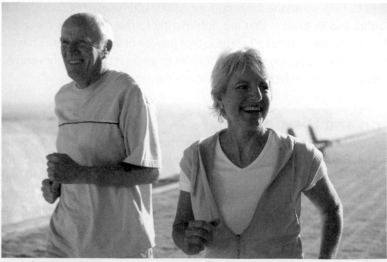

© Pixland/Thinkstock

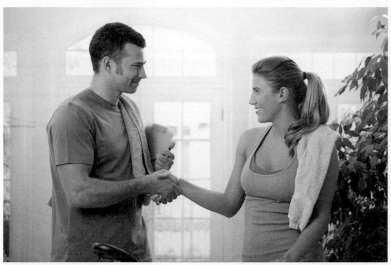

© StockLite/Shutterstock

CHECK IT OUT

Fitness professionals can offer their clients a number of different types of social support:

- *Instrumental support*: This is the perception that someone is listening without giving advice or being judgmental. In addition to being able to communicate fitness information, fitness professionals also need to be good listeners.
- *Emotional support*: This is the perception that another person is providing comfort and caring and is there to help. Oftentimes fitness professionals and clients develop close bonds, especially when clients' experience tough times. Fitness professionals need to be there comfort their clients and express sympathy when they complain of sore muscles.
- *Personal assistance support*: This is the perception that a person is providing services of help. In the case of the fitness professional, it might be helping to arrange for transportation or a babysitter so the client can attend the training session.
- *Task appreciation support*: This is the perception that another person is acknowledging one's efforts and expressing appreciation for the work that has been done. For fitness professionals, this means providing feedback and rewards based on the client's accomplishments.

and praises attendance and maintenance of exercise, adherence improves. Fitness professionals can, and do, make a difference in exercise adherence, depending on the type and amount of social support provided.

Self-Monitoring

The strategy of **self-monitoring** has been used as a tool in changing several health-related behaviors (e.g., smoking cessation, alcohol recovery). It involves identifying the cues and consequences of the target health behavior. Thoughts, feelings, and aspects of the situation before and after successful attempts at the target behavior are recorded and reviewed. Self-monitoring

Self-monitoring

Ability to recognize and regulate one's behavior.

Day: (Monday) Tuesday Wednesday Thursday Friday Saturday Sunday						
Date: 1/1/20XX						

Time	Food	Carbohydrates(g)	Fats(g)	Protein(g)	Calories	Mood
8:30 AM	Cereal w/ skim milk	58 g	3.4 g	13 g	293	anxious
11:30 AM	Tacos	51 g	21.5 g	43.5 g	590	irritated
5:30 PM	Spaghetti with meatballs	67 g	35 g	41 g	740	happy
		Total: 176 g	Total: 59.9	Total: 91.5 g	Total: 1623	

FIGURE 16.4 A self-monitoring nutrition journal.

is a practical way to collect information about behavior patterns that can be used to identify cues and barriers to exercise (**Figure 16.4**).

Information gained from self-monitoring can help to identify the best times in a client's schedule for an exercise routine and any accommodations that may be necessary, such as picking up a child from day care an hour later to accommodate exercising after work. Self-monitoring may be particularly useful for people who have been active in the past as a strategy to identify factors that contributed to their lapse in regular exercise. Similarly, for clients who have gone off their nutrition plan, self-monitoring can identify the kinds of situations that led to going off their plan in the first place (e.g., eating out with friends, eating at an all-you-can-eat restaurant).

The use of electronic devices (e.g., smartphones) for self-monitoring also opens up the opportunity for prompting behavior. Periodic evaluation of behavioral records by fitness professionals can provide meaningful positive feedback and help clients monitor their goals.

Cognitive Restructuring

Cognitive restructuring

Psychotherapeutic process of learning to identify and dispute irrational or maladaptive thoughts.

Cognitive distortions

The mind's way of convincing itself that something true is actually untrue to reinforce negative thinking or emotions.

Cognitive restructuring is a popular technique that focuses on changing the way an individual thinks, which should also change the way he or she behaves. More specifically, it is a psychotherapeutic process of learning to identify and dispute irrational or maladaptive thoughts, known as **cognitive distortions**. In most cases, cognitive restructuring has to do with the way individuals think to themselves, which is called *self-talk*. People talk to themselves all the time (either internally or aloud), but sometimes what they say to themselves is negative and self-defeating, or even irrational. These types of thoughts or self-statements can cause emotional distress and interfere with performance, as well as adherence to physical activity (Cousins & Gillis, 2005). In essence, it is the self-talk that often determines a person's reactions to an event, rather than the event itself.

Consider the situation of an exerciser who has a setback in rehabilitating a knee injury. He might say to himself, "I'll never get back to exercising hard again," and this would likely lead to feelings of hopelessness, frustration, and anger. Take the same situation but with different self-talk: "This type of injury just takes time to heal, so I need to continue to work hard." This would likely lead to optimism, motivation, and increased effort. Similarly, reflect on the situation of being on a nutrition plan, and then eating way too much at a restaurant. This might cause the individual to say, "Here we go again, I never can follow a meal plan," and this might lead to depression, anger, and frustration. Conversely, the individual might say, "It's only one night, I just need to get back on the program tomorrow," which would likely lead to optimism and increased effort. By restructuring clients' thoughts and self-statements, fitness professionals can keep them motivated even when things are not going as planned.

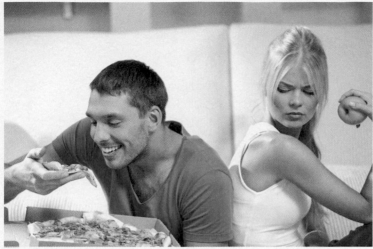

© Syda Productions/Shutterstock

Coping Strategies

Coping is a process of managing specific internal (i.e., self-expectations) or external (e.g., demands from an employer) conflicts that tax or exceed one's resources. The two most widely accepted coping strategies are problem-focused coping and emotion-focused coping. **Problem-focused coping** involves efforts to alter or manage the problem that is causing the stress for the individual concerned. It includes such specific behaviors as information gathering, making pre-competition and competition plans, goal setting, time management, problem solving, and increasing effort. **Emotion-focused coping** entails regulating the emotional responses to the problem that is causing the stress for the individual through tools such as meditation, relaxation, wishful thinking, reappraisal, mental and behavioral withdrawal, and cognitive efforts to change the meaning of the situation (but not the actual problem or environment). Generally, problem-focused coping is used when the problem is amenable to change, whereas emotion-focused coping is used when the problem is not amenable to change. For example, if a client knows that she has a vacation is coming up, and in the past this has caused a lapse in her exercise regimen, then she might use time management as a coping technique to organize the vacation time to make room for regular exercise bouts. Similarly, if a client on a nutrition plan binged at a party and was feeling stressed and depressed because of it, he might use some relaxation or meditation strategies to reduce the stress, because there is nothing that can be done to change the fact that he ate too much last night. By reducing stress and depression, the client can start to focus on continuing with the nutrition plan. Fitness professionals can use these coping strategies to help clients get through difficult periods or barriers to continuing their exercise regimen, but they should always remain within their scope of practice, referring the client to other professionals when necessary.

Intrinsic Approach

Most of the previous approaches relied on some sort of knowledge, feedback, or reward system for enhancing exercise behavior. Although these helpful cues, knowledge, and rewards can certainly help improve exercise adherence, the best and most long-lasting motivation comes from

Coping
Process of managing specific internal or external demands that tax or exceed one's resources.

Problem-focused coping
Targets an issue causing stress to reduce the effects of the stress.

Emotion-focused coping
Distracts from negative feelings associated with stress.

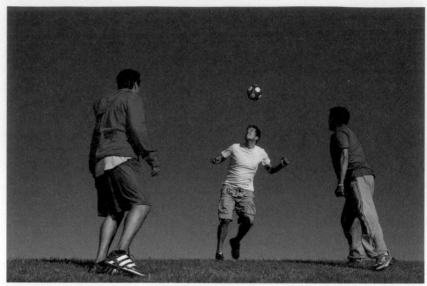

© Donald Miralle/Photodisc/Thinkstock

Intrinsic approach

An inside-out approach to exercise that emphasizes the enjoyment and fun of exercise and making it something to look forward to, not just a means to goal accomplishment.

within. Thus, despite the emphasis on health and fitness, eating properly, and maintaining an active lifestyle, the large majority of people still fall short in achieving regular physical activity. Along these lines, people should take an **intrinsic approach** to exercise, emphasizing the enjoyment and fun of exercise, and making it something to look forward to, not just as a means to an external goal such as weight loss (Kimiecik, 2002).

Fitness professionals should help clients find activities they enjoy, whether it is sport and competition oriented (e.g, tennis, golf, racquetball) or more physical activity and exercise oriented (e.g, cycling, swimming, walking on the treadmill, resistance training). Just enjoying the experience regardless of the outcome is focusing on the process. It is enjoying the movement or sport for itself, and not for any extrinsic reason.

A number of different behavior change strategies are available to help fitness professionals in their attempts to make positive behavior changes with their clients. Note that different strategies will be more effective for different individuals, so the fitness professional needs to apply the best strategy for each client. The environment in which the client is in as well as the client's personal attributes need to be considered before selecting the most appropriate strategy. As the situation changes, different strategies may be used on the same client.

Principles and Practices of Effective Goal Setting

People often set goals for one thing or another. The problem is not getting people to set goals; rather it is getting them to set the *right kinds* of goals. The right goals are those that provide direction and enhance motivation. As many learn from their New Year's resolutions, it is much easier to set a goal than to follow through on it. Seldom are goals for weight loss or exercise set realistically in terms of commitment, difficulty, evaluation of progress, and specific strategies for achieving them.

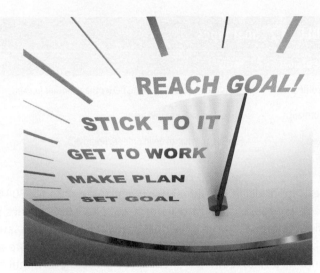

© Hemera/Thinkstock

Definition of Goals

By definition, an **objective goal** is something that an individual is trying to accomplish; it is the object or aim of an action. For example, in most goal-setting studies, the term *goal* refers to attaining a specific level of proficiency on a task, usually within a specified time limit (Locke, Shaw, Saari, & Latham, 1981). From a practical point of view, goals focus on standards of excellence or improvement, such as lowering one's time in a 10K race by 30 seconds, swimming continuously for an extra 10 minutes, or reducing caloric intake by 500 calories per day. In addition, objective goals should have to be reached in a given timeframe, such as a certain number of days, weeks, or months.

In contrast, **subjective goals**, such as having more fun while exercising, are based on experience or expectations. Because they are less tangible than objective goals, they are not as easily measured. However, these types of goals can be measured. For example, clients can rate how much fun they had exercising on a numeric scale ranging from 1 ("least") to 10 ("most"). To determine how much fun was had, the clients would define components that make participation fun, such as positive comments from the fitness professional, spending more social time with other exercisers, and seeing improvement in performance. Similarly, a fitness professional might have a client who quit once before, because exercise and training were boring, difficult, and painful. Therefore, the fitness professional could set a subjective goal to enjoy the exercise experience more this time around. Then, to help makes things more enjoyable this time, the fitness professional might have the client exercise at lower intensities, find out what type of activities the client likes, and provide lots of positive reinforcement.

Types of Goals

Three types of goals have been identified: outcome, performance, and process (Weinberg & Gould, 2015; **Table 16.2**). An **outcome goal** is usually concerned with winning or losing. In exercise settings, however, an outcome goal is usually seen as the end result of some behavior. For example, an outcome goal might be to win a step competition with coworkers, or to be the first person in a group of friends to lose 10 pounds. A **performance goal** specifies the end product of performance, but it is usually expressed in terms of personal achievement.

Objective goal

Something an individual is trying to accomplish; the object or aim of an action.

Subjective goal

Goal based on experience or expectations; less tangible than an objective goal.

Outcome goal

A goal that is usually about winning or losing; in exercise settings, it is the end result of some behavior.

Performance goal

A goal that specifies the end products of performance expressed in terms of personal achievement.

TABLE 16.2 Goal Types

Type of Goal	Focus
Outcome	Focus is on winning or being better than another person.
Performance	Focus is on self-improvement.
Process	Focus is on what to do in order to improve.

Process goals

A goal that specifies the processes the individual wants to perform in a satisfactory manner (however that is defined).

For example, to lose 10 pounds an individual may want to exercise for 30–40 minutes, three or four times per week, or reduce caloric intake from 2,500 to 2,000 calories per day. Finally, a **process goal** specifies the processes the individual wants to perform in a satisfactory manner. An example might be keeping the heart rate above 130 beats per minute for 20 minutes of each exercise session. Similarly, to reduce caloric intake, a process goal might be to eat only one serving of food at meals if an individual usually goes back for seconds.

Outcome goals are important, but they should not be the main focus of a wellness or fitness program because they are out of an individual's control. Rather, the focus should be on performance and process goals. These types of goals are under a person's direct control and can be used to achieve the outcome goals.

Goal-Setting Principles

Recall that some of the statistics related to physical activity, weight, and health are staggering—and dispiriting. One potential strategy that can help improve fitness and health is goal setting (**Figure 16.5**). As will be shown later in the chapter, a great deal of research, as well as anecdotal reports, support the idea that goals can enhance performance and productivity, change behavior, and boost personal growth. However, the mere fact that a goal is set does not in any way ensure that the goal will actually be achieved.

Specific and Measurable Goals

One of the most consistent findings from the goal-setting literature is that specific goals produce higher levels of task performance than having no goals or general "do your best" goals; leading to the overwhelming conclusion that specific goals consistently enhance performance. It is hypothesized that goal specificity works by providing individuals with specific feedback relating to their progress in meeting their goals (Locke & Latham, 1990).

GOAL-SETTING PRINCIPLES

- Set specific and measurable goals.
- Set realistic but challenging goals.
- Set both short- and long-term goals.
- Focus on performance and process goals.
- Develop goal commitment.
- Develop goal achievement strategies.
- Get goal feedback and evaluation.
- Set timelines to achieve goals.

FIGURE 16.5 Goal-setting principles.

CHECK IT OUT

Approximately half the people who start an exercise program drop out in the first 6 months (Dishman & Chambliss, 2010). Millions of people set goals, especially at the beginning of the year, but in many cases these goals are not set effectively, leading to the huge dropout rate, as has already been noted.

One important key to lowering this dropout rate is to structure goal-setting programs so that they are consistent with the basic principles derived from the organizational, sport, and exercise literatures, as well as from the professional practice knowledge of professionals working in these fields.

Realistic, but Challenging Goals

Another consistent finding from the literature is that goals should be challenging and difficult, yet attainable (Locke & Latham, 2002). Goals that are too easy do not present enough of a challenge to the individual, which often leads to less than maximum effort. This, in turn, might result in being satisfied with mediocre performance instead of striving to reach one's maximum potential and the goal. For example, say that a client sets a goal of increasing the amount of time spent exercising from 15 minutes a week to 30 minutes a week over 2 months. The client may reach this goal in 1 month, but then not be motivated to improve any further, because the goal has already been achieved. The client also may like the fact that it was easy and then set the next goal too low so it, too, can be easily reached. This results in a much slower rate of improvement, and possibly being satisfied with less than maximal effort. Conversely, setting goals that are too difficult or unrealistic will often result in failure. This can lead to frustration, decreased self-confidence, and less motivation, making it less likely the individual will continue to strive to reach the goal.

Short-Term vs. Long-Term Goals

Another area that has received a lot of attention with regard to goal setting is **goal proximity**. Although there is some inconsistency when comparing the effectiveness of short-term versus long-term goals, researchers do agree that a combination of **short-term** and **long-term goals** produces enhanced performance and productivity, and positive changes in behavior (Weinberg, 2010). Both short-term and long-term goals provide important information to individuals as they attempt to reach their goals. Suppose an individual has a long-term goal of losing 50 pounds in a year. This goal provides the direction and the final destination as to what the person is trying to accomplish, and keeps the focus on where the person wants to end up. However, short-term goals are important as well, because they can provide feedback concerning progress toward the long-term goal. Such feedback can serve a motivational function and allow for adjustment of goals either upward or downward, depending on the situation. Thus, if the individual has lost only 5 pounds after 4 months, then perhaps a change in the long-term goal from 50 pounds to 25 pounds might be in order. Oftentimes, when people are performing below their expectations, it is not unusual for them to lose motivation and even give up. Weight loss is extremely difficult for many people; when faced with failure to lose weight, the result is often to simply stop trying. Resetting the goal, in such a case, can keep motivation at a reasonable level so that the individual will continue striving to meet this new goal. **Table 16.3** provides an example of a long-term goal and the short-term goals that are required to achieve it.

TRAINER TIPS

Your clients will want to "see the numbers" with regard to their hard work. Ensure that the goals and milestones you and your client decide on are measurable. An easy way to determine this is to ask your client, "How do we know whether or not you have reached this goal/milestone?" If the client cannot give you a definitive answer, the goal is not specific.

Goal proximity
The relative nearness of a goal in terms of time frame.

Short-term goal
A goal that is set to be achieved within the near future.

Long-term goal
A large goal that is set to be achieved over a long period of time.

TABLE 16.3 Example Long-Term Goal and Short-Term Goals to Achieve It

Goal Proximity	Example
Long-term goal	Increase moderate-intensity physical activity from zero times per week to 150 minutes per week in 6 months.
Short-term goals	Short-term goals needed to achieve above long-term goal: Exercise for 25 minutes after 1 month. Exercise for 50 minutes after 2 months. Exercise for 75 minutes after 3 months. Exercise for 100 minutes after 4 months. Exercise for 125 minutes after 5 months.

FIGURE 16.6 SMART goals.

CHECK IT OUT

The acronym SMART—Specific, Measurable, Attainable, Realistic, and Time oriented/Timely—is widely used in health and fitness settings, as well as in business and industry (Figure 16.6). It is a way of simplifying the goal-setting process. Although this is a straightforward and clear way of creating goals, it is important to take into consideration all of the goal-setting principles discussed in this chapter, because research on goal setting has consistently demonstrated its importance in changing behavior.

Goal Commitment

Fitness professionals can include all of the other principles of goal setting when developing a goal-setting program, but if the client is not committed to achieving the goals that have been set, then goal attainment probably will not happen. Without goal commitment, individuals are not likely to put forth the effort required to achieve their goal, especially if that goal is challenging.

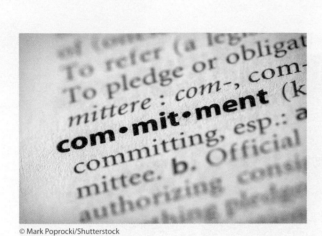
© Mark Poprocki/Shutterstock

To increase commitment as much as possible, clients should develop their own goals. If individuals are not knowledgeable about exercise and dietary standards, they may have to rely on their fitness professional (or other health professional) to provide guidance. However, regardless of who develops the goals, it is important that clients "own" and embrace them and be invested in achieving them.

Research from many different fields has demonstrated the importance of writing down goals in a systematic way (Burton & Raedeke, 2008). However, research has also found that most individuals do not write down their goals, and that even if they do, they often fail to document their goals in a systematic fashion. Accountability is also increased when individuals share their goals with others, such as by posting them on a locker.

Goal Achievement Strategies

Once a client has set specific, measurable goals, it is necessary to develop some strategies so that the client can reach these goals. In developing action plans, the fitness professional should be prepared for potential barriers that might be encountered. For example, when trying to increase healthy eating, a barrier might be the fact that the client travels a great deal for work and, therefore, must eat out a lot. Preparing for this eventuality might include checking out the different amounts of calories and macronutrients contained in the types of foods usually consumed when dining out, which may require a change in the food that is chosen or the portion size.

Goal Feedback and Evaluation

Combining goals with feedback appears to be extremely important in the achievement of goals. In one study, adding feedback to goals raised performance by just under 20% (Matthews, 2007). Feedback can come from a fitness professional, wellness professional, dietitian, coach, friend, or teammate, depending on the goal.

Although feedback provides individuals with information on how they are doing, goal evaluation provides specific information on how they are progressing toward their goal. For example, a client who has lost 15 pounds in 6 months, with a goal to lose 50 pounds in 12 months, is not likely to achieve this goal. This might produce frustration and disappointment, in turn leading to a lack of motivation and a lack of trying. In response, the client might change the 12-month goal to losing 30 pounds, which is still a realistic and challenging goal. Fitness professionals

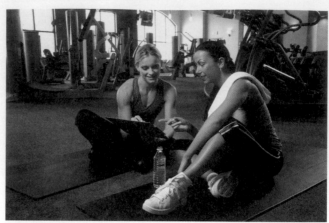
© iofoto/Shutterstock

need to help their clients understand why they might have fallen short of their goal (e.g., injury, motivation, work pressure, unrealistic goal), and then work with them to offer some solutions on how to reach it. For example, say a client fell short of her goal because she was feeling pressured to spend more time at work. The solution might be to just set a more realistic goal, or perhaps help her manage her time more effectively, so she can fit in her workout (e.g., getting up a little earlier so she can work out before going to work) and still spend the time she needs to at work. The main point is that goals are starting points, not ending points, and individuals should reevaluate their goals regularly.

Timelines to Achieve Goals

When individuals set goals, they should include the dates by which they want to achieve those goals. Oftentimes, individuals set goals without a specific, explicitly expressed timeframe for meeting them. Research has revealed that establishing a timeline provides information to individuals regarding what they must do to reach their goal by the date specified (Locke & Latham, 2002). Determining a timeline for goals may be one of the most challenging parts of the goal-setting process. Although it is difficult to pinpoint the exact date when a goal may be achieved, it is important not to skip this part of the process. A timeline can help individuals achieve a goal faster than they would in the absence of one (**Figure 16.7**). When there is a date by which a goal needs to be met, the deadline provides extra motivation and sets the client's focus on reaching the goal. Without a definitive timeline, it is difficult to gauge the progress being made toward achieving the goal.

Progress Evaluation Practices

It is important to assess the effectiveness of any program that has been implemented. In essence, did the program achieve its objectives in an efficient manner? Evaluating progress toward the eventual goal is also important for motivational reasons, as well as to determine if any changes need to be made.

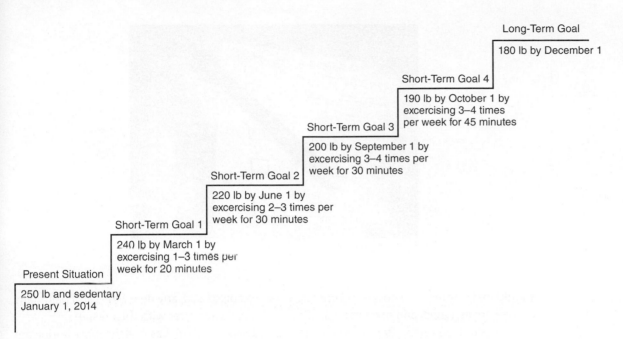

FIGURE 16.7 Goal staircase.

Progress Reviews

When fitness professionals effectively monitor and support their clients, progress reviews are a great tool to celebrate their success. These reviews not only help to identify factors that have helped or hindered client success, but they can assist clients in *understanding* what makes them successful. They can also help clients to recognize and eliminate barriers that may have gotten in the way of the accomplishment of the goal. In essence, progress reviews give fitness professionals a formal opportunity to "dig around" with a client, and determine why the training approach is working or what needs to be improved upon. The fitness professional can provide the client with data during these program reviews, perhaps displaying information in chart format. Every client is different, so the data reviews for each client will also be somewhat different. The number of reviews, the scheduling of reviews, and the type of data to be reviewed will all need to be worked out with clients to best help accomplish their goals. In order to perform successful reviews, fitness professionals need to be systematic in collecting data and keeping records.

Record Keeping

Keeping accurate records is an important part of a fitness professional's job both for business purposes and for designing and implementing workouts. Details matter in running a successful long-lasting business. Fitness professionals should plan all workouts ahead of time. Depending on the fitness professional's level of experience, as this could take anywhere from an hour or two for beginners, to a few minutes for those who are very experienced. The longer the relationship with a client the easier this process becomes. However, a fitness professional should never start a workout with a client without having a predetermined written plan for the session. Taking the time to write down specific goals for the session and the order of the exercises will allow the session to go a lot smoother. In addition, after the session the fitness professional

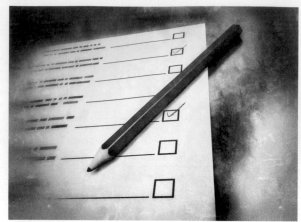

© JNT Visual/Shutterstock

should make notes as to how the client felt, what was discussed, any new aches and pains, any homework assigned, and of course specific exercises and activities with their results.

Fitness professionals often see several clients in a row, which makes it all the more important to write down an outline for the workout in each person's file. With all the other responsibilities of the job, it can be tough to leave everything to memory. Having a chart/folder to refer to, and making notes during or soon after the session, makes for better and more efficient fitness professionals. It is important that fitness professionals record not only clients' objective workout results, but also what was discussed during the workout. How did they feel? What are their goals for the week or month? Do they have any new aches and pains? For clients who are seen only once a month or every few weeks, these notes help the fitness professional to remember exactly what went on during their last session. Clients will recognize this as professional behavior, which will help to establish and maintain the fitness professional's credibility.

Along these lines, every client must have a separate file where detailed records of each workout are kept. This file should be an integral part of how fitness professionals' conduct their business and train their clients. Useful information should be printed on the flap of every file, including the client's name, phone number, e-mail, and start date. In fact, in this digital age it is a good idea to keep a paper copy file as well as a computer file as a backup system. Keeping accurate training records is an important administrative task, because keeping track of clients' sessions is also an important part of billing.

Fitness professionals should keep two types of records. The first type is concerned with clients' progress. Clients come in with different abilities, needs, and goals; these should be individualized and tracked on a daily, weekly, or monthly basis, depending on what is most germane to the client. This will allow both the fitness professional and the client to understand the progress (or lack of it) made, and make appropriate adjustments (when reevaluating goals).

The other type of records that professionals should keep is concerned with the business aspect of the job. It is important to keep good records from a business perspective, because they can be used to show how successful the fitness professional has been. It also allows fitness professionals to see where they have been spending their professional time.

The specific items recorded will vary based on the job responsibilities, but the following are some typical records that are kept on a daily, weekly, monthly, or yearly basis:

- Number of days worked
- Average income (per hour)
- Number of days off

- Client hours cancelled/rescheduled
- Percentage of cancellations that were paid
- Mileage driven (to in-home clients)
- Average number of sessions
- Average time spend in the gym not getting paid

Conclusion

Fitness professionals should apply evidence-based goal-setting principles, especially when setting short- and long-term goals and in assessing progress (which might require resetting goals). By recognizing the stages of the TTM, fitness professionals can use behavior change strategies, combined with coaching and communication to motivate their clients to meet, or even exceed, their fitness goals. Fitness professionals should keep detailed records, so that they can assess their clients' progress as they strive to reach their goals. Having periodic progress reviews is imperative to demonstrate to clients that they are improving, which is very motivating. Clients need this motivation, as many clients do not sustain their exercise programs over time. In addition, records should be kept from a financial point of view, as personal training is, indeed, a business, and therefore one must keep accurate records of time spent and payments made by clients.

Case in Review

Looking back at your client's progress, you see that Mary has only lost 3.5 pounds over the past month, and is slipping on the progress required to reach her 20-pound weight loss goal. Before meeting with Mary to go over her progress, you analyze where she falls within the stages of change, and it is evident that she remains in the preparation stage. Although she might feel as though she is making the effort necessary to lose those 20 pounds, her progress does not match up with her intentions and goals. Mary is preparing to lose the weight by obtaining a gym membership and purchasing sessions with a trainer, but action would be demonstrated by complying with all your recommendations, which would yield undeniable results.

Educating Mary on the specific influences she may come into contact with should begin with further evaluation. You interview Mary to determine the influences that might be serving as barriers to her achieving her goals, discuss who makes up her social support network, and identify what they do to have fun and interact with one another. Based on her response, it seems they engage in habits that are not supportive of Mary's goals. You and Mary brainstorm alternative ways to have fun with friends and family. In addition, you pay special attention to the things Mary says on a casual basis, because it might be reflective of self-talk that needs cognitive restructuring. For example, if Mary shows up to a workout and says she doesn't think her goal is realistic anymore, it might be an indicator that Mary is telling herself that she can't accomplish a goal that she has set for herself.

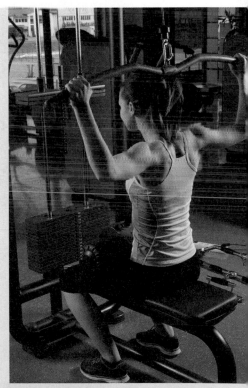
© fotoinfot/Shutterstock

To help Mary get back on track to losing the weight needed to meet her goal, you work with her to create the following action plan that will help promote favorable changes in her behavior:

- *Schedule an evaluation session*: Devote a session to reevaluating the progress Mary has made toward her goal and the barriers she feels like she is encountering.

- *Reestablish short-term goals*: You work backwards with her to determine short-term, process-oriented goals that will support the long-term outcome goal of losing 20 pounds.

- *Tracking*: Mary should also take ownership of tracking her progress through the use of self-monitoring and journaling. This will help Mary identify the influences that are affecting her work toward her goal.

- *Affirm commitment:* You gain buy-in from Mary by having her write a future testimonial, in the present tense, of all the things in her life that have changed as a result of her accomplishing her goals. This will help Mary imagine a successful self, and it will be written in her own words, along with her plan of how all of it can be accomplished. This will bring Mary into the process as a collaborator, rather than as a client just following recommendations.

References

Bandura, A. (1997). *Self-efficacy: The exercise of control*. New York, NY: Freeman.

Berger, B., & Tobar, D. (2011). Exercise and quality of life. In T. Morris & P. Terry (Eds.), *The new sport and exercise psychology companion* (pp. 483–505). Morgantown, WV: Fitness Information Technology.

Breckon, J. (2002). Motivational interviewing and exercise prescription. In D. Lavellee & I. Cockerill (Eds.), *Counseling in sport and exercise contexts* (pp. 48–60). Leicester, England: British Psychological Society.

Burton, D., & Raedeke T. (2008). *Sport psychology for coaches*. Champaign, IL: Human Kinetics.

Carron, A. V., Hausenblas, H. A., & Mack, D. (1996). Social influence and exercise: A meta-analysis. *Journal of Sport and Exercise Psychology, 18,* 1–16.

Consumer Reports. (2013, February). Best diet plans to lose weight. Available at: http://www.consumerreports.org/cro/magazine/2013/02/lose-weight-your-way/index.htm

Cousins, S., & Gillis, M. (2005). "Just do it . . . before you talk yourself out of it": The self-talk of adults thinking about physical activity. *Psychology of Sport and Exercise, 6,* 313–334.

Dishman, R. K., & Buckworth, J. (1997). Adherence to physical activity. In W. P. Morgan (Ed.), *Physical activity and mental health* (pp. 63–80). Englewood, NJ: Taylor & Francis.

Dishman, R., & Chambliss, H. (2010). Exercise psychology. In J. Williams (Ed.), *Applied sport psychology: Personal growth to peak performance* (6th ed., pp. 563–595). New York, NY: McGraw-Hill, 563–595.

Estabrooks, P., Smith-Ray, R., Almeida, F., Hill, J., Gonzales, M., Schreiner, P., & Van Den Berg, R. (2011). Move more: Translating an efficacious group dynamics physical activity intervention into effective clinical practice. *International Journal of Sport and Exercise Psychology, 42*, 461–479.

Gauvin, L., Levesque, L., & Richard, L. (2001). Helping people initiate and maintain a more active lifestyle: A public health framework for physical activity promotion research. In R. Singer, H. Hausenblas, & C. Janelle (Eds.), *Handbook of sport psychology* (2nd ed., pp. 695–717). New York, NY: John Wiley.

Kanfer, F., & Gaelick, L. (1986). Self-management methods. In F. Kanfer & A. Goldstein (Eds.), *Helping people change: A textbook of methods* (pp. 283–345). New York, NY: Pergamon Press.

Kimiecik, J. C. (2002). *The intrinsic exerciser: Discovering the joy of exercise.* Wilmington, MA: Mariner Books.

Lind, E., Welch, A., & Ekkekakis, P. (2009). Do "mind over muscle" strategies work? *Sports Medicine, 39*, 743–764.

Locke, E., & Latham, G. (1990). *A theory of goal setting and task performance.* Englewood Cliffs, NJ: Prentice Hall.

Locke, E., & Latham, G. (2002). Building a practically useful theory of goal setting and task motivation. *American Psychologist, 57*, 705–715.

Locke, E., Shaw, K., Saari, L., & Latham, G. (1981). Goal setting and task performance: 1969–1980. *Psychological Bulletin, 90*, 125–152.

Marcus, B., Banspach, S., Lefebvre, R., Rossi, J., Carelton, R., & Abrams, D. (1992). Using the changes of stage model to increase the adoption of physical activity among community participants. *American Journal of Applied Social Psychology, 24*, 489–508.

Marcus, B., Rossi, J., Selby, V., Niaur, R., & Adams, D. (1992). The stages and processes of exercise adoption and maintenance in a worksite sample. *Health Psychology, 11*, 386–395.

Martin, J., Dubbert, P., Katell, A., Thompson, J., Raczynski, J., Lsake, M., & Cohen, R. (1984). The behavioral control of exercise in In sedentary adults: Studies 1–6. *Journal of Consulting and Clinical Psychology, 52*, 795–811.

Matthews, G. (2007). The impact of commitment, accountability, and written goals on goal achievement. 87th Convention of the Western Psychological Association, Vancouver, BC, Canada.

Ntoumanis, N., & Standage, M. (2009). Morality in sport: A self-determination theory perspective. *Journal of Applied Sport Psychology, 2*, 365–380.

Ortís, L., Maymí, I., Feliu, J., Vidal, J., Romero, E., Bassets, M., & Brosa, J. (2007). Exercise motivation in university community members: A behavioral intervention. *Psicothema, 19*, 250–255.

Phillippe, P., & Seiler, R. (2006). Closeness, co-orientation and complementarity in coach–athlete relationships. What male swimmers say about male coaches. *Psychology of Sport and Exercise, 7*, 159–171.

Positive Coaching Alliance. (2013, October 8). *Keep emotional tanks full.* Available at: http://www .positivecoach.org/our-story/pca-in-the-news/news-detail/294/keep-emotional-tanks-full-%3E%3E

Prochaska, J., & DiClemente, C. (1983). Stages and processes of self-change of smoking: Toward an integrative model of change. *Journal of Consulting and Clinical Psychology, 51*, 390–395.

Prochaska, O., DiClemente, C., & Norcross, J. (1992). In search of how people change: Applications to addictive behaviors. *American Psychologist, 47*, 1102–1114.

Prochaska, O., & Velicer, W. (1997). Misinterpretation and misapplication of the transtheoretical model. *American Journal of Health Promotion, 12*, 11–12.

Raglin, J. (2001). Factors in exercise adherence: Influence of spouse participation. *The Academy Papers: Adherence to Exercise and Physical Activity, 53*, 356–361.

Rollnick, S., Miller, W., & Butler, C. (2007). *Motivational interviewing in health care: Helping patients change behavior.* New York, NY: Guilford Press.

Rosenfeld, L., & Wilder, I. (1990). Communication fundamentals: Active listening. *Sport Psychology Training Bulletin, 1*, 1–8.

Rovniak, L., Sallis, J., Saelens, D., Frank, L., Marshall, S., Norman, G. . . . Hovell, M. F. (2010). Adults' physical activity patterns across the life domains: Cluster analysis with repetition. *Health Psychology, 29*, 496–505.

Smith, R. (2006). Positive reinforcement, performance feedback, and performance enhancement. In J. Williams (Ed.). *Applied sport psychology: Personal growth to peak performance* (5th ed., pp. 40–56). Mountain View, CA: Mayfield.

Sonstroem, R. (1988). Psychological models. In R. Dishman (Ed.), *Exercise adherence* (pp. 125–154). Champaign, IL: Human Kinetics.

Thayer, R., Newman, R., & McClain, T. (1994). Self-regulation of mood: Strategies for changing a bad mood, raising energy, and reducing tension. *Journal of Personality and Social Behavior, 67,* 910–925.

Trost, S., Owen, N., Bauman, A., Sallis, J., & Brown, W. (2002). Correlates of adults' participation in physical activity: Review and update. *Medicine and Science in Sport and Exercise, 34,* 1996–2001.

U.S. Department of Health and Human Services. (1996). *Physical activity and health: A report of the Surgeon General.* Atlanta, GA: Author.

Vanden Auweele, Y., Boen, P., Schapendonk, W., & Dornez, K. (2005). Promoting stair use among female employees: The effects of a health sign followed by an e-mail. *Journal of Sport and Exercise Psychology, 27,* 188–196.

Wankel, L. (1984). Decision-making and social support structures for increasing exercise adherence. *Journal of Cardiac Rehabilitation, 4,* 124–128.

Weinberg, R. (2010). "Making goals effective: A primer for coaches." *Journal of Sport Psychology in Action, 1,* 57–65.

Weinberg, R., & Gould, D. (2015). *Foundations of sport an exercise psychology* (6th ed.). Champaign, IL: Human Kinetics.

Wilson, P. M., & Rodgers, W. (2004). The relationships between autonomy support, exercise motives, and behavioral intentions in females. *Psychology of Sport and Exercise, 5,* 229–242.

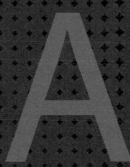

APPENDIX A

EXERCISE LIBRARY

Flexibility

Self-Myofascial Release

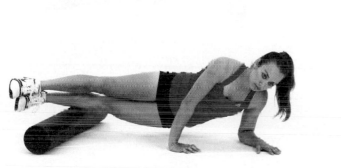

Peroneals

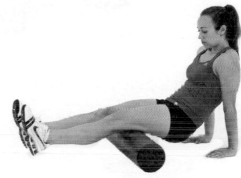

Hamstrings

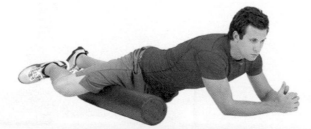

Adductors

Flexibility *continued*

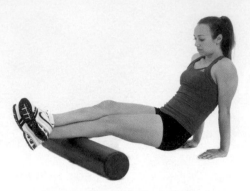

Gastrocnemius/Soleus (Calves)

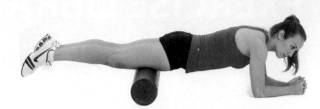

Quadriceps

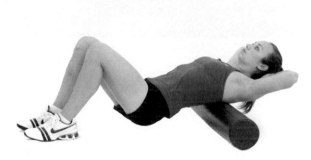

Thoracic spine

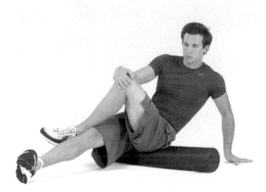

Piriformis

Static Stretching

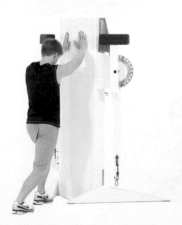

Static soleus stretch

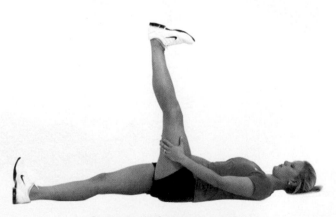

Static 90/90 hamstring stretch

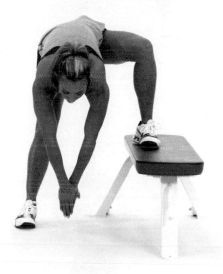

Static supine biceps femoris stretch

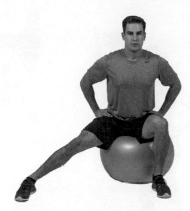

Static seated ball adductor stretch

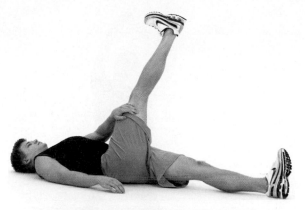

Static adductor magnus stretch

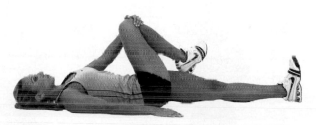

Static supine piriformis stretch

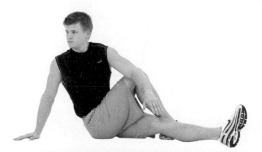

Static erector spinae stretch

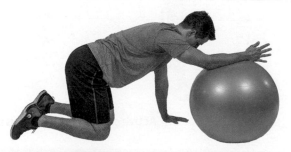

Static latissimus dorsi ball stretch

Flexibility *continued*

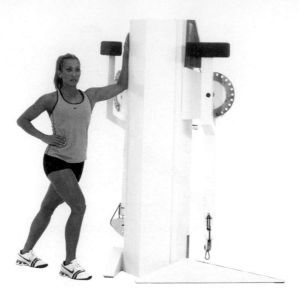

Static pectoral stretch

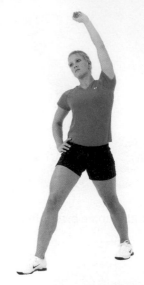

Static standing TFL stretch

Active-Isolated Stretching

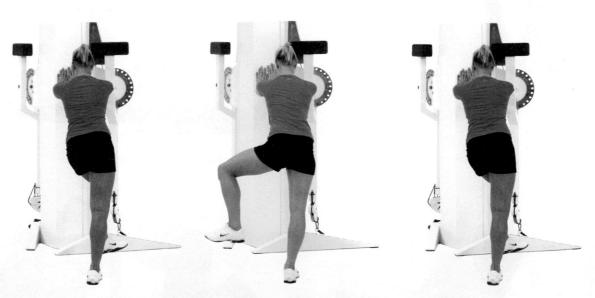

Active gastrocnemius stretch with pronation and supination

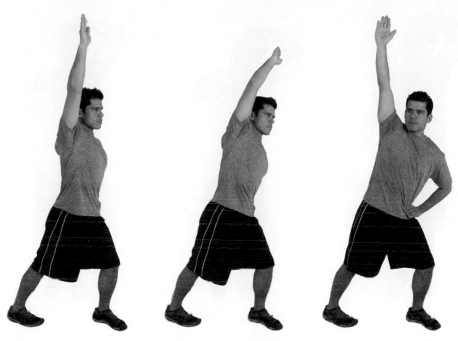

Active standing TFL stretch

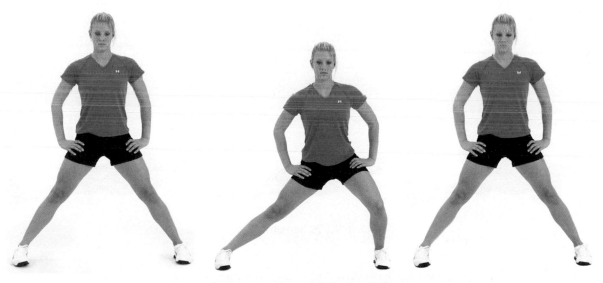

Active standing adductor stretch

Flexibility *continued*

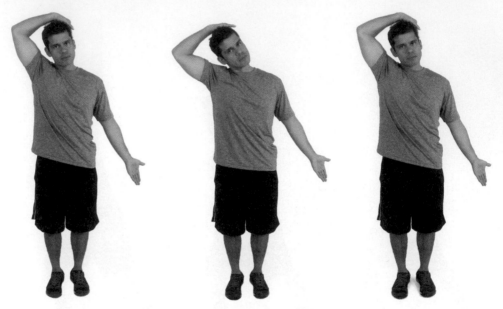

Active upper trapezius/scalene stretch

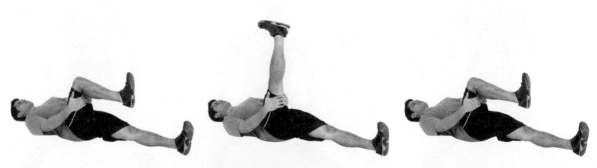

Active 90/90 hamstring stretch

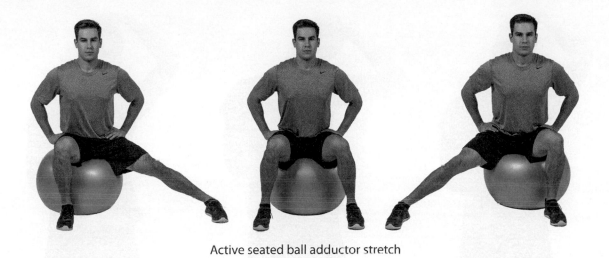

Active seated ball adductor stretch

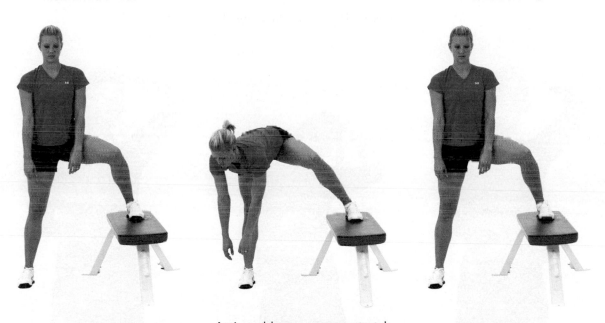

Active adductor magnus stretch

Flexibility *continued*

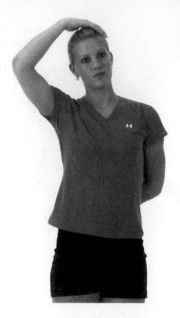 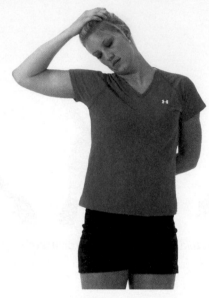 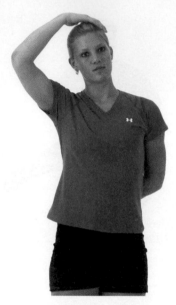

Active levator scapulae stretch

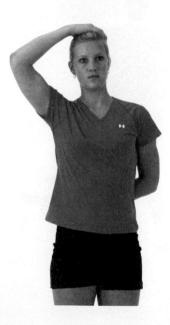 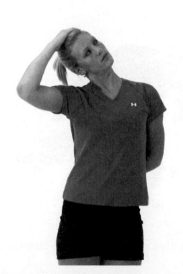 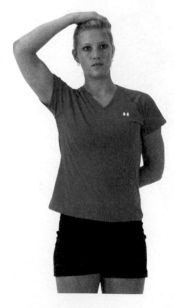

Active sternocleidomastoid stretch

Dynamic Stretching

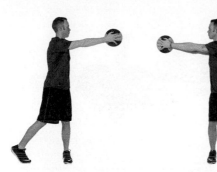

Medicine ball rotation

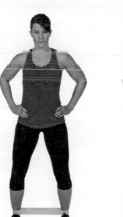
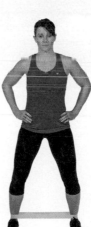

Leg swings: front to back

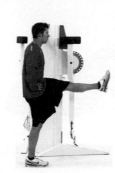

Leg swings: side to side

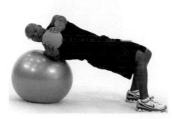

Russian twist

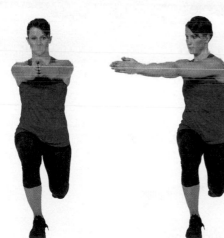

Lunge with rotation

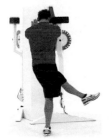
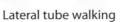

Lateral tube walking

Core Exercises

Core-Stabilization

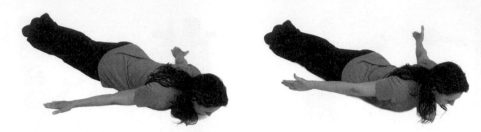

Floor cobra

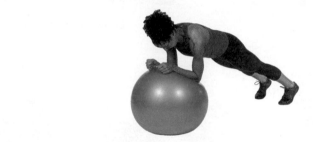

Ball Iso-abs

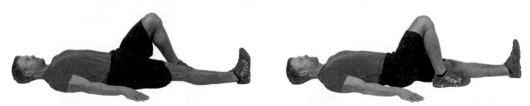

Heel slides

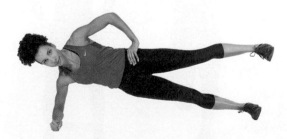

Side Iso-abs with hip abduction

Core-Strength

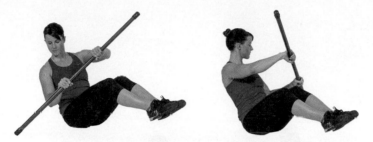

Rolling active resistance row

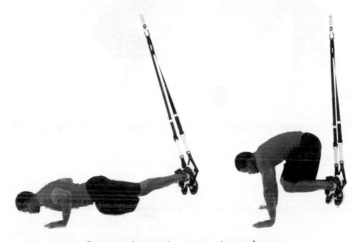

Suspension trainer atomic push-up

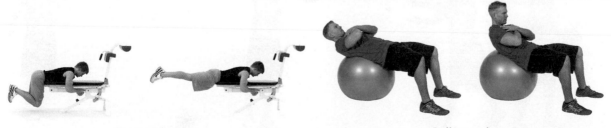

Reverse hypers

Ball crunch

Core Exercises *continued*

Core-Power

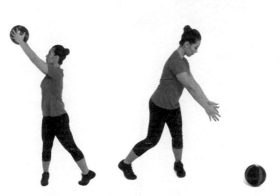

Overhead rotational medicine ball slam

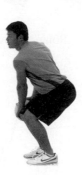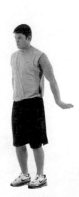

Medicine ball overhead throw with rotation

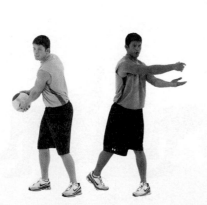

Front medicine ball oblique

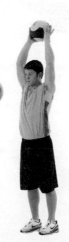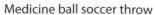

Medicine ball soccer throw

Balance Exercises

Balance-Stabilization

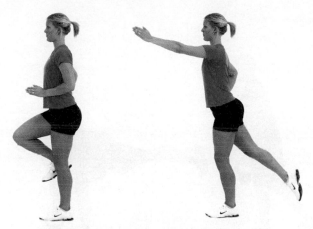

Single leg opposite arm opposite leg reach

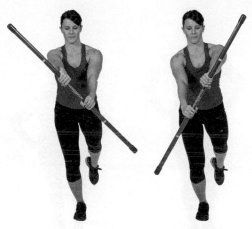

Rolling active resistance single leg balance

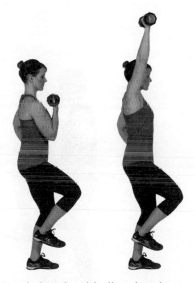

Single leg dumbbell curl and press

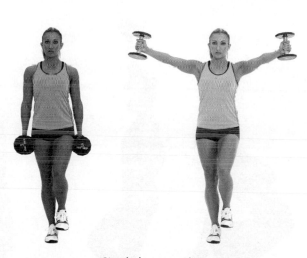

Single leg scaption

Balance Exercises *continued*

Balance-Strength

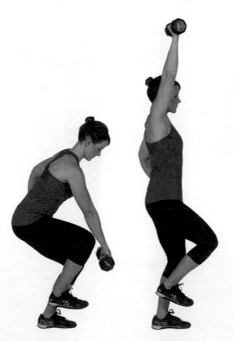

Single leg squat

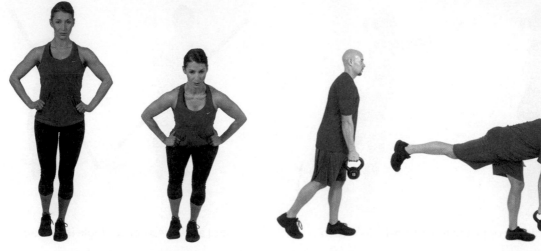

Single leg Kettlebell romanian deadlift

Single leg dumbbell squat to overhead press

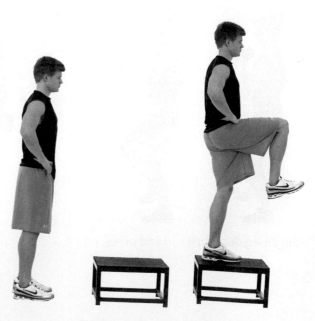

Single leg step-up to balance

Balance-Power

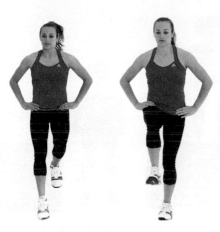

Sagittal plane single leg hop with stabilization

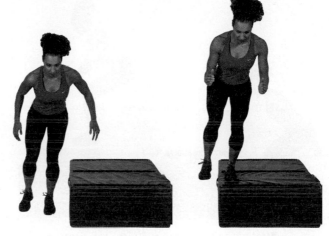

Frontal plane single leg box hop up with stabilization

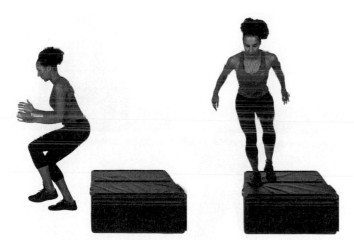

Transverse plane single leg box hop down with stabilization

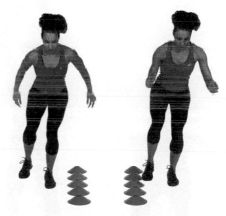

Frontal plane single leg cone hops with stabilization

Reactive Exercises

Reactive-Stabilization

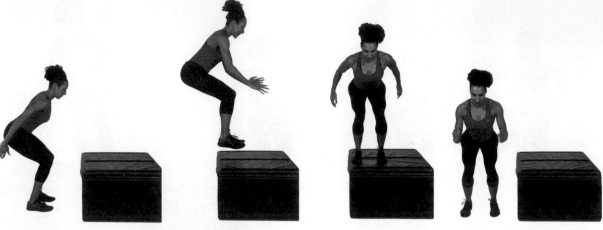

Sagittal plane box jump up with stabilization   Frontal plane box jump down with stabilization

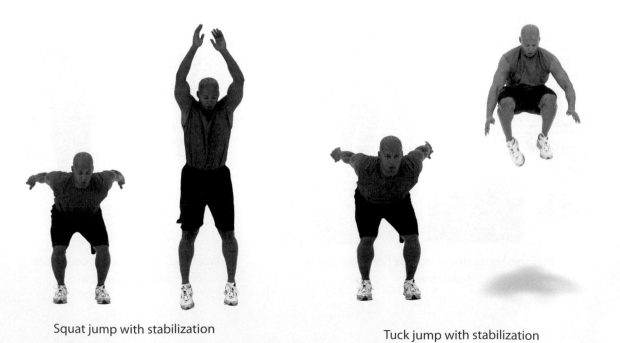

Squat jump with stabilization   Tuck jump with stabilization

Reactive-Strength

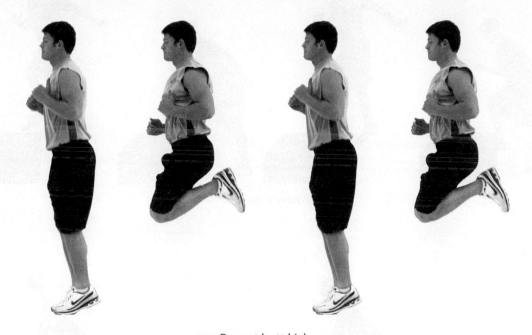

Repeat butt kicks

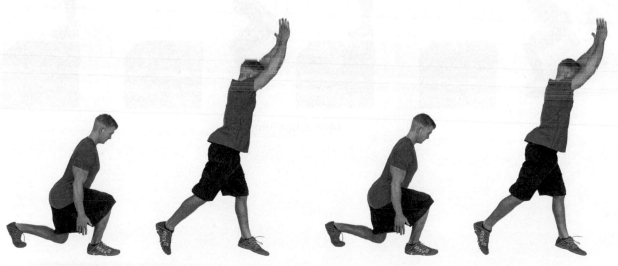

Jumping lunges

Reactive Exercises *continued*

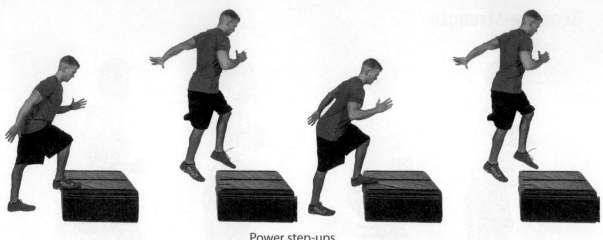

Power step-ups

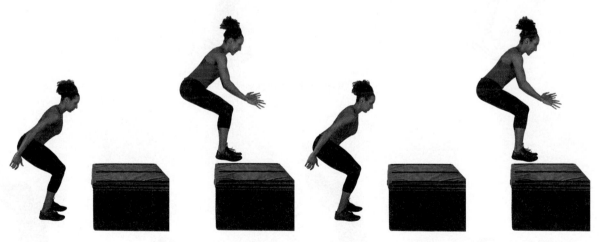

Repeat box jump

Reactive-Power

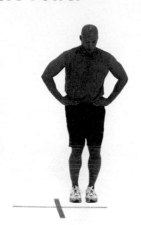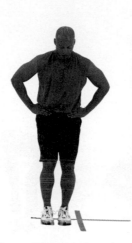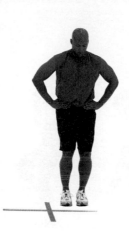

Two-leg proprioceptive plyometrics

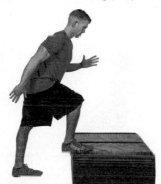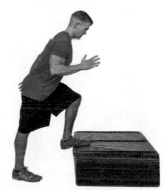

Box run steps

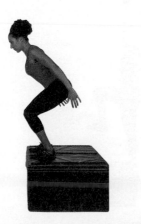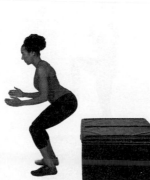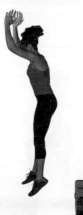

Depth jump to jump

Resistance Exercises

Total Body-Stabilization

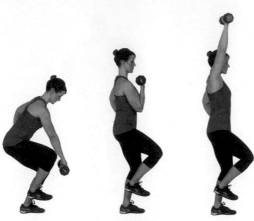

Single-leg squat touchdown, curl , to overhead press

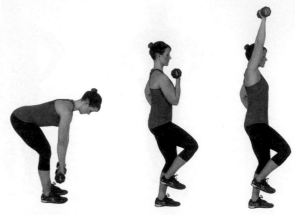

Single Leg Romanian deadlift, curl, to overhead press

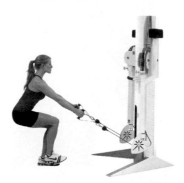

Single-leg squat to row

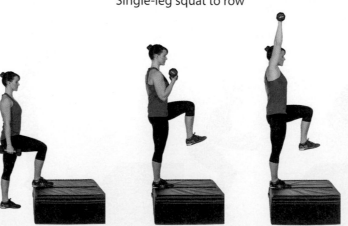

Step-up to balance curl to overhead press

Total Body-Strength

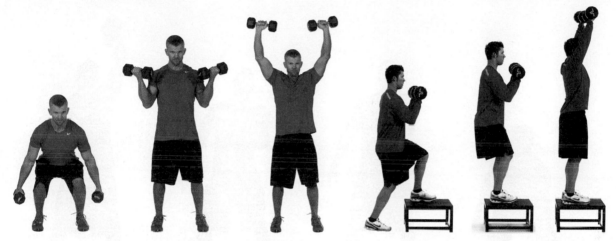

Dumbbell squat, curl to overhead press

Dumbbell step-up overhead press

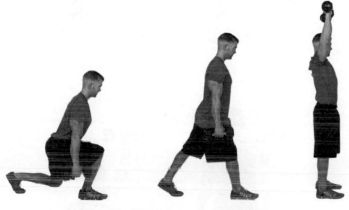

Dumbbell lunge to overhead press

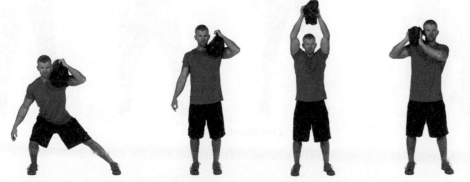

Frontal plane sandbag lunge to arc press

Resistance Exercises *continued*

Total Body-Power

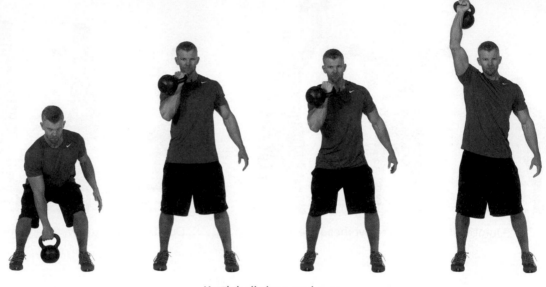

Kettlebell clean and press

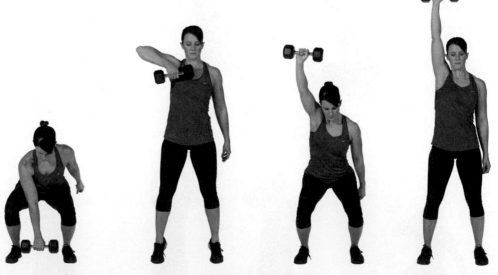

Dumbbell snatch

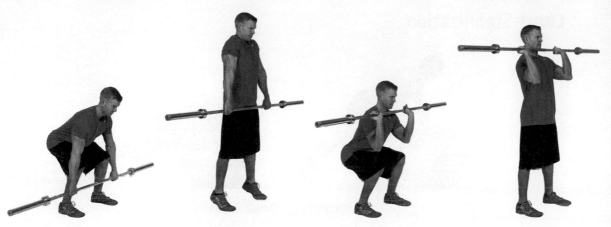

Barbell hang clean

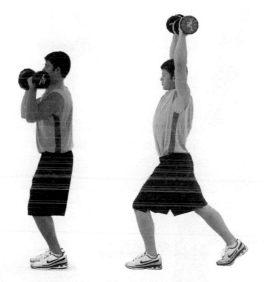

Dumbbell split jerk

Resistance Exercises *continued*

Chest-Stabilization

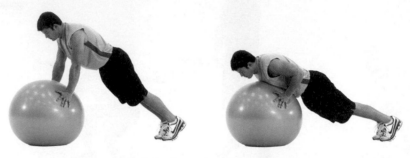

Ball push-up: hands on ball

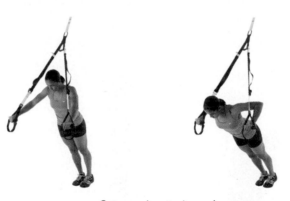

Suspension trainer chest press

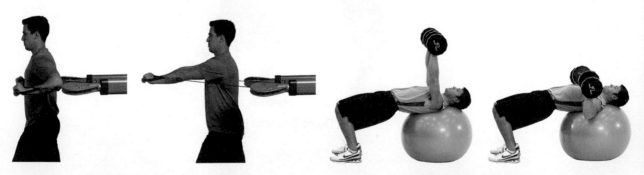

Standing cable chest press

Ball dumbbell chest press

Chest-Strength

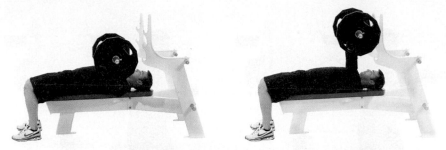

Bench press

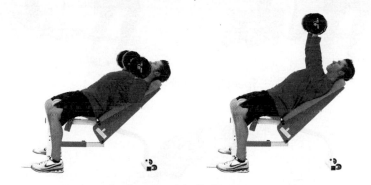

Incline dumbbell chest press

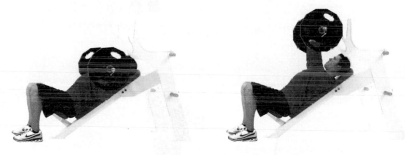

Incline bench press

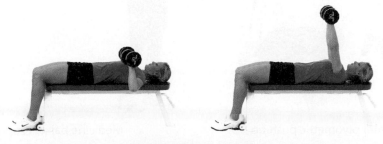

Dumbbell chest press

Resistance Exercises *continued*

Chest-Power

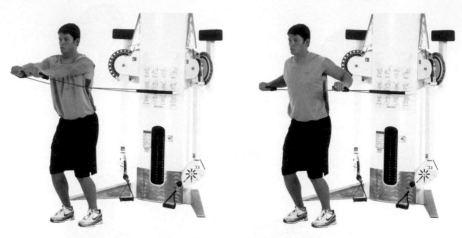

Speed tubing chest press

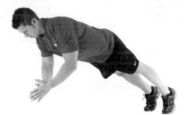

Plyometric push-up

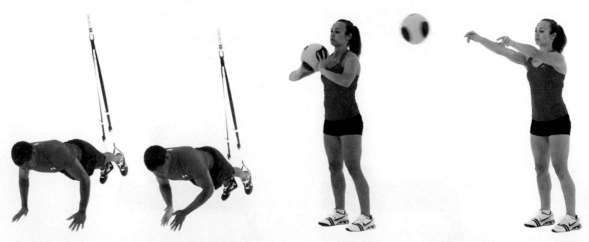

Suspension trainer plyometric push-up   Medicine ball chest pass

Back-Stabilization

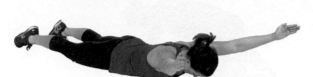

Prone Ys

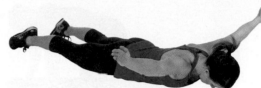

Prone Ts

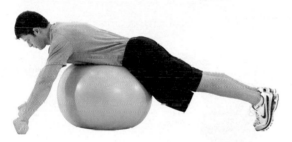

Ball dumbbell rows

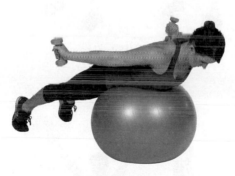

Ball cobra

Resistance Exercises *continued*

Back-Strength

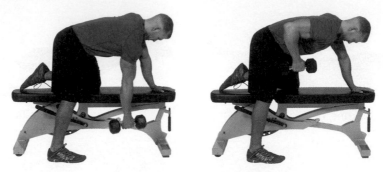

Supported dumbbell row

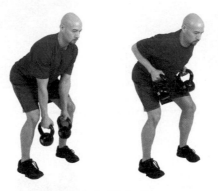

Standing kettlebell row

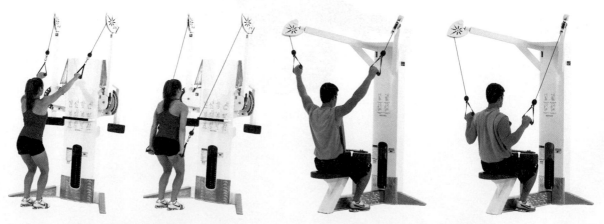

Straight-arm pulldown   Seated lat pulldown

Back-Power

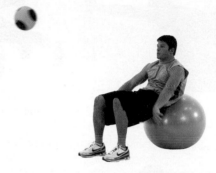

Ball medicine ball pullover throw

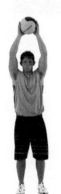
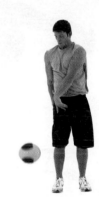

Woodchop throw

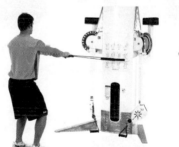
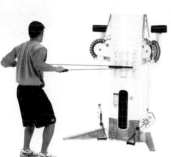

Speed tubing row

Shoulder-Stabilization

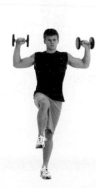
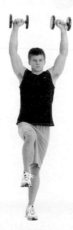

Single-leg dumbbell overhead press

Resistance Exercises *continued*

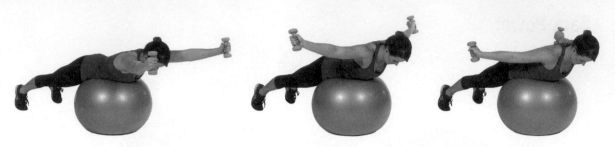

Ball combo I

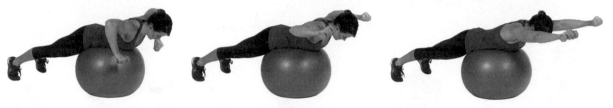

Ball combo II

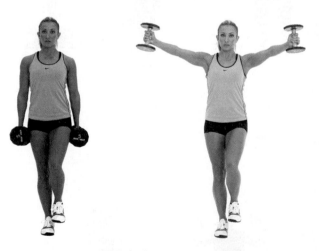

Single-leg scaption

Shoulder-Strength

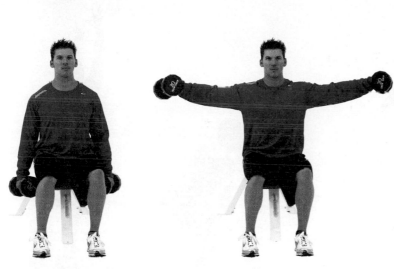

Dumbbell lateral raise

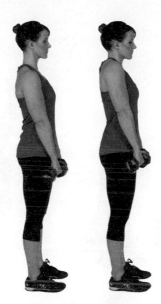

Dumbbell shrug

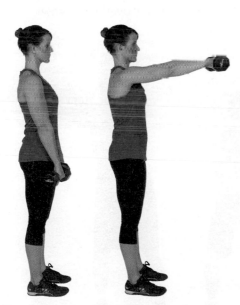

Dumbbell front raise

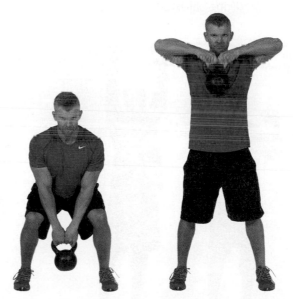

Kettlebell high pull

Resistance Exercises *continued*

Shoulder-Power

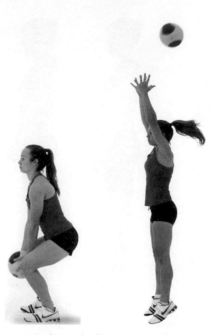

Medicine ball overhead throw

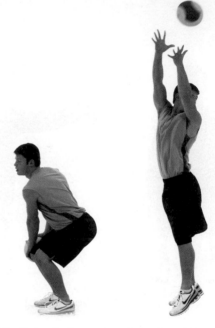

Medicine ball rotational overhead throw

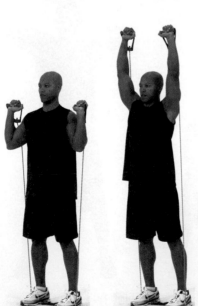

Speed tubing shoulder press

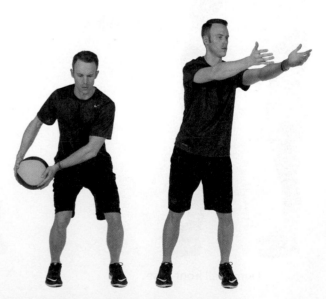

Side medicine ball oblique throw

Biceps-Stabilization

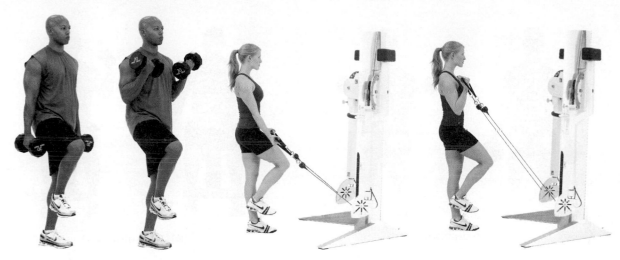

Single-leg dumbbell biceps curl

Single-leg cable curl

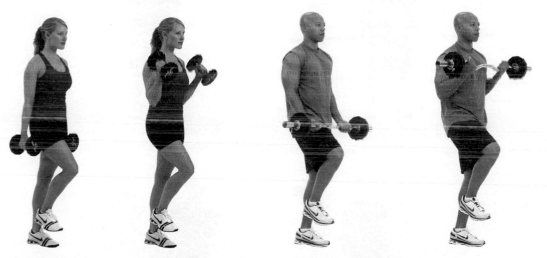

Single-leg dumbbell hammer curl

Single-leg barbell curl

Resistance Exercises *continued*

Biceps-Strength

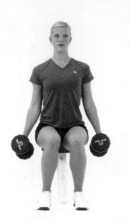
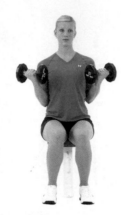

Seated dumbbell curl

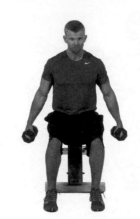
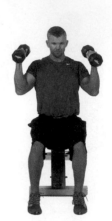

Seated hammer curl

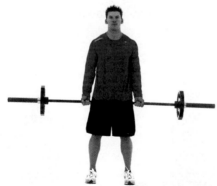
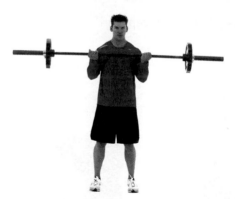

Standing barbell curl

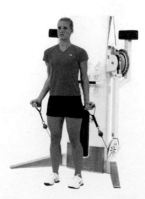
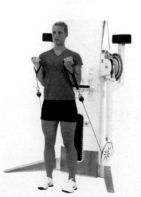

Standing cable curl

Triceps-Stabilization

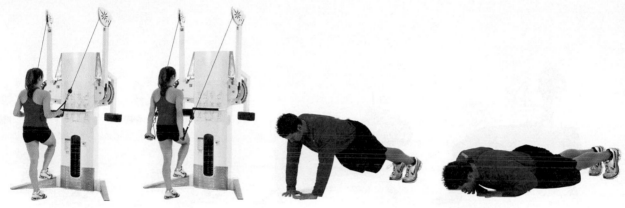

Single leg cable pressdown

Narrow grip push-up

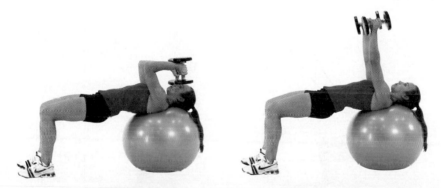

Supine ball dumbbell triceps extension

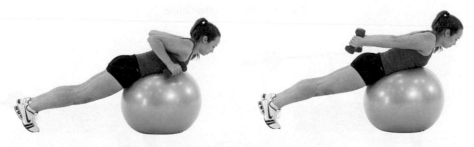

Prone dumbbell triceps extension

Resistance Exercises *continued*

Triceps-Strength

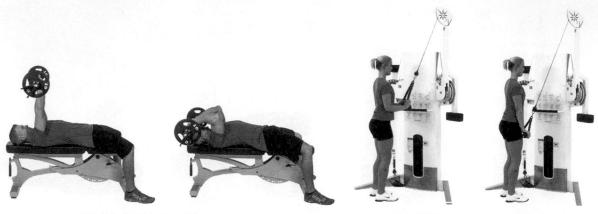

Supine bench barbell triceps extension

Standing cable pressdowns

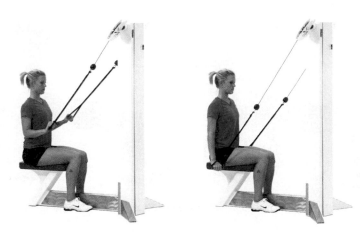

Triceps extension machine

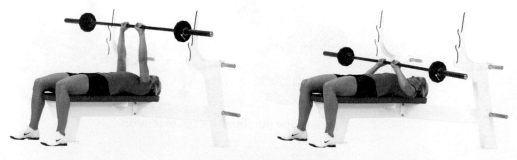

Close-grip bench press

Legs-Stabilization

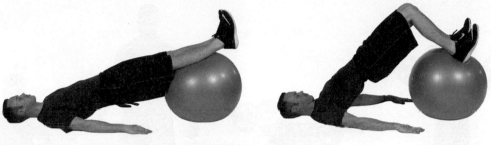

Ball hamstring curl

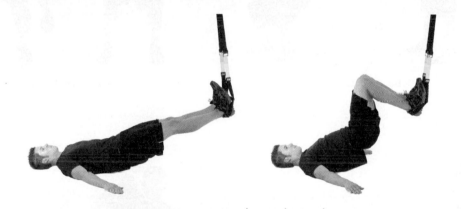

Suspension trainer hamstring curl

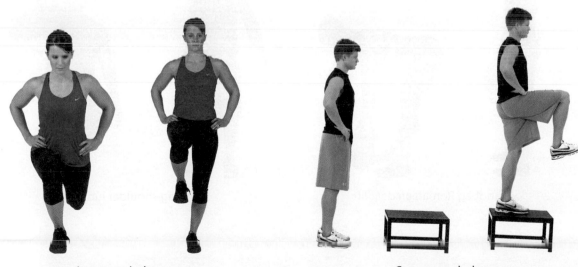

Lunge to balance

Step-up to balance

Resistance Exercises *continued*

Legs-Strength

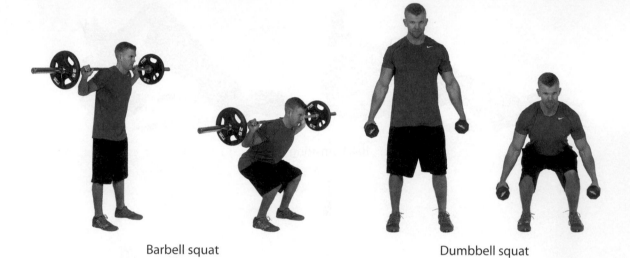

Barbell squat

Dumbbell squat

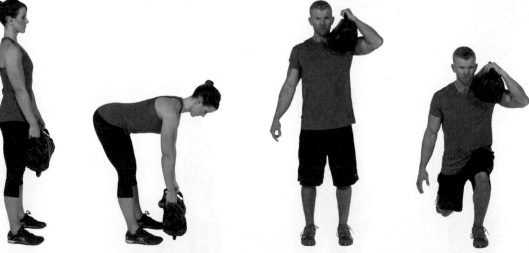

Sandbag Romanian deadlift

Sandbag shoulder lunges

Legs-Power

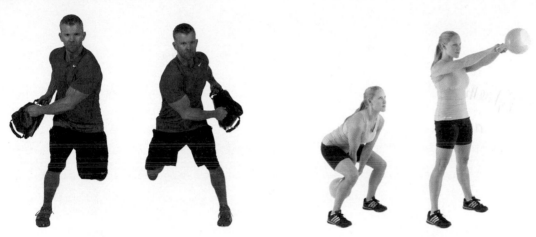

Sandbag ice skaters

Kettlebell swings

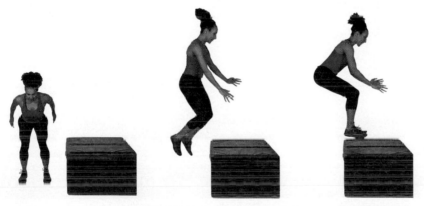

Transverse plane box jump ups

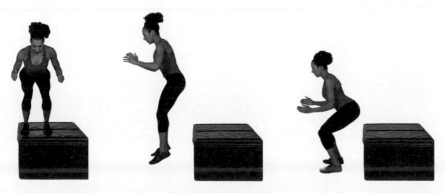

Transverse plane box jump downs

APPENDIX B

NUTRITIONAL CONCEPTS

The Digestive System

Protein Digestion, Absorption, and Utilization

Proteins must be broken down into their constituent amino acids before the body can use them to build or repair tissue, or as an energy substrate. The fate of the amino acids after digestion and absorption by the intestines depends on the body's homeostatic needs, which can range from tissue replacement or addition, to a need for energy.

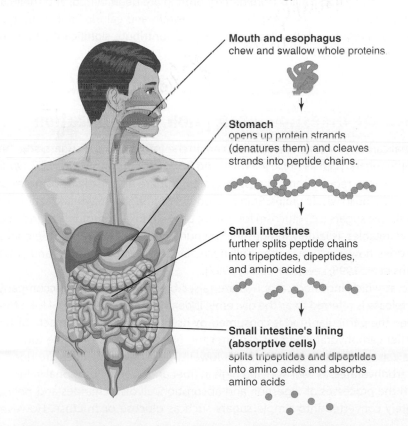

Mouth and esophagus
chew and swallow whole proteins

Stomach
opens up protein strands
(denatures them) and cleaves
strands into peptide chains.

Small intestines
further splits peptide chains
into tripeptides, dipeptides,
and amino acids

**Small intestine's lining
(absorptive cells)**
splits tripeptides and dipeptides
into amino acids and absorbs
amino acids

As ingested proteins enter the stomach, they encounter hydrochloric acid (HCl), which uncoils (i.e., denatures) the protein so that digestive enzymes can begin dismantling the peptide bonds. In addition, the enzyme pepsin begins to cleave the protein strand into smaller polypeptides (strands of several amino acids) and single amino acids. As these protein fragments leave the stomach and enter the small intestine, pancreatic and intestinal proteases (enzymes that aid in protein digestion) continue to dismantle the protein fragments.

The resulting dipeptides, tripeptides, and single amino acids are then absorbed through the intestinal wall into the enterocytes and released into the blood supply to the liver. Once in the bloodstream, the free-form amino acids have several possible fates: they can be used for protein synthesis (building and repairing tissues or structures), immediate energy, or potential energy (fat storage).

Amino Acids for Immediate Energy

The body has a constant need for energy, and the brain and nervous system, in particular, have a constant need for glucose. If carbohydrate or total energy intake is too low, the body has the ability to use amino acids (from dietary or body proteins) to provide energy (Berdanier, 1995; Martineau et al., 1985). This process is typically known as gluconeogenesis. The amino acids are first deaminated (i.e., stripped of their amine group), allowing the remaining carbon skeleton to be used for the production of glucose or ketones to be used for energy. The removed amine group produces ammonia, a toxic compound, which is converted to urea in the liver and excreted as urine by the kidneys.

Amino Acids for Potential Energy (Fat)

If protein intake exceeds the amount needed for tissue synthesis and the body's energy needs have been met, then amino acids from dietary protein are deaminated, and their carbon fragments may be stored as fat. Among Americans, protein and caloric intakes are typically well above the body's requirements, allowing protein to contribute significantly to individuals' fat stores (Seagle et al., 2009).

Carbohydrate Digestion, Absorption, and Utilization

The principal carbohydrates present in food are in the form of simple sugars, starches, and cellulose. Simple sugars, such as those in honey and fruits, are very easily digested. Double sugars, such as table sugar, require some digestive action, but are not nearly as complex as starches, such as those found in whole grains. Starches require prolonged enzymatic action to be broken down into simple sugars (i.e., glucose) for utilization. Cellulose, commonly found in the skins of fruits and vegetables, is largely indigestible by humans and contributes little energy value to the diet. It does, however, provide the bulk necessary for intestinal motility and aids in elimination (Jenkins et al., 1998; Lewis & Heaton, 1997).

The rate at which ingested carbohydrate raises blood sugar and its accompanying effect on insulin release is referred to as the glycemic index (GI; **Table B.1**). The GI for a food is determined when the particular food is consumed by itself on an empty stomach. Mixed meals of protein, other carbohydrate, and fat can alter the glycemic effect of single foods (Järvi et al., 1995). One can see in **Table B.2** that foods lower on the glycemic index are good sources of complex carbohydrates, as well as being high in fiber and overall nutritional value.

Through the processes of digestion and absorption, all disaccharides and polysaccharides are ultimately converted into simple sugars such as glucose or fructose. However, fructose

TABLE B.1 Glycemic Index

High	>70
Moderate	56–69
Low	>55

TABLE B.2 Glycemic Index for Assorted Foods

Low		Moderate		High	
Food	**GI**	**Food**	**GI**	**Food**	**GI**
Peanuts	14	Apple juice	40	Life Savers	70
Plain yogurt	14	Snickers	41	White bread	70
Soy beans	18	Peach	42	Bagel	72
Peas	22	Carrots	47	Watermelon	72
Cherries	22	Brown rice	50	Popcorn	72
Barley	25	Strawberry jam	51	Graham crackers	74
Grapefruit	25	PowerBar	53	French fries	75
Link sausage	28	Orange juice	53	Grape-Nuts	75
Black beans	30	Honey	55	Shredded wheat	75
Lentils	30	Pita bread	57	Gatorade	78
Skim milk	32	Oatmeal plain	58	Corn flakes	81
Fettuccine	32	Pineapple	59	Rice cakes	82
Chickpeas	33	Sweet potato	61	Pretzels	83
Chocolate milk	32	Coca Cola	63	Baked white potato	85
Whole-wheat spaghetti	37	Raisins	64	Instant rice	87
Apple	38	Cantaloupe	65	Gluten-free bread	90
Pinto beans	39	Whole-wheat bread	67	Dates	103

must be converted to glucose in the liver before it can be used for energy. Some of the glucose (or blood sugar) is used as fuel by tissues of the brain, nervous system, and muscles. Because humans are periodic eaters, a small portion of the glucose is converted to glycogen after a meal and stored within the liver and muscles. Any excess is converted to fat and stored throughout the body as a reserve source of energy. When total caloric intake exceeds output, any excess carbohydrate, dietary fat, or protein may be stored as body fat until energy expenditure once again exceeds energy input.

Role of Fiber in Health

One of the greatest contributions made by complex carbohydrates is fiber. Higher intakes of dietary fiber are associated with lower incidence of heart disease and certain types of cancer (Anderson, Smith, & Gustafson, 1994; Wolk et al., 1999). Fiber is an indigestible carbohydrate. Dietary fiber is either soluble or insoluble. Soluble fiber is dissolved by water and forms a gel-like substance in the digestive tract. Soluble fiber has many benefits, including moderating blood glucose levels and lowering cholesterol. Good sources of soluble fiber include oats and oatmeal, legumes (e.g., peas, beans, lentils), barley, and many uncooked fruits and vegetables (especially oranges, apples, and carrots).

Insoluble fiber does not absorb or dissolve in water. It passes through the digestive tract close to its original form. Insoluble fiber offers many benefits to intestinal health, including a reduction in the risk of colorectal cancer and occurrence of hemorrhoids and constipation. Most insoluble fibers come from the bran layer of cereal grains. The recommended intake of fiber is set at 38 grams per day and 25 grams per day for young men and women respectively (Ryan-Harshman & Aldoori, 2006). Additional benefits of fiber include the following (Aldoori et al., 1998; Anderson et al., 1994; Fernstrom & Miller, 1994; Howe et al., 1992; Rimm et al., 1996):

- ◆ Provides bulk in the diet, thus increasing the satiety value of foods.
- ◆ Delays emptying of the stomach, further increasing satiety.
- ◆ Prevents constipation and establishes regular bowel movements.
- ◆ May reduce the risks of heart and artery disease by lowering blood cholesterol.
- ◆ Regulates the body's absorption of glucose (diabetics included), perhaps because fiber is believed to be capable of controlling the rate of digestion and assimilation of carbohydrates.
- ◆ High-fiber meals have been shown to exert regulatory effects on blood glucose levels for up to 5 hours after eating.

Fat Digestion, Absorption, and Utilization

Digestion of dietary fat starts in the mouth, moves to the stomach, and is completed in the small intestine. In the intestine, the fat interacts with bile to become emulsified so that pancreatic enzymes can break the triglycerides down into two fatty acids and a monoglyceride. Absorption of these constituents occurs through the intestinal wall into the blood. In the intestinal wall, they are reassembled into triglycerides that are then released into the lymph in the form of a lipoprotein called chylomicron. Chylomicrons from the lymph move to the blood. The triglyceride content of the chylomicron is removed by the action of the enzyme lipoprotein lipase (LPL), and the released fatty acids are taken up by the tissues. Throughout the day, triglycerides are constantly cycled in and out of tissues, including muscles, organs, and adipose tissue.

Dietary Reference Intake

TABLE B.3   Dietary Reference Intake Terminology

Term	Definition
Estimated Average Requirement (EAR)	The average daily nutrient intake level that is estimated to meet the requirement of half the healthy individuals who are in a particular life stage and gender group.
Recommended Dietary Allowance (RDA)	The average daily nutrient intake level that is sufficient to meet the nutrient requirement of nearly all (97–98%) healthy individuals who are in a particular life stage and gender group.
Adequate Intake (AI)	A recommended average daily nutrient intake level, based on observed (or experimentally determined) approximations or estimates of nutrient intake that are assumed to be adequate for a group (or groups) of healthy people. This measure is used when RDA cannot be determined.
Tolerable Upper Intake Level (UL)	The highest average daily nutrient intake level likely to pose no risk of adverse health affects to almost all individuals in a particular life stage and gender group. As intake increases above the UL, the potential risk of adverse health effects increases.

TABLE B.4   Comparison of Dietary Reference Intake Values for Adult Men and Women and Daily Values for Micronutrients with the Tolerable Upper Intake Levels, Safe Upper Levels, and Guidance Levels[a]

Nutrient	RDA/AI (Men/ Women) ages 31–50	Daily Value (Food Labels)	UL	SUL or Guidance Level	Selected Potential Effects of Excess Intake
Vitamin A (μg)	900/700	1,500 (5,000 IU)	3,000	1,500[c] (5,000 IU)	Liver damage, bone and joint pain, dry skin, loss of hair, headache, vomiting.
β-carotene (mg)				7 (11,655 IU)	Increased risk of lung cancer in smokers and those heavily exposed to asbestos.
Vitamin D (μg)	5[b]	10 (400 IU)	50	25 (1,000 IU)	Calcification of brain and arteries, increased blood calcium, loss of appetite, nausea.
Vitamin E (mg)	15	20 (30 IU)	1,000	540 (800 IU)	Deficient blood clotting.
Vitamin K (μg)	120/90[b]	80	–	1,000[c]	Red blood cell damage or anemia, liver damage.
Thiamin (B_1) (mg)	1.2/1.1	1.5	–	100[c]	Headache, nausea, irritability, insomnia, rapid pulse, weakness (7,000+ mg dose).
Riboflavin (B_2) (mg)	1.3/1.1	1.7	–	40[c]	Generally considered harmless; yellow discoloration of urine.
Niacin (mg)	16/14	20	35	500[c]	Liver damage, flushing, nausea, gastrointestinal problems.
Vitamin B_6 (mg)	1.3	2	100	10	Neurologic problems, numbness and pain in limbs.
Vitamin B_{12} (μg)	2.4	6	–	2,000[c]	No reports of toxicity from oral ingestion.
Folic acid (μg)	400	400	1,000	1,000[c]	Masks vitamin B_{12} deficiency (which can cause neurologic problems).

(continued)

TABLE B.4 Comparison of Dietary Reference Intake Values for Adult Men and Women and Daily Values for Micronutrients with the Tolerable Upper Intake Levels, Safe Upper Levels, and Guidance Levels (*continued*)

Nutrient	RDA/AI (Men/Women) ages 31–50	Daily Value (Food Labels)	UL	SUL or Guidance Level	Selected Potential Effects of Excess Intake
Pantothenic acid (mg)	5^b	10	–	200^c	Diarrhea and gastrointestinal disturbance (10,000+ mg/day).
Biotin (μg)	30^b	300	–	900^c	No reports of toxicity from oral ingestion.
Vitamin C (mg)	90/75	60	2,000	$1,000^c$	Nausea, diarrhea, kidney stones.
Boron (mg)			20	9.6	Adverse effects on male and female reproductive systems.
Calcium (mg)	$1,000^b$	1,000	2,500	$1,500^c$	Nausea, constipation, kidney stones.
Chromium (μg)	35^b	120	–	$10,000^c$	Potential adverse effects on liver and kidneys; picolinate form possibly mutagenic.
Cobalt (mg)				1.4^c	Cardiotoxic effects; not appropriate in a dietary supplement except as vitamin B_{12}.
Copper (μg)	900	2,000	10,000	10,000	Gastrointestinal distress, liver damage.
Fluoride (mg)	$4/3^b$		10		Bone, kidney, muscle, and nerve damage; supplement only with professional guidance.
Germanium				$zero^c$	Kidney toxin; should not be in a dietary supplement.
Iodine (μg)	150	150	1,100	500^c	Elevated thyroid hormone concentration.
Iron (mg)	8/18	18	45	17^c	Gastrointestinal distress, increased risk of heart disease, oxidative stress.
Magnesium (mg)	420/320	400	350^d	400^c	Diarrhea.
Manganese (mg)	$2.3/1.8^b$	2	11	4c	Neurotoxicity.
Molybdenum	45	75	2,000	$zero^c$	Goutlike symptoms, joint pains, increased uric acid.
Nickel (μg)				260^c	Increased sensitivity of skin reaction to nickel in jewelry.
Phosphorus (mg)	700	1,000	4,000	250^c	Alteration of parathyroid hormone levels, reduced bone mineral density.
Potassium (mg)				$3,700^c$	Gastrointestinal damage.
Selenium (μg)	55	70	400	450	Nausea, diarrhea, fatigue, hair and nail loss.
Silicon (mg)				700	Low toxicity, possibility of kidney stones.
Vanadium (mg)			1.8	zero	Gastrointestinal irritation; fatigue.
Zinc (mg)	11/8	15	40	25	Impaired immune function, low HDL-cholesterol.

[a]Food and Nutrition Board, Institute of Medicine (U.S.). Dietary Reference Intake Tables. Available at [www4.nationalacademies.org/IOM/IOMHome.nsf/Pages/Food+and+Nutrition+Board].
[b]Indicates adequate intake (AI).
[c]Indicates guidance levels, set by the Expert Group on Vitamins and Minerals of the Food Standards Agency, United Kingdom. These are intended to be levels of daily intake of nutrients in dietary supplements that potentially susceptible individuals could take daily on a lifelong basis without medical supervision in reasonable safety. When the evidence base was considered inadequate to set an SUL, guidance levels were set based on limited data. SULs and guidance levels tend to be conservative, and it is possible that for some vitamins and minerals, greater amounts could be consumed for short periods without risk to health. The values presented are for a 60-kg (132-lb) adult. Consult the full publication for values expressed per kilogram of body weight. This FSA publication, *Safe Upper Levels for Vitamins and Minerals*, is available at: [http://www.foodstandards.gov.uk/multimedia/pdfs/vitmin2003.pdf].
[d]The UL for magnesium represents intake specifically from pharmacologic agents and dietary supplements in addition to dietary intake.
RDA, recommended dietary allowance; *UL*, tolerable upper intake level; *AI*, adequate intake; *SUL*, safe upper level.

References

Aldoori, W. H., Giovanucci, E. L., Rockett, H. R., Sampson, L., Rimm, E. B., & Willett, W. C. (1998). A prospective study of dietary fiber types and symptomatic diverticular disease in men. *Journal of Nutrition, 128*(4), 714–719.

Anderson, J. W., Smith, B. M., & Gustafson, N. J. (1994). Health benefits and practical aspects of high-fiber diets. *American Journal of Clinical Nutrition, 59*(5 Suppl), 1242S–1247S.

Berdanier, C. D. (1995). *Advanced nutrition: Macronutrients.* Boca Raton, FL: CRC Press.

Fernstrom, J. D., & Miller, G. D. (1994). *Appetite and body weight regulation.* Boca Raton, FL: CRC Press.

Howe, G. R., Benito, E., Castelleto, R., Cornée, J., Estève, J., Gallagher, R. P … Shu, Z. (1992). Dietary intake of fiber and decreased risk of cancers of the colon and rectum: Evidence from the combined analysis of 13 case-control studies. *Journal of the National Cancer Institute, 84*(24), 1887–1896.

Järvi, A. E., Karlström, B. E., Granfeldt, Y. E., Björck, I. M., Vessby, B. O., & Asp, N. G. (1995). The influence of food structure on postprandial metabolism in patients with non-insulin-dependent diabetes mellitus. *American Journal of Clinical Nutrition, 61*(4), 837–842.

Jenkins, D. J., Vuksan, V., Kendall, C. W., Würsch, P., Jeffcoat, R., Waring, S., & Wong, E. (1998). Physiological effects of resistant starches on fecal bulk, short chain fatty acids, blood lipids and glycemic index. *Journal of the American College of Nutrition, 17*(6), 609–616.

Lewis, S. J., & Heaton, K. W. (1997). Increasing butyrate concentration in the distal colon by accelerating intestinal transit. *Gut, 41*(2), 245–251.

Martineau, A., Lecavalier, L., Falardeau, P., & Chiasson, J. L. (1985). Simultaneous determination of glucose turnover, alanine turnover, and gluconeogenesis in human using a double stable-isotope-labeled tracer infusion and gas chromatography-mass spectrometry analysis. *Analytical Biochemistry, 151*(2), 495–503.

Rimm, E. B., Ascherio, A., Giovanucci, E., Spiegelman, D., Stampfer, M. J., & Willett, W. C. (1996). Vegetable, fruit, and cereal fiber intake and risk of coronary heart disease among men. *Journal of the American Medical Association, 275*(6), 447–451.

Ryan-Harshman, M., & Aldoori, W. (2006). New dietary reference intakes for macronutrients and fibre. *Canadian Family Physician, 52*, 177–179.

Seagle, H. M., Strain, G. W., Makris, A., Reeves, R. S., & American Dietetic Association. (2009). Position of the American Dietetic Association: Weight management. *Journal of the American Dietetic Association, 109*, 330–346.

Wolk, A., Manson, J. E., Stampfer, M. J., Colditz, G. A., Speizer, F. E., Hennekens, C. H., & Willett, W. C. (1999). Long-term intake of dietary fiber and decreased risk of coronary heart disease among women. *Journal of the American Medical Association, 281*(21), 1998–2004.

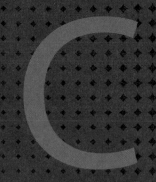

ADDITIONAL OBJECTIVE ASSESSMENT INFORMATION

Gait: Treadmill Walking

Purpose

Assessment of dynamic posture during ambulation.

Procedure

1. Have the individual walk on a treadmill at a comfortable pace at a 0-degree incline.
2. From an anterior view, observe the feet and knees. The feet should remain straight, with the knees in line with the toes. From a lateral view, observe the low back, shoulders, and head. The low back should maintain a neutral lordotic curve. The shoulders and head should also be in neutral alignment. From a posterior view, observe the feet and lumbo-pelvic-hip complex (LPHC). The feet should remain straight and the LPHC should remain level.

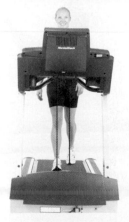

Gait treadmill walking assessment:
Anterior view.

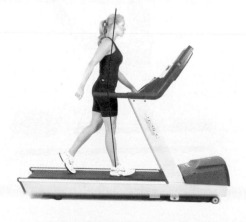

Gait treadmill walking assessment:
Lateral view.

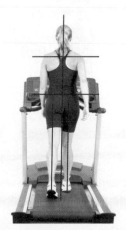

Gait treadmill walking assessment:
Posterior view.

737

Compensations: Anterior View

1. Feet: Do the feet flatten and/or turn out?
2. Knees: Do the knees move inward?

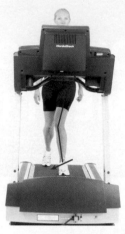

Gait treadmill walking assessment compensations:
Feet flatten/knees move inward.

Compensations: Lateral View

1. LPHC: Does the low back arch?
2. Shoulders and head:
   a. Do the shoulders round?
   b. Does the head migrate forward?

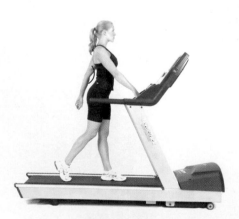

Gait treadmill walking assessment
compensations: Low back arches.

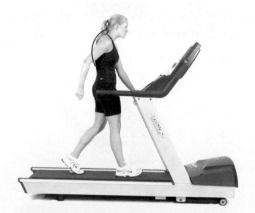

Gait treadmill walking assessment
compensations: Shoulders round.

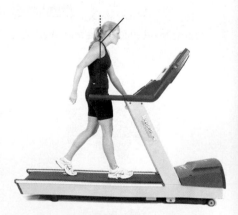

Gait treadmill walking assessment
compensations: Head forward.

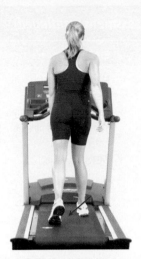

Gait treadmill walking assessment compensations: Feet flatten and/or turn out.

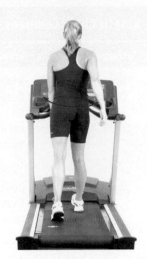

Gait treadmill walking assessment compensations: Pelvic rotation.

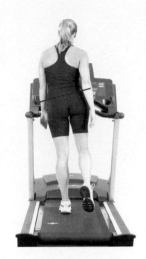

Gait treadmill walking assessment compensations: Hip hikes.

Compensations: Posterior View

1. Feet: Do the feet flatten and/or turn out?
2. LPHC:
   a. Is there excessive pelvic rotation?
   b. Do the hips hike?

When performing the assessment, record all of your findings. You can then refer to the following **Table C.1** to determine potential overactive and underactive muscles that will need to be addressed through corrective flexibility and strengthening techniques to improve the individual's quality of movement, decreasing the risk for injury and improving overall performance.

TABLE C.1 Kinetic Chain Compensations for the Gait Assessment

Checkpoint	Compensation	Probable Overactive Muscles	Probable Underactive Muscles
Feet	Flatten	Peroneal complex Lat. Gastrocnemius Biceps femoris (short head) TFL	Anterior tibialis Posterior tibialis Med. Gastrocnemius Gluteus medius
	Turn out	Soleus Lat. Gastrocnemius Biceps femoris (short head) Tensor fascia lata (TFL)	Med. Gastrocnemius Med. Hamstring Gluteus medius/maximus Gracilis Sartorius Popliteus

(continued)

TABLE C.1 Kinetic Chain Compensations for the Gait Assessment (*continued*)

Checkpoint	Compensation	Probable Overactive Muscles	Probable Underactive Muscles
Knees	Move inward (Valgus)	Adductor complex Biceps femoris (short head) TFL Lat. Gastrocnemius Vastus lateralis	Med. Hamstring Med. Gastrocnemius Gluteus medius/maximus Vastus medialis oblique Anterior tibialis Posterior tibialis
LPHC	Low back arches	Hip flexor complex Erector spinae Latissimus dorsi	Gluteus maximus Intrinsic core stabilizers Hamstrings
	Excessive rotation	External obliques Adductor complex Hamstrings	Gluteus medius/maximus Intrinsic core stabilizers
	Hip hike	Quadratus lumborum (opposite side) TFL/ Gluteus minimus (same side)	Adductor complex (same side) Gluteus medius (same side)
Shoulders	Rounded	Pectorals Latissimus dorsi	Middle and lower trapezius Rotator cuff
Head	Forward	Upper trapezius Levator scapulae Sternocliedomastoid	Deep cervical flexors

Landing Error Scoring System (LESS) Test

Purpose

The LESS test is a dynamic movement assessment tool for identifying improper movement patterns during jump-landing tasks (DiStefano et al., 2009; Padua et al., 2009). This test evaluates landing technique based on 9 jump-landing concepts using 14 different yes or no questions.

Procedure

1. The individual stands on a 30-cm (12-inch) box. A target line is drawn on the floor at a distance of half the individual's height.
2. The individual is instructed to "jump forward from the box with both feet so that you land with both feet just after the line" and "as soon as you land, jump up for maximum height and land back down."

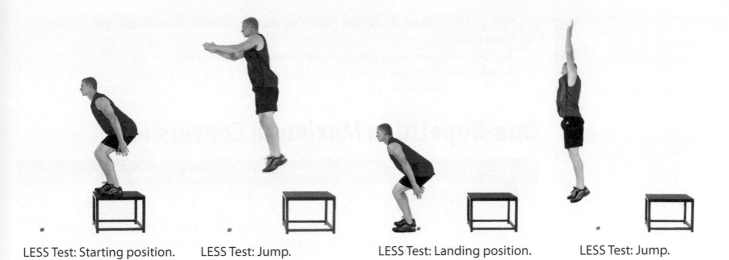

LESS Test: Starting position. LESS Test: Jump. LESS Test: Landing position. LESS Test: Jump.

3. The individual views a demonstration performed by the fitness professional, and then gets the opportunity to practice.
4. Ideally, video cameras are placed 10 feet in front and to the right of the landing area.
5. The videos are evaluated as follows:
   a. Knee flexion angle at initial contact >30 degrees: 0 = yes, 1 = no
   b. Knee valgus at initial contact, knees over midfoot: 0 = yes, 1 = no
   c. Trunk flexion angle at contact: 0 = yes, 1 = no
   d. Lateral trunk flexion at contact: 0 = yes, 1 = no
   e. Ankle plantar flexion at contact: 0 = yes, 1 = no
   f. Foot position at initial contact, toes 30 degrees external rotation: 0 = yes, 1 = no
   g. Foot position at initial contact, toes 30 degrees internal rotation: 0 = yes, 1 = no
   h. Stance width at initial contact, shoulder width: 0 = yes, 1 = no
   i. Initial foot contact symmetric: 0 = yes, 1 = no
   j. Knee flexion displacement (knee position before jumping) 45 degrees: 0 = yes, 1 = no
   k. Knee valgus displacement (knee position before jumping), knee inside great toe: 0 = yes, 1 = no
   l. Trunk flexion at maximal knee angle, trunk flexed more than at initial contact: 0 = yes, 1 = no
   m. Hip flexion angle at initial contact, hips flexed: 0 = yes, 1 = no
   n. Hip flexion at maximal knee angle, hips flexed more than at initial contact: 0 = yes, 1 = no
   o. Joint displacement, sagittal plane: 0 = soft, 1 = average, 2 = stiff
   p. Overall impression: 0 = excellent, 1 = average, 2 = poor
6. A higher LESS score indicates a greater number of landing errors committed and therefore a higher risk for injury.

Although the LESS test will provide the fitness professional with the most comprehensive analysis of a person's functional status, this assessment may be difficult to perform in some settings in which video cameras are not an option. In this case, a modified version of this assessment can be used to assess some of the primary compensations that can be indicators of potential injury. In the modified version, the fitness professional would view the individual from an anterior view. The primary compensations to look for would include the foot and knee positions:

1. Foot position: At initial contact, toes > 30 degrees external rotation: 0 = yes, 1 = no
2. Knee position:
   a. Knee valgus at initial contact, knees over midfoot: 0 = yes, 1 = no
   b. Knee valgus displacement, knee inside great toe: 0 = yes, 1 = no

One-Repetition Maximum Conversion

Pounds	10 reps	9 reps	8 reps	7 reps	6 reps	5 reps	4 reps	3 reps	2 reps
5	7	6	6	6	6	6	6	5	5
10	13	13	13	12	12	11	11	11	11
15	20	19	19	18	18	17	17	16	16
20	27	26	25	24	24	23	22	22	21
25	33	32	31	30	29	29	28	27	26
30	40	39	38	36	35	34	33	32	32
35	47	45	44	42	41	40	39	38	37
40	53	52	50	48	47	46	44	43	42
45	60	58	56	55	53	51	50	49	47
50	67	65	63	61	59	57	56	54	53
55	73	71	69	67	65	63	61	59	58
60	80	77	75	73	71	69	67	65	63
65	87	84	81	79	76	74	72	70	68
70	93	90	88	85	82	80	78	76	74
75	100	97	94	91	88	86	83	81	79
80	107	103	100	97	94	91	89	86	84
85	113	110	106	103	100	97	94	92	89
90	120	116	113	109	106	103	100	97	95
95	127	123	119	115	112	109	106	103	100
100	133	129	125	121	118	114	111	108	105
105	140	135	131	127	124	120	117	114	111
110	147	142	138	133	129	126	122	119	116
115	153	148	144	139	135	131	128	124	121
120	160	155	150	145	141	137	133	130	126
125	167	161	156	152	147	143	139	135	132

(continued)

Pounds	10 reps	9 reps	8 reps	7 reps	6 reps	5 reps	4 reps	3 reps	2 reps
130	173	168	163	158	153	149	144	141	137
135	180	174	169	164	159	154	150	146	142
140	187	181	175	170	165	160	156	151	147
145	193	187	181	176	171	166	161	157	153
150	200	194	188	182	176	171	167	162	158
155	207	200	194	188	182	177	172	168	163
160	213	206	200	194	188	183	178	173	168
165	220	213	206	200	194	189	183	178	174
170	227	219	213	206	200	194	189	184	179
175	233	226	219	212	206	200	194	189	184
180	240	232	225	218	212	206	200	195	189
185	247	239	231	224	218	211	206	200	195
190	253	245	238	230	224	217	211	205	200
195	260	252	244	236	229	223	217	211	205
200	267	258	250	242	235	229	222	216	211
205	273	265	256	248	241	234	228	222	216
210	280	271	263	255	247	240	233	227	221
215	287	277	269	261	253	246	239	232	226
220	293	284	275	267	259	251	244	238	232
225	300	290	281	273	265	257	250	243	237
230	307	297	288	279	271	263	256	249	242
235	313	303	294	285	276	269	261	254	247
240	320	310	300	291	282	274	267	259	253
245	327	316	306	297	288	280	272	265	258
250	333	323	313	303	294	286	278	270	263
255	340	329	319	309	300	291	283	276	268
260	347	335	325	315	306	297	289	281	274
265	353	342	331	321	312	303	294	286	279
270	360	348	338	327	318	309	300	292	284
275	367	355	344	333	324	314	306	297	289

(continued)

Pounds	10 reps	9 reps	8 reps	7 reps	6 reps	5 reps	4 reps	3 reps	2 reps
280	373	361	350	339	329	320	311	303	295
285	380	368	356	345	335	326	317	308	300
290	387	374	363	352	341	331	322	314	305
295	393	381	369	358	347	337	328	319	311
300	400	387	375	364	353	343	333	324	316
305	407	394	381	370	359	349	339	330	321
310	413	400	388	376	365	354	344	335	326
315	420	406	394	382	371	360	350	341	332
320	427	413	400	388	376	366	356	346	337
325	433	419	406	394	382	371	361	351	342
330	440	426	413	400	388	377	367	357	347
335	447	432	419	406	394	383	372	362	353
340	453	439	425	412	400	389	378	368	358
345	460	445	431	418	406	394	383	373	363
350	467	452	438	424	412	400	389	378	368
355	473	458	444	430	418	406	394	384	374
360	480	465	450	436	424	411	400	389	379
365	487	471	456	442	429	417	406	395	384
370	493	477	463	448	435	423	411	400	389
375	500	484	469	455	441	429	417	405	395
380	507	490	475	461	447	434	422	411	400
385	513	497	481	467	453	440	428	416	405
390	520	503	488	473	459	446	433	422	411
395	527	510	494	479	465	451	439	427	416
400	533	516	500	485	471	457	444	432	421
405	540	523	506	491	476	463	450	438	426
410	547	529	513	497	482	469	456	443	432
415	553	535	519	503	488	474	461	449	437
420	560	542	525	509	494	480	467	454	442
425	567	548	531	515	500	486	472	459	447
430	573	555	538	521	506	491	478	465	453

(continued)

Pounds	10 reps	9 reps	8 reps	7 reps	6 reps	5 reps	4 reps	3 reps	2 reps
435	580	561	544	527	512	497	483	470	458
440	587	568	550	533	518	503	489	476	463
445	593	574	556	539	524	509	494	481	468
450	600	581	563	545	529	514	500	486	474
455	607	587	569	552	535	520	506	492	479
460	613	594	575	558	541	526	511	497	484
465	620	600	581	564	547	531	517	503	489
470	627	606	588	570	553	537	522	508	495
475	633	613	594	576	559	543	528	514	500
480	640	619	600	582	565	549	533	519	505
485	647	626	606	588	571	554	539	524	511
490	653	632	613	594	576	560	544	530	516
495	660	639	619	600	582	566	550	535	521
500	667	645	625	606	588	571	556	541	526
505	673	652	631	612	594	577	561	546	532
510	680	658	638	618	600	583	567	551	537
515	687	665	644	624	606	589	572	557	542
520	693	671	650	630	612	594	578	562	547
525	700	677	656	636	618	600	583	568	553
530	707	684	663	642	624	606	589	573	558
535	713	690	669	648	629	611	594	578	563
540	720	697	675	655	635	617	600	584	568
545	727	703	681	661	641	623	606	589	574
550	733	710	688	667	647	629	611	595	579
555	740	716	694	673	653	634	617	600	584
560	747	723	700	679	659	640	622	605	589
565	753	729	706	685	665	646	628	611	595
570	760	735	713	691	671	651	633	616	600
575	767	742	719	697	676	657	639	622	605
580	773	748	725	703	682	663	644	627	611

(continued)

Pounds	10 reps	9 reps	8 reps	7 reps	6 reps	5 reps	4 reps	3 reps	2 reps
585	780	755	731	709	688	669	650	632	616
590	787	761	738	715	694	674	656	638	621
595	793	768	744	721	700	680	661	643	626
600	800	774	750	727	706	686	667	649	632
605	807	781	756	733	712	691	672	654	637
610	813	787	763	739	718	697	678	659	642
615	820	794	769	745	724	703	683	665	647
620	827	800	775	752	729	709	689	670	653
625	833	806	781	758	735	714	694	676	658
630	840	813	788	764	741	720	700	681	663
635	847	819	794	770	747	726	706	686	668
640	853	826	800	776	753	731	711	692	674
645	860	832	806	782	759	737	717	697	679
650	867	839	813	788	765	743	722	703	684
655	873	845	819	794	771	749	728	708	689
660	880	852	825	800	776	754	733	714	695
665	887	858	831	806	782	760	739	719	700
670	893	865	838	812	788	766	744	724	705
675	900	871	844	818	794	771	750	730	711
680	907	877	850	824	800	777	756	735	716
685	913	884	856	830	806	783	761	741	721
690	920	890	863	836	812	789	767	746	726
695	927	897	869	842	818	794	772	751	732
700	933	903	875	848	824	800	778	757	737
705	940	910	881	855	829	806	783	762	742
710	947	916	888	861	835	811	789	768	747
715	953	923	894	867	841	817	794	773	753
720	960	929	900	873	847	823	800	778	758
725	967	935	906	879	853	829	806	784	763
730	973	942	913	885	859	834	811	789	768
735	980	948	919	891	865	840	817	795	774

(continued)

Pounds	10 reps	9 reps	8 reps	7 reps	6 reps	5 reps	4 reps	3 reps	2 reps
740	987	955	925	897	871	846	822	800	779
745	993	961	931	903	876	851	828	805	784
750	1000	968	938	909	882	857	833	811	789
755	1007	974	944	915	888	863	839	816	795
760	1013	981	950	921	894	869	844	822	800
765	1020	987	956	927	900	874	850	827	805
770	1027	994	963	933	906	880	856	832	811
775	1033	1000	969	939	912	886	861	838	816
780	1040	1006	975	945	918	891	867	843	821
785	1047	1013	981	952	924	897	872	849	826
790	1053	1019	988	958	929	903	878	854	832
795	1060	1026	994	964	935	909	883	859	837
800	1067	1032	1000	970	941	914	889	865	842
805	1073	1039	1006	976	947	920	894	870	847
810	1080	1045	1013	982	953	926	900	876	853
815	1087	1052	1019	988	959	931	906	881	858
820	1093	1058	1025	994	965	937	911	886	863
825	1100	1065	1031	1000	971	943	917	892	868
830	1107	1071	1038	1006	976	949	922	897	874
835	1113	1077	1044	1012	982	954	928	903	879
840	1120	1084	1050	1018	988	960	933	908	884
845	1127	1090	1056	1024	994	966	939	914	889
850	1133	1097	1063	1030	1000	971	944	919	895
855	1140	1103	1069	1036	1006	977	950	924	900
900	1200	1161	1125	1091	1059	1029	1000	973	947
905	1207	1168	1131	1097	1065	1034	1006	978	953
910	1213	1174	1138	1103	1071	1040	1011	984	958
915	1220	1181	1144	1109	1076	1046	1017	989	963
920	1227	1187	1150	1115	1082	1051	1022	995	968
925	1233	1194	1156	1121	1088	1057	1028	1000	974

(continued)

Pounds	10 reps	9 reps	8 reps	7 reps	6 reps	5 reps	4 reps	3 reps	2 reps
930	1240	1200	1163	1127	1094	1063	1033	1005	979
935	1247	1206	1169	1133	1100	1069	1039	1011	984
940	1253	1213	1175	1139	1106	1074	1044	1016	989
945	1260	1219	1181	1145	1112	1080	1050	1022	995
950	1267	1226	1188	1152	1118	1086	1056	1027	1000
955	1273	1232	1194	1158	1124	1091	1061	1032	1005
960	1280	1239	1200	1164	1129	1097	1067	1038	1011
965	1287	1245	1206	1170	1135	1103	1072	1043	1016
970	1293	1252	1213	1176	1141	1109	1078	1049	1021
975	1300	1258	1219	1182	1147	1114	1083	1054	1026
980	1307	1265	1225	1188	1153	1120	1089	1059	1032
985	1313	1271	1231	1194	1159	1126	1094	1065	1037
990	1320	1277	1238	1200	1165	1131	1100	1070	1042
995	1327	1284	1244	1206	1171	1137	1106	1076	1047
1000	1333	1290	1250	1212	1176	1143	1111	1081	1053

References

DiStefano, L. J., Padua, D. A., DiStefano, M. J., & Marshall, S. W. (2009). Influence of age, sex, technique, and exercise program on movement patterns after an anterior cruciate ligament injury prevention program in youth soccer players. *The American Journal of Sports Medicine, 37*(3), 495–505.

Padua, D. A., Marshall S. W., Boling, M. C., Thigpen, C. A., Garrett, Jr., W. E., & Beutler, A. I. (2009). The Landing Error Scoring System (LESS) is a valid and reliable clinical assessment tool of jump-landing biomechanics: The JUMP-ACL study. *The American Journal of Sports Medicine, 37*(10), 1996–2002.

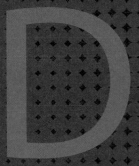

APPENDIX D

THE KINETIC CHAIN

The Nervous System

The Neuron

The functional unit of the nervous system is the neuron (**Figure D.1**). Billions of neurons make up the complex structure of the nervous system and provide it with the ability to communicate internally with itself, as well as externally with the outside environment. A neuron is a specialized cell that processes and transmits information through both electrical and chemical signals. Neurons form the core of the nervous system, which includes the brain, spinal cord, and peripheral ganglia. Collectively, the merging of many neurons together forms the nerves of the body. Neurons are composed of three main parts: the cell body, axon, and dendrites (Fox, 2006; Milner-Brown, 2001; Tortora, 2001; Vander, Sherman, & Luciano, 2001).

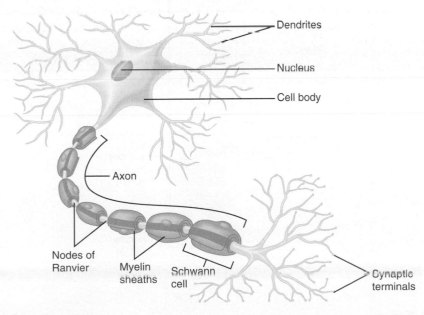

FIGURE D.1 The Neuron.

The cell body (or soma) of a neuron contains a nucleus and other organelles, including lysosomes, mitochondria, and a Golgi complex. The axon is a cylindrical projection from the cell body that transmits nervous impulses to other neurons or effector sites (i.e., muscles, organs, other neurons). The axon is the part of the neuron that provides communication from the brain and spinal cord to other parts of the body. The dendrites gather information from other structures and transmit it back into the neuron (Fox, 2006; Milner-Brown, 2001; Tortora, 2001; Vander et al., 2001).

The Central Nervous System

The nervous system is composed of two interdependent divisions: the central nervous system (CNS) and the peripheral nervous system (PNS). The CNS consists of the brain and the spinal cord; its primary function is to coordinate the activity of all parts of the body (**Figure D.2**; Cohen, 1999; Fox, 2006; Milner-Brown, 2001; Tortora, 2001; Vander et al., 2001).

The Peripheral Nervous System

The PNS consists of nerves that connect the CNS to the rest of the body and the external environment. The nerves of the PNS are how the CNS receives sensory input and initiates responses.

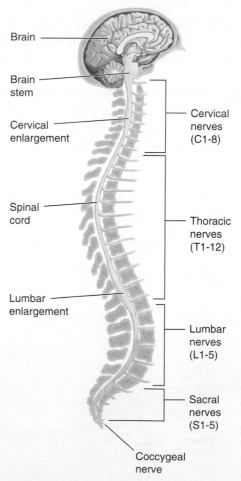

Brain

Brain stem

Cervical enlargement

Cervical nerves (C1-8)

Spinal cord

Thoracic nerves (T1-12)

Lumbar enlargement

Lumbar nerves (L1-5)

Sacral nerves (S1-5)

Coccygeal nerve

FIGURE D.2 The central nervous system.

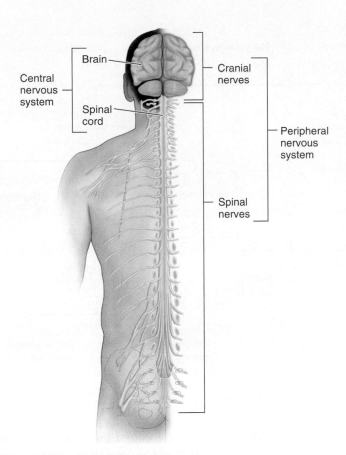

FIGURE D.3 The peripheral nervous system.

The PNS consists of 12 cranial nerves, 31 pairs of spinal nerves (which branch out from the brain and spinal cord), peripheral nerves, and sensory receptors (**Figure D.3**). The peripheral nerves serve two main functions. First, they provide a connection for the nervous system to activate different effector sites, such as muscles (motor function). Second, peripheral nerves relay information from the effector sites back to the brain via sensory receptors (sensory function), thus providing a constant update on the relation between the body and the environment (Fox, 2006; Milner-Brown, 2001; Tortora, 2001; Vander et al., 2001).

Two further subdivisions of the PNS include the somatic and autonomic nervous systems (**Figure D.4**). The somatic nervous system consists of nerves that serve the outer areas of the body and skeletal muscle, and are largely responsible for the voluntary control of movement. The autonomic nervous system supplies neural input to the involuntary systems of the body (e.g., heart, digestive systems, and endocrine glands; Tortora, 2001; Vander et al., 2001).

The autonomic system is further divided into the sympathetic and parasympathetic nervous systems. During exercise, both of these systems serve to increase levels of activation in preparation for activity (sympathetic) or to decrease levels of activation during rest and recovery parasympathetic; Tortora 2001; Vander et al., 2001).

The Muscular System

The traditional perception of muscles is that they work concentrically and predominantly in one plane of motion. However, to more effectively understand motion it is imperative to view

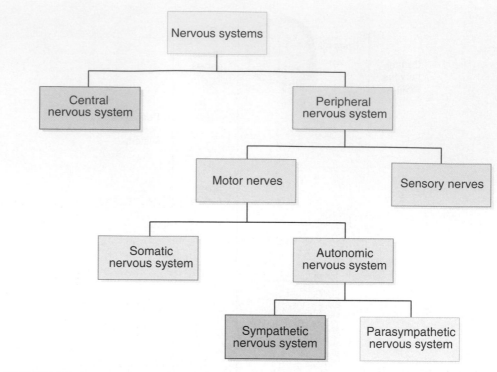

FIGURE D.4 Nervous system structure.

muscles functioning in all planes of motion and through the entire muscle action spectrum. This section describes the isolated (concentric) and integrated (isometric, eccentric) actions of the major muscles of the human movement system.

This section also describes the origin, insertion, and function of each muscle. The origin and insertion refer to the anatomic locations of where a muscle attaches (usually a bone). The origin refers to the proximal attachment site that remains relatively flexed during contraction. The insertion refers to the muscle's distal attachment site to a moveable bone.

Lower Leg Musculature

Anterior Tibialis

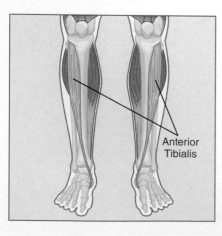

Anterior Tibialis

Origin
- Lateral condyle and proximal two-thirds of the lateral surface of the tibia.

Insertion
- Medial and plantar aspects of the medial cuneiform and the base of the first metatarsal.

Isolated Function
- Concentrically accelerates dorsiflexion and inversion.

Integrated Function
- Eccentrically decelerates plantarflexion and eversion.
- Isometrically stabilizes the arch of the foot.

Posterior Tibialis

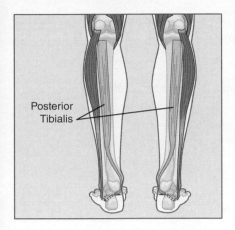

Origin
- Proximal two-thirds of posterior surface of the tibia and fibula.

Insertion
- Every tarsal bone (naviular, cuneiform, cuboid) but the talus plus the bases of the second through the fourth metatarsal bones.
- The main insertion is on the navicular tuberosity and the medial cuneiform bone.

Isolated Function
- Concentrically accelerates plantarflexion and inversion of the foot.

Integrated Function
- Eccentrically decelerates dorsiflexion and eversion of the foot.
- Isometrically stabilizes the arch of the foot.

Soleus

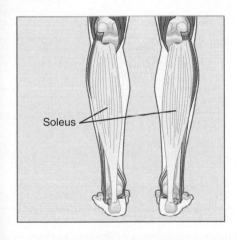

Origin
- Posterior surface of the fibular head and proximal one-third of its shaft and from the posterior side of the tibia.

Insertion
- Calcaneus via the Achilles tendon.

Isolated Function
- Concentrically accelerates plantarflexion.

Integrated Function
- Decelerates ankle dorsiflexion.
- Isometrically stabilizes the foot and ankle complex.

Gastrocnemius

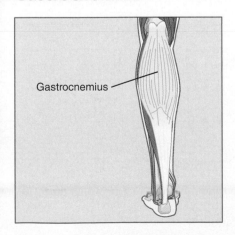

Origin
- Posterior aspect of the lateral and medial femoral condyles.

Insertion
- Calcaneus via the Achilles tendon.

Isolated Function
- Concentrically accelerates plantarflexion.

Integrated Function
- Decelerates ankle dorsiflexion.
- Isometrically stabilizes the foot and ankle complex.

Peroneus Longus

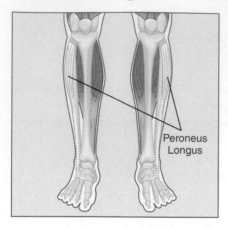

Origin
- Lateral condyle of tibia, head, and proximal two-thirds of the lateral surface of the fibula.

Insertion
- Lateral surface of the medial cuneiform and lateral side of the base of the first metatarsal.

Isolated Function
- Concentrically plantarflexes and everts the foot.

Integrated Function
- Decelerates ankle dorsiflexion.
- Isometrically stabilizes the foot and ankle complex.

Hamstring Complex

Biceps Femoris: Long Head

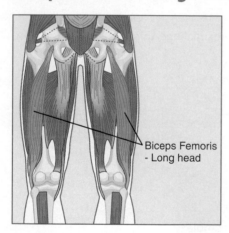

Origin
- Ischial tuberosity of the pelvis, part of the sacrotuberous ligament.

Insertion
- Head of the fibula.

Isolated Function
- Concentrically accelerates knee flexion and hip extension.
- Tibial external rotation.

Integrated Function
- Eccentrically decelerates knee extension.
- Eccentrically decelerates hip flexion.
- Eccentrically decelerates tibial internal rotation at midstance of the gait cycle.
- Isometrically stabilizes the lumbo-pelvic-hip complex (LPHC) and knee.

Biceps Femoris: Short Head

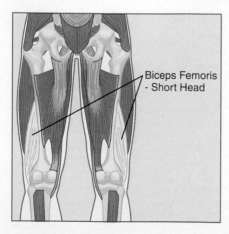

Origin
- Lower one-third of the posterior aspect of the femur.

Insertion
- Head of the fibula.

Isolated Function
- Concentrically accelerates knee flexion and tibial external rotation.

Integrated Function
- Eccentrically decelerates knee extension.
- Eccentrically decelerates tibial internal rotation.
- Isometrically stabilizes the knee.

Semimembranosus

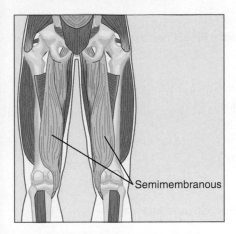

Origin
◆ Ischial tuberosity of the pelvis.

Insertion
◆ Posterior aspect of the medial tibial condyle of the tibia.

Isolated Function
◆ Concentrically accelerates knee flexion, hip extension, and tibial internal rotation.

Integrated Function
◆ Eccentrically decelerates knee extension.
◆ Eccentrically decelerates hip flexion.
◆ Eccentrically decelerates tibial external rotation.
◆ Isometrically stabilizes the LPHC and knee.

Semitendinosus

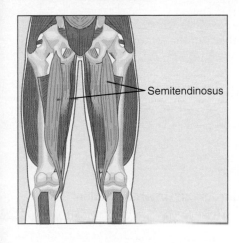

Origin
◆ Ischial tuberosity of the pelvis and part of the sacrotuberous ligament.

Insertion
◆ Proximal aspect of the medial tibial condyle of the tibia (pes anserine).

Isolated Function
◆ Concentrically accelerates knee flexion, hip extension, and tibial internal rotation.

Integrated Function
◆ Eccentrically decelerates knee extension.
◆ Eccentrically decelerates hip flexion.
◆ Eccentrically decelerates tibial external rotation.
◆ Isometrically stabilizes the LPHC and knee.

Quadriceps

Vastus Lateralis

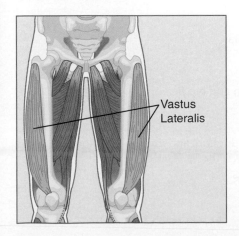

Origin
◆ Anterior and inferior border of the greater trochanter, lateral region of the gluteal tuberosity, lateral lip of the linea aspera of the femur.

Insertion
◆ Base of patella and tibial tuberosity of the tibia.

Isolated Function
◆ Concentrically accelerates knee extension.

Integrated Function
◆ Eccentrically decelerates knee flexion, adduction, and internal rotation.
◆ Isometrically stabilizes the knee.

Vastus Medialis

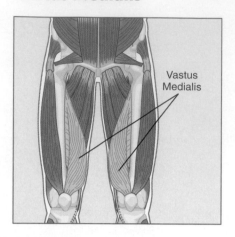

Origin
- Lower region of intertrochanteric line, medial lip of linea aspera, proximal medial supracondylar line of the femur.

Insertion
- Base of patella, tibial tuberosity of the tibia.

Isolated Function
- Concentrically accelerates knee extension.

Integrated Function
- Eccentrically decelerates knee flexion, adduction, and internal rotation.
- Isometrically stabilizes the knee.

Vastus Intermedius

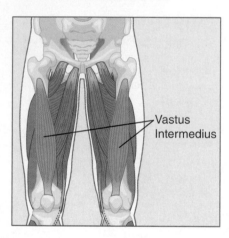

Origin
- Anterior-lateral regions of the upper two-thirds of the femur.

Insertion
- Base of patella, tibial tuberosity of the tibia.

Isolated Function
- Concentrically accelerates knee extension.

Integrated Function
- Eccentrically decelerates knee flexion, adduction, and internal rotation.
- Isometrically stabilizes the knee.

Rectus Femoris

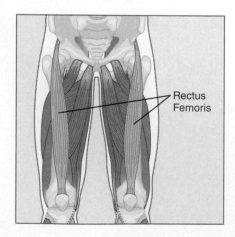

Origin
- Anterior-inferior iliac spine of the pelvis.

Insertion
- Base of patella, tibial tuberosity of the tibia.

Isolated Function
- Concentrically accelerates knee extension and hip flexion.

Integrated Function
- Eccentrically decelerates knee flexion, adduction, and internal rotation.
- Decelerates hip extension.
- Isometrically stabilizes the LPHC and knee.

Hip Musculature

Adductor Longus

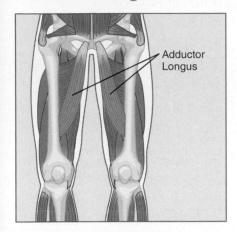

Origin
- Anterior surface of the inferior pubic ramus of the pelvis.

Insertion
- Proximal one-third of the linea aspera of the femur.

Isolated Function
- Concentrically accelerates hip adduction, flexion, and internal rotation.

Integrated Function
- Eccentrically decelerates hip abduction, extension, and external rotation.
- Isometrically stabilizes the LPHC.

Adductor Magnus: Anterior Fibers

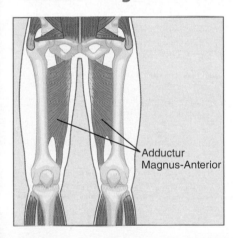

Origin
- Ischial ramus of the pelvis.

Insertion
- Linea aspera of the femur.

Isolated Function
- Concentrically accelerates hip adduction, flexion, and internal rotation.

Integrated Function
- Eccentrically decelerates hip abduction, extension, and external rotation.
- Dynamically stabilizes the LPHC.

Adductor Magnus: Posterior Fibers

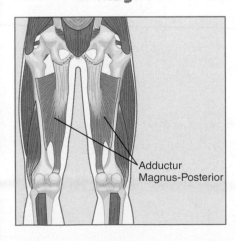

Origin
- Ischial tuberosity of the pelvis.

Insertion
- Adductor tubercle on femur.

Isolated Function
- Concentrically accelerates hip adduction, extension, and external rotation.

Integrated Function
- Eccentrically decelerates hip abduction, flexion, and internal rotation.
- Isometrically stabilizes the LPHC.

Adductor Brevis

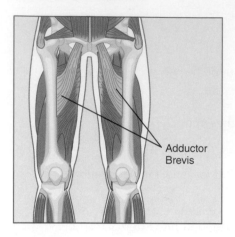

Origin

- Anterior surface of the inferior pubic ramus of the pelvis.

Insertion

- Proximal one-third of the linea aspera of the femur.

Isolated Function

- Concentrically accelerates hip adduction, flexion, and internal rotation.

Integrated Function

- Eccentrically decelerates hip abduction, extension, and external rotation.
- Isometrically stabilizes the LPHC.

Gracilis

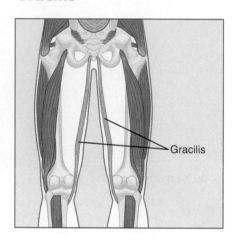

Origin

- Anterior aspect of lower body of pubis.

Insertion

- Proximal medial surface of the tibia (pes anserine).

Isolated Function

- Concentrically accelerates hip adduction, flexion, and internal rotation.
- Assists in tibial internal rotation.

Integrated Function

- Eccentrically decelerates hip abduction, extension, and external rotation.
- Isometrically stabilizes the LPHC and knee.

Pectineus

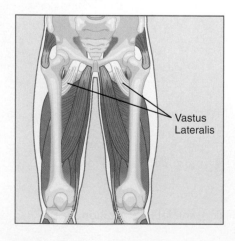

Origin

- Pectineal line on the superior pubic ramus of the pelvis.

Insertion

- Pectineal line on the posterior surface of the upper femur.

Isolated Function

- Concentrically accelerates hip adduction, flexion, and internal rotation.

Integrated Function

- Eccentrically decelerates hip abduction, extension, and external rotation.
- Isometrically stabilizes the LPHC.

Gluteus Medius

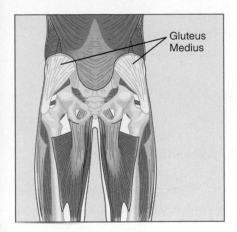

Origin
- Outer surface of the ilium of the pelvis.

Insertion
- Lateral surface of the greater trochanter on the femur.

Isolated Function
- Concentrically accelerates hip abduction and internal rotation (anterior fibers).
- Concentrically accelerates hip abduction and external rotation (posterior fibers).

Integrated Function
- Eccentrically decelerates hip adduction and external rotation (anterior fibers).
- Eccentrically decelerates hip adduction and internal rotation (posterior fibers).
- Isometrically stabilizes the LPHC.

Gluteus Minimus

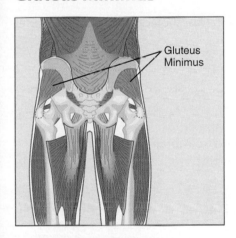

Origin
- Ilium of the pelvis between the anterior and inferior gluteal line.

Insertion
- Greater trochanter of the femur.

Isolated Function
- Concentrically accelerates hip abduction and internal rotation.

Integrated Function
- Eccentrically decelerates hip adduction and external rotation.
- Isometrically stabilizes the LPHC.

Gluteus Maximus

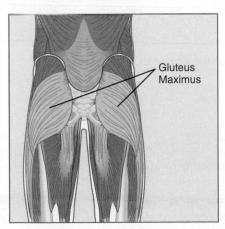

Origin
- Outer ilium of the pelvis, posterior side of sacrum and coccyx, and part of the sacrotuberous and posterior sacroiliac ligament.

Insertion
- Gluteal tuberosity of the femur and iliotibial tract.

Isolated Function
- Concentrically accelerates hip extension and external rotation.

Integrated Function
- Eccentrically decelerates hip flexion and internal rotation.
- Decelerates tibial internal rotation via the iliotibial band.
- Isometrically stabilizes the LPHC.

Tensor Fascia Latae (Including the Iliotibial Band)

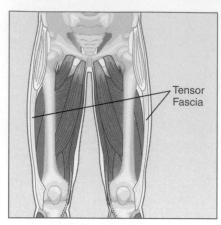

Origin
- Outer surface of the iliac crest just posterior to the anterior-superior iliac spine of the pelvis.

Insertion
- Proximal one-third of the iliotibial band.

Isolated Function
- Concentrically accelerates hip flexion, abduction, and internal rotation.

Integrated Function
- Eccentrically decelerates hip extension, adduction, and external rotation.
- Isometrically stabilizes the LPHC.

Psoas

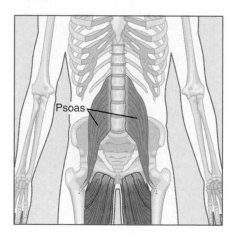

Origin
- Transverse processes and lateral bodies of the last thoracic and all lumbar vertebrae including intervetebral disks.

Insertion
- Lesser trochanter of the femur.

Isolated Function
- Concentrically accelerates hip flexion and external rotation.
- Concentrically extends and rotates lumbar spine.

Integrated Function
- Eccentrically decelerates hip internal rotation.
- Eccentrically decelerates hip extension.
- Isometrically stabilizes the LPHC.

Iliacus

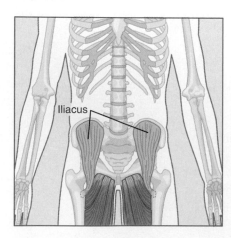

Origin
- Superior two-thirds of iliac fossa, inner lip of the iliac crest.

Insertion
- Lesser trochanter of femur.

Isolated Function
- Concentrically accelerates hip flexion and external rotation.

Integrated Function
- Eccentrically decelerates hip extension and internal rotation.
- Isometrically stabilizes the LPHC.

Sartorius

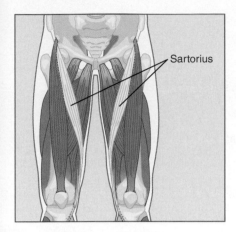

Origin
- Anterior-superior iliac spine of the pelvis.

Insertion
- Proximal medial surface of the tibia.

Isolated Function
- Concentrically accelerates hip flexion, external rotation, and abduction.
- Concentrically accelerates knee flexion and internal rotation.

Integrated Function
- Eccentrically decelerates hip extension and internal rotation.
- Eccentrically decelerates knee extension and external rotation.
- Isometrically stabilizes the LPHC and knee.

Piriformis

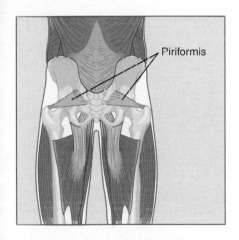

Origin
- Anterior side of the sacrum.

Insertion
- The greater trochanter of the femur.

Isolated Function
- Concentrically accelerates hip external rotation, abduction, and extension.

Integrated Function
- Eccentrically decelerates hip internal rotation, adduction, and flexion.
- Isometrically stabilizes the hip and sacroiliac joints.

Abdominal Musculature

Rectus Abdominis

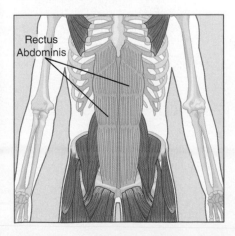

Origin
- Pubic symphysis of the pelvis.

Insertion
- Ribs 5–7.
- Xiphoid process of the sternum.

Isolated Function
- Concentrically accelerates spinal flexion, lateral flexion, and rotation.

Integrated Function
- Eccentrically decelerates spinal extension, lateral flexion, and rotation.
- Isometrically stabilizes the LPHC.

External Oblique

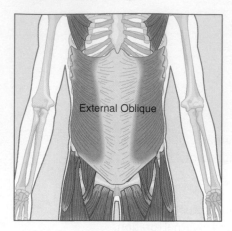

Origin
- External surface of ribs 4–12.

Insertion
- Anterior iliac crest of the pelvis, linea alba, and contralateral rectus sheaths.

Isolated Function
- Concentrically accelerates spinal flexion, lateral flexion, and contralateral rotation.

Integrated Function
- Eccentrically decelerates spinal extension, lateral flexion, and rotation.
- Isometrically stabilizes the LPHC.

Internal Oblique

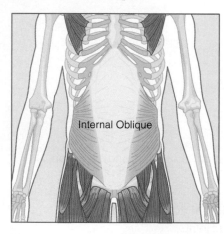

Origin
- Anterior two-thirds of the iliac crest of the pelvis and thoracolumbar fascia.

Insertion
- Ribs 9–12, linea alba, and contralateral rectus sheaths.

Isolated Function
- Concentrically accelerates spinal flexion, lateral flexion, and ipsilateral rotation.

Integrated Function
- Eccentrically decelerates spinal extension, rotation, and lateral flexion.
- Isometrically stabilizes the LPHC.

Transverse Abdominis

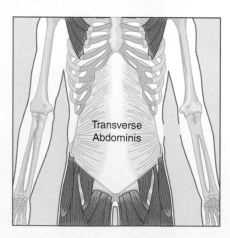

Origin
- Ribs 7–12, anterior two-thirds of the iliac crest of the pelvis, and thoracolumbar fascia.

Insertion
- Lineae alba and contralateral rectus sheaths.

Isolated Function
- Increases intra-abdominal pressure.
- Supports the abdominal viscera.

Integrated Function
- Isometrically stabilizes the LPHC.

Diaphragm

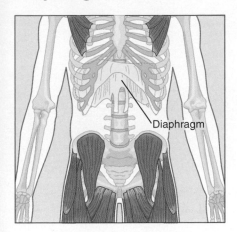

Origin
- ◆ Costal part: Inner surfaces of the cartilages and adjacent bony regions of ribs 6–12.
- ◆ Sternal part: Posterior side of the xiphoid process.
- ◆ Crural (lumbar) part: (1) Two aponeurotic arches covering the external surfaces of the quadratus lumborum and psoas major; (2) right and left crus, originating from the bodies of L1–L3 and their intervertebral disks.

Insertion
- ◆ Central tendon.

Isolated Function
- ◆ Concentrically pulls the central tendon inferiorly, increasing the volume in the thoracic cavity.

Integrated Function
- ◆ Stabilizes the LPHC.

Back Musculature

Superficial Erector Spinae: Iliocostalis, Longissimus, and Spinalis

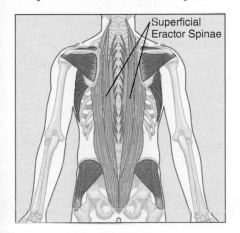

Division in the Group
- ◆ Lumborum (lumbar).
- ◆ Thoracis (thoracic).
- ◆ Cervicis (cervical).

Common Origin
- ◆ Iliac crest of the pelvis.
- ◆ Sacrum.
- ◆ Spinous and transverse process of T11–L5.

Insertion
Iliocostalis
- ◆ Lumborum: Inferior border of ribs 7–12.
- ◆ Thoracis: Superior border of ribs 1–6.
- ◆ Cervicis: Transverse process of C4–C6.

Longissimus
- ◆ Thoracis: Transverse process T1–T12; ribs 2–12.
- ◆ Cervicis: Transverse process of C6–C2.
- ◆ Capitis: Mastoid process of the skull.

Spinalis
- ◆ Thoracis: Spinous process of T7–T4.
- ◆ Cervicis: Spinous process of C3–C2.
- ◆ Capitis: Between the superior and inferior nuchal lines on occipital bone of the skull.

Isolated Function
- ◆ Concentrically accelerates spinal extension, rotation, and lateral flexion.

Integrated Function
- ◆ Eccentrically decelerates spinal flexion, rotation, and lateral flexion.
- ◆ Dynamically stabilizes the spine during functional movements.

Quadratus Lumborum

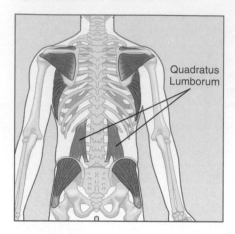

Origin
- Iliac crest of the pelvis.

Insertion
- 12th rib.
- Transverse process L2–L5.

Isolated Function
- Spinal lateral flexion.

Integrated Function
- Eccentrically decelerates contralateral lateral spinal flexion.
- Isometrically stabilizes the LPHC.

Multifidus

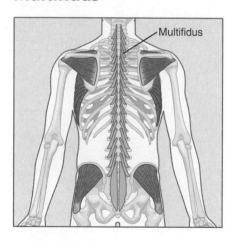

Origin
- Posterior aspect of the sacrum.
- Processes of the lumbar, thoracic, and cervical spine.

Insertion
- Spinous processes one to four segments above the origin.

Isolated Function
- Concentrically accelerates spinal extension and contralateral rotation.

Integrated Function
- Eccentrically decelerates spinal flexion and rotation.
- Isometrically stabilizes the spine.

Latissimus Dorsi

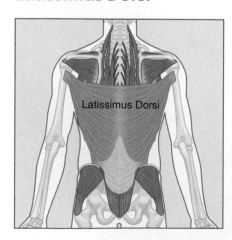

Origin
- Spinous processes of T7–T12.
- Iliac crest of the pelvis.
- Thoracolumbar fascia.
- Ribs 9–12.

Insertion
- Inferior angle of the scapula.
- Intertubercular groove of the humerus.

Isolated Function
- Concentrically accelerates shoulder extension, adduction, and internal rotation.

Integrated Function
- Eccentrically decelerates shoulder flexion, abduction, and external rotation.
- Eccentrically decelerates spinal flexion.
- Isometrically stabilizes the LPHC and shoulder.

Shoulder Musculature

Serratus Anterior

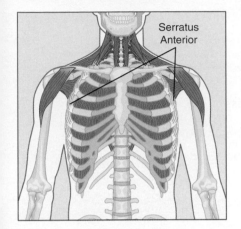

Origin
◆ Ribs 4–12.

Insertion
◆ Medial border of the scapula.

Isolated Function
◆ Concentrically accelerates scapular protraction.

Integrated Function
◆ Eccentrically decelerates dynamic scapular retraction.
◆ Isometrically stabilizes the scapula.

Rhomboid Major

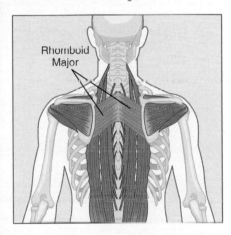

Origin
◆ Spinous processes C7–T5.

Insertion
◆ Medial border of the scapula.

Isolated Function
◆ Concentrically produces scapular retraction and downward rotation.

Integrated Function
◆ Eccentrically decelerates scapular protraction and upward rotation.
◆ Isometrically stabilizes the scapula.

Rhomboid Minor

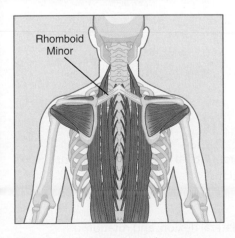

Origin
◆ Spinous processes C7–T1.

Insertion
◆ Medial border of the scapula superior to spine.

Isolated Function
◆ Concentrically produces scapular retraction and downward rotation.

Integrated Function
◆ Eccentrically decelerates scapular protraction and upward rotation.
◆ Isometrically stabilizes the scapula.

Lower Trapezius

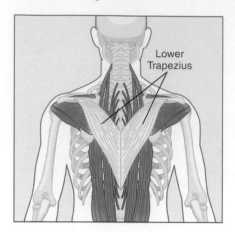

Origin

- Spinous processes of T6–T12.

Insertion

- Spine of the scapula.

Isolated Function

- Concentrically accelerates scapular depression.

Integrated Function

- Eccentrically decelerates scapular elevation.
- Isometrically stabilizes the scapula.

Middle Trapezius

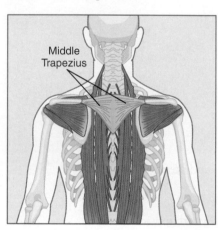

Origin

- Spinous processes of T1–T5.

Insertion

- Acromion process of the scapula.
- Superior aspect of the spine of the scapula.

Isolated Function

- Concentrically accelerates scapular retraction.

Integrated Function

- Eccentrically decelerates scapular elevation.
- Isometrically stabilizes the scapula.

Upper Trapezius

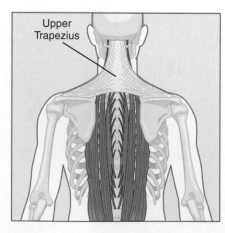

Origin

- External occipital protuberance of the skull.
- Spinous process of C7.

Insertion

- Lateral third of the clavicle.
- Acromion process of the scapula.

Isolated Function

- Concentrically accelerates cervical extension, lateral flexion, and rotation.
- Concentrically accelerates scapular elevation.

Integrated Function

- Eccentrically decelerates cervical flexion, lateral flexion, and rotation.
- Eccentrically decelerates scapular depression.
- Isometrically stabilizes the cervical spine and scapula.

Pectoralis Major

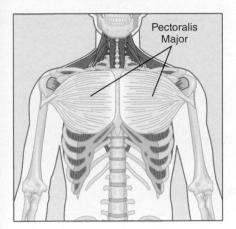

Origin
- ◆ Clavicular: Anterior surface of the clavicle.
- ◆ Sternocostal: Anterior surface of the sternum, cartilage of ribs 1–7.

Insertion
- ◆ Greater tubercle of the humerus.

Isolated Function
- ◆ Concentrically accelerates shoulder flexion (clavicular fibers), horizontal adduction, and internal rotation.

Integrated Function
- ◆ Eccentrically decelerates shoulder extension, horizontal abduction, and external rotation.
- ◆ Isometrically stabilizes the shoulder girdle.

Pectoralis Minor

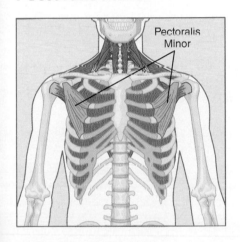

Origin
- ◆ Ribs 3–5.

Insertion
- ◆ Coracoid process of the scapula.

Isolated Function
- ◆ Concentrically protracts the scapula.

Integrated Function
- ◆ Eccentrically decelerates scapular retraction.
- ◆ Isometrically stabilizes the shoulder girdle.

Anterior Deltoid

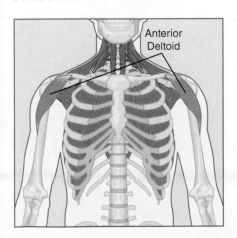

Origin
- ◆ Lateral third of the clavicle.

Insertion
- ◆ Deltoid tuberosity of the humerus.

Isolated Function
- ◆ Concentrically accelerates shoulder flexion and internal rotation.

Integrated Function
- ◆ Eccentrically decelerates shoulder extension and external rotation.
- ◆ Isometrically stabilizes the shoulder girdle.

Medial Deltoid

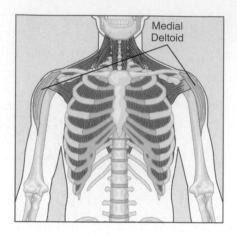

Origin
◆ Acromion process of the scapula.

Insertion
◆ Deltoid tuberosity of the humerus.

Isolated Function
◆ Concentrically accelerates shoulder abduction.

Integrated Function
◆ Eccentrically decelerates shoulder adduction.
◆ Isometrically stabilizes the shoulder girdle.

Posterior Deltoid

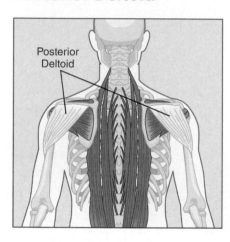

Origin
◆ Spine of the scapula.

Insertion
◆ Deltoid tuberosity of the humerus.

Isolated Function
◆ Concentrically accelerates shoulder extension and external rotation.

Integrated Function
◆ Eccentrically decelerates shoulder flexion and internal rotation.
◆ Isometrically stabilizes the shoulder girdle.

Teres Major

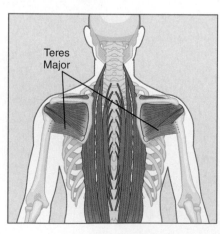

Origin
◆ Inferior angle of the scapula.

Insertion
◆ Lesser tubercle of the humerus.

Isolated Function
◆ Concentrically accelerates shoulder internal rotation, adduction, and extension.

Integrated Function
◆ Eccentrically decelerates shoulder external rotation, abduction, and flexion.
◆ Isometrically stabilizes the shoulder girdle.

Rotator Cuff

Teres Minor

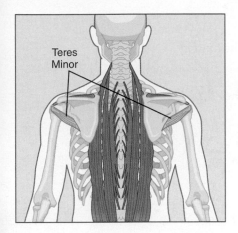

Origin
◆ Lateral border of the scapula.

Insertion
◆ Greater tubercle of the humerus.

Isolated Function
◆ Concentrically accelerates shoulder external rotation.

Integrated Function
◆ Eccentrically decelerates shoulder internal rotation.
◆ Isometrically stabilizes the shoulder girdle.

Infraspinatus

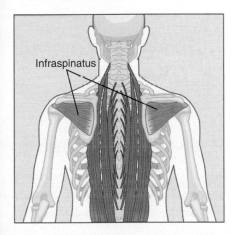

Origin
◆ Infraspinous fossa of the scapula.

Insertion
◆ Middle facet of the greater tubercle of the humerus.

Isolated Function
◆ Concentrically accelerates shoulder external rotation.

Integrated Function
◆ Eccentrically decelerates shoulder internal rotation.
◆ Isometrically stabilizes the shoulder girdle.

Subscapularis

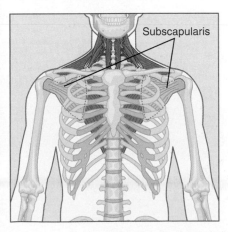

Origin
◆ Subscapular fossa of the scapula.

Insertion
◆ Lesser tubercle of the humerus.

Isolated Function
◆ Concentrically accelerates shoulder internal rotation.

Integrated Function
◆ Eccentrically decelerates shoulder external rotation.
◆ Isometrically stabilizes the shoulder girdle.

Supraspinatus

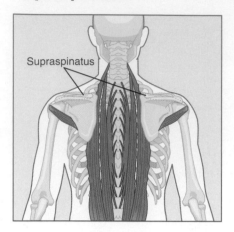

Origin
- Supraspinous fossa of the scapula.

Insertion
- Superior facet of the greater tubercle of the humerus.

Isolated Function
- Concentrically accelerates abduction of the arm.

Integrated Function
- Eccentrically decelerates adduction of the arm.
- Isometrically stabilizes the shoulder girdle.

Arm Musculature

Biceps Brachii

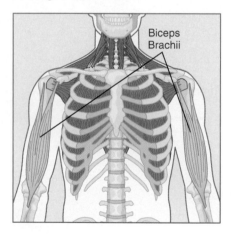

Origin
- Short head: Coracoid process of the scapula.
- Long head: Tubercle above glenoid cavity on the humerus.

Insertion
- Radial tuberosity of the radius.

Isolated Function
- Concentrically accelerates elbow flexion, supination of the radioulnar joint, and shoulder flexion.

Integrated Function
- Eccentrically decelerates elbow extension, pronation of the radioulnar joint, and shoulder extension.
- Isometrically stabilizes the elbow and shoulder girdle.

Triceps Brachii

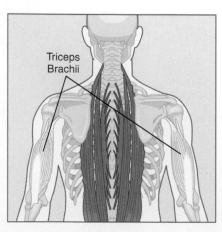

Origin
- Long head: Infraglenoid tubercle of the scapula.
- Short head: Posterior humerus.
- Medial head: Posterior humerus.

Insertion
- Olecranon process of the ulna.

Isolated Function
- Concentrically accelerates elbow extension and shoulder extension.

Integrated Function
- Eccentrically decelerates elbow flexion and shoulder flexion.
- Isometrically stabilizes the elbow and shoulder girdle.

Brachioradialis

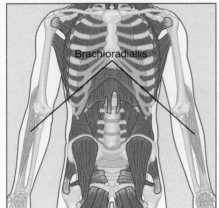

Origin
◆ Lateral supracondylar ridge of the humerus.

Insertion
◆ Lateral surface of distal radius, immediately above styloid process.

Isolated Function
◆ Concentrically accelerates elbow flexion.

Integrated Function
◆ Eccentrically decelerates elbow extension.
◆ Isometrically stabilizes the elbow.

Brachialis

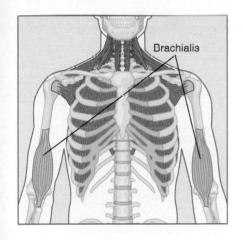

Origin
◆ Lower half of the anterior surface of the humerus.

Insertion
◆ Tuberosity and coronoid process of the ulna.

Isolated Function
◆ Concentrically accelerates elbow flexion.

Integrated Function
◆ Eccentrically decelerates elbow extension.
◆ Isometrically stabilizes the elbow.

Neck Musculature

Levator Scapulae

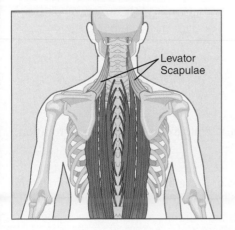

Origin
◆ Transverse processes of C1–C4.

Insertion
◆ Superior vertebral border of the scapulae.

Isolated Function
◆ Concentrically accelerates cervical extension, lateral flexion, and ipsilateral rotation when the scapulae is anchored.
◆ Assists in elevation and downward rotation of the scapulae.

Integrated Function
◆ Eccentrically decelerates cervical flexion and contralateral cervical rotation and lateral flexion.
◆ Eccentrically decelerates scapular depression and upward rotation when the neck is stabilized.
◆ Stabilizes the cervical spine and scapulae.

Sternocleidomastoid

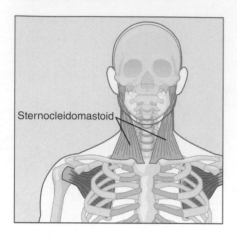

Origin
- Sternal head: Top of manubrium of the sternum.
- Clavicular head: Medial one-third of the clavicle.

Insertion
- Mastoid process, lateral superior nuchal line of the occiput of the skull.

Isolated Function
- Concentrically accelerates cervical flexion, rotation, and lateral flexion.

Integrated Function
- Eccentrically decelerates cervical extension, rotation, and lateral flexion.
- Isometrically stabilizes the cervical spine and acromioclavicular joint.

Scalenes

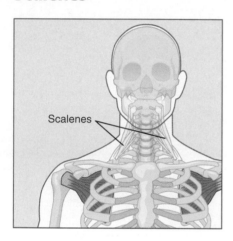

Origin
- Transverse processes of C3–C7.

Insertion
- First and second ribs.

Isolated Function
- Concentrically accelerates cervical flexion, rotation, and lateral flexion.
- Assists rib elevation during inhalation.

Integrated Function
- Eccentrically decelerates cervical extension, rotation, and lateral flexion.
- Isometrically stabilizes the cervical spine.

Longus Coli

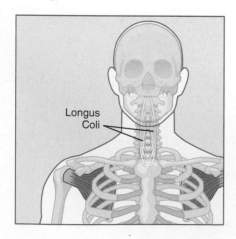

Origin
- Anterior portion of T1–T3.

Insertion
- Anterior and lateral C1.

Isolated Function
- Concentrically accelerates cervical flexion, lateral flexion, and ipsilateral rotation.

Integrated Function
- Eccentrically decelerates cervical extension, lateral flexion, and contralateral rotation.
- Isometrically stabilizes the cervical spine.

Longus Capitis

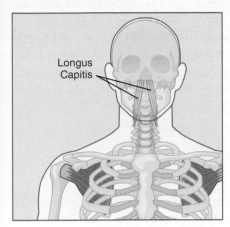

Origin

◆ Transverse processes of C3–C6.

Insertion

◆ Inferior occipital bone.

Isolated Function

◆ Concentrically accelerates cervical flexion and lateral flexion.

Integrated Function

◆ Eccentrically decelerates cervical extension.
◆ Isometrically stabilizes the cervical spine.

The Skeletal System

Bone Growth

Throughout life, bone is constantly renewed through a process called remodeling. This process consists of resorption and formation. During resorption, old bone tissue is broken down and removed by special cells called osteoclasts. During bone formation, new bone tissue is laid down to replace the old. This task is performed by special cells called osteoblasts.

During childhood and through adolescence, new bone is added to the skeleton faster than old bone is removed. As a result, bones become larger, heavier, and denser. For most people,

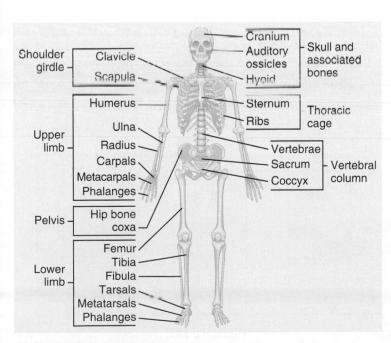

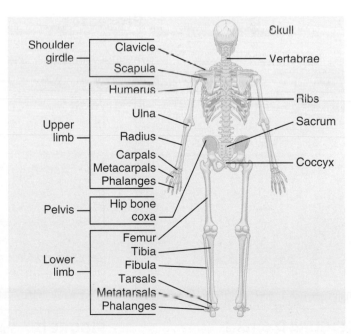

FIGURE D.5 The skeletal system.

bone formation continues at a faster pace than removal until bone mass peaks, usually by the time individuals reach their 30s (National Institute of Arthritis and Musculoskeletal and Skin Diseases, 2015).

It is also worth noting that remodeling tends to follow the lines of stress placed on the bone (Watkins, 1999). Exercise and habitual posture, therefore, have a fundamental influence on the health of the skeletal system. Incorrect exercise technique, coupled with a generally poor alignment, will lead to a remodeling process that may reinforce the predominating bad posture.

Bone Markings

The majority of all bones have specific distinguishing structures known as surface markings. These structures are necessary for joint stability as well as for providing attachment sites for muscles. Some of the more prominent and important ones will be discussed here. These surface markings can be divided into two simple categories: depressions and processes (Tortora, 2001).

Depressions

Depressions are simply flattened or indented portions of the bone. A fossa is a common type of depression. An example is the supraspinous or infraspinous fossa located on the scapulae (**Figure D.6**). These are attachment sites for the supraspinatus and infraspinatus muscles, respectively (Tortora, 2001).

A sulcus is another type of depression. A sulcus is simply a groove in a bone that allows soft tissue (i.e., tendons) to pass through. An example is the intertubercular sulcus located between the greater and lesser tubercles of the humerus (**Figure D.7**). This is commonly known as the groove for the biceps tendon (Tortora, 2001).

Processes

Processes are projections that protrude from the bone to which muscles, tendons, and ligaments can attach (**Figure D.8**). Processes include condyles, epicondyles, tubercles, and

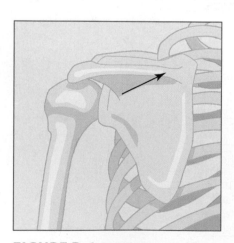

FIGURE D.6 Fossa.

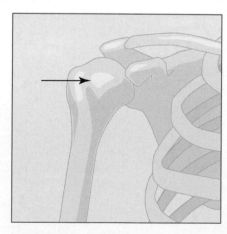

FIGURE D.7 Sulcus.

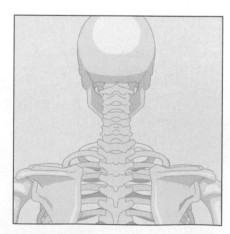

FIGURE D.8 Process.

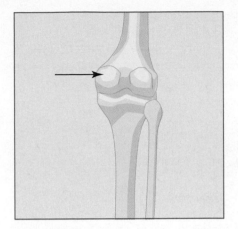

FIGURE D.9 Condyle.

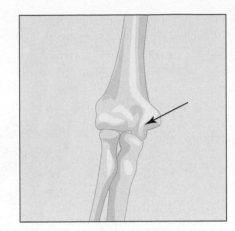

FIGURE D.10 Epicondyle.

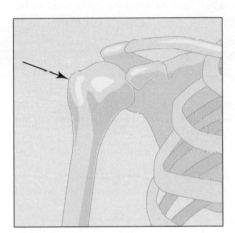

FIGURE D.11 Tubercle.

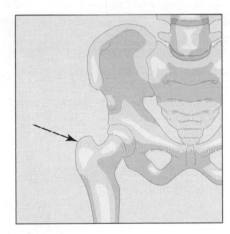

FIGURE D.12 Trochanter.

trochanters. Examples of processes include the spinous processes found on the vertebrae and the acromion and coracoid processes found on the scapulae (Tortora, 2001).

Condyles are located on the inner and outer portions at the bottom of the femur and top of the tibia to form the knee joint (**Figure D.9**). Epicondyles are located on the inner and outer portions of the humerus to help form the elbow joint (**Figure D.10**).

The tubercles are located at the top of the humerus at the glenohumeral joint (**Figure D.11**). There are the greater and lesser tubercles, which are attachment sites for shoulder musculature.

Finally, the trochanters are located at the top of the femur and are attachment sites for the hip musculature (**Figure D.12**). The greater trochanter is commonly called the hipbone (Tortora, 2001).

Vertebral Column

The first seven vertebrae starting at the top of the spinal column (**Figure D.13**) are called the cervical vertebrae (cervical spine, C1–C7). These bones form a flexible framework and provide support and motion for the head.

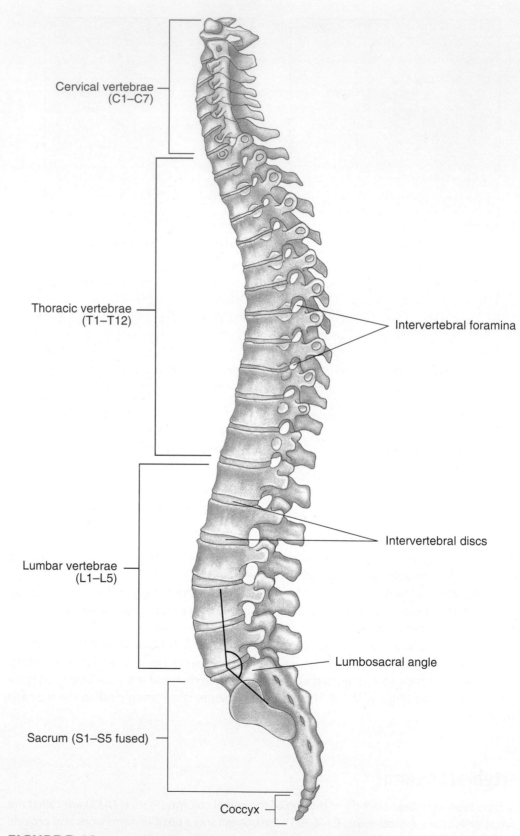

Cervical vertebrae
(C1–C7)

Thoracic vertebrae
(T1–T12)

Intervertebral foramina

Intervertebral discs

Lumbar vertebrae
(L1–L5)

Lumbosacral angle

Sacrum (S1–S5 fused)

Coccyx

FIGURE D.13 The vertebral column.

The next 12 vertebrae located in the upper and middle back are called the thoracic vertebrae (thoracic spine, T1–T12). These bones articulate with the ribs to form the rear anchor of the rib cage. Thoracic vertebrae are larger than cervical vertebrae and increase in size from top to bottom.

Below the thoracic spine are the five vertebrae comprising the lumbar vertebrae (lumbar spine, L1–L5). These bones are the largest in the spinal column. These vertebrae support most of the body's weight and are attached to many of the back muscles. The lumbar spine is often a location of pain for individuals because these vertebrae carry the most amount of body weight and are subject to the largest forces and stresses along the spine.

The sacrum is a triangular bone located just below the lumbar vertebrae. It consists of four or five sacral vertebrae in a child, which become fused into a single bone during adulthood.

The bottom of the spinal column is called the coccyx or tailbone. It consists of three to five bones that are fused together in an adult. Many muscles connect to the coccyx.

In between the vertebrae are intervertebral discs made of fibrous cartilage that act as shock absorbers and allow the spine to move. In addition to allowing humans to stand upright and maintain their balance, the vertebral column serves several other important functions. It helps to support the head and arms, while permitting freedom of movement. It also provides attachment for many muscles, the ribs, and some of the organs and protects the spinal cord, which controls most bodily functions (National Institute of Neurological Disorders and Stroke, 2010).

The optimal arrangement of curves is referred to as a neutral spine and represents a position in which the vertebrae and associated structures are under the least amount of load. The adult human spine has three major curvatures:

- ◆ *Posterior cervical curvature*: The posterior concavity of the cervical spine.
- ◆ *Anterior thoracic curvature*: The posterior convexity of the thoracic spine.
- ◆ *Posterior lumbar curvature*: The posterior concavity of the lumbar spine.

References

Cohen, H. (1999). *Neuroscience for rehabilitation* (2nd ed.). Philadelphia, PA: Lippincott Williams & Wilkins.

Fox, S. I. (2006). *Human physiology* (9th ed.). New York, NY: McGraw-Hill.

Milner-Brown, A. (2001). *Neuromuscular physiology.* Thousand Oaks, CA: National Academy of Sports Medicine.

National Institute of Arthritis and Musculoskeletal and Skin Diseases. (2015). What is bone? Accessed April 1, 2016. Available at: www.niams.nih.gov/Health_Info/bone/Bone_Health/default.asp

National Institute of Neurological Disorders and Stroke. (2014). Low back pain fact sheet. Accessed April 1, 2016. Available at: www.ninds.nih.gov/disorders/backpain/detail_backpain.htm#102183102

Tortora, G. J. (2001). *Principles of human anatomy* (9th ed.). New York, NY: John Wiley & Sons.

Vander, A., Sherman, L., & Luciano, D. (2001). *Human physiology: The mechanisms of body function* (8th ed.). New York, NY: McGraw-Hill.

Watkins, J. (1999). *Structure and function of the musculoskeletal system*. Champaign, IL: Human Kinetics.

Glossary

A

Abduction   A body segment is moving away from the midline of the body.

Abductors   A muscle that produces abduction of a limb or joint.

Acceleration   The speed of an object.

Acceptable Macronutrient Distribution Range (AMDR)   Recommendations for intake of carbohydrates, fats, and proteins.

Acetyl-CoA   An important molecule in metabolism that is formed as an intermediate in the oxidation of carbohydrates, fats, and proteins. After glucose has become pyruvate, and if there is enough oxygen available, it enters the mitochondria for aerobic metabolism and becomes acetyl-CoA.

Acidosis   The accumulation of excessive hydrogen ions in the body, causing increased acidity of the blood and muscle.

Action Stage   The stage of change in the TTM where individuals have made specific, overt modifications in their lifestyle within the past 6 months.

Active Force   Muscle tension that is generated by its contractile elements.

Active Listening   A listening technique that requires the listener to provide feedback to the speaker by restating what the listener heard in his or her own words.

Active-Isolated Stretching   Flexibility exercises in which agonists move a limb through a full range of motion, allowing the antagonists to stretch.

Acute Variables   The components that specify how each exercise is to be performed.

Adaptation Phase   The second stage of the GAS in which physiological changes take place in order to meet the demands of the newly imposed stress.

Adduction   A body segment is moving toward the midline of the body.

Adductors   A muscle that produces adduction of a limb or joint.

Adenosine Triphosphate (ATP)   Energy storage and transfer unit within the cells of the body.

Adequate Intake (AI)   Estimated amount of a nutrient per day consumed by people assumed to be maintaining adequate nutrition.

Adipose Tissue   One of the main types of connective tissue where fat is stored.

Aerobic Metabolism   Chemical reactions in the body that require the presence of oxygen to extract energy from carbohydrates, fatty acids, and amino acids.

Affective Influence   Influence resulting from emotions.

Afferent Neurons   Nerve impulses that move toward the spinal cord and brain from the periphery of the body and are sensory in nature.

Agility   The ability to maintain center of gravity over a changing base of support while changing direction at various speeds.

Agonists   Muscles that works as the prime mover of a joint exercise.

Alarm Phase   The first stage of the GAS; the initial phase of response to a new stimuli within the Human Movement System.

Altered Arthrokinematics   Altered joint motion caused by altered length–tension relationships and force-couple relationships that affects the joints and causes poor movement efficiency.

Altered Neuromuscular Efficiency   Occurs when the kinetic chain is not performing optimally to control the body in all three planes of motion.

Altered Reciprocal Inhibition   Process by which a short muscle, a tight muscle, and/or myofascial adhesions in the muscle cause decreased neural drive of its functional antagonist.

Amino Acid Pool   A mixture of amino acids available in the cell derived from dietary sources or the degradation of protein.

Amino Acids   The building blocks of proteins; composed of a central carbon atom, a hydrogen atom, an amino group, a carboxyl group, and an R-group.

Amortization Phase   The second phase of the integrated performance paradigm requiring an isometric muscle contraction.

Anabolism   A metabolic process that builds molecules.

Anaerobic Metabolism   Chemical reactions in the body that do not require the presence of oxygen to create energy through the combustion of carbohydrates.

Anaerobic Power   Maximum power (work per unit time) that is the result of all-out, high-intensity, physical output without the use of oxygen. It is a reflection of the short-term effects of the intramuscular high-energy phosphates—adenosine triphosphates (ATP) and phosphocreatine (PCr).

Anaerobic Threshold   The point during high-intensity activity when the body can no longer meet its demand for oxygen and anaerobic metabolism predominates; also called the *lactate threshold*.

Anatomic Position   Standard posture wherein the body stands upright with the arms beside the trunk, the palms face forward, and the head faces forward.

Ancillary Revenue   Revenue beyond the sale of memberships and services generated by the direct sale of products to customers.

Antagonists   Muscles that oppose the prime mover.

Anterior Cruciate Ligament (ACL)   One of the four ligaments in the knee that connects the femur to the tibia.

Anterior Oblique Subsystem (AOS)   Subsystem of the global movement system composed of the internal and external obliques, the adductor complex, and the hip external rotators. The synergistic coupling of the AOS creates stability from the trunk, through the pelvic floor, and to the hips. It contributes to rotational movements, leg swing, and stabilization. The AOS and POS work together in enabling rotational force production in the transverse plane.

Anterior-Posterior Axis   A straight line that cuts through the body from front to back.

Aponeurosis   A white tendinous sheet that attaches muscle to bone.

Appendicular Skeleton   Portion of the skeleton that includes the bones that connect to the spinal column including the upper extremities and lower extremities.

Arginine   Conditionally essential amino acid that the body can normally synthesize in sufficient amounts; however, in some disorders the body cannot make enough, and it becomes essential.

Arteries   Vessels that transport blood away from the heart.

Arthrokinematics   The motions of the joints in the body.

Association   Focus on internal body feedback (e.g., how muscles or breathing feels).

Ataxia   The loss of control of body movements.

Atom   The basic, and smallest, unit of a chemical element.

Atrioventricular (AV) Node   Small mass of specialized cardiac muscle fibers located on the wall of the right atrium of the heart that receives impulses from the sinoatrial (SA) node and directs them to the walls of the ventricles.

Atrioventricular (AV) Valves   Valves that allow for proper blood flow from the atria to the ventricles.

Autogenic Inhibition   The process by which neural impulses that sense tension are greater than the impulses that cause muscles to contract, providing an inhibitory effect to the muscle.

Autonomy-Supportive Style   A coaching style that focuses on creating an environment that emphasizes self-improvement, rather than competing against others.

Axial Skeleton   Portion of the skeletal system that consists of the bones of the skull, rib cage, and vertebral column.

Axon   A cylindrical projection from the cell body that transmits nerve impulses to other neurons or effector sites.

B

Balance   Ability to maintain the body's center of gravity within its base of support.

Barbells   Common free weight modality found in most gyms. Allows for greater amounts of resistance through the addition of plates. Useful for high-load training in exercises such as squats, deadlifts, and bench presses.

Behavior Influences   Influences that are created as a result of an individual's own behavior.

Best Practices   Professional procedures that are considered to be correct, safe, or most effective.

Beta-Oxidation   The breakdown of triglycerides into smaller subunits called free fatty acids (FFAs) to convert FFAs into acetyl-CoA molecules, which are then available to enter the Krebs cycle and ultimately lead to the production of additional ATP.

Biomechanics   The study of how forces affect a living body.

Biotensegrity   The examination of how biological structural integrity may occur.

Blood Glucose   Also referred to as "blood sugar"; the sugar that is transported in the body to supply energy to the body's cells, including fueling the brain and other cells in the body that cannot use fat as a fuel.

Blood Pressure   The pressure of circulating blood against the walls of the blood vessels after blood is ejected from the heart.

Body Composition   The relative percentage of body weight that is fat versus fat-free tissue.

Body Mass Index (BMI)   A rough assessment metric based on the concept that a person's weight should be proportional to his or her height.

Bodyweight Exercise   Form of resistance training where the source of resistance is the weight of the body.

Bone Mineral Density (BMD)   Mineral matter per square centimeter of bone. It is an indirect indicator of osteoporosis and fracture risk.

Branched-Chain Amino Acids (BCAAs)   Essential amino acids, including leucine, isoleucine, and valine, that can be used for energy directly in the muscle and do not have to go to the liver to be broken down during exercise.

C

Cable Resistance Machines   Machine that offers protection and ease of load adjustments without a fixed movement path through the use of a cable.

Calisthenics   A form of bodyweight training that uses rhythmic full-body movements.

Calorie   A scientific unit of energy.

Capillaries   The smallest blood vessels and the site of water and gas exchange between the blood and tissues.

Carbon Skeleton   The skeletal structure of an organic compound; it is the series of atoms bonded together that form the essential structure of the compound.

Carboxyl Group (–COOH)   A carbon atom joined to a hydroxyl group by a single bond and to an oxygen atom by a double bond.

Cardiac Output ($\dot{Q}$)   Heart rate multiplied by stroke volume; a measure of the overall performance of the heart.

Cardiac Rehabilitation   A specialized medical process that helps individuals suffering from various cardiac conditions to return to full function and fitness.

Cardiorespiratory System System of the body composed of the cardiovascular and respiratory systems.

Cardiovascular System System of the body composed of the heart, blood, and blood vessels.

Carotid Pulse Pulse obtained from the carotid artery of the neck.

Casein Protein commonly found in mammalian milk.

Catabolism A metabolic process that breaks down molecules.

Cell Body The portion of the neuron that contains the nucleus, lysosomes, mitochondria, and Golgi complex.

Center of Gravity (COG) The area within an object at which the weight is equally balanced in all directions. In a person, this is generally around the umbilicus, but can change depending on the posture/movement of the body.

Centers for Disease Control and Prevention (CDC) Federal agency that conducts and supports activities related to public health.

Central Nervous System (CNS) The division of the nervous system comprising the brain and the spinal cord. Its primary function is to coordinate activity of all parts of the body.

Chemical Energy Energy contained in a molecule that has not yet been released in carbohydrates, fats, and proteins.

Chronic Contemplation Individuals who constantly weigh the pros and cons of changing a particular behavior (e.g., exercising).

Chronic Disease A persistent disease lasting 3 months or longer.

Circuit Training A series of exercises performed in order to ensure a full-body resistance training session combined with cardiorespiratory exercise.

Cognitive Distortions The mind's way of convincing itself that something true is actually untrue to reinforce negative thinking or emotions.

Cognitive Restructuring Psychotherapeutic process of learning to identify and dispute irrational or maladaptive thoughts.

Commitment The state or quality of being dedicated to a cause or activity.

Competitive Season The period that consists of regulated games or competitions of a particular sport; the period of time featuring the most competitive activity.

Complementary Goods and Services Goods and services that are similar and share a beneficial relationship with another product or service offering, but are not viewed by the consumer as an alternative or direct competition.

Complementary Proteins Consuming two or more incomplete proteins together to provide needed amino acids.

Complete Protein A protein that provides all of the essential amino acids in the amount the body needs and is also easy to digest and absorb; also called a *high-quality protein*.

Complex Carbohydrate A carbohydrate with more than 10 carbon/water units. Includes the fiber and starch found in whole grains and vegetables.

Concentric Activation The production of an active force when a muscle develops tension while shortening in length.

Concurrent Training Training designed to maintain or improve multiple fitness components in the same training phase.

Conditionally Essential Amino Acids Nonessential amino acids that cannot be produced due to disease and as a result must be acquired in dietary sources.

Confidence Feeling or belief of certainty.

Contemplation Stage The stage of change in the TTM where individuals are contemplating making a change within the next 6 months.

Continuing Education Any of a variety of course offerings that serve the purpose to keeping professionals up-to-date with their knowledge and skills.

Continuing Education Unit (CEU)   A measure used in continuing education courses that is designed for professionals to maintain a certification or licensure.

Contracts   Agreements between two or more parties that specify expectations, responsibilities, and contingencies for behavior change.

Coping   Process of managing specific internal or external demands that tax or exceed one's resources.

Corporate Fitness   Implementation of health and fitness programming by a fitness professional within a company structure.

Corrective Exercise   The programming process that identifies neuromuscular dysfunction, develops a plan of action, and implements a corrective strategy as a part of an exercise training program.

Corrective Flexibility   Flexibility training that is applied with the goal of improving muscle imbalances and correcting altered joint mechanics.

Creatine   Compound made in the body but that can also be consumed in the diet, mostly from meat and fish. Involved in the supply of energy for muscular contraction.

Cueing   Verbal and nonverbal communication used to evoke an action response from participants.

Cumulative Injury Cycle   A cycle whereby an injury will induce inflammation, muscle spasm, adhesions, altered neuromuscular control, and muscle imbalances. Muscle imbalance can lead to more inflammation, and the cycle repeats.

D

Daily Value   Guide to nutrients found within one serving of food.

Davis' Law   Soft tissue will align along the lines of stress that are placed upon it.

Deamination   The first step in the breakdown of amino acids; it includes the removal of the nitrogen group.

Deconditioned   A state of lost physical fitness, which may include muscle imbalances, decreased flexibility, and a lack of core and joint stability.

Deep Longitudinal Subsystem (DLS)   Subsystem of the global movement system that includes the peroneus longus, anterior tibialis, long head of the biceps femoris, sacrotuberous ligament, thoracolumbar fascia, and erector spinae. These muscles work together to create a contracting tension to absorb and control ground reaction forces during gait.

Demographics   Statistical data relating to the population and the particular groups in it.

Dendrite   The portion of a neuron that is responsible for gathering information from other structures.

Diastolic Pressure   The bottom number of a blood pressure measurement that represents the pressure within the arterial system when the heart is resting and filling with blood.

Dietary Reference Intakes (DRIs)   A general term for a set of reference values used to plan and assess nutrient intakes of healthy individuals.

Dietary Standards   Recommended intakes for specific nutrients.

Dietary Supplement Health and Education Act of 1994 (DSHEA)   Act that defines and regulates dietary supplements. Enacted by Congress following public debate concerning the role of dietary supplements in promoting health.

Diminishing Returns   As the systems of the body become more developed, the rate of improvement in fitness slows.

Disassociation   Focus on the external environment (e.g., noticing the scenery or listening to music).

Driver of Sales   Activities that create opportunities for future sales.

Drop Jump   This plyometric drill consists of stepping off a box typically 18–24 inches high and immediately jumping up after landing. This is the most stressful and technically demanding plyometric drill. It is also known as a depth jump.

Dumbbells   Common handheld free weight modality found in most gyms. Beneficial when coordination and mobility are desired during an exercise.

Dynamic   A trait that changes over time.

Dynamic Balance   Ability to maintain equilibrium through the intended path of motion when external forces are present.

Dynamic Stretching   Multiplanar extensibility with optimal neuromuscular control through a full range of motion.

Dyspnea   Difficulty or troubled breathing.

E

Eccentric Activation   The production of an active force when a muscle develops tension while lengthening.

Eccentric Function   Action of a muscle when it is generating an eccentric contraction.

Eccentric Strength   One of the three phases in the movement of a muscle. Refers to the action of a muscle while lengthening under load.

Efferent Neurons   Efferent neurons are motor neurons that send a message for muscles to contract.

Electrolytes   Minerals in blood and other body fluids that carry an electrical charge.

Electron Transport Chain   A series of compounds that transfer electrons from electron donors to electron acceptors, generating ATP in the process.

Emotion-Focused Coping   Distracts from negative feelings associated with stress.

Empty Calories   Calories that provide little or no nutrients.

Emulsification   The ability of a fat to mix with water.

Ergogenic Aids   Supplements used to benefit athletic performance or exercise.

Essential Amino Acids   Amino acids that cannot be produced by the body and must be acquired by food.

Estimated Average Requirement (EAR)   Estimated amount of a nutrient per day at which the needs of 50% of the population will be met.

Estimated Energy Requirement (EER)   General recommendation for calorie intake based on formulas designed to include individual characteristics such as age, gender, height, weight, and level of physical activity.

Exercise Selection   The process of choosing exercises that allow for achievement of the desired adaptation.

Exercise Tolerance   Increased ability to perform more exercise in less time, without undue fatigue or excessive soreness.

Exhaustion Phase   The third stage of GAS in which stress continues beyond the body's ability to adapt, leading to potential physiological and structural breakdown.

Extended Healthcare Providers   Professionals in the healthcare system such as physicians, physical therapists, and cardiac rehabilitation therapists who provide specialized guidance to patients suffering from various physical illnesses or impairments.

Extension   A bending at a joint where the relative angle between two adjoining segments increases.

Extensors   A muscle that produces extension of a limb or joint.

External Rotation   Rotation of a limb or body segment away from the midline of the body.

Extrinsic   Located from outside yet act on a structure being considered.

F

Fascia   A web of connective tissue that wraps and surrounds muscle fibers, bones, nerves, and blood vessels. The myofascial system covers individual muscles as well as connecting groups of larger muscles together.

Fat-Free Mass (FFM)   Total body mass, without the fat. It is the lean or nonfat components of the body.

Fatty Acid   A chain of carbons linked or bonded together, and the building blocks of fat within the human body.

Firing Frequency   The number of activation signals sent to a single motor unit in 1 second.

First Law of Thermodynamics   Energy can neither be created nor destroyed, only transferred from one form to another.

Fitness Coaching   The application of various behavior change and communications strategies with clients that leads to increased accountability and motivation, thus supporting their desire to achieve fitness goals.

Fixed-Isolated Machines   Resistance training machines that provide a fixed range of motion.

Flavin Adenine Dinucleotide (FAD)   A redox cofactor, more specifically a prosthetic group, involved in several important metabolic reactions.

Flexibility   The normal extensibility of soft tissue, which allows a joint to be moved through its full range of motion.

Flexion   A bending at a joint where the relative angle between two adjoining segments decreases.

Flexors   A muscle that produces flexion of a limb or joint.

Force   **(1)** A push or a pull that can create, stop, or change movement. **(2)** Force = Mass × Acceleration.

Force-Couple Relationship   Muscle groups moving together to produce movement around a joint.

Forecasting   Process whereby trainers and/or managers apply specific percentages based on previous performance to predict future sales or other measurable outcomes, such as sessions serviced.

Formative Assessment   An informal, quick assessment of movement proficiency during a workout to gauge progress and screen for any new areas of concern.

Free Weights   Unrestricted objects of various weights that can be used as resistance for exercise movements.

Frontal Plane   An imaginary plane that bisects the body into equal halves, producing a front half and a back half.

Fructose   Known as fruit sugar; found in fruits, honey, syrups, and certain vegetables.

Function   Integrated, multiplanar movement that involves acceleration, stabilization, and deceleration.

Functional Efficiency   The ability of the neuromuscular system to perform functional tasks with the least amount of energy, decreasing stress on the body's structure.

Functional Movements   Movements based on real-world biomechanics and activities.

G

Galactose   Combines with glucose in lactose.

General Adaptation Syndrome (GAS)   **(1)** How the kinetic chain responds and adapts to imposed demands. **(2)** How the body responds and adapts to stress.

Gland   An organ that secretes hormones into the bloodstream to regulate a variety of bodily functions, such as mood, growth and development, tissue function, or metabolism.

Global Muscular System System composed of four subsystems that are designed for larger muscles to work synergistically in larger movement patterns, such as a combination squat to row exercise.

Gluconeogenesis Formation of glucose from noncarbohydrate sources, such as amino acids.

Glucose A simple sugar manufactured by the body from carbohydrates, fat, and (to a lesser extent) protein that serves as the body's main source of fuel.

Glycerol A simple polyol (sugar alcohol) compound. It is a colorless, odorless, viscous liquid. The glycerol backbone is central to all lipids known as triglycerides.

Glycogen A complex carbohydrate that is stored in the liver and muscle cells. When carbohydrate energy is needed, glycogen is converted into glucose for use by the muscle cells.

Glycolysis A catabolic process that breaks down glucose to a usable form of energy, ATP.

Goal Proximity The relative nearness of a goal in terms of time frame.

Golgi Tendon Organs (GTOs) Receptors sensitive to the change in tension of the muscle, and the rate of that change.

Gravity A force that accelerates an object or mass downward toward the earth's center.

Ground Reaction Force An equal and opposite external force that is exerted back onto the body by the ground.

Group Personal Training Exercise setting in which one trainer provides tailored exercise guidance to two or more individuals simultaneously.

H

Heart Palpitations Heart flutters or rapid beating of the heart.

Heart Rate (HR) The rate at which the heart pumps; usually measured in beats per minute (bpm).

Heart Rate Reserve (HRR) Method A method of establishing training intensity based on the difference between a client's predicted maximal heart rate and his or her resting heart rate.

Heart Rate Variability Variations in the time interval between heartbeats.

Henneman's Size Principle Motor units which are under load are recruited from smallest to largest

High-Fructose Corn Syrup (HFCS) A sweetener made from cornstarch and converted to fructose in food processing.

HMB (Beta-Hydroxy Beta-Methylbutyrate) A metabolite of the essential amino acid leucine that is synthesized in the human body. Used as a supplement to increase muscle mass and decrease muscle breakdown.

Homeostasis The ability or tendency of an organism or a cell to maintain internal equilibrium by adjusting its physiological processes.

Horizontal Loading Performing all sets of an exercise or body part before moving on to the next exercise or body part.

Hormones Chemical messengers that enter the bloodstream to attach to target tissues and target organs.

Hypertrophy Enlargement of skeletal muscle fibers in response to overcoming force from high volumes of tension.

Hypertrophy Training The chronic enlargement of muscles.

Hypokalemia Loss of significant amounts of potassium, resulting in weakness, fatigue, constipation, and muscle cramping.

Hypomobility Decrease in normal movement and functionality of a joint, which affects range of motion.

Hyponatremia Loss of significant amounts of sodium, resulting in an increase in the body's water levels.

I

Imagine Action   Program designed to help people through the different stages of change.

Implement   A unique, free-standing object that can be used as resistance.

Incomplete Protein   Food that does not contain all of the essential amino acids in the amount needed by the body.

Insensible Water Loss   Water lost through mild daily sweating and exhalation of air humidified by the lungs, as well as other minor water losses, such as secretions from the eyes, that generally go unnoticed.

Insertion   The relatively mobile attachment site.

Integrated Function   The coordination of muscles to produce, reduce, and stabilize forces in multiple planes for efficient and safe movement.

Integrated Performance Paradigm (Stretch–Shortening Cycle)   A forceful cycle of muscle contraction that involves eccentric loading of the muscle, isometric muscle contraction, and concentric muscle contraction.

Integrated Training   A comprehensive training approach that combines all the components necessary to help a client achieve optimum performance.

Intermuscular Coordination   The ability of the neuromuscular system to allow all muscles to work together with proper activation and timing.

Internal Rotation   Rotation of a limb or body segment toward the midline of the body.

Interneurons   Only located within the spinal cord and brain; receive impulses from afferent (sensory) neurons and conduct back out to provide a motor (efferent) response.

Interpersonal Influences   Influences from those individuals or groups one interacts with regularly.

Interval Training   Training that alternates between intense exertion and periods of rest or lighter exertion.

Intervention   Strategies within a fitness professional's scope of practice that are aimed at disrupting unhealthy habits and/or promoting healthy behaviors.

Intramuscular Coordination   The ability of the neuromuscular system to allow optimal levels of motor unit recruitment and synchronization within a muscle.

Intrinsic   Located from within and acting directly on a structure being considered.

Intrinsic Approach   An inside-out approach to exercise that emphasizes the enjoyment and fun of exercise and making it something to look forward to, not just a means to goal accomplishment.

Intrinsic Core Stabilizers   Deep inner muscles behind the superficial abdominals that have a direct effect on stabilizing the lumbo-pelvic-hip complex.

Isolated Function   **(1)** A muscle's primary function. **(2)** A muscle action produced at a joint when a muscle is being concentrically activated to produce acceleration of a body segment.

Isometric Activation   The production of an active force when a muscle develops tension while maintaining a constant length.

J

Joint Receptors   Receptors in and around a joint that respond to pressure, acceleration, and deceleration of the joint.

Joint Stability   Ability to prepare, maintain, anticipate, and restore stability at each joint.

Journaling   A type of self-monitoring and a practical way to collect information about behavior patterns that can be used to identify cues and barriers to exercise and nutrition plans.

K

Ketone Bodies   Two molecules, acetoacetate and β-hydroxybutyrate, that are synthesized in the liver from acetyl-CoA.

Kettlebell   A cast-iron, cannonball-like weight with a handle used to perform ballistic exercises.

Kilocalorie   A unit of energy equal to 1,000 calories. It is the amount of heat energy required to raise the temperature of a kilogram or liter of water by 1 degree Celsius.

Kinesiology   The study of human movement.

Kinetic Chain   The combination and interrelation of the actions of the nervous, muscular, and skeletal systems to create movement.

Kinetics   Biomechanics term that involves the study of forces.

Knee Valgus   The process where the knees move forward and in, known as "knock knees."

Krebs Cycle   Central metabolic pathway in all aerobic organisms. The cycle is a series of eight reactions that occur in the mitochondrion. These reactions take a two-carbon molecule (acetate) and completely oxidize it to carbon dioxide.

Kyphotic Curve   Outward curvature of the thoracic spine by which the spine is bent forward.

L

Lactate   A byproduct of anaerobic metabolism that occurs when oxygen delivery to the working muscles cannot meet the demands of the tissue.

Lactose   A sugar present in milk that is composed of glucose and galactose.

Lateral Subsystem (LS)   Composed of the gluteus medius, tensor fascia, latae, adductor complex, and quadratus lumborum, all of which participate in frontal plane and pelvofemoral stability.

Leads   Individuals who have shown a certain level of interest in personal training services.

Length–Tension Relationship (LTR)   The resting length of a muscle and the tension the muscle can produce at that resting length.

Lever   A relatively rigid rod or bar that rotates around a fulcrum.

Ligament   Strong connective tissue that connects bone to bone.

Line of Pull   The direction in which a muscle is pulled.

Linear Periodization   Classic or traditional strength and power programming that begins with high-volume, low-intensity training and progresses toward low-volume, high-intensity training.

Lipids   A group of compounds that includes triglycerides (fats and oils), phospholipids, and sterols.

Lipogenesis   The metabolic pathway responsible for formation of fat.

Load   The amount of weight lifted or resistance used during training.

Long-Term Goal   A large goal that is set to be achieved over a long period of time.

Longitudinal Axis   An imaginary long, straight line that cuts through the body from top to bottom.

Low-Density Lipoprotein (LDL)   The molecule that carries lipids throughout the body and delivers cholesterol that can accumulate on artery walls.

Lower Crossed Syndrome   A postural distortion syndrome characterized by an anterior tilt to the pelvis (arched lower back).

M

Macronutrients   Nutrients that provide calories.

Maintenance   Sustaining developed levels of muscular fitness without improvement.

Maintenance Stage   The stage of change in the TTM that begins 6 months after the criterion has been reached until such time that the risk of returning to the old behavior has been terminated.

Malalignment   The incorrect or improper alignment of the joints in a body without movements.

Maltose   Sugar produced in the breakdown of starch. Rare in our food supply.

Mass   The amount of matter in an object or physical body.

Matter   A substance that has mass and takes up space.

Maximal Oxygen Consumption ($\dot{V}O_{2max}$)   The highest rate of oxygen transport and utilization achieved at maximal physical exertion.

Maximal Strength   The maximum force a muscle can produce in a single voluntary effort, regardless of the rate of force production.

Mechanical Specificity   **(1)** The specific muscular requirements using different weights and movements that are performed to increase strength or endurance in certain body parts. **(2)** The weights and movements placed on the body.

Mechanoreceptors   Sensory receptors responsible for sensing distortion in body tissues.

Medicine Ball   An implement used to add external resistance to bodyweight exercises (similar to dumbbells and kettlebells) and for reactive exercises such as rotational throws.

Mentor   A trusted advisor in a specific area.

Metabolic Conditioning   Exercise that improves effective and efficient energy storage and delivery for physical activity.

Metabolic Conditioning Circuit   A high-intensity exercise circuit designed to increase the storage and delivery of energy for any activity. It primarily conditions the phosphagen and glycolytic pathways.

Metabolic Pathway   A series of chemical steps or reactions that either break down or build up compounds in the body.

Metabolic Resistance Training   The use of high work-rate resistance activities with few or no recovery intervals.

Metabolic Specificity   Energy demand placed on the body.

Metabolism   All of the chemical reactions that occur in the body that are required for life. It is the process by which nutrients are acquired, transported, used, and disposed of by the body.

Methyl Group ($-CH_3$)   An alkyl derived from methane that has one carbon atom bonded to three hydrogen atoms.

Midline   That which is contained within an imaginary line that splits the body into equal halves.

Mitochondria   Organelle found in the cytoplasm of eukaryotic cells that contains genetic material and enzymes necessary for cell metabolism, converting food to energy.

Modality   A form or mode of exercise that presents a specific stress to the body.

Motivational Interviewing   A collaborative person-centered form of guiding to elicit and strengthen motivation for change.

Motor Behavior   Motor response to internal and external environmental stimuli.

Motor Control   How the central nervous system integrates internal and external sensory information with pervious experiences to produce a motor response.

Motor Development   The change in motor skill behavior over time throughout the lifespan.

Motor Learning   The integration of motor control processes with practice and experience that leads to relatively permanent changes in the body's capacity to produce skilled movements.

Motor Output   Response to stimuli that activates movement in organs or muscles.

Motor Unit Activation   Increased recruitment of motor units and/or recruitment of motor units rapidly and repeatedly.

Motor Unit   One motor neuron and the muscle fibers it connects (innervates) with.

Motor Unit Recruitment   The activation of motor units in a successive manner to produce more strength.

Motor Unit Synchronization The simultaneous recruitment of multiple motor units resulting in more muscle tissue contracting at the same time.

Movement Preparation The systematic implementation of flexibility, core, balance, reactive, and SAQ (as applicable) training principles prior to completing the remaining majority portion of the workout (e.g., resistance training).

Multiplanar Occurring in more than one plane of motion.

Muscle Belly The mid-region in between the origin and insertion.

Muscle Coordination Complex neurological control of motor units, ensuring effective contraction and relaxation of muscle tissue across agonist and antagonist muscle groups.

Muscle Imbalance Alteration of muscle length surrounding a joint.

Muscle Spindles Receptors sensitive to change in length of the muscle, and the rate of that change.

Muscular Endurance **(1)** A muscle's ability to contract for an extended period. **(2)** The ability to produce and maintain force production over prolonged periods of time.

Muscular Failure A training approach that involves the completion of as many reps as possible until the individual is unable to complete a repetition due to fatigue.

Musculoskeletal System The combined, interworking system of all muscles and bones in the body.

N

Nerve Impulses The consecutive linking of neurons by electrochemical signals that travel throughout the nerve fiber.

Nervous System A conglomeration of billions of cells specifically designed to provide a communication network within the human body.

Neural Drive The frequency of activation signals sent to muscle fibers via motor neurons.

Neuromuscular Efficiency When the neuromuscular system allows agonists, antagonists, and stabilizers to synergistically produce muscle actions in all three planes of motion.

Neuromuscular Specificity The specific muscular contractions using different speeds and patterns that are performed to increase neuromuscular efficiency.

Neuron The functional unit of the nervous system.

New Business A new client who has purchased personal training services as a result of the fitness professional's prospecting activities.

Nicotinamide Adenine Dinucleotide (NAD) A coenzyme found in all living cells that is a carrier in the electron transport chain.

Nonessential Amino Acids Amino acids that are produced by the body and do not need to be consumed in dietary sources.

Nonsynovial Joints Joints that do not have a joint cavity, connective tissue, or cartilage.

Nutrient Density The nutrient content of a food relative to its calories.

O

Obesity The condition of being considerably overweight; a person who is at least 30 pounds over the recommended weight for his or her height.

Objective Assessments Assessments that address observations that can be directly measured and quantified by the fitness professional.

Objective Goal Something an individual is trying to accomplish; the object or aim of an action.

Off-Season The period of the sports year when an activity or sport is not engaged in; the period of time when the most training can be performed.

Omega-3 Fatty Acids   Fatty acids that have anti-inflammatory effects and help to decrease blood clotting.

Omega-6 Fatty Acids   Fatty acids that promote blood clotting and cell membrane formation.

Open-Chain Exercises   Exercises where the foot or hand is free to move and usually not in contact with the ground. These exercises, such as a leg extension on a machine, are not as functional as closed-chain exercises such as squats.

Open-Ended Question   A question that cannot be answered with a simple "yes" or "no." It gives the person answering the scope to provide more detailed information.

Operations   Activities involved in the day-to-day functions of a business that do not directly generate revenue.

Origin   The relatively stationary attachment site where skeletal muscle attaches begins.

Outcome Goal   A goal that is usually about winning or losing; in exercise settings, it is the end result of some behavior.

Overactive   Referring to a state of having disrupted neuromuscular recruitment patterns that lead a muscle to be more active during a joint action.

Overhead Squat Assessment   A transitional movement assessment designed to assess dynamic flexibility, core strength, balance, and overall neuromuscular control.

Overload Principle   States that in order to create physiological changes an exercise stimulus must be applied at an intensity greater than the body is accustomed to receiving.

Overtraining Syndrome (OTS)   Excessive frequency, volume, or intensity of training, resulting in fatigue; also caused by a lack of proper rest and recovery.

Oxaloacetate (OAA)   A crystalline organic compound that is a metabolic intermediate in many metabolic processes.

P

Parallel Muscle   Muscle with fibers that are oriented parallel to that muscle's longitudinal axis.

Parasympathetic Nervous System   Stimulates rest and digestion physiological processes.

Pattern Overload   Repetitive physical activity that moves through the same patterns of motion, placing the same stresses on the body over time.

Pelvo-Ocular Reflex   The neuromotor response of the pelvic girdle and lower extremity that serves to orient the body region in response to head position and visual cues.

Pennate Muscle   Muscle with fibers that are oriented at an angle to the muscle's longitudinal axis.

Performance Goal   A goal that specifies the end products of performance expressed in terms of personal achievement.

Periodization   Division of a training program into smaller, progressive stages.

Perturbation   A disturbance of equilibrium; shaking.

Phospholipid   Type of lipid in which one fatty acid has been replaced by a phosphate group and one of several nitrogen-containing molecules.

Phytochemicals   Biologically active compounds found in plants.

Point-of-Sale Client   A client who has purchased a personal training package or program at the time that he or she enrolled in a membership program.

Polyunsaturated Fatty Acids   Fatty acids that have several spots where hydrogens are missing.

Positive Reinforcement   The practice of offering a reward following a desired behavior to encourage repetition of the behavior.

Post Rehab   A period of time following general physical therapy before a patient returns to full fitness and function following an injury or surgery.

Posterior Oblique Subsystem (POS)   Subsystem of the global movement system composed of the latissimus dorsi and the contralateral gluteus maximus, with the thoracolumbar fascia creating a fascial bridge for the cross body connection. These muscles create a nearly straight line with each other across the sacroiliac joint, and when they both contract they produce a pulling force across the thoracolumbar fascia and stabilization force at the sacroiliac joint (force closure). This system works concurrently with the DLS during gait.

Postural Distortion Patterns   Common postural malalignments and muscle imbalances that individuals develop based on a variety of factors.

Postural Stability   Ability to prepare, maintain, anticipate, and restore stability of the entire Human Movement System.

Posture   Position and bearing of the body for alignment and function of the kinetic chain.

Power   The ability to produce a large amount of force in a short amount of time.

Precontemplation Stage   Stage of change in the TTM where individuals do not intend to change their high-risk behaviors in the foreseeable future.

Preparation Stage   The stage of change in the TTM where individuals intend to take action in the near future, usually within the next month.

Preseason   The period immediately before the beginning of a new competitive season.

Principle of Variation   Rationale for challenging the kinetic chain with a wide variety of exercises and stimuli.

Problem-Focused Coping   Targets an issue causing stress to reduce the effects of the stress.

Process Goals   A goal that specifies the processes the individual wants to perform in a satisfactory manner (however that is defined).

Profit Center   A part of an organization with assignable revenues and costs, and hence ascertainable profitability.

Progressive Resistance Exercise (PRE)   A method of increasing the ability of muscles to generate force. The progressions within the OPT model are divided up to support each component of integrated fitness training (flexibility, cardio, core, balance, reactive, SAQ, and resistance training) and each level (Stabilization, Strength, and Power).

Prompting   Promoting an action through encouragement, persuasion, or reminding.

Pronation   A triplanar movement that is associated with force reduction.

Pronation Distortion Syndrome   A postural distortion syndrome characterized by foot pronation (flat feet) and adducted and internally rotated knees (knock knees).

Pronation of the Foot   A combination of dorsiflexion, eversion, and abduction.

Pronators   A muscle that produces pronation of a limb or body segment.

Prone   Body position where one is lying with the face downward.

Proprioception   The ability to recognize bodily movement and position

Proprioception   The cumulative sensory input to the central nervous system from all mechanoreceptors that sense body position and limb movements.

Proprioceptively Enriched Environments   Unstable, yet controllable environments.

Proprioceptors   Sensors in muscles and tendons that provide information about joint angle, muscle length, and muscle tension (i.e., muscle spindles, GTOs).

Prospecting   Activities designed to search for potential customers or clients.

Protein   Long chains of amino acids linked by peptide bonds. Serve several essential functional roles in the body.

Protein Synthesis   An anabolic process that results in the building of muscle.

Psychographics   The study of personality, values, opinions, attitudes, interests, and lifestyles.

Pulse   The force created by blood moving or pulsating through the arteries each time the heart contracts.

Pyruvate   A byproduct of anaerobic glycolysis that is an intermediate in several metabolic pathways.

Q

Qualitative Analysis   Applying principles of proper technique and combining them with observations in order to make an educated evaluation.

Quantitative Analysis   Taking physical measurements and making mathematical computations to reach a conclusion.

Quickness   The ability to react to a stimulus with an appropriate muscular response without hesitation.

R

Radial Pulse   Pulse obtained on the forearm, just below the wrist.

Range of Motion (ROM)   **(1)** The range through which a joint may be freely moved with no resistance or pain. **(2)** The amount of movement produced by one or multiple joints.

Rapport   The aspect of a relationship characterized by similarity, agreement, or congruity.

Rate of Force Production   Ability of muscles to exert maximal force output in a minimal amount of time.

Rating of Perceived Exertion (RPE)   A technique used to express or validate how hard a client feels he or she is working during exercise.

Re-Sign   An existing client who has elected to continue training and purchases additional personal training services or commits contractually to training for a longer period of time.

Reactive Training   Exercises that use quick, powerful movements involving an eccentric contraction immediately followed by an explosive concentric contraction.

Reciprocal Inhibition   The simultaneous contraction of one muscle and the relaxation of its antagonist to allow movement to take place.

Recommended Dietary Allowance (RDA)   Estimated amount of a nutrient per day considered necessary for good health.

Relative Flexibility   The human movement system's way of finding the path of least resistance during movement.

Relaxin   Hormone produced during pregnancy that loosens and softens ligaments.

Repetition   One complete movement of a single exercise.

Repetition Tempo   The speed at which each repetition is performed.

Repetitive Lack of Motion   Frequent immobility, which holds the potential for repetitive stress injuries.

Repetitive Stress Injury (RSI)   Injury due to pattern overload.

Resistance Training Machines   Machines that enable novice exercisers to engage in resistance training without needing to be, or become, experts in lifting techniques.

Respiratory System   System of the body composed of the lungs and respiratory passages that collect oxygen from the external environment and transport it to the bloodstream.

Rest Period   The time taken between sets or exercises to rest or recover.

Resting Heart Rate (RHR)   The number of contractions of the heart occurring in 1 minute while the body is at rest.

Retraction   Adduction of the shoulder blades where the shoulder blades move toward the spine.

S

Sagittal Plane   An imaginary plane that bisects the body into equal halves, producing a left half and a right half.

Sarcopenia   The loss of muscle tissue as a natural result of the aging process.

Saturated Fat   A chain of carbons that is saturated with all of the hydrogens that it can hold; there are no double bonds.

Scapular Winging   The scapula protrudes from the back in an abnormal position.

Scope of Practice   The actions, procedures, and processes that a professional is allowed to undertake in keeping with the terms of the professional's license or credential.

Self-Confidence   The belief in one's ability to execute a certain behavior.

Self-Efficacy   Belief regarding one's ability to succeed or perform in a specific situation.

Self-Monitoring   Ability to recognize and regulate one's behavior.

Self-Talk   One's internal dialogue.

Sensation Influences   Physical feelings an individual experiences as it relates to behaviors involved in establishing a healthy lifestyle.

Sensorimotor Control   A complex interaction involving the muscular system, PNS, and CNS to obtain balance or postural control.

Sensorimotor Integration   The ability of the nervous system to gather and interpret information to anticipate and execute the proper motor response.

Set   A group of consecutive repetitions.

Short-Term Goal   A goal that is set to be achieved within the near future.

Shoulder Impingement   When the space between the bone on top of the shoulder (acromion) and the tendons of the rotator cuff rub against each other during arm elevation.

Simple Carbohydrate   A carbohydrate with fewer than 10 carbon/water units. Includes glucose, sucrose, lactose, galactose, maltose, and fructose.

Single-Leg Squat Assessment   A transitional assessment performed on one leg to assess dynamic flexibility, core strength, balance, and overall neuromuscular control.

Sinoatrial (Sa) Node   A specialized area of cardiac tissue located in the right atrium of the heart that initiates the electrical impulses that determine the heart rate; often termed the "pacemaker for the heart."

Social Support   An individual's favorable attitude toward another person's involvement in an exercise program.

Spasticity   An increase in muscle tone or stiffness that impairs movement.

Special Population   **(1)** A group of people who have similar conditions or characteristics that require alterations to the general exercise plan. **(2)** Individuals who will require modifications or specialized training.

Specific Adaptation to Imposed Demands (SAID) Principle   States that the type of exercise stimulus placed on the body will determine the expected physiological outcome.

Speed   The straight-ahead velocity of an individual.

Stabilization System   The muscles whose primary function is to provide joint support and stabilization; also known as the *local muscular system*.

Stabilizers   Muscles that minimize unwanted movement while the agonist and synergists work to provide movement at the joint.

Stable   A trait that does not change over time.

State   A temporary change in one's personality, such as an emotion.

Static Balance   Ability to maintain equilibrium in place with no external forces.

Static Posture   The starting point from which an individual moves.

Sterols   A subgroup of the steroids and an important class of organic molecules.

Strength   Ability of the neuromuscular system to provide internal tension and exert force against external resistance.

Strength Endurance   The ability of the body to repeatedly produce high levels of force for prolonged periods.

Stride Length   The distance covered with each stride.

Stride Rate   The number of strides taken in a given amount of time (or distance).

Stroke Volume (SV)   The amount of blood pumped out of the heart with each contraction.

Structural Efficiency   The structural alignment of the muscular and skeletal systems that allows the body to maintain balance in relation to its center of gravity.

Subjective Assessment   Assessment used to obtain information about a client's personal history, as well as his or her occupation, lifestyle, and medical background.

Subjective Goal   Goal based on experience or expectations; less tangible than an objective goal.

Suboptimal Positioning   Less than optimal body positioning that when repeated reinforces poor motor patterns and can lead to abnormal stress and pattern overload.

Sucrose   Often referred to as table sugar, it is a molecule made up of glucose and fructose.

Superset   One exercise immediately followed by another exercise with no rest.

Supination   A triplanar motion that is associated with force production.

Supination of the Foot   A combination of plantar flexion, inversion, and adduction.

Supinators   A muscle that produces supination of a limb or body segment.

Supine   Body position where one is lying on the back and face is upward.

Suspension Training   The combined use of straps and body weight to place a stress load on the neuromuscular system.

Symmetry   Proportion and balance between two items or two sides.

Synergistic Dominance   When synergists take over function for a weak or inhibited prime movers.

Synergists   Muscles that assist the prime mover in a joint action.

Synovial Joints   Joints that are held together by a joint capsule and ligaments; type of joint most associated with movement in the body.

Systolic Pressure   The top number of a blood pressure measurement that represents the pressure within the arterial system after the heart contracts.

T

Target Cells   Cells that have hormone specific receptors, ensuring that each hormone will communicate only with specific target cells.

Tempo   The amount of time that muscle is actively producing tension during exercise movements.

Tendon   Connectivetissue that attaches muscle to bone.

Tendons   Connective tissues that attach muscle to bone and provide an anchor for muscles to produce force.

Tensegrity   Term coined by Buckminster Fuller that refers to a skeletal structure in which compression and tension are used to give a structure its form, providing stability and efficiency in mass and movement.

Termination Stage   The stage of change in the TTM in which individuals have zero temptation to engage in the old behavior and exhibit 100% self-efficacy in all previously tempting situations.

Time Under Tension (TUT)   The amount of time from the beginning of one resistance training set to the end without breaking.

Timed Hold An acute variable where the requirement is to hold a specific pose or posture for a specified period of time.

Tolerable Upper Intake Level (UL) Highest level of a nutrient per day that is unlikely to pose a risk of adverse health effects.

Top-Line A company's overall sales or revenues, before any discounts or returns.

Torque The rotary or rotational effect that a force has around an axis.

Toxicity The degree to which a substance can cause damage to an organism.

Training Age Refers to the number of years a client has been training. A 12-year-old client who started training at 9 years old would have a training age of 3, whereas a 23-year-old who started training at age 22 would have a younger training age of 1.

Training Duration (1) Length of workout from beginning to end. (2) Amount of time spent in a particular phase of training.

Training Frequency The number of training sessions performed during a given period, usually 1 week.

Training Intensity An individual's level of effort, compared with his or her maximal effort; usually expressed as a percentage.

Training Volume The total amount of work performed within a specified time; typically the number of repetitions multiplied by the number of sets in a training session.

Trait A part of an individual's behavior that shapes his or her personality.

Transitional Movement Assessment A type of assessment that evaluates dynamic posture.

Transtheoretical Model (TTM) States that individuals progress through a series of stages of behavior change and that movement through these stages is cyclical, not linear, because many do not succeed in their efforts at establishing and maintaining lifestyle changes.

Transverse Plane An imaginary plane that bisects the body into equal halves, producing a top half and a bottom half.

Tricarboxylic Acid (TCA) Cycle Another term for the Krebs cycle. A tricarboxylic acid is an organic carboxylic acid whose chemical structure contains three carboxyl functional groups (–COOH). The best known example of a tricarboxylic acid is citric acid.

Triglyceride The chemical or substrate form in which most fat exists in food as well as in the body.

Triple Extension A multijoint exercise that involves extension at the hip, knee, and ankle.

Triple Flexion A multijoint exercise that involves flexion at the hip, knee, and ankle.

Turn-Key A complete product or service that is ready for immediate use.

U

Underactive Referring to the state of having disrupted neuromuscular recruitment patterns that lead a muscle to be relatively less active during a joint action.

Undulating Periodization A form of periodization that provides changes in the acute variables of workouts to achieve different goals on a daily or weekly basis.

Unsaturated Fatty Acids Fatty acids that have areas that are not completely saturated with hydrogens, and therefore have double bonds where the hydrogen is missing.

Upper Crossed Syndrome A postural distortion syndrome characterized by a forward head and rounded shoulders.

V

$\dot{V}O_{2max}$ The highest rate of oxygen transport and utilization achieved at maximal physical exertion.

Valsalva Maneuver   Movement in which a person tries to exhale forcibly with a closed glottis (windpipe) so that no air exits through the mouth or nose as, for example, in lifting a heavy weight. The Valsalva maneuver impedes the return of venous blood to the heart.

Veins   Vessels that transport blood from the capillaries toward the heart.

Ventilatory Threshold (T_{VENT})   The point during graded exercise at which ventilation increases disproportionately to oxygen uptake, signifying a switch from predominately aerobic energy production to anaerobic energy production.

Ventricles   The inferior chambers of the heart that receive blood from their corresponding atrium and, in turn, force blood into the arteries.

Vertical Loading   Circuit applied to more conditioned clients allowing alternating body parts to be trained from set to set, starting from the upper extremity and moving to the lower extremity with little to no rest in between.

Vibration Exercise   The use of rapid oscillations of a platform or implement to stimulate and challenge the neuromuscular system.

Viscoelastic   Ability to stretch linearly.

W

Wearable Technology   Devices that are worn during exercise and collect/transmit information regarding performance and physiological variables relating to the workout.

Weekend Warriors   Clients who work busy jobs or live sedentary lifestyles during the week but try to maintain participation in moderate to aggressive weekend recreational activities.

Weight   The amount of force that gravity has on the body.

Whey Protein   A mixture of globular proteins isolated from whey, the liquid material created as a byproduct of cheese production.

Whey Protein Concentrate (WPC)   Dietary supplement obtained by removal of sufficient nonprotein constituents from pasteurized whey.

Whey Protein Isolate (WPI)   Dietary supplement obtained by separating components from milk.

Index

Page numbers followed by f and t indicate material in figures and tables, respectively.

A

abdominal bracing, 194–195, 195f, 195t
abdominal musculature
    diaphragm, 763
    external oblique, 762
    internal oblique, 762
    rectus abdominis, 761
    transverse abdominis, 762
abduction, 48
abductors, 51
acceleration, definition of, 59
acceptable macronutrient distribution range
        (AMDR), 167, 168
acetyl-CoA, 155–156
achilles tendon, 117
acidosis, 399
active force, 58
active-isolated stretching, 188, 546–553,
        692–696
    active kneeling hip flexor stretch, 547–548
    active latissimus dorsi, 551–552
    active pectoral stretch, 552–553
    active piriformis stretch, 548–550
    active supine biceps femoris stretch,
        550–551
active listening, 665–667, 667t
activity trackers, 517–518
acute variables, 180, 181, 327–331
    exercise selection, 330
    load and intensity, 329, 329t
    order of exercises, 331
    rest periods, 329–330, 330t
    tempo, 328–329, 329t
    volume, 327–328
Adam's apple. *See* thyroid hormones
adduction, 48, 49
adductor brevis, 758
adductor longus, 757
adductor magnus
    anterior fibers, 757
    posterior fibers, 757
adductors, 51, 535, 541
adenosine triphosphate (ATP), 154
adequate intake (AI), 167, 733t
adipose issue, 157, 158
adrenaline. *See* epinephrine
aerobic exercise, 501
aerobic metabolism, 155

affective influences, on exercise behavior,
        659–661
afferent neurons, 87, 89
age
    older adult training, 493t, 496–497,
        497f, 498f
    youth training, 493t, 494–496, 495f, 496f
agility, definition of, 201
agonists, 92, 93t
alcohol, 153–154
alimentary canal, 135
altered arthrokinematics, 283
altered neuromuscular efficiency, 283
altered reciprocal inhibition, 115
American Heart Association (AHA), 3
amino acids, 145, 146t
    conditionally essential, 147
    essential, 145, 147
    for immediate energy, 730
    pool, 157, 159
    for potential energy, 730
amortization phase, 198
anabolic hormone. *See* growth hormone
anabolism, 154
anaerobic metabolism, 155
anaerobic power, 445
anaerobic threshold, 192
anatomic locations, 41–42, 41f
anatomic position, 41
ancillary revenue, 220
ankle stretch, 540–541
antagonist, 92–93, 93t
anterior cruciate ligament (ACL) injuries,
        182–183, 183f, 445, 445f
anterior deltoid, 767
anterior oblique subsystem (AOS), 106, 107f
anterior-posterior axis, 43
anterior tibialis, 752
aponeurosis, 65
appendicular skeletons, 96
arginine, 171
arm machine row, alternate, 620–621
arm musculature
    biceps brachii, 770
    brachialis, 771
    brachioradialis, 771
    triceps brachii, 770
arteries, 123, 124

arthrokinematics, 99
assessment considerations, 351–357
    balance, 356
    cardio, 351–354, 352–354f
    core, 355–356, 356f
    flexibility, 354–355, 355f
    reactive training, 357
    resistance, 357
assessment modifications, 318–321
    for common injuries, 320–321
    for obese population, 320
    for pregnant population, 318
    for senior population, 319, 319t
    for youth population, 318
assessment outcomes
    assessment considerations, 351–357
    communication with
        client, 360–361
    exercise selection and movement
        dysfunction, 358–360
    movement and muscle balance, 350
    and program design, 350–361
association strategies, for exercise behavior,
        671–672
ataxia, 508
atherosclerosis, 493t, 504
athletic trainer, 20–22
atlas, 94, 95f
atoms, 158, 159
atrioventricular (AV) nodes, 122
atrioventricular valves, 123
atrium, 123
autogenic inhibition, 186
autonomic nervous system, 751
autonomy-supportive style, 667–668
axial skeletons, 94–96
axon, 87, 88, 749f, 750

B

back
    power, 717
    stabilization, 715
    strength, 716
back musculature
    latissimus dorsi, 764
    multifidus, 764
    quadratus lumborum, 764
    superficial erector spinae, 763

balance
definition of, 196
single-leg, 566–567
stabilization, 387–390, 387–388t, 389–390f, 701
balance ball
dumbbell press, 600–602
leg curls/bridge, 580–581
balance protocols
in power level, 459–460, 459–460f, 460t, 703
in stabilization level, 387–390, 387–388t, 389–390f
in strength level, 421–423, 422–423f, 422t, 702
ball-and-socket joint, 101, 102f, 102t
ball dumbbell chest press, 600–602
ballistic stretching, 553
barbell Russian deadlift, 595–597
barbell squat, 599–600
barbells, 479, 479f
battling rope exercise, 485, 485f
behavior change strategies
coaching and communication strategies, 663–668
human behavior, influences of, 656–663
introduction to, 652–653, 653f
principles and practices of goal setting, 676–682
progress evaluation practices, 682–685
transtheoretical model (TTM), 653–656
behavior influences, 122–663
journaling, 662–663, 662f
positive reinforcement, 662
behavior modification approaches, 669–671
charting attendance and participation, 670
contracting, 669–670
prompting, 669
providing feedback on progress, 670–671
bench press test, 306–307, 307f
best practices, definition of, 29
beta-hydroxy beta-methylbutyrate, 173
beta-oxidation, 156, 157
biceps
brachii, 770
curl machine, 616–617
stabilization, 721
strength, 722
biceps femoris
active supine stretch, 550–551
long head, 754
short head, 754
static stretch, 542–543

biomechanics, 39–81, 40
as a language, 63–69
application of, 51–57
basics of, 40–44
and kinetic chain disruption, 77–81
muscles that become dysfunctional, 70–76
muscular function and application, 57–63
role of, 40–50
biotensegrity, 112
bird dogs, 572–573
blood glucose, 143, 144
blood pressure, 261
blood vessels, 124–127, 126f
functions of blood, 124–127
support mechanisms of blood, 127, 127t
body composition, 262
body fat, measuring, 262–264, 263–264t, 265–266t
body mass index (BMI), 269, 270t
bodyweight exercise, 476–477, 476f
floor bridge, 569–570
floor cobra, 568–569
floor crunch, 573–574
horizontal jump with stabilization, 586–587
ice skaters, 590–591
knee-up, 576–578
multiplanar jump, 587–590
multiplanar lunge to balance, 581–584
prone iso-abs, 567–568
push-up with plus, 578–579
quadruped opposite arm and opposite leg raise, 572–573
reverse crunch, 575–576
sagittal plane hop with stabilization, 584–585
sagittal plane proprioceptive reactives, 592–593
single-leg balance, 566–567
single-leg floor bridge, 570–572
stability ball hamstring curl, 580–581
bone markings, 774–775
depressions, 774, 774f
processes, 774–775, 774–775f
bone mass effects, 103–104
bone mineral density (BMD), 450
bones, 96–98
flat bones, 98, 98f
irregular bones, 98, 98f
long bones, 97, 97f
sesamoid bones, 98
short bones, 97, 98f
of spinal column, 94–96, 95f

boutique and high-end fitness facilities, 227–228
common clientele, 228
organizational setting, 228
brachialis, 771
brachioradialis, 771
branched-chain amino acids (BCAAs), 171
breathing, 128

C
cable machines, 606–616
cable chop, 612–614
cable leg extension, 606–608
cable lift, 614–616
cable pushdown, 608–610
cable rotation, 610–612
cable resistance machines, 484–485, 485f
caffeine, 171–172, 172t
calisthenics, 476
calorie, definition of, 143
cancer, 493t, 508–509
exercise guidelines, 509f
sample Phase 1 program, 508f
capillaries, 124
carbohydrates, 143–145
digestion, 730–732, 732t
function of, 143–144
high-fructose corn syrup, 144
importance of, 145–146, 146t
recommended intake of, 144–145
structure of, 143, 144t
carbon skeleton, 156, 158
carboxyl group (–COOH), 148
cardiac output (Q̇), 124
cardiac rehabilitation process, 512–513
cardiorespiratory assessment, for fitness professional, 311–314
Rockport walk test, 312–314, 313t
YMCA 3-minute step test, 311–312, 312t
cardiorespiratory disease, 504–506
exercise guidelines for lung disease training, 505f
sample Phase 1 program, 506f
cardiorespiratory system, 121, 130–131
cardiorespiratory training.
See also integrated cardiorespiratory training
in power level, 452–454, 453f
in stabilization level, 380–382
in strength level, 414–416, 415f, 416f
cardiovascular system, 121–127, 122f

careers
    directions, for fitness professionals, 17–37
        educational responsibilities, 28–33
        employment opportunities, 19–20
        introduction to, 18
        professional growth, 33–35
        profiles of adjacent careers, 20–28
        scope of practice and professional
            limitations, 35–37
    opportunities, for fitness
            professional, 10–11
        adjacent fitness careers, 10
        fitness careers, 10
        places of employment, 10–11
carotid pulse, 260, 260f
casein, 170–171
catabolic hormone. *See* cortisol
catabolism, 154
catecholamines, 133
cell body, 87, 88, 749f, 750
center of gravity (CoG), 387
Centers for Disease Control and
        Prevention (CDC), 162
central nervous system (CNS), 87, 750, 750f
cervical spine, 94, 95f
cervical vertebrae, 94, 95f, 775, 776f
chemical energy, 154
chest
    power, 714
    stabilization, 712
    strength, 713
chronic contemplation, 654
chronic disease, 162
chylomicron, 732
circuit training, 208, 491
circumference measurements, 266–268,
        267–268f, 412, 413f
client acquisition and consultations,
        237–278
    building rapport, 252–257
    formal consultations, 257–259
    introduction to, 238–239
    objective assessments, 260–270
    overcoming objections, techniques
        for, 274–278
    prospective clients and marketing,
        240–251
    sales presentation, 271–274
client-specific goals, 361–364
    improve sports performance, 363–364
    increase lean body mass, 362
    weight loss goal, 361–362
club/gym, management of, 26

coaching and communication
        strategies, 663–668
    active listening, 665–667
    coaching styles, 667–668
    level of personal disclosure, 668
    motivational interviewing, 663–664
    verbal communication, 664–665
coccyx, 95f, 96, 776f, 777
cognitive-behavioral
        approaches, 671–674
    association and dissociation, 671–672
    cognitive restructuring, 674
    self-monitoring, 673–674
    social support, 672–673
cognitive distortions, 674
cognitive influences, 657–658
    confidence, 657–658
    self-confidence, 657
    self-talk, 658
cognitive restructuring, 674
commitment, definition of, 272
common gym movements, 53, 54t
competitive season, 364
complementary goods and
        services, 251
complementary proteins, 147
complete protein, 147
concentric activation, 58
concurrent training, 416
condyles, 775, 775f
condyloid joint, 100, 101f, 102t
congestive heart failure, 493t, 504
continuing education unit (CEU), 29
contracts, definition of, 670
coping strategies, 675
    emotion-focused, 675
    problem-focused, 675
core protocols
    in power level, 457–458, 457–458f, 458t
    in stabilization level, 384–387, 384–385t,
        386f, 698
    for strength level, 419–421, 420f, 421t, 699
coronary heart disease, 493t, 504
corporate fitness, 513–514
corrective exercise, 81
corrective flexibility, 188, 382, 401
cortisol, 134
creatine, 172–173
crunches
    floor, 573–574
    reverse, 575–578
cueing, 492
cumulative injury cycle, 113

D

daily value, 168
Davies test, 304–305, 304–305f
Davis' law, 382
deamination, 156, 158
deconditioned a person, 8
deep longitudinal subsystem (DLS),
        105–106, 106f
deformation, 88
deltoid
    anterior, 767
    medial, 768
    posterior, 768
demographics, 216
dendrites, 87, 88, 749f, 750
depressions, 774, 774f
diaphragm, 763
diastolic pressure, 261
dietary fiber, 732
dietary reference intakes (DRIs), 167
    comparison of DRI values for men and
        women, 733–734t
    terminology, 733t
dietary standards, 167
Dietary Supplement Health and Education
        Act (DSHEA) of 1994, 169
digestive system, 135–136, 729–732
    carbohydrate digestion, 730–732, 732t
    fat digestion, 732
    large intestine, 136
    mouth, 135
    overview, 135
    pharynx and esophagus, 135
    protein digestion, 729–730
    small intestine, 136
    stomach, 135–136
diminishing returns, 413, 414f
dissociation strategies, for exercise behavior,
        671–672
drawing-in maneuver, 194, 194f, 195t
driver of sales, 219
drop jump, 448
dumbbells, 479, 479f
dynamic balance, 196
dynamic state, 654
dynamic stretching, 188, 454, 553–565, 697
    inchworms, 564–565
    iron cross, 561–562
    lateral tube walking, 558–559
    multiplanar lunge with reach, 555–557
    prisoner squat, 554–555
    push-up with rotation, 559–561
    scorpion, 562–563

dynamic stretching (*Continued*)
single-leg squat touchdown, 557–558
straight-leg march, 563–564
dyspnea, 505

E

eccentric activation, 58
eccentric function, 58
eccentric strength, 452
educational responsibilities, for fitness professionals, 28–33
CEU courses, 30
live events, 31
overview, 28–29
publications, 32–33
traditional advanced education, 31
efferent neurons, 88, 89
electrolytes, 159
electron transport chain, 156, 158
employment opportunities, for fitness professionals, 19–20, 229–232
clinical settings, 20
interviewing, 230–232
in large-scale facilities, 19, 229
in medium-sized and small facilities, 19, 229
resume writing, 230, 231*f*
sports performance, 20
empty calories, 165
emulsification, 149, 150
endocrine glands, 133
endocrine system, 131–135, 132*f*
catecholamines, 133
cortisol, 134
effects of exercise on, 134–135
endocrine glands, 133
growth hormone, 134
overview, 131–133
testosterone and estrogen, 133
thyroid hormones, 134
endurance/stabilization, 206
endurance athletes, 364
epicondyles, 775, 775*f*
epinephrine, 133
ergogenic aids, 168
esophagus, 135
estimated average requirement (EAR), 167, 733*t*
estimated energy requirement (EER), 167
estrogen, 133
evidence-based practice, 8
excitation–contraction coupling, 205

exercise naming conventions, 53–57
body position, 54, 55*t*
joint action, 56, 56*t*
planes of motion, 54, 54*t*
primary muscle targeted, 56, 56*t*
putting it all together, 56–57, 57*t*
resistance modality exercises, 55, 55*t*
exercise selection, 330
exercise technique
flexibility exercises, 532–565
introduction, 531
resistance training, 566–648
exercise tolerance, 409
exhalation. *See* expiration
expiration, 128
extended healthcare providers, 511–513
extension, 47
extensors, 51
external oblique, 762
external rotation, 49
extrinsic muscles, 70

F

facility owner, 24–25
fascia, 382
fat, 148–150, 730
digestion, 732
food sources of, 149*t*, 150, 150*t*
functions of, 149
recommended intake of, 149
structure of, 148–149
types of, 149*t*
fat-free mass (FFM), 173
fatty acids, 148
fiber, in health, 732
firing frequency, 197
first law of thermodynamics, 154, 155
fitness assessments, 281–321
modifications for specific populations, 318–321
postural assessments, 286–314
pre-assessment information, 284–285
robust goal plan for client, 314–318
scientific components of, 282–284
fitness-based nutrition, 142–143
alcohol, 153–154
carbohydrates, 143–145
fat, 148–150
protein, 145–148
vitamins and minerals, 150–153
fitness coaching, 367

fitness environment, navigation of, 215–234
boutique and high-end facilities, 227–228
facility comparison in, 235*t*
getting hired, 229–232
independent fitness professionals, 232–234
introduction to, 216–217
large-scale facilities and national chains, 217–221
medium-sized fitness centers, 221–224
small group training facilities, 224–227
fitness industry, 1–14
fitness professional, 5–14
history of, 4–5
modern state of health and fitness, 3–4
National Academy of Sports Medicine (NASM), 7–10
overview, 2–3
succeeding in, 11–13
fitness professional
career opportunities for, 10–11
evolution of, 6–7
role of, 5–7
scope of practice for, 13–14
fitness technologies and trends, 516–520
activity trackers, 517–518
emerging technologies, 519–520
smartphone apps, 516–517
social media, 518–519
tracking fitness with mobile technology, 516*f*
fixed-isolated machines, 483–484, 484*f*
flat bones, 98, 98*f*
flavin adenine dinucleotide (FAD), 156, 158
flexibility
continuum, 186*f*, 188
definition of, 81, 185
exercises
active-isolated stretching, 546–553, 692–696
dynamic stretching, 553–565, 697
self-myofascial release (SMR), 532–539, 689–690
static stretching, 539–546, 690–692
improvement, 186–187
in golgi tendon organs, 186, 187*f*
in muscle spindles, 186, 186*f*
multiplanar extensibility, 187
flexion, 44
flexors, 51
floor bridge, 569–570
single-leg, 570–572
floor cobra, 568–569
floor crunch, 573–574

foam-rolling, 382
  front of the upper leg, 534–535
  hip flexor, 536
  inside of the upper leg, 535
  outside of the leg, 538
  outside of the upper leg, 535–536
  piriformis, 537
  posterior lower leg, 533–534
  side of the upper torso, 537–538
  upper back, 538–539
food labels, 168
force, 59
  force-couple relationships, 110, 111*f*
  force-velocity curve, 446, 446*f*
forecasting technique, 240
formal consultations, 257–259
formative assessment, 468
fossa, 774, 774*f*
40-yard dash, 309, 309*f*
free weights and implements,
      478–483, 593–606
  ball dumbbell chest press, 600–602
  barbell Russian deadlift, 595–597
  barbell squat, 599–600
  barbells, 479, 479*f*
  dumbbells, 479, 479*f*
  kettlebells, 480, 480*f*
  medicine balls, 480–481, 481*f*
  other implements, 482–483
  sagittal plane step-up, balance, curl to
      one-arm overhead press, 604–606
  sandbags, 482, 482*f*
  squat, curl to one-arm overhead press,
      602–604
  standing two-arm hammer curl, 593–595
  stationary dumbbell lunge, 597–598
front, side, and turning lunge to balance,
      581–584
front hip stretch, 547–548
front neck stretch, 544–545
front plank, 567–568
front-to-back hop with balance, 584–585
frontal plane jump with stabilization,
      586–587
frontal plane motions, 42, 47–49, 48–49*f*
fructose, 143
function, definition of, 179
functional efficiency, 283
functional movements, 481

G

gait treadmill walking assessment, 737–740
galactose, 143

gastrocnemius/soleus (calves), SMR, 533–534,
      540–541, 649, 753
gastrointestinal (GI) tract, 135
general adaptation syndrome
      (GAS), 179–180, 179*t*, 446
  adaptation phase, 180
  alarm phase, 180
  exhaustion phase, 180
  intermuscular coordination, 180
  overtraining syndrome (OTS), 180
glands, 131
gliding joint, 100, 100*f*, 102*t*
global muscular system, 105
gluconeogenesis, 157, 158, 730
glucose, 143
gluteus maximus, 759
gluteus medius, 759
gluteus minimus, 759
glycemic index, 730, 731*t*
  for assorted foods, 731*t*
glycerol, 149
glycogen, 143, 144
glycolysis, 154, 155
goals
  achievement strategies, 681
  commitment, 680–681
  definition and types, 677–678, 678*t*
  feedback and evaluation, 681–682
  principles and practices of, 676–682, 678*f*
  short-term *vs.* long-term, 679–680, 680*t*
  timelines to achieve, 682, 683*f*
golgi tendon organs (GTOs), 88, 90, 382
government nutrition
      guidelines, 166–168
  dietary guidelines for Americans, 166–167
  dietary reference intakes (DRIs), 167
  energy and macronutrient requirements,
      167–168
  food labels, 168
  MyPlate, 168
gracilis, 758
gravity, definition of, 59
groove, 774
ground reaction force, 41
group fitness, 25–26
group personal training, 488–489
  assessments, 490, 490*f*
  common mistakes fitness professionals
      make in, 492–493
  determining program needs in, 489–490
  implementing OPT™ model in, 491
growth hormone, 134
gymnastics, 476

H

hamstring complex
  biceps femoris
      long head, 754
      short head, 754
  semimembranosus, 755
  semitendinosus, 755
heart, 121–122
  cardiac muscle contraction, 122–123, 123*f*
  function of, 124, 125*f*
  path of blood through, 124
  structure of, 123
heart palpitations, 506
heart rate (HR), 124
  variability, 517
heart rate reserve (HRR) method, 189, 191*t*
Henneman's size principle, 447, 447*f*
high blood pressure, 493*t*, 502–504
  exercise guidelines, 504*f*
  sample Phase 1 program, 504*f*
high-fructose corn syrup (HFCS), 144
hinge joint, 100, 101*f*, 102*t*
hip musculature
  adductor brevis, 758
  adductor longus, 757
  adductor magnus
      anterior fibers, 757
      posterior fibers, 757
  gluteus maximus, 759
  gluteus medius, 759
  gluteus minimus, 759
  gracilis, 758
  iliacus, 760
  pectineus, 758
  piriformis, 761
  psoas, 760
  sartorius, 761
  tensor fascia latae, 760
hipbone, 775
HMB (beta-hydroxy beta-methylbutyrate), 173
homeostasis, 181, 182
horizontal jump with stabilization,
      586–587
horizontal loading, 379
hormones, 132
human behavior, 656–663
  affective influences, 659–661
  behavior influences, 122–663
  cognitive influences, 657–658
  interpersonal influences, 659
human movement system, 85–136
  cardiorespiratory system, 121, 130–131
  cardiovascular system, 121–127

human movement system (*Continued*)
  digestive system, 135–136
  endocrine system, 131–135
  flexibility in, 111–112
  kinetic chain, interactions of, 104–112
  kinetic chain dysfunction, 112–121
  kinetic chain movement, 85–136
  muscular system, 89–93
  nervous system, 87–89
  overview, 86
  respiratory system, 127–130
  skeletal system, 93–104
hypertension, 493t, 502–504
hypertrophy, 178, 206, 410
  training, 362
hypokalemia, 161
hypomobility, 114–115
hyponatremia, 161

I

ice skaters, 590–591
iliacus, 760
iliotibial (IT) band, 535–536
imagine action, 656
implements, 478
inchworms, 564–565
independent fitness professionals, 232–234
  common clientele, 233
  organizational setting, 233–234
infraspinatus, 769
ingestion, 135
inhalation. *See* inspiration
inner hip stretch, 541–542
insensible water losses, 159
insertion, definition of, 65
insoluble fiber, 732
inspiration, 128
integrated balance training, 195–197
  importance of, 196
  science of balance, 196–197
integrated cardiorespiratory training,
      188–193
  common goals of, 188
  exercise intensity, methods for
      prescribing, 189–191, 191t
  heart rate reserve (HRR) method, 189, 191t
  interval training and zone training,
      benefits of, 191–192
  maximal heart rate (HR) method, 189, 191t
  peak V̇o₂ method, 189, 191t
  rating of perceived exertion (PRE) method,
      190, 190f, 191t
  talk test, 190, 191t

integrated core training, 193–195
  abdominal bracing, 194–195, 195f, 195t
  activating the core, 193–194, 195t
  drawing-in maneuver, 194, 194f, 195t
  structure and function of the core, 193, 193f
integrated flexibility training, 185–188
  flexibility continuum, 188
  flexibility improvement, 186–187
  multiplanar extensibility, 187
integrated function, 59
integrated performance paradigm, 198, 199f
integrated reactive training, 197–200
  desensitization of golgi tendon organ, 199
  enhanced muscle spindle activity, 199
  enhanced neuromuscular efficiency,
      199–200
  importance of, 199–200
  science behind, 198–199
integrated resistance training, 202–207
  endurance/stabilization, 206
  excitation–contraction coupling, 205
  hypertrophy, 206
  muscle fibers and their contractile
      elements, 203
  neural activation, 203–205, 204f
  power, 206–207
  sliding filament theory, 205, 205f
  strength, 206
integrated training, 8–10, 177–209
  balance training, 195–197
  cardiorespiratory training, 188–193
  components of, 179–182
  core training, 193–195
  definition of, 178
  flexibility training, 185–188
  introduction to, 178–179
  rationale to support, 182–185
  reactive training, 197–200
  resistance training, 202–207
      systems, 207–209
  speed, agility, and quickness (SAQ)
      training, 200–202
internal oblique, 762
internal rotation, 49
interneurons, 88, 89
interpersonal influences, 659
interval training, benefits of, 191–192
intervention, definition of, 669
intramuscular coordination, 195
intrinsic approach, for exercise behavior,
      675–676
intrinsic core stabilizers, 72
intrinsic muscles, 70

iron cross, 561–562
irregular bones, 98, 98f
isolated function, of muscle, 58, 65
isometric activation, 58

J

joints, 99–103
  ball-and-socket joint, 101, 102f, 102t
  classification of, 99–101, 102t
  condyloid joint, 100, 101f, 102t
  function of, 101–103
  gliding joint, 100, 100f, 102t
  hinge joint, 100, 101f, 102t
  joint connective tissue, 103
  movements naming conventions, 44–50
      frontal plane motions, 47–49, 48–49f
      sagittal plane motions, 44–47, 45–47f
      transverse plane motions, 49–50, 50f
  nonsynovial joint, 101, 102f, 102t
  pivot joint, 100, 101f, 102t
  receptors, 88–89, 90
  rolling joint, 99, 99f
  saddle joint, 100, 101f, 102t
  sliding joint, 99, 99f
  spinning joint, 99, 100f
  stability, 196, 197
  synovial joints, 99–101, 100–101f, 102t
journaling, 662–663, 662f
jump, multiplanar, 587–590

K

ketone bodies, 156, 157
kettlebells, 480, 480f
kilocalories, definition of, 143
kinesiology, 40
kinetic chain, interactions of, 104–112
  anterior oblique subsystem (AOS), 106, 107f
  deep longitudinal subsystem
      (DLS), 105–106, 106f
  efficient movement, creation
      of, 110–111
  force-couple relationships, 110, 111f
  global muscular system, 105
  human movement, flexibility in, 111–112
  lateral subsystem (LS), 108, 108f
  length–tension relationship,
      109–110, 109f
  local muscular system, 104–105, 105f
  posterior oblique subsystem (POS),
      106, 107f
  reciprocal inhibition, 108–109
kinetic chain compensations for gait
      assessment, 739–740t

kinetic chain disruption
  biomechanics and, 77–81, 77–78f, 79t
  neuromuscular efficiency, 81
kinetic chain dysfunction, 112–121
  altered reciprocal inhibition, 115
  areas of, 116–121
  in cervical spine, 120–121
  contributors of, 113–115
  culture and lifestyle, 113–114
  in foot and ankle, 117–118
  injury, 114–115
  in knee, 118
  lumbo-pelvic-hip complex (LPHC), 118–119
  medical issues, 115
  overview, 112–113
  pattern overload, 113
  repetitive lack of motion, 114
  scientific concepts related to, 115–116
  in shoulder, 119–120
  suboptimal positioning, 114
  synergistic dominance, 115–116
  unbalanced training, 114
kinetic chain movement, 85–136
  cardiorespiratory system, 121, 130–131
  cardiovascular system, 121–127
  digestive system, 135–136
  endocrine system, 131–135
  flexibility in, 111–112
  kinetic chain dysfunction, 112–121
  kinetic chain, interactions of, 104–112
  muscular system, 89–93
  nervous system, 87–89
  overview, 86
  respiratory system, 127–130
  skeletal system, 93–104
kinetics, definition of, 59
knee injuries, 182–184, 183–184f
knee stretch, 547–548
knee-up, 576–578
knee valgus, 293
kneeling medicine ball chest pass, 630–631
Krebs cycle, 156
kyphotic curve, 290

L

lactate, 156
lactose, 143, 144
landing error scoring system (LESS) test, 740–742
large intestine, 136
large scale fitness facility, 217–221
  child care and additional services, 220
  common clientele, 218

fitness department, 219
front desk and operations, 220
maintenance, 221
management, 220
organizational setting, 219–221
sales department, 219–220
sports and aquatics, 220
lateral hamstring stretch, 542–543, 550–551
lateral rotation. *See* external rotation
lateral subsystem (LS), 108, 108f
lateral tube walking, 558–559
latissimus dorsi, 537–538, 551–552, 764
leads, definition of, 239
LEFT test, 310, 310f
leg press machine, 624–625
legs
  power, 727
  stabilization, 725
  strength, 726
length–tension relationship, 109–110, 109f
levator scapulae, 771
levers, 59–60, 60f, 62f
licensed massage therapist, 28
lifestyle considerations, 514–516
ligaments, 93, 103, 103f
line of pull, 63
linear periodization, 331–333, 332f
lipids, 148
lipogenesis, 157, 158
load and intensity, 329, 329t
local muscular system, 104–105, 105f
long bones, 97, 97f
long-term goal, 679
longitudinal axis, 43
longus capitis, 773
longus coli, 772
low back pain, 182, 183f
low-density lipoprotein (LDL), 149–150
lower crossed syndrome, 286, 287f, 288t, 292t
lower leg musculature
  anterior tibialis, 752
  gastrocnemius, 753
  peroneus longus, 754
  posterior tibialis, 753
  soleus, 753
lower trapezius, 766
lumbar spine, 95f, 96
lumbar vertebrae, 95f, 96, 776f, 777
lumbo-pelvic-hip complex (LPHC), 77f, 92, 118–119, 193f, 315, 375, 384, 407
lunge to balance in all planes of motion, 581–584

M

machines, 616–625
  alternate arm machine row, 620–621
  biceps curl, 616–617
  cable machines, 606–616
  cable resistance machines, 484–485, 485f
  fixed-isolated machines, 483–484, 484f
  leg press, 624–625
  machine chest press, 622–623
  machine pull-down, 618–619
macronutrients, definition of, 143
malalignment, 70
mass, definition of, 59
master gland. *See* pituitary glands
matter, definition of, 59
maximal heart rate (HR) method, 189, 191t
maximal oxygen consumption ($\dot{V}o_{2max}$), 131, 189
maximal strength, definition of, 206
mechanical specificity, 181
mechanoreceptors, 88–89
medial deltoid, 768
medial rotation. *See* Internal rotation
medicine balls, 480–481, 481f, 626–638
  kneeling chest pass, 630–631
  lift and chop, 626–627
  oblique throw, 635–637
  one-hand push-up, 628–629
  overhead throw, 637–638
  pullover (power) throw, 633–635
  rotation chest pass, 631–633
medium-sized fitness centers, 221–224
  common clientele, 222
  fitness department, 223
  front desk and operations, 224
  management, 224
  organizational setting, 222–224
mentor, definition of, 33
metabolic conditioning, 407
  circuit, 448
metabolic pathways, 154, 155
metabolic resistance training, 491
metabolic specificity, 181
metabolism, 154–157
  building and storing energy, 156–157
  carbohydrates and glucose, 155–156
  creation of glucose, 157
  creation of new proteins, 157
  fat storage, 157
  fats and triglycerides, 156
  forms of energy, 154
  glucose storage, 157
  pathways to energy, 155–156, 155f

metabolism (*Continued*)
protein and amino acids, 156
site of ATP creation, 156
methyl group, 148
micronutrients, 150
middle trapezius, 766
midline, 42
mitochondria, 154, 155
modalities and OPT™ model, 475–488
bodyweight training, 476–477, 476f
free weights and implements, 478–483,
479–482f
resistance training machines, 483–485,
484f, 485f
rolling active resistance training, 488, 488f
ropes, 485–486, 485f
suspension training, 477–478, 478f
whole body vibration training,
486–487, 486f
monounsaturated fatty acid, 148
motivational interviewing, 663–664
motor behavior, 111
motor control, 87, 111
motor development, 87, 111
motor function, 751
motor learning, 87, 111
motor outputs, 110–111
motor unit, 204
activation, 411, 412f
recruitment, 197
synchronization, 197
movement assessments, for fitness
professional, 292–303
overhead squat assessment, 293–297,
293–294f, 295t, 296–297f
pulling assessment, 301–303,
302–303f, 302t
pushing assessment, 299–301, 299t,
300–301f
single-leg squat assessment, 297–298,
298f, 298t
movement preparation, 382
in power level, 454–462
in stabilization level, 382–395
in strength level, 417–426
movement system. *See* global
muscular system
multifidus, 764
multiplanar extensibility, 187
multiplanar jump, 587–590
multiplanar lunge
to balance, 581–584
with reach, 555–557

multiplanar movements, 52
muscle action spectrum, 57–58
muscle belly, 67
muscle-building athletes, 364
muscle contraction, 91
muscle coordination, 409
muscle fibers, 89–90, 90t
type I, 89, 90t
type II, 89–90, 90t
muscle spindles, 88, 89
muscles
imbalances, 8, 116–117, 117f
common, 70
and injury, 283–284
isolated function, 65
location of, 63–65, 65t
name analyzing based on, 65–69
action, 66, 67t
attachment, 66
direction, 67, 67t
location, 67, 68t
shape, 69, 69t
size, 68, 69t
structure, 67–68, 68t
overactive and underactive
muscles, 70–76
of foot and ankle, 70–71, 71f
of head and neck, 75–76, 76f
of knee, 71–72, 72f
of LPHC, 72–74, 73f
of shoulder, 74–75, 74f
muscular endurance, 375–376
muscular failure, 430
muscular function and application, 57–63
application of tempo, 62–63
force, torque, and levers, 59–62
muscle action spectrum, 57–58
muscle function, 58–59
muscular system, 89–93, 751–773
abdominal musculature, 761–763
arm musculature, 770–771
back musculature, 763–764
behavioral properties of muscle, 90–92
global, 105
hamstring complex, 754–755
hip musculature, 757–761
local, 104–105, 105f
lower leg musculature, 752–754
muscle fibers, 89–90, 90t
muscles as movers, 92–93
neck musculature, 771–773
overview, 89
quadriceps, 755–756

rotator cuff, 769–770
shoulder musculature, 765–768
musculoskeletal system, 8
myoglobin, 89
MyPlate, 168

N
National Academy of Sports Medicine
(NASM), 7–10, 18
Certified Personal Trainer (CPT)
certification, 8
evidence-based practice, 8
integrated training and OPT™ model,
8–10, 9f
neck musculature
levator scapulae, 771
longus capitis, 773
longus coli, 772
scalenes, 772
sternocleidomastoid, 772
nerve impulses, 87, 88
nervous system
central nervous system (CNS), 87, 750,
750f
golgi tendon organs (GTOs), 88, 90
joint receptors, 88–89, 90
mechanoreceptors, 88–89
muscle spindles, 88, 89
neurons, 87–88, 749–750, 749f
overview, 87
peripheral nervous system, 750–751, 751f
proprioceptors, 88–89
structure, 752f
neural activation, 203–205, 204f
neural drive, 411
neuromuscular efficiency, 81
neuromuscular specificity, 181
neurons, 87–88
neurotransmitters, 133
new business client, 240
nicotinamide adenine dinucleotide (NAD),
156, 158
nonessential amino acids, 147
nonsynovial joint, 101, 102f, 102t
norepinephrine, 133
nutrient density, 145
nutrition apps, 517

O
obesity, 4, 162, 500–502
exercise guidelines for training, 502f
prevalence of, 4
sample Phase 2 program, 503f

objective assessments, 260–270
  additional information, 737–748
  blood pressure, 261
  body composition, 262
  body fat, measuring, 262–264, 263–264t, 265–266t
  body mass index (BMI), 269, 270t
  circumference measurements, 266–268, 267–268f
  pulse, 260–261
  waist-to-hip measurements, 268–269
oblique, external/internal, 762
oblique medicine ball throw, 635–637
occupational positioning, 114
off-season, 364
older adults
  exercise guidelines for, 497f
  resistance training among, 493t, 496–497
  sample Phase 3 program, 498f
omega-3 fatty acids, 148, 149
omega-6 fatty acids, 148, 149
one-hand medicine ball push-up, 628–629
one-repetition maximum conversion, 742–748
open-chain exercises, 464
open-ended question, 270
operations, definition of, 217
Optimum Performance Training™ (OPT™) model, 8–10, 9f, 184–185, 185f, 473–521
  and client-specific goals, 361–364
  fitness technologies and trends, 516–520
  group training and, 488–493
  modalities and, 475–488
  populations with special considerations, 493–511
  power level, 441–468
  program design and, 326–331, 327f
  programming for specific populations, 511–516
  stabilization level, 373–401
  strength level, 405–433
  templates for programming, 334–339
  using every day, 474–475
order of exercises, 331
origin, definition of, 65
osteoblasts, 773
osteoporosis, 493t, 509–511
  exercise guidelines, 510f
  sample Phase 2 program, 511f
outcome goals, 677, 678t
overactive muscle imbalances, 70
overhead medicine ball throw, 637–638

overhead squat assessment, 293–297, 293–294f, 295t, 296–297f
overload principle, 181–182, 410–411
overtraining syndrome (OTS), 180
oxaloacetate (OAA), 156, 157

P

palms-down superman, 568–569
parallel muscle, 64, 64f
parasympathetic nervous system, 452, 751
pattern overload, 113
peak V̇o₂ method, 189, 191t
pectineus, 758
pectoral stretch, 552–553
pectoralis major, 767
pectoralis minor, 767
pelvo-ocular reflex, 120
pennate muscle, 64, 64f
performance assessments, for fitness professional, 303–311
  bench press test, 306–307, 307f
  Davies test, 304–305, 304–305f
  40-yard dash, 309, 309f
  LEFT test, 310, 310f
  pro shuttle test, 309–310, 309f
  push-up test, 303–304, 304f
  shark skill test, 305–306, 306f
  squat test, 307–308, 307f
  standing broad jump, 310–311
  vertical jump test, 308, 308f
performance goals, 677–678, 678t
periodization, 331
peripheral artery disease, 493t, 504
peristalsis, 135
peroneals, 538
peroneus longus, 754
perturbation, 196
pharynx, 135
phospholipids, 148
Physical Activity Readiness Questionnaire (PAR-Q), 258, 259f
physical therapist, 22–23
phytochemicals, 150
piriformis, 537, 549, 761
pituitary glands, 133
pivot joint, 100, 101f, 102t
plane stability, 387t
planes and axes of motion, 42–44, 43f, 44t
plyometric training, 390
point-of-sale client, 240
polyunsaturated fatty acid, 148–149
positive reinforcement, 662
post rehab, 512

posterior deltoid, 768
posterior oblique subsystem (POS), 106, 107f
posterior tibialis, 753
postural assessments, for fitness professional, 9–10, 286–314
  cardiorespiratory assessment, 311–314
  movement assessments, 292–303
  performance assessments, 303–311
  static postural assessment, 286–292
postural distortion patterns, 286–287, 287f
postural stability, 196
posture, 112, 283
power, defined, 206–207
power level, OPT™ model, 441–468
  balance protocols for, 459–460, 459–460f, 460t
  benefits of, 449–452
  cardiorespiratory training protocols for, 452–454, 453f
  common mistakes made in, 465–467
  core protocols for, 457–458, 457–458f, 458t
  corrective strategies for clients, 468
  criteria for participation in, 449
  goals and adaptations in, 443–452
  integrating with other phases, 467–468
  introduction to, 443, 443f
  movement preparation in, 454–462
  problems related to avoiding/rushing, 448
  reactive protocols for, 460, 460t, 461f, 462f
  resistance training protocols in, 462–465, 465t
  SAQ protocols for, 461–462, 462t
  scientific principles for training, 446–447
  SMR and flexibility protocols for, 454–457, 455–457f, 457t
  tracking progress in, 447–448
pre-assessment, for fitness professional, 284–285
pregnancy
  benefits of exercise during, 497–500
  exercise guidelines, 500f
  sample Phase 1 program, 501f
preseason, 363–364
price determination, 273–274
prisoner squat, 554–555
pro shuttle test, 309–310, 309f
process goals, 678, 678t
processes, 774–775, 774–775f
professional growth, for fitness professionals, 33–35
  mentors, 33–34
  networking, 34–35
profit center, 221

program design, 325–369
  assessment outcomes and, 350–361
  and OPT™ model, 326–331, 327f
    and client-specific goals, 361–364
  session structure and flow, 364–369
  starting, 331–334
  templates for OPT programming, 334–349
progress evaluation practices, 682–685
  progress reviews, 683
  record keeping, 683–685
progression, principle of, 411
progressive resistance exercise (PRE), 327
prohormones and anabolic steroids, 173
prompting, definition of, 669
pronation, 49, 117
pronation distortion syndrome, 286, 287f,
    288t, 292t
pronation of the foot, 79
pronators, 51
prone, 51, 51f
prone iso-abs, 567–568
proprioception, 88, 89, 376
proprioceptively enriched environments, 195
proprioceptors, 88–89, 444
  role in power production, 447
prospecting activities, 239
prospective clients and marketing,
    240–251
  additional prospecting activities,
    243–244
  creating a plan, 240
  cross-departmental interaction and
    promotion, 245–247
  face-to-face prospecting, 241–243
  former prospects and follow-ups, 248–250
  independent professional, promoting,
    250–251, 251t
  professional networking, 244–245
protein, 145–148
  digestion, 729–730
  food sources of, 147–148, 148t
  functions of, 147
  incomplete, 147
  recommended intake of, 147
  structure of, 145–147
  supplements, 170–171
  synthesis, 154, 155
psoas, 760
psychographics, 216
pulling assessment, 301–303, 302–303f, 302t
pulse, 260–261
  carotid, 260, 260f
  radial, 260, 260f

push-ups, 477
  with plus/shoulder raise, 578–579
  with rotation, 559–561
  test, 303–304, 304f
pushing assessment, 299–301, 299t, 300–301f
pyruvate, 155, 156

Q

quadratus lumborum (QL), 108, 764
quadriceps, 534–535, 547
  rectus femoris, 756
  vastus intermedius, 756
  vastus lateralis, 755
  vastus medialis, 756
quadruped opposite arm and opposite leg
    raise, 572–573
qualitative analysis, 41
quantitative analysis, 41
quickness, definition of, 201

R

radial pulse, 260, 260f
range of motion (ROM), 44, 112–113
rapport, 239
  barriers to establishing, 254–255
  building, 252–257
  characteristics of professionalism, 255–257
rate of force production, 197
rating of perceived exertion (PRE) method,
    190, 190f, 191t
re-sign client, 240, 249–250
reactive protocols
  in power level, 460, 460t, 461f, 462f, 707
  in stabilization level, 390–393, 391–392f,
    392–393t, 704
  in strength level, 423–424, 423–424f, 424t,
    705–706
rear hip stretch, 548–550
rear neck stretch, 545–546
reciprocal inhibition, 108–109
recommended dietary allowance (RDA),
    167, 733t
rectus abdominis, 761
rectus femoris, 756
registered dietician, 23–24
relative flexibility, 81, 284
relaxin, 218
remodeling process, 773
repetition tempo, 62
repetitions, definition of, 181
repetitive lack of motion, 114
repetitive stress injury (RSI), 113
resistance modality exercises, 55, 55t

resistance training
  bodyweight exercise, 566–593
  cable machines, 606–616
  circuit-training system, 208–209
  free weights, 593–606
  machines, 483–485, 616–625
    cable resistance machines, 484–485, 485f
    fixed-isolated machines, 483–484, 484f
  medicine ball, 626–638
  multiple-set system, 208
  peripheral heart-action system, 209
  in power level, 462–465, 465t
  pyramid system, 208, 208f
  single-set system, 207
  split-routine system, 209
  in stabilization level, 395–397,
    396–397f, 396t
  in strength level, 426–429, 427–428f, 427t
  superset system, 208
  tri-set system, 209
  whole body vibration (WBV) exercises,
    639–648
respiratory system, 121, 127–130
  abnormal breathing patterns, 131
  oxygen consumption, 130–131
  respiratory airways, 129f, 129–130, 129t
  structures of respiratory pump, 128t
rest periods, 329–330, 330t
resting heart rate (RHR), 192
retraction, 75
reverse ball throw, 637–638
reverse crunch, 575–576
  with straight legs, 576–578
rhomboid major, 765
rhomboid minor, 765
robust goal plan, for clients, 314–318
  foot, ankle, and knee, 314–315
  lumbo-pelvic-hip complex (LPHC), 315
  prioritizing compensations, 315–317
  reassessing clients and evaluating
    progress, 317–318
  shoulder complex and cervical spine, 315,
    316t
Rockport walk test, 312–314, 313t
rolling active resistance training, 488, 488f
rolling joint, 99, 99f
Romanian deadlift, WBV exercise, 641–642
ropes, 485–486, 485f
rotator cuff
  infraspinatus, 769
  subscapularis, 769
  supraspinatus, 770
  teres minor, 769

S

sacrum, 95f, 96, 776f, 777
saddle joint, 100, 101f, 102t
sagittal plane hop with stabilization, 584–585
sagittal plane motions, 42, 44–47, 45–47f
sagittal plane proprioceptive reactives, 592–593
sagittal plane step-up, balance, curl to one-arm overhead press, 604–606
sandbags, 482, 482f
sarcomere, 203, 203f
sarcopenia, 444
sartorius, 761
saturated fat, 148, 149
saturation, 148
scalenes, 772
scapular winging, 315
scientific components, of fitness assessments, 282–284
   muscle imbalances and injury, 283–284
   posture, importance of, 283
scientific principles of training
   in power level, 446–447
   in stabilization level, 376–380, 378t
   in strength level, 410–412
scope of practice, for fitness professionals, 13–14, 35–37
scorpion, 562–563
seated chest press, 622–623
seated lat pull-down, 618–619
seated machine row, 620–621
self-efficacy/self-confidence, 655, 657
self-monitoring strategy, 673–674, 674f
self-myofascial release (SMR), 532–539, 689–690
   adductors, 535
   gastrocnemius/soleus (calves), 533–534
   iliotibial (IT) band, 535–536
   latissimus dorsi, 537–538
   peroneals, 538
   piriformis, 537
   quadriceps, 534–535
   tensor fasciae latae (TFL), 536
   thoracic spine, 538–539
self-myofascial release and flexibility protocols
   in power level, 454–457, 455–457f, 457t
   in stabilization level, 382–384, 382t, 383–384f
   in strength level, 417–419, 418t

semimembranosus, 755
semitendinosus, 755
sensorimotor
   control, 196
   integration, 197
sensory function, 751
sensory receptors, 87–89
serratus anterior, 765
sesamoid bones, 98
session structure and flow, program design, 364–369
   coaching combo sessions, 368–369
   coaching sessions, 367–368
   corrective combo sessions, 369
   60-minute traditional training session, 365–366
   training vs. coaching, 365
   25 to 30-minute traditional training session, 366–367
set, definition of, 182
shark skill test, 305–306, 306f
short bones, 97, 98f
short-term goal, 679
shoulder
   impingement, 78, 78f
   power, 720
   stabilization, 717–718
   strength, 719
   stretch, 551–553
shoulder musculature
   anterior deltoid, 767
   lower trapezius, 766
   medial deltoid, 768
   middle trapezius, 766
   pectoralis major, 767
   pectoralis minor, 767
   posterior deltoid, 768
   rhomboid major, 765
   rhomboid minor, 765
   serratus anterior, 765
   teres major, 768
   upper trapezius, 766
side medicine ball toss, 635–637
single-arm machine row, 620–621
single-arm squat, curl to military press, 602–604
single-leg balance, 566–567
single-leg floor bridge, 570–572
single-leg shoulder scaption, WBV exercise, 646–648
single-leg squat assessment, 297–298, 298f, 298t

single-leg squat touchdown, 557–558
sinoatrial (SA) node, 122
skeletal system, 93–104, 773f
   appendicular skeletons, 96
   axial skeletons, 94–96
   bone growth, 773–774
   bone markings, 774–775, 774–775f
   bone mass, effects on, 103–104
   bones, types of, 96–98
   joints, 99–103
   roles of, 93–94
   vertebral column, 775, 776f, 777
sliding filament theory, 205, 205f
sliding joint, 99, 99f
small group training fitness facility, 224–227
   common clientele, 225
   fitness, sales, and operations, 227
   management, 226
   organizational setting, 225–227
small intestine, 136
smart goals, 680f
smartphone apps, 516–517
social media, 518–519
social support, 672–673
soleus, 753
soluble fiber, 732
soma, of a neuron, 87
somatic nervous system, 751
spasticity, 507
special populations, 29, 493–511, 493t
specific adaptation to imposed demands (SAID) principle, 180, 181
specificity, principle of, 180
spectator prospects, 243
speed, agility, and quickness (SAQ) training, 200–202
   importance of, 201
   in power level, 461–462, 462t
   science of agility, 201
   science of quickness, 201
   science of speed, 200
   in stabilization level, 393–395, 394–395t
   in strength level, 424–426, 425t
speed, definition of, 200
spinning joint, 99, 100f
sports coach, 27
squat
   curl to one-arm overhead press, 602–604
   pattern, 449
   test, 307–308, 307f
stability ball hamstring curl, 580–581

stabilization level, OPT™ model, 373–401
  balance protocols in, 387–390, 387–388t, 389–390f
  cardiorespiratory training protocols in, 380–382
  common mistakes made in, 397–400, 400t
  core protocols in, 384–387, 384–385t, 386f
  corrective strategies for clients, 401
  goals and adaptations in, 375–380
  horizontal jump with, 586–587
  integrating with other phases, 400–401
  introduction to, 374–375, 375f
  movement preparation in, 382–395
  reactive protocols in, 390–393, 391–392f, 392–393t
  resistance training protocols in, 395–397, 396–397f, 396t
  sagittal plane hop with, 584–585
  SAQ protocols in, 393–395, 394–395t
  scientific principles of training, 376–380, 378t
  SMR and flexibility protocols in, 382–384, 382t, 383–384f
  tracking progress in, 380
stabilization system. *See* local muscular system
stabilizers, 92, 93t
stable state, 654
standing broad jump, 310–311
standing cable lift, 614–616
standing cable trunk rotation, 610–612
standing leg extension, 606–608
standing two-arm hammer curl, 593–595
state, definition of, 653–654
static balance, 196
static postural assessment, for fitness professional, 286–292, 290–291f
  observing static posture, 287–289
  performing, 289–292
  postural distortion patterns, 286–287, 287f
static posture, 52
static stretching, 383, 539–546, 690–692
  static biceps femoris stretch, 542–543
  static gastrocnemius/soleus (calves) stretch, 540–541
  static standing adductor stretch, 541–542
  static sternocleidomastoid stretch, 544–545
  static upper trapezius/scalenes stretch, 545–546
stationary dumbbell lunge, 597–598
step-up, balance, curl to one-arm overhead press, 604–606, 649
step-up to balance, WBV exercise, 644–646

sternocleidomastoid, 544–545, 772
sterols, 148
stomach, 135–136
straight-leg deadlift, 595–597
straight-leg march, 563–564
strength, 206
  conditioning coach, 27–28
  endurance, 410
strength level, OPT™ model, 405–433
  balance protocols in, 421–423, 422–423f, 422t
  cardiorespiratory training protocols in, 414–416, 415f, 416f
  common mistakes made in, 429–431
  core protocols for, 419–421, 420f, 421t
  corrective strategies for clients, 432–433
  goals and adaptations in, 407–414
  integrating with other phases, 431–432, 432f
  introduction to, 407, 407f
  movement preparation in, 417–426
  reactive training protocols for, 423–424, 423–424f, 424t
  resistance training protocols in, 426–429, 427–428f, 427t
  SAQ protocols for, 424–426, 425t
  scientific principles of training, 410–412
  SMR and flexibility protocols for, 417–419, 418t
  tracking progress in, 412–414
stretching. *See also specific entries*
  active-isolated, 188, 546–553, 692–696
  dynamic, 188, 553–565, 697
  static, 188, 539–546, 690–692
stride length, 200
stride rate, 200
stroke, 493t, 506–507
  sample Phase 1 program, 507f
  training guidelines for exercise and strength training after, 506, 507f
stroke volume (SV), 124
structural efficiency, 87
subjective assessment, 258
subjective goals, 677
suboptimal positioning, 114
subscapularis, 769
sucrose, 143
sulcus, 774, 774f
superficial erector spinae, 763
supersets, 444
supination, 49
  foot, 79
supinators, 51

supine, 51, 51f
supplementation concepts, 168–173
  dietary supplement, 169
  supplement types, 170–173
  before taking a supplement, 169–170
supraspinatus, 770
surface markings, 774
  depressions, 774, 774f
  processes, 774–775, 774–775f
suspension training, 477–478, 478f
symmetry, definition of, 289
sympathetic nervous system, 751
synergistic dominance, 115–116
synergists, 92, 93t
synovial joints, 99–101, 100–101f, 102t
systolic pressure, 261

T
tailbone, 95f, 96, 776f, 777
talk test, 190, 191t
target cells, 132
templates
  for clients, 345, 347–349
    monthly programming, 349, 349f
    yearly programming, 347, 348f
  for fitness professionals, 339–345
    completed training sessions, 345
    daily programming, 344–345, 346–347f
    monthly programming, 341, 342f
    weekly programming, 341, 343f, 344
    yearly programming, 339–341, 340f
  for OPT programming, 334–349
    client homework, 337, 338f
    trainer templates and record keeping, 337–339
tempo, 328–329, 329t
  application of, 62–63
tendons, 65, 93
tensegrity, 116
tensor fascia latae (TFL), 108, 536, 760
teres major, 768
teres minor, 769
testosterone (TST), 133
thoracic spine, 94, 95f, 538–539
thoracic vertebrae, 94, 95f, 776f, 777
thyroid hormones, 134
time under tension (TUT), 377
timed hold variable, 378
tolerable upper intake level (UL), 167, 733t
top-line revenue, 219
torque, 61, 61f

total body
  power, 710–711
  stabilization, 708
  strength, 709
toxicity, 150
training age, 448
training duration, 380
training frequency, 380
training volume, 327–328
trait, definition of, 653
transitional movement assessment, 293
transtheoretical model
    (TTM), 653–656, 653f
  action stage, 654–655
  applications of, 655–656
  contemplation stage, 654
  maintenance stage, 655
  precontemplation stage, 654
  preparation stage, 654
  termination stage, 655
transverse abdominis, 762
transverse plane motions, 42,
    49–50, 50f
trapezius
  lower, 766
  middle, 766
  upper, 766
treadmill walking assessment, 737–740
tricarboxylic acid (TCA) cycle, 156
triceps
  brachii, 770
  dips, 639–640
  pushdown, 608–610
  stabilization, 723
  strength, 724
triglycerides, 148
triple extension, 51, 52f
triple flexion, 51, 52f
trochanters, 775, 775f
tubercles, 775, 775f
turn-key business solutions, 21

twist pass, 631–633
two-arm bent-over row, WBV exercise,
    643–644

U

underactive muscle imbalances, 70
undulating periodization, 333
    applying to OPT™ model, 333–334,
      335–336f
unsaturated fatty acids, 148–149
unstable resistance training, 477
upper crossed syndrome, 286, 287f, 288t,
    292t
upper trapezius, 766
  and scalenes, 545

V

Valsalva maneuver, 499
variation, principle of, 182
vastus intermedius, 756
vastus lateralis, 755
vastus medialis, 756
vastus medialis oblique (VMO), 105
veins, 123, 124
ventilation. See breathing
ventilatory threshold (T$_{vent}$), 190
ventricles, 123
verbal communication, 255t
vertebral column, 775, 776f, 777
vertical jump test, 308, 308f
vertical loading, 379
vibration exercise, 486–487, 486f
vibration plate deadlift, 641–642
vibration plate dips, 639–640
viscoelastic property, of muscle, 91
vitamins and minerals, 150–153, 151–153t

W

waist-to-hip measurements, 268–269
walking kick, 563–564
water, 157–162

balance, 158–159, 159t
dehydration, 159–160, 160t
electrolytes, 161
function of, 158
guidelines for intake, 158, 158t
hydration status, monitoring,
    160–161, 161f
loss, 159
sports drinks, 161–162
structure of, 158
wearable technology, 519–520
weekend warriors, 515
weight, definition of, 59
weight loss/gain, 142–166
  better eating, strategies for, 164–166
  diets, 162–163, 163t
  environment of eating, 164
whey protein concentrate (WPC), 171
whey protein isolate (WPI), 171
whey proteins, 170
whole body vibration (WBV) exercises,
    486–487, 486f, 639–648
  Romanian deadlift, 641–642
  single-leg shoulder scaption, 646–648
  step-up to balance, 644–646
  triceps dips, 639–640
  two-arm bent-over row, 643–644
World Health Organization (WHO), 3

Y

YMCA 3-minute step test,
    311–312, 312t
youth
  exercise guidelines for, 495f
  sample Phase 2 program, 496f
  training, 493t, 494–496

Z

zone training
  benefits of, 191–192
  preventing overtraining during, 192